CORPVS MEDICORVM GRAECORVM

EDIDERVNT

ACADEMIAE BEROLINENSIS HAVNIENSIS LIPSIENSIS

XI 1,2

STEPHANI PHILOSOPHI

IN HIPPOCRATIS PROGNOSTICVM COMMENTARIA III

EDIDIT ET IN LINGVAM ANGLICAM VERTIT

JOHN M. DUFFY

BEROLINI IN AEDIBVS ACADEMIAE SCIENTIARVM MCMLXXXIII

STEPHANUS THE PHILOSOPHER

A COMMENTARY ON THE PROGNOSTICON OF HIPPOCRATES

EDITION AND TRANSLATION

BY

JOHN M. DUFFY

THEORIA CUM PRAXI

AKADEMIE-VERLAG · BERLIN 1983

Erschienen im Akademie-Verlag, DDR - 1086 Berlin, Leipziger Str. 3—4

Lizenznummer: 202 · 100/262/83
Printed in the German Democratic Republic
Gesamtherstellung: IV/2/14 VEB Druckerei »Gottfried Wilhelm Leibniz«,
4450 Gräfenhainichen · 5558
LSV 0886
Bestellnummer: 753 748 9 (2028/24)

08000

VORWORT

Mit der vorliegenden Edition des Stephanos-Kommentars zum Prognostikon des Hippokrates wird die Reihe der spätalexandrinischen Hippokrateskommentare eröffnet, deren Publikation bereits von H. Diels als vordringliche Aufgabe des Corpus Medicorum Graecorum bezeichnet worden ist, da sie als sekundäre Überlieferungsträger wichtiger Hippokratestexte eine wesentliche Voraussetzung für die Aufarbeitung der Überlieferungsgeschichte dieser Hippokratesschriften darstellen. Für die Textkonstituierung des Prognostikonkommentars, der in vollständiger Fassung bislang nur in der 1834 erschienenen Ausgabe von F. R. Dietz zugänglich war, hat J. M. Duffy zum erstenmal alle heute noch greifbaren griechischen Handschriften mit dem Text dieses Kommentars ausgewertet und somit eine den Anforderungen der modernen Textkritik entsprechende Edition erstellt, die dem künftigen Herausgeber des hippokratischen Prognostikon in der geforderten Weise als zuverlässiges Arbeitsinstrument zu dienen vermag. Die dem griechischen Text beigegebene englische Übersetzung ist die erste modernsprachige Übersetzung dieses Textes überhaupt, die den Zugang zu der Sprache des frühbyzantinischen Autors, die sich sowohl im Formenbestand als auch in der Syntax von dem nachklassischen Griechisch beträchtlich unterscheidet, wesentlich erleichtert und den Kommentar darüber hinaus erstmals auch dem des Griechischen unkundigen Medizinhistoriker voll erschließt.

Als medizinhistorisches Dokument verdient der Kommentar des Stephanos vor allem deswegen Beachtung, weil er wertvolle Aufschlüsse sowohl über den Lehrbetrieb an den medizinischen Ausbildungsstätten der Spätantike, speziell in Alexandria, als auch über den Wissensstand auf dem Gebiet der Medizin zu dieser Zeit gibt. Bei dem Kommentar handelt es sich um Nachschriften einer Vorlesung, die Stephanos, der in der Zeit zwischen 550 und 650 als Lehrer der Medizin und der Philosophie in Alexandria tätig gewesen ist, über das Prognostikon des Hippokrates gehalten hat. Aus Hinweisen des Stephanos erfahren wir, daß seine medizinische Vorlesungstätigkeit sehr umfangreich gewesen sein muß: außer dem Prognostikon und den Aphorismen des Hippokrates sowie der Galenischen Therapeutik an Glaukon standen zumindest noch drei physiologische Werke Galens und ein oder mehrere – vermutlich auch von Galen stammende – Pulstraktate auf seinem Lehrprogramm.

Medizinhistorisch bedeutsam ist aber ebenso auch die Tatsache, daß Stephanos in seinen Erläuterungen zum Prognostikon, in denen er sich

weitgehend an den Prognostikonkommentar des Galen anlehnt, immer wieder den Versuch unternimmt, seinen Hörern über die eigentliche Hippokrateserklärung hinaus auch die Kenntnis der zu seiner Zeit gültigen medizinischen Theorie nahezubringen. In dem Bild, das Stephanos uns auf diese Weise von der zeitgenössischen Medizin vermittelt, zeigt sich diese infolge der für jene Zeit charakteristischen Neigung zum Schematisieren als eine stark vereinfachende Zusammenfassung des durch seine Vielfalt bestechenden medizinischen Wissens vorangegangener Jahrhunderte.

Die Redaktion des
Corpus Medicorum Graecorum
Jutta Kollesch

CONTENTS

LITERATURE CITED

Agnellus, Commentaries on Galen's De sectis, Ars, De pulsibus ad Teuthram, De methodo medendi ad Glauconem I, in: cod. Ambrosianus G 108 inf., fol. 22r–130r

Alexander von Tralles, ed. Th. Puschmann, vol. II, Vienna 1879

B. Alexanderson, Die hippokratische Schrift Prognostikon, Studia Graeca et Latina Gothoburgensia 17, Göteborg 1963

Appianus, Historia Romana, vol. I, ed. P. Viereck, A. G. Roos, E. Gabba, Leipzig 1962

G. Baffioni, Scolii inediti di Palladio al De sectis di Galeno, Bollettino del Comitato per la Preparazione della Edizione Nazionale dei Classici Greci e Latini, N. S. 6 (1958), pp. 61–78

A. M. Bandini, Catalogus codicum Graecorum Bibliothecae Laurentianae, vol. II, Florence 1768

W. H. Bond-C. U. Faye, Supplement to the Census of Medieval and Renaissance Manuscripts in the United States and Canada, New York 1962

W. Bräutigam, De Hippocratis Epidemiarum Libri Sexti Commentatoribus, Diss. Königsberg 1908

CAG = Commentaria in Aristotelem Graeca

R. Charterius, Opera Hippocratis Coi et Galeni Pergameni, vol. XII, Paris 1679

CMG = Corpus Medicorum Graecorum

David, Prolegomena Philosophiae et in Porphyrii Isagogen Commentarium, ed. A. Busse, CAG XVIII 2, Berlin 1904

F. R. Dietz, Apollonii Citiensis, Stephani, Palladii, Theophili, Meletii, Damascii, Joannis, aliorum Scholia in Hippocratem et Galenum, vol. I–II, Königsberg 1834 (reprint Amsterdam 1966)

Elias, Prolegomena Philosophiae, ed. A. Busse, CAG XVIII 1, Berlin 1900

Galenus, Opera omnia, ed. C. G. Kühn, vol. I–XX, Leipzig 1821–1833 (= K.)

– De elementis ex Hippocratis sententia libri duo, ed. G. Helmreich, Erlangen 1878

– Scripta minora, vol. III, ed. G. Helmreich, Leipzig 1893

– De usu partium libri XVII, ed. G. Helmreich, vol. I–II, Leipzig 1907/1909

– In Hippocratis Prorrheticum I comm. III, De comate secundum Hippocratem, In Hippocratis Prognosticum comm. III, ed. H. Diels, J. Mewaldt, J. Heeg, CMG V 9, 2, Leipzig and Berlin 1915

– De sanitate tuenda, ed. K. Koch, in: CMG V 4,2, Leipzig and Berlin 1923, pp. 1–198

– In Hippocratis Epidemiarum libr. III comm. III, ed. E. Wenkebach, CMG V 10,2,1, Leipzig and Berlin 1936

– De placitis Hippocratis et Platonis, ed., transl., comm. Ph. De Lacy, CMG V 4,1,2 (part I), Berlin 1978, (part II), Berlin 1980

– De praecognitione, ed., transl., comm. V. Nutton, CMG V 8,1, Berlin 1979

Ch. Graux-A. Martin, Notices sommaires des manuscrits grecs d'Espagne et de Portugal, in: Nouvelles Archives des Missions scientifiques et littéraires, vol. II, Paris 1892

Heeg see Galenus

Hermogenes, Opera, ed. H. Rabe, Leipzig 1913

Œuvres complètes d'Hippocrate, ed. E. Littré, vol. I–X, Paris 1839–1861 (= L.)

Hippocrates, Opera quae feruntur omnia, ed. H. Kühlewein, vol. I–II, Leipzig 1894/1902 (= Kw.)

Hippocrates, Lex, De arte, De decente habitu, De alimento, ed. J. L. Heiberg, in: CMG I 1, Leipzig and Berlin 1927, pp. 7f.; 9–19; 25–29; 79–84
– Die hippokratische Schrift „Über die heilige Krankheit", ed., transl., comm. H. Grensemann, Ars Medica II 1, Berlin 1968
– De natura hominis, ed., transl., comm. J. Jouanna, CMG I 1,3, Berlin 1975
H. Hunger (-O. Kresten), Katalog der griechischen Handschriften der Österreichischen Nationalbibliothek, vol. II, Vienna 1969
Joannes of Alexandria, Commentary on Galen's De sectis, in: Galeni Omnes libri (Latin edition, R. Placentinus), vol. I, Pavia 1515, fol. 6^r–12^v
– Scholia in Hippocratis De natura pueri, in: Dietz II, pp. 205–235
– Commentaria in sextum librum Hippocratis Epidemiarum, ed. C. D. Pritchet, Leiden 1975
Julianus, Opera, ed. W. C. Wright, vol. II, London and New York 1913
Lucianus, Opera, ed. C. Jacobitz, vol. III, Leipzig 1904
A. Mai, Spicilegium Romanum, vol. V, Rome 1841
A. Martini-D. Bassi, Catalogus codicum Graecorum Bibliothecae Ambrosianae, vol. I–II, Milan 1906
G. Mercati, Minuzie, Bessarione 33 (1917), pp. 334–340 (=Opere Minori, vol. IV, Vatican City 1937, pp. 38ff.)
M. Meyerhof, Von Alexandrien nach Bagdad, Sitzungsberichte d. Preuß. Akademie d. Wiss., Phil.-hist. Kl. 23, Berlin 1930, pp. 389–429
S. A. J. Moorat, Catalogue of Western Manuscripts on Medicine and Science in the Wellcome Historical Medical Library, London 1962
Olympiodorus, In Platonis Gorgiam Commentaria, ed. L. G. Westerink, Leipzig 1970
H. Omont, Inventaire sommaire des manuscrits grecs de la Bibliothèque nationale, Paris, vol. II 1888, vol. IV 1898
Palladius, Scholia in librum Hippocratis De fracturis, in: Charterius XII, pp. 270–286
– Commentarium in Hippocratis librum sextum De morbis popularibus, in: Dietz II, pp. 1–204
– Scholia in Galeni De sectis see Baffioni
A. I. Papadopoulos-Kerameus, Ἔκθεσις παλαιογραφικῶν καὶ φιλολογικῶν ἐρευνῶν ἐν Θράκῃ καὶ Μακεδονίᾳ, in: Ὁ ἐν Κωνσταντινουπόλει Ἑλληνικὸς φιλολογικὸς σύλλογος. Ἀρχαιολογικὴ ἐπιτροπή. Παράρτημα τοῦ ιζ' τόμου, Constantinople 1886
Plutarchus, Vitae Parallelae, ed. K. Ziegler, vol. III 1, Leipzig 1971
Pritchet see Joannes of Alexandria
Pseudo-Elias, Lectures on Porphyry's Isagoge, ed. L. G. Westerink, Amsterdam 1967
M. Richard, Ἀπὸ φωνῆς, Byzantion 20 (1950), pp. 191–222
– Répertoire des bibliothèques et des catalogues de manuscrits grecs, Supplément I, Paris 1964
R. Sabbadini, Classici e Umanisti da Codici Ambrosiani, Florence 1933
F. Sezgin, Geschichte des arabischen Schrifttums, vol. III, Leiden 1970
Soranus, Vita Hippocratis, ed. J. Ilberg, in: CMG IV, Leipzig and Berlin 1927, pp. 175–178
Stephanus, Commentary on the Aphorisms of Hippocrates, in: cod. Escorialensis Σ. II. 10, fol. 1^r–149^v; cod. Ambrosianus S 19 sup., fol. 1^r–58^r; extracts in: Dietz II, pp. 238ff.
– Commentary on Galen's Therapeutics to Glaucon I, in: Dietz I, pp. 233–344
O. Temkin, Geschichte des Hippokratismus im ausgehenden Altertum, Kyklos 4 (1932), pp. 1–80
M. Ullmann, Die Medizin im Islam (Handbuch der Orientalistik, 1. Abt.), Leiden 1970
L. G. Westerink, Anonymous Prolegomena to Platonic Philosophy, Amsterdam 1962
– Philosophy and Medicine in Late Antiquity, Janus 51 (1964), pp. 169–177

INTRODUCTION

I. Author and work

The history of the medical school of Alexandria in the sixth and seventh centuries is not well known in detail; nevertheless, as research continues, more information can be expected on some of the leading personalities and their work. As in the case of philosophy at this period, the main source of our knowledge is the body of commentaries based on the lectures of the school professors. In addition to revealing the method and style of instruction, such texts can shed light on the curriculum followed and sometimes provide enough evidence to establish the succession of teachers.[1] Unfortunately, few of the medical commentaries have survived and of these some remain in poor editions, while others exist only in Latin translations which have not been explored to the full.[2] The sole external description of the school and its activities is contained in the accounts of certain Arab writers, who are not always in complete agreement. However, the main point of interest is their claim that the Alexandrians established for teaching purposes a canon of sixteen works of Galen and, according to one authority, twelve works of Hippocrates; with this selection they associate a number of individuals, varying between four and seven. The evidence available so far from the texts seems to corroborate these statements.[3]

Of the seven physicians mentioned by the Arabs four can almost certainly be identified with the commentators Gesius, Palladius, Joannes and Stephanus. With the exception of Gesius, a small number of the works of these men are extant and have been partly published by Dietz in his collection.[4] They are all lecture notes recorded by students and edited on the same pattern as the commentaries on Plato and Aristotle of the sixth and seventh centuries. The original oral presentation is

[1] For the philosophers see Westerink's introduction to his edition of Anonymous Prolegomena to Platonic Philosophy, pp. X–XXV.

[2] Notably the commentaries of Joannes on Galen's De sectis (in the Latin edition of Galen printed at Pavia in 1515, fol. 6^r–12^v) and on the sixth book of the Epidemics (included in the so-called Articella collection of medical works, Venice 1483 etc.), newly edited by C. D. Pritchet, Leiden 1975.

[3] The sources are discussed by Bräutigam, pp. 35–45; Meyerhof, pp. 394ff.; Temkin, pp. 51ff. See also Sezgin, pp. 140–150; Ullmann, pp. 65–67. Of particular value on the question of the "canonization" of Galen are the many references, to works read or scheduled to be read, in Stephanus' commentary on the Aphorisms; the first complete edition of this text, by L. G. Westerink, will appear in the CMG.

[4] F. R. Dietz, Scholia in Hippocratem et Galenum, 2 vols., Königsberg 1834 (reprint Amsterdam 1966).

reflected in the expression ἀπὸ φωνῆς[1] which frequently appears in the titles. The first lecture (πρᾶξις) is devoted to a discussion of the eight points traditional in the Alexandrian schools of the time, the author's intention, the usefulness of the work, its order on the reading list, and so on; each subsequent lecture consists of a general discussion (θεωρία) of a portion of the text, followed by an explanation of individual words or phrases, if needed. Since the time of Olympiodorus, who was still teaching in 565, it became customary to separate each lecture by a heading and number, and to mark the end of both the theoria and the lecture itself with more or less regular formulas, such as ταῦτα ἔχει ἡ θεωρία and ἐν οἷς σὺν θεῷ ἡ πρᾶξις.[2] Such external marks, then, can be used as a means of approximate dating. Because they appear in the works of Joannes and Stephanus, it is safe to posit c. 550 as the terminus post quem.[3] It is not possible to establish a second terminus with the same assurance, though the fact that no text of this type can be firmly dated to the period following the Arab takeover of the city (642) suggests c. 650 as the outside limit.[4]

The three main extant works of Stephanus are his commentaries on the Prognosticon, the Aphorisms and Galen's Therapeutics to Glaucon I.[5] From their titles we learn that he is always described as a philosopher and once as a philosopher and physician. That he may have been also a teacher of philosophy, which the term usually implies at this time, would not be surprising, since the combination seems to have become common during the final stages of Alexandrian science.[6] It would also account for the knowledge of philosophy and its methods which he displays. The title of the commentary on Galen calls him an Athenian and this is how he is usually distinguished in the handbooks. He may have been born at Athens, but there can be no doubt that he taught in Alexandria.[7] Apart from the name, there is no other indication that Stephanus might have been a Christian.[8]

The commentary on the Prognosticon, as might be expected, owes a good deal of its matter to Galen, though the lecturer does not always acknowledge the dependence or is not aware of it. On the other hand,

[1] The meaning and history of the phrase have been thoroughly examined by Richard, Ἀπὸ φωνῆς, pp. 191–222.

[2] Sometimes they are not well preserved. In the commentary on the Prognosticon only a trace is left, at 34,11 (cf. 70,4; 74,14; 112,22).

[3] See Westerink, Philosophy and Medicine, pp. 169–177.

[4] It remains uncertain whether Stephanus is to be identified with the philosophy teacher of the same name who was still active late in the sixth century.

[5] A few shorter treatises bear his name in some manuscripts, though in others they are ascribed to different authors (e. g. to Palladius and Theophilus). The problem awaits solution.

[6] Westerink, Philosophy and Medicine, p. 169.

[7] Commentary on the Aphorisms Escor. Σ. II. 10, fol. 28^r (Professor Westerink kindly provided me with a copy of his text); Dietz I, p. 335,5.

[8] The doxology at the end of the work is likely to reflect the piety of a Byzantine copyist.

it is strongly influenced in substance and method by the long exegetical tradition of the school, of which Stephanus is perhaps the last representative. The earlier commentators are referred to several times, but never by name, as οἱ ἐξηγηταί or τινες. The ἐξηγητής mentioned at 184,8 is Stephanus himself, the note-taker having changed from first to third person narrative, a not unusual occurrence in these texts. On the other hand, the νέος ἐξηγητής twice quoted (126,1; 256,32) as supporting the Aristotelian doctrine that the heart is the seat of the soul's governing principle cannot be Stephanus who elsewhere in his works always takes the opposite, i. e. Galenic, view that the brain is the primary organ. Dietz is inclined to identify him with the medical professor Asclepius.[1]

Variant readings from manuscripts of the Prognosticon are cited three times (48,2; 124,2; 282,26) but, as Alexanderson has argued[2], two are probably due to misunderstandings and the third already appears in Galen. At any rate, it is highly unlikely that Stephanus consulted other copies of the text.

On two occasions he refers to previous lectures, on pulses (106,4) and on the part of the syllabus known as Physics (132,17).[3]

The alternative explanations appearing in the second and third lectures have been subordinated to the main commentary, since there is no good reason to suppose that they were included by Stephanus. They were probably inserted by a later user of the text, and from the fact that in most instances two comments (and not more) are supplied it can reasonably be concluded that two works were drawn upon. The wording and style have the familiar ring of lecture notes.[4]

II. The sources for the text

A. The manuscripts

The text is preserved entirely or in part by the following manuscripts[5], which fall into two distinct groups: 1. Laurentianus Plut. 59,14, Vindobonensis med. Gr. 15 (= β) and 2. Ambrosianus L 30 sup., Parisinus Gr. 2296, Vaticanus Gr. 2154, Yale Medical Library 50, Ambrosianus A 27 inf., Wellcome Historical Medical Library 354 (= γ).

[1] Dietz II, pp. IX–X; Westerink, Philosophy and Medicine, p. 172, suggests that Asclepius was the teacher of Stephanus.

[2] Alexanderson, p. 66.

[3] For physics (or physiology) the following works of Galen were read: Περὶ τῶν καθ' Ἱπποκράτην στοιχείων, Περὶ κράσεων and Περὶ φυσικῶν δυνάμεων.

[4] The idea expressed at 46,25ff., that Hippocrates practiced the dialectic method, could be a point of contact with Joannes, since he says the same thing three times in his commentary on the Epidemics (134a5; 146c11; 149b57).

[5] Cf. H. Diels, Die Handschriften der antiken Ärzte, II, Abh. d. Königl. Preuß. Akademie d. Wiss. 1906, Phil.-hist. Kl. 1, Berlin 1906, p. 96.

1.

L Laurentianus Plut. 59,14[1] (= L), 15th cent., folios 244. It contains these works: Hippocrates Προγνωστικόν (beginning missing); a fragment of Gregory Thaumaturgus; Stephanus on the Prognosticon; Galen Περὶ τύπων; (Theophilus) on the Aphorisms (incomplete); Galen on Περὶ φύσεως ἀνθρώπου; Galen on Περὶ διαίτης ὑγιεινῆς (fragment); Philaretus, tract on pulses; Galen, synopsis of his own work on pulses; Galen Περὶ τῆς τῶν κυουμένων διαπλάσεως; Joannes on Περὶ παιδίου φύσεως (incomplete). The commentary on the Prognosticon (fol. 12r–97r) is entitled σχόλια σὺν θεῷ εἰς τὸ προγνωστικὸν ἱπποκράτους ἀπὸ φωνῆς στεφάνου φιλοσόφου. Within this section of the codex the order of the pages has become disturbed at a number of places. In addition, some leaves have been lost giving rise to gaps at 32,27 ἤγουν – 36,2 δυνήσηται (1 folio) and 50,14 τὸ νόσημα – 52,18 τοιούτῳ (1 folio). There are two further lacunas of much greater extent, namely 78,1 ὅπερ – 96,6 περιπνευμονία and 174,27 αὕτη – 202,39 πνεύμονα, both of which were already in the exemplar, since they occur also in Vindobonensis med. Gr. 15. In general the writing is careful and the scribe went over the work to correct his own errors; there remains, however, a number of the usual mistakes in spellings (e. g. those due to iotacism and confusion of ο/ω), accents and breathings. For errors in L see below.

S Vindobonensis med. Gr. 15[2] (= S), 16th cent. (first half), folios 257. Most of the codex consists of extracts from a large number of the writings of Galen (26) and Hippocrates (35); it also contains excerpts from the following: Galen and others on fevers; Marcellinus Περὶ σφυγμῶν; [Aristotle] Προβλήματα; an anonymous medical treatise; the commentary of Stephanus (fol. 182r–201v) under the title ἐν τοῖς σχολίοις προγνωστικοῦ ἱπποκράτου (sic). The extracts begin at 48,28 ἰστέον and end at 292,31 ἐποιήσατο, comprising in all less than a third of the whole. In common with L this version has the two lacunas at 78,1–96,6 and 174,27–202,39, but despite the affinity of the two copies S is an extremely poor witness, being full of all sorts of errors and misunderstandings which often reduce the Greek to nonsense. Besides, the excerptor has taken considerable liberty with the text and in addition to the inevitable abridging and omitting of sentences he frequently resorts to rewording, in order to facilitate the transition from one extract to the next. In view of the manuscript's general unreliability use has been made of only those readings which serve to isolate the peculiarities of L. The instances are:

74,34 ἀτροφοῦνται SMPVY: -οῦντα L
100,29 ὅτι SMPVY: om. L
108,34 ἡμᾶς εἰπεῖν SMPVY: εἰπεῖν ἡμᾶς L
130,7 ὀψιαίτερον SMPVY: πρωιαίτερον L

[1] See Bandini, pp. 524–526.
[2] See Hunger (-Kresten), pp. 55–59.

132,23 καὶ^VI SMPVY: om. L
150,4 κἂν SMPV: κἂν καὶ L
152,21 ἐν^II SMPV: ἐν τῇ L
160,21 τῶν SMPV: ταῖς τῶν L
164,23 τότε SMPV: ποτὲ L
240,13 ἐν SMP: ἐν τῷ L
254,20 ἢ SMP: om. L

2.

Ambrosianus L 30 sup.[1] (= M), 16th cent. (1524), folios III[2] and 265. Contents: (Theophilus) on the Aphorisms, (Stephanus) on the Prognosticon (fol. 127r–261r), and an index to the Aphorisms. The inscription on fol. 1, Φιλοθέου ἐξήγησις εἰς τοὺς ἀφορισμοὺς Ἱπποκράτους καὶ ἀνωνύμου (over this Στεφάνου Ἀθηναίου) ἐξήγησις εἰς τὸ προγνωστικὸν Ἱπποκράτους, is a later addition. The lemmas from Hippocrates are normally distinguished by κείμενον and the comments by ἐξήγ(ησις), and there are numerous short omissions mostly due to homoeoteleuton. The cases where M differs from PV(Y) are often to be explained as efforts to correct the exemplar, e. g. M

48,2 πολλὰ M: παρὰ PVY
50,36 ἀποθνήσκει M: -ουσιν PVY
134,19 εὐκράσεως M: εὐκράτου PVY
182,2 ὅτε M: ὅτι PV
182,14 ὁ ἄρρωστος ἑκὼν M: ὁ ἑκὼν ἄρρωστος PV
186,38 ἄγεται M: ἅλεται P, ἄλεται V
200,34 εἴτε M: καὶ PV
222,28 τιτάνου (τι supra lin.) M: τάνου PV[3]

Parisinus Gr. 2296[4] (= P), 16th cent., folios 278. It contains (Theophilus)[5] on the Aphorisms and (Stephanus) on the Prognosticon (fol. 131v–278r). The handwriting is very careless and the scribe committed many mistakes, some of which he righted in a revision, when he also restored in the margins several of the passages left out the first time because of homoeoteleuton. He also managed to correct the exemplar in a few places; e. g. P

[1] See Martini-Bassi I, p. 566; Dietz I, pp. XVIII–XIX.
[2] fol. IIIv: "Hic codex fuit Hieronymi Mercurialis illiusque manu notis adspersus et Pisis emptus a Gratia Maria Gratia ... anno 16X1."
[3] This correcting activity will also account for the occasional coincidence (in minor matters) of LM against the rest, e. g. 40,16 μείζονος LM: μείζονος καὶ PVY; 40,34 πρόγνωσιν καὶ πρόρρησιν LM: πρόρρησιν καὶ πρόγνωσιν PVY; 48,28 ταῦτα τὰ LM: ταῦτα PVY; 150,6 εὐθὺς LM: εὐθὺς οἱ PV; 156,5 ἐλάχιστος LM: -ον PV; 170,5 τοιοῦτός LM: -όν PV; 222,20 τραφῆναι LM: στροφῆναι PV.
[4] See Omont II, p. 232; IV, p. 397; Dietz I, pp. XVII–XVIII.
[5] The title written by the scribe was σχόλια εἰς τοὺς ἱπποκράτους ἀφορισμοὺς κατὰ σύνοψιν. A later hand has deleted the word σχόλια, replacing it with Θεοφίλου φιλοσόφου ἐξήγησις. For the Stephanus commentary neither author nor title is given.

98,10 παραφρονῆ P: -ει MVY
100,13 δὲ P: om. MVY
124,33 ἡ P: ἢ MVY
184,1 στεχθῶσιν P: τεχθῶσιν M: στερχθῶσιν V
218,12 μέσης P: μέσως MV

Sample peculiar readings:

30,11 γίνεται P: γενήσεται MVY
34,4 παραβάσεις P: παρέμβασεις MVY
50,21 τοῦτο P: τούτου MVY
52,2 καλέσαι P: ἐκκαλέσαι MVY
78,12 τρυφῆ P: τροφῆ MVY
88,20 σφαλίζεσθαι P: ἀσφαλίζεσθαι MVY
90,1 καὶ P: ὁ MVY
178,30 ζωμένων P: ζωμευομένων MV
196,29 ἄπνους P: εὔπνους MV

V Vaticanus Gr. 2154[1] (= V), 16th cent., folios 174. The manuscript was written and signed by Andreas Darmarios[2] and consists of the commentary on the Prognosticon of which it contains only the first two sections, ending at 236,25 πεπλήρωται. It is supplied with the title δαμασκίου φιλοσόφου ἐξήγησις εἰς τὸ προγνωστικὸν τοῦ ἱπποκράτους which Mercati rightly suspects to have been forged by this notoriously fraudulent copyist.

Some peculiar readings:

38,28 γὰρ om. V
44,13 ἰητρῷ V: ἰατρῷ cett.
80,26 ἐν^{II} om. V
88,8 μὲν γὰρ V: γὰρ MPY
96,33 καὶ^{I} om. V
104,3 ἐν^{II} om. V
114,11 σωτήριός – 13 νοσημάτων om. V
120,21 εἰσὶ V: εἰ δὲ cett.
136,28 πύγιον V: πύον cett.

Y Yale Medical Library 50[3] (= Y) (formerly Saragossa, Cabildo de la Santa Iglesia Mayor del Pilar, 1427[4]), 16th cent., folios 94. Also in the hand of Darmarios, with the same title as V. Both are based on a common

[1] See Mai, pp. XXII–XXIII; Mercati, pp. 334–335 (= Opere Minori IV, pp. 38–39).
[2] fol. 174^{r}: ὑπὸ ἀνδρέου δαρμαρίου τοῦ ἐπιδαυρίου.
[3] See Bond-Faye, p. 63.
[4] See Graux-Martin, p. 218; cf. Richard, Répertoire, Supplément I, pp. 54–55.

exemplar (= ζ), but this time Darmarios has copied much less of the text, stopping without explanation at 146,2 γίνεσθαι. In view of the practices of the scribe here (see below, p. 18) and with other texts it should not be taken for granted that ζ contained less than the whole commentary. The extra headings at 34,13–15 (see apparatus) also may be confidently attributed to him.

Examples of conjunctive errors:

66,36 διὰ VY: δηλοῖ cett.
68,26 κόσμου VY: κόσμιον cett.
72,15 κοινὸν VY: μόνον cett.
76,20 καὶ διαστέλλεται VY: ἀντιδιαστέλλεται cett.
78,19 ἀκολασία VY: ἀκολουθία MP
78,20 ἡμερινή VY: θερινή MP
88,3 συνίσταται VY: συνίστασθαι MP
92,35 κρατούσης VY: κρατυνούσης MP

The scribe of ζ had already corrected the readings of its exemplar (= γ) not a few times, as the following cases will show:

28,29 παρὰ VY: περὶ MP
30,12 ὅτι VY: τί M: τι P
56,11 τὸ VY: om. MP
60,29 διέγνων μὲν VY: διέγνω μὲν P: διέγνομεν M
82,2 νομίζειν VY: -ει MP
92,34 ἔχων VY: -ειν MP
116,6 τὸ VY: τῷ MP
138,16 τείνονται VY: γείν- M: γίν- P

The two remaining manuscripts of this group have not been used for establishing the text, since they are not independent.

Ambrosianus A 27 inf.[1] (= A), 16th cent., folios I, 83. It consists of the commentary on the Prognosticon copied directly from P, and besides reproducing the many peculiarities of that codex (see above, p.16) it has a legion of its own. A

Sample peculiar errors:

28,32 καὶ om. A
32,22 μέν om. A
36,12 ἀδέοντα A: τὰ δέοντα cett.
46,32 αὐτῶν A: ἐκ τῶν cett.
64,9 καὶ] καλῶς A
114,24 μὴ κινούμενα A: μηκυνόμενα cett.

[1] See Martini-Bassi II, pp. 881–882.

132,30 ἐκείνων A: οἰκείων cett.
134,30 τὴν om. A

W Wellcome Historical Medical Library 354[1] (= W), 15th and 16th cent., folios 107. As presently bound the codex contains three works, each written by a different hand: 1. anonymous commentary on the Aphorisms and 2. the Prognosticon (both late 15th cent.?); 3. folios 22v–107v the commentary on the Prognosticon in the hand of Darmarios (c. 1582). This is an immediate copy of Y, ending at the same spot (see above, p. 17), but with the telltale marginal comment ἐλλιπὲς ἦν τὸ τέλος ὑπὸ τῆς ἀρχαιότητος.

Some shared errors:

32,10 κατὰ τὰ YW: τὰ κατὰ cett.
44,19 ἑτέρα YW: ἄλλη cett.
60,4 ἔβαλε YW: ἐπέβαλε cett.
64,4 πατικῶς YW: πλατικῶς cett.
66,4 σύνοδος YW: σύνοχος cett.

Two examples will suffice to highlight the dependency: 60,26 βούλομαι αὐτὸν θεραπεῦσαι, οὐ θέλω δέ et in mg. γρ'. δύναμαι αὐτὸν θεραπεῦσαι οὐ βούλομαι Y: δύναμαι αὐτὸν θεραπεῦσαι, οὐ βούλομαι οὐ θέλω δέ in textu W; 80,25 καυσώδης] καιδυσώδης (sic) Y: καὶ δυσώδης W (καισώδης V).

It looks as if MP and ζ (= VY) are related directly to the archetype of the group (γ) and not through intermediaries. Thus, when any two of MPζ agree in an error against the third, it means that those two have transmitted the reading of γ, while the third has corrected it; several examples of such correcting have already been given with the descriptions of those copies. γ will have been a codex containing at least (Theophilus) on the Aphorisms and (Stephanus) on the Prognosticon. It must have had numerous compendia, especially for verbs, which would explain the many cases where each of MPζ shows a variant; e. g. 44,24 θαυμάσει M: -η, ει sscr., Y: ambig. V: θαυμάσιον P; 44,26 ἀκούση M: -σει ζ: -οῦσαι P; 66,16 ἐμπέσεις M: -ης P: ambig. ζ; 80,33 σημειώση P: -σεις M: ambig. ζ; 88,14 ἀντιστρέφειν M: -έφον P: -έφει Y: -έφουσιν V; 134,32 ἀπορήσει P: -ήσοι ζ: ambig. M. The state of γ will also account for other discrepancies between the three; e. g. 28,14 ξένα M: ἑνα P: ἐ ζ; 32,31 δὲ M: supra lin. inscr. P: om. ζ; 34,26 νοσήματος] νοσώματος, ut vid., P: σώματος Mζ; 48,23 ἡ ἀκοὴ ζ: ἀκοὴ P: ἡ κοὴ M; 52,7 μεμπταίος P: μεμπτὸς M: μεμπτοῖ ζ; 102,35 δύναμις M: δύναμις αὕτη P: αὕτη δύναμις ζ.

Another manuscript containing the commentary belonged at one G time to the Church of St. Nicholas in Gallipoli (= G), but its present

[1] See Moorat, pp. 225–226.

whereabouts are not known.[1] However, Papadopoulos-Kerameus in his description[2] has preserved the title – Σχόλια σὺν Θεῷ εἰς τὸ Προγνωστικὸν Ἱπποκράτους ἀπὸ φωνῆς Στεφάνου τοῦ φιλοσόφου –, and the opening words. He dates the book to the 14th cent. and lists the rest of the contents as: anonymous treatises on medical topics, botany and pulses; a medical poem; the letter of Hippocrates to Ptolemy; two tracts of Galen on pulses and two on urines; Magnus Emesenus on urines; Theophilus on urines; Aetius on urines and pulses; the Prognosticon (followed by the commentary). The contrast in age and contents suggests that G is not closely related to L, which would tend to bolster their joint authority for the title.

In late 1447 or early 1448, Cyriacus of Ancona, while visiting Mistra in the Morea, apparently got his hands on a manuscript of the commentary, for he quotes the whole story of Erasistratus and Antiochus (58,18 ταῦτα δὲ πάντα – 62,4 ἀπηλλάγη).[3] The copy belonged to the γ group, as the following readings show: 58,19 τινός om.; 58,23 γοῦν; 58,35 ἐμνημόνευσεν Εὐρυδίκης ante τις trsp.; 58,36 αὐτῷ; 58,36 ὁ om.; 60,21 ἐθεώρησεν] ἐχώρησεν; 60,21 ante γέγονεν add. καὶ. In spite of a multitude of spelling errors, the extract is the only witness to have the correct reading ὧν at 58,22.

In a fourteenth century copy of Galen's commentary on the Prognosticon, Vaticanus Reginensis Gr. 175, the scribe has written in the margins with red ink a number of scholia which, as Heeg rightly observed[4], are largely based on the work of Stephanus. They have no value for the text, but are an interesting example of how a Byzantine writer (of unknown date) made use of the Stephanus commentary. In one passage Holy Scripture is quoted several times (p. 205).

The overall relationship of the manuscripts may be seen from the following stemma:

[1] An unsuccessful attempt to locate it was made in recent years. See Alexanderson, pp. 73–74.

[2] Papadopoulos-Kerameus, pp. 8–9.

[3] Cod. Ambrosianus-Trotti 373, fol. 117r–119v. See Sabbadini, p. 33, who gives a list of the variants. Thanks to the kindness of Fr. E. Bodnar I was able to examine a photocopy of the original; the Stephanus extract is in the autograph part of the manuscript (fol. 101–124).

[4] CMG V 9,2, pp. XX–XXI. Heeg has included the scholia in his edition, printing them under the parts of Galen's text to which they refer.

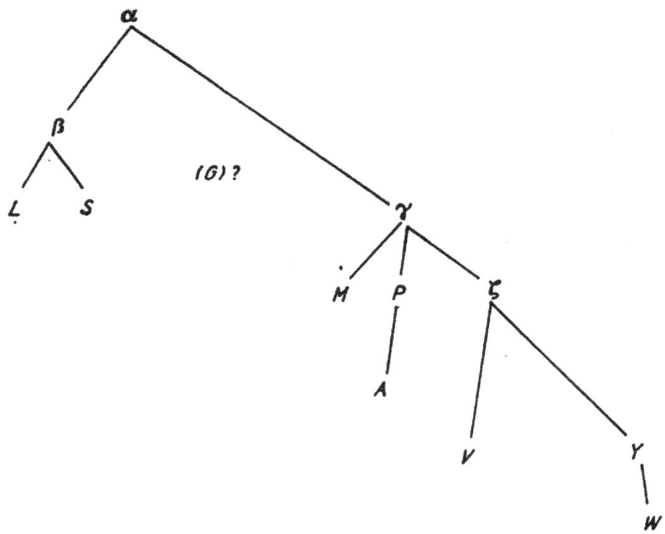

B. The editions

The first and only edition of the entire text was that published by Dietz in 1834. The manuscripts known to him were LMPA and he based his text on three of these, having decided to discard P on the grounds that its readings agreed with those of M. He corrected many of the obvious errors and made a number of sound conjectures, but his apparatus gives a very incomplete picture of the manuscript readings.

In 1841, unaware of Dietz's work, A. Mai reproduced almost without critical comment the curtailed version of V, in Spicilegium Romanum V, pp. 1–160. He did not hesitate, however, to oust Damascius from the title and restore the name of Stephanus, when his initial suspicions were confirmed by, among other things, the catalog descriptions of L and M.

III. Editorial conventions

A. The text

Because the tradition separates clearly into two branches, we are never faced with more than two real variants. The differences are often minor and linguistic in nature (involving word order, verb tenses and moods, choice of prepositions, adverbs, particles etc.) and it is sometimes possible to make a decision on the basis of usage in the immediate surroundings or elsewhere in the commentary. In cases where the readings appear of equal value the practical procedure has been adopted of giving preference to L, since it on the whole presents a more accurate text. Where there are gaps in L a rather full account is given of MPVY.

In the matter of grammar it has seemed best to be conservative.

The instances of loose or careless syntax, ungrammatical use of participles and so on, are so numerous that a great many of them must be original. Of course the note-taker may have had a hand in shaping the language of the text, but it is not possible to distinguish his influence. Some accents and spellings have been silently corrected or normalized.

The original division into lectures has been reconstructed; where there is some doubt, this has been indicated by brackets.

B. The lemmas

There is considerable variation in detail between the versions of L and γ; apart from this, L frequently gives longer extracts, while γ tends to preserve more Ionic forms. There is ample indication that both have been tampered with during transmission and in some cases it is probable that the lecturer himself manipulated the text for his own purposes. Neither branch on its own nor the common version of both is very close to any single witness of the Prognosticon, though overall there are slightly more similarities with the lemmas in Galen's commentary and manuscripts YSX of Hippocrates. Most of the readings of Lγ are to be found in the tradition of the Prognosticon. Of those not attested elsewhere some are obvious deteriorations and none of the rest is likely to be a true variant from an unknown corner of the tradition. Hence it is safe to conclude, as Alexanderson does[1], that they have no interest for the text of Hippocrates. The instances in question are:

72,30 χλωρόν – ἐόν] sic nullus test. Hipp.; 156,12 ὑδέρων] ὑδρώπων Hipp.; 158,23 ὅλον σῶμα] ἄλλο σῶμα codd. Hipp. praeter X (σῶμα πᾶν); 220,1 ἐπύρεξεν ὁ ἄνθρωπος] ὁ ἄνθρωπος ἐπύρεξεν Hipp.; 248,32 sq. ξυνεχεῖ – δεινὸν] hic nullus test. Hipp.; 268,1 sq. αἱ τοιαῦται ἀποστάσιες post χρόνῳ trsp. Hipp.; 276,3 δὲ non habet Hipp.; 280,18 τὰ τοιαῦτα] ταῦτα Hipp.; 282,19 sq. τριάκοντα ἐτέων] τριηκονταετέσι Hipp.; 286,14 χλωρὸν] καὶ χλωρὸν Hipp.; 286,35 ξύμπασι τοῖς] τοῖσι ξύμπασι Hipp.; 290,29 Ἐπειδὴ] ἐπεὶ Hipp.

Occasionally one can decide which reading is more likely to have appeared originally with the commentary, if the lemma is quoted again in the same lecture (e.g. 74,17; 130,28; 146,4; 158,33). When this criterion is not available and there are no other means of choosing, the version of L has generally been accepted.

In an earlier and less complete form this edition served as a doctoral dissertation in Classical Philology for the State University of New York at Buffalo in 1975. In addition to other improvements made in the meantime, the translation has been thoroughly overhauled, going from a fairly free version to one that may well err at the other extreme; however, it seemed best to keep uppermost in mind the needs of the

[1] Alexanderson, p. 67.

Greekless medical historian, and this will account for the rather scrupulous effort to distinguish anything that, strictly speaking, does not appear in the Greek. The intervening years have also seen new publications of a few of the works mentioned in the footnotes and bibliography, which may be noted here.[1]

Setting out on the road to Graduate School I was kindly advised and helped by John J. O'Meara of University College, Dublin. George L. Kustas at Buffalo always showed a keen interest in my work for which I am grateful. In Buffalo, too, it was my great good fortune to study under the direction of Leendert G. Westerink and each passing year makes me only more aware of what a privileged apprenticeship that was. It is saying the very least to record that Professor Westerink suggested this edition, fostered its preparation at every stage, and with characteristically deft strokes removed all kinds of blemishes in the transmitted text of Stephanus and in my translation of it.

For several years I enjoyed the facilities of the Dumbarton Oaks Library where Mrs. Irene Vaslef and her staff were models of courtesy and helpfulness. At the National Library of Medicine in Bethesda Mrs. Hanks and her fellow Librarians made me feel very welcome.

I wish to thank the Zentralinstitut für Alte Geschichte und Archäologie of the Akademie der Wissenschaften der DDR for accepting the edition into the Corpus Medicorum Graecorum. Special thanks go to Dr. sc. Jutta Kollesch and Dr. Diethard Nickel. They have devoted a considerable amount of time to bringing my work into line with the requirements of the series and have made numerous improvements in both text and translation.

The work I dedicate to my wife Pilar.

University of Maryland St. Patrick's Day, 1982

John M. Duffy

[1] The Agnellus commentary on Galen's De sectis has been edited and translated for the first time by Seminar Classics 609, Arethusa Monographs VIII, Buffalo N. Y. 1981. Incidentally, the Buffalo scholars tell us (p. X) that the work on De sectis attributed to Joannes of Alexandria is in reality a rewritten version of the Agnellus text.

Dieter Irmer has published a new edition of Palladius on De fracturis, Hamburg 1977.

ΣΤΕΦΑΝΟΥ ΦΙΛΟΣΟΦΟΥ

ΣΧΟΛΙΑ
ΕΙΣ ΤΟ ΠΡΟΓΝΩΣΤΙΚΟΝ ΙΠΠΟΚΡΑΤΟΥΣ

STEPHANUS THE PHILOSOPHER

A COMMENTARY
ON THE PROGNOSTICON OF HIPPOCRATES

CONSPECTVS SIGLORVM

L = Laurentianus Plut. 59,14
S = Vindobonensis med. Gr. 15
M = Ambrosianus L 30 sup.
P = Parisinus Gr. 2296
V = Vaticanus Gr. 2154
Y = Yale Medical Library 50 (olim Saragossa, Cabildo de la Santa Iglesia Mayor del Pilar, 1427)

ζ = consensus VY

γ = consensus MPζ (MPV post p. 146,2)

G = Gallipoli, 'Εκκλησία ἁγίου Νικολάου, 38

Wk. = L. G. Westerink

ΣΧΟΛΙΑ
ΣΥΝ ΘΕΩΙ ΕΙΣ ΤΟ ΠΡΟΓΝΩΣΤΙΚΟΝ ΙΠΠΟΚΡΑΤΟΥΣ
ΑΠΟ ΦΩΝΗΣ
ΣΤΕΦΑΝΟΥ ΦΙΛΟΣΟΦΟΥ

I

I 51 Dietz Τὰ εἰωθότα ἐπὶ ἑκάστου συγγράμματος προλέγεσθαι η' κεφάλαια καὶ νῦν προ[σ]λάβωμεν, τὸν σκοπόν, τὸ χρήσιμον καὶ τὰ ἑξῆς.

Σκοπὸς τοίνυν ἐστὶ τῷ Ἱπποκράτει περὶ τῶν ὀξέων νοσημάτων διαλαβεῖν, οὐχὶ τῶν ἁπλῶς ὀξέων, ἀλλὰ τῶν μετὰ πυρετοῦ ὀξέων· εἰσὶ γὰρ ὀξέα νοσήματα καὶ ἄνευ πυρετοῦ, ὥσπερ ἀποπληξία καὶ ἐπιληψία καὶ σπασμὸς καὶ τέτανος. τριττὴ δὲ ἡ σημείωσις· ἢ γὰρ τῶν παρῳχηκότων 52 ἢ τῶν ἐνεστώτων ἢ τῶν μελλόν|των. καὶ τῶν μὲν παρῳχηκότων ἡ σημείωσις λέγεται ἀνάμνησις· ἡ δὲ τῶν ἐνεστώτων λέγεται διάγνωσις· ἡ δὲ τῶν μελλόντων λέγεται πρόγνωσις. ἁπλῶς γοῦν περὶ τῶν ὀξέων νοσημάτων τῶν μετὰ πυρετοῦ διαλέγεται, ἐπειδὴ ταῦτα ταράσσει τὴν φύσιν καὶ τὴν τέχνην ἐφέλκεται. καὶ ὅτι τοῦτο ἀληθὲς δηλοῦσι τρία τινά.

Πρῶτον μὲν τὸ ὀξὺ τῆς κινήσεως καὶ ἡ σφοδρότης τῆς θερμασίας ταράσσει τὴν φύσιν, ἐπειδὴ πολλὰ περιττώματα γεννῶσι καὶ τὸ τηνικαῦτα ἡ φύσις κατεπείγει τὸ τάχος καὶ τὴν πυκνότητα τῶν σφυγμῶν, εἶτα καὶ τὴν ἀναπνοήν· οὐ μὴν ἀλλὰ καὶ τὴν συστολὴν καὶ τὴν διαστολὴν κατεπείγει ἡ φύσις, τὴν μὲν διὰ τὸ ἐξάξαι τὰ λιγνυώδη περιττώματα, τὴν δὲ διὰ τὸ εἰσάξαι καθαρὸν καὶ ψυχρὸν ἀέρα πρὸς τὸ ἐμψῦξαι τὸ ἔμφυτον θερμόν. ἀλλὰ καὶ ἡ τέχνη κατεπείγεται εἰς βοήθειαν τῆς φύσεως.

Δεύτερον δὲ καὶ διὰ τὸ συνεχὲς τῆς θερμασίας ταράσσεται ἡ φύσις, καὶ διὰ τὸ μὴ ἔχειν ἀνακωχὴν καταβάλλονται αἱ δυνάμεις αὐτῆς καὶ ἐν πολλῷ ἀγῶνι καὶ ταραχῇ ἐστιν ἡ φύσις. ἀλλὰ καὶ ὁ τεχνίτης ταράσσεται διὰ τὸ μὴ εὑρίσκειν καιρὸν τοῦ δοῦναι τροφὴν καὶ ἀνακομίσασθαι τὴν δύναμιν διὰ τὴν συνέχειαν τῆς θερμασίας.

Τρίτον δὲ διὰ τὸν ξενισμὸν καὶ τὸ ἀλλότριον τῶν συμβαινόντων ταράττεται ἡ φύσις καὶ τὴν τέχνην ἐφέλκεται. δεῖ γὰρ εἰδέναι ὅτι τῶν ἐν τοῖς

6 Τὰ – κεφάλαια] *cf.* Steph. Comm. in Hipp. Aph.: II pp. 238–240 Dietz Pall. Schol. in Hipp. De fract.: XII pp. 270–272 Chart. Comm. in Hipp. De morb. pop. VI: II pp. 1–4 Dietz Ioann. Comm. in Hipp. De morb. pop. VI: 120a1–120b38 Pritchet Comm. in Gal. De sect.: I fol. 7^r–7^v ed. Pav. Schol. in Hipp. De nat. pueri: II pp. 205–208 Dietz Agnell. Comm. in Gal. De sect.: Ambros. G 108 inf. fol. 27^v–28^v Comm. in Gal. Artem: ibid. fol. 48^v–49^r Comm. in Gal. De puls.: ibid. fol. 92^r–93^r 11–14] *cf.* [Gal.] Introd. s. med. 7: XIV p. 690 K. Gal. Ars med. 3: I p. 313 K.

1–4 ἐν τοῖς σχολίοις προγνωστικοῦ ἱπποκράτου *(sic)* S: *tit. non praebent* MP: δαμασκίου φιλοσόφου ἐξήγησις εἰς τὸ προγνωστικὸν τοῦ ἱπποκράτους ζ 4 *ante* φιλοσόφου *add.* τοῦ G *(v. supra, p. 19)* 6 sq. καὶ νῦν *om.* γ 7 προσλάβωμεν *codd.*: *correxi* 8 ἐστὶ *om.* γ 9 ὀξέων$^{I\ et\ II}$ *om.* γ εἰσὶ γὰρ] διαλέγεται εἰς τὰ L 10 ἀποπληξία] ἐπιπληξία L 21 λιτρώδη L 24 καὶ^{I} *om.* γ 26 ταράττεται γ 29 *post* συμβαινόντων *add.* συμπτωμάτων γ 30 τῇ τέχνῃ *codd.*: *corr. Wk.*

A COMMENTARY, WITH GOD'S HELP, ON THE PROGNOSTICON OF HIPPOCRATES, BASED ON THE LECTURES OF STEPHANUS THE PHILOSOPHER

I

Let us now begin with the eight preliminary points usual for each work, the intention, the usefulness, and so on.

Now Hippocrates intends to deal with acute diseases, not acute without distinction, but those attended by fever; for there are acute diseases without fever, such as apoplexy, epilepsy, spasm and tetanus. And there are three kinds of symptom interpretation, of past or present or future (symptoms). For past it is called anamnesis, for present diagnosis, and for future prognosis. In general, then, he discusses the acute diseases which are attended by fever, since these upset nature and involve the art. And three things show that this is true.

In the first place, the violence of the movement and the severity of the heat disturb nature, because they give rise to a lot of residues; then nature forces the speed and frequency of the pulses, then respiration also; on top of this nature puts pressure on systole and diastole, on the former by expelling the sooty residues, on the latter by driving in clean, cold air to cool the innate heat. The art, too, is rushed to the aid of nature.

Secondly, nature is also harassed by the constant heat and, getting no rest, its faculties are overcome and it is involved in a great struggle and disturbance. And the doctor too is harassed because, due to the constant heat, he does not find an opportunity to administer nutriment and restore strength.

Thirdly, when the symptoms which appear are strange and unusual, nature is disturbed and brings in the art. For it should be noted that of

νοσήμασι θεωρουμένων συμπτωμάτων τὰ μὲν οἰκεῖά εἰσι καὶ γνώριμα καὶ συνήθη, τὰ δὲ ξένα. καὶ οἰκεῖα μέν, καθάπερ ἐπὶ τῆς πλευρίτιδος, τὰ τέσσαρα ἐκεῖνα, ἡ βήξ, ἡ δύσπνοια, ὁ ὀξὺς πυρετὸς καὶ τὸ νυγματῶδες ἄλγημα. ξένα δέ ἐστι συμπτώματα ὥσπερ ἐπὶ τῆς πλευρίτιδος ἐὰν γένηται κῶμα καὶ παραφροσύνη καὶ αἵματος ἀναγωγὴ καὶ λύγξ. πλευρῖτις δέ ἐστι φλεγμονὴ τοῦ τὰς πλευρὰς ὑπεζωκότος ὑμένος, ἀλλὰ διὰ τὸ ἔνδον εἶναι τὴν φλεγμονὴν ἐκ τῶν τεσσάρων
53 συμπτωμάτων διαγινώσκει ὁ ἰατρὸς τὴν | πλευρῖτιν. τὰ οὖν ἴδια συμπτώματα τὸ εἶδος δηλοῦσι τοῦ νοσήματος, τὰ δὲ ξένα τὸ ἦθος τοῦ νοσήματος, καὶ τοῦτο διχῶς· ἢ γὰρ μέτριά εἰσιν ἢ ἄμετρα. καὶ εἰ μὲν μέτρια ὦσιν, ὥσπερ ἐπὶ τῆς πλευρίτιδος μετρία ἐκτάραξις γαστρός, ὅπερ ξένον ἐστὶ σύμπτωμα, ἐπειδὴ ἀλλαχοῦ ἐστιν ἡ ὕλη, καὶ δηλοῖ εὔηθες τὸ νόσημα. εἰ δὲ ἄμετρα ὦσι τὰ συμπτώματα, ἅπερ εἰρήκαμεν ἐπὶ τῆς πλευρίτιδος, τὸ κῶμα λέγω καὶ ἡ παραφροσύνη καὶ ἡ ἀναγωγὴ τοῦ αἵματος καὶ ὁ σπασμός, κακόηθες δηλοῦσι τὸ νόσημα. τὰ τοιαῦτα οὖν ξένα συμπτώματα πάντως ταράττουσι τὴν φύσιν καὶ τὴν τέχνην ἐφέλκονται.

Ὡς οὖν ἐν συντόμῳ εἰπεῖν, ὅτι σκοπός ἐστι τῷ Ἱπποκράτει σημείωσιν ἡμῖν παραδοῦναι τῶν ὀξέων νοσημάτων, ἐπειδὴ ταῦτα ταράσσουσι τὴν φύσιν καὶ τὴν τέχνην ἐφέλκονται διὰ τοὺς τρεῖς τρόπους οὓς εἰρήκαμεν. εἰ δέ τις λέγοι ὅτι «Περὶ χρονίων νοσημάτων προϊὼν διαλέγεται· περὶ γὰρ ὑδέρου καὶ σπληνὸς κακωθέντος καὶ περὶ ἐμπυημάτων διαλέγεται, ταῦτα δὲ χρόνιά εἰσι», πρὸς ὃ λέγομεν ὅτι καὶ περὶ τούτων διαλεγόμενος ἔτι πλείονα σπουδὴν ποιεῖται τῶν ὀξέων· οὐχ ὡς χρονίων γὰρ περὶ τούτων διαλέγεται, ἀλλ' ὡς ἐκ μεταπτώσεως ὀξέων νοσημάτων γεγονότων.

Τὸ δὲ χρήσιμον διττόν ἐστιν· οὐ μόνον γὰρ χρησιμεύει τῷ ἀναγινώσκοντι, ἀλλὰ καὶ ἀναγκαῖόν ἐστιν, ἐπειδὴ τὸ παρὸν σύγγραμμα ἐπὶ τὴν ἀρίστην ὁδὸν ἡμᾶς παιδεῦον ἀπάγει, λέγω δὴ ἐπὶ τὴν θεραπευτικὴν κατὰ τὸ εἰρημένον «Ὁ ἄριστα διαγνοὺς ἄριστα καὶ θεραπεύει.» καὶ ἰστέον ὅτι τὸ θεραπευτικὸν εἰς τρία διαιρεῖται, εἰς προφυλακτικόν, παρηγορικὸν καὶ θεραπευτικόν, ἐπειδὴ καὶ τὰ παρὰ φύσιν τριττά εἰσιν· ἢ γὰρ νοσήματά εἰσιν ἢ συμπτώματα ἢ αἴτια. καὶ πρὸς μὲν τὰ αἴτια ἐνιστάμενοι προφυλακτικοὶ λεγόμεθα, πρὸς δὲ τὰ νοσήματα θεραπευτικοί, πρὸς δὲ τὰ συμπτώματα παρηγορικοί. ἐντεῦθεν καὶ ἡ σημείωσις τριττή ἐστι, προγνωστική,
54 διαγνωστική, ἀναμνηστική. καὶ διὰ μὲν τῆς προγνώσεως | προφυλαττόμεθα θεραπευτικῶς, διὰ δὲ τῆς διαγνώσεως τὰ νοσήματα θεραπεύομεν, διὰ δὲ τῆς ἀναμνήσεως ⟨τὰ συμπτώματα παρηγοροῦμεν. ἀλλὰ περὶ τῆς ἀναμνήσεως⟩ ἄπορος δοκεῖ εἶναι ὁ λόγος, ⟨εἰ⟩ ἡ παρηγορία τῶν συμπτωμάτων τῶν ἐνεστώτων ἐστίν, ἡ δὲ ἀνάμνησις τῶν παρῳχηκότων·

2 sq.] *cf.* Gal. De cris. I 3: IX p. 554 K. 27 τὸ εἰρημένον] *cf.* Steph. Comm. in Hipp. Aph.: Escor. Σ. II. 10 fol. 13r Pall. Schol. in Hipp. De fract.: XII p. 271 Chart. Alex. Trall. IX 3: II p. 415 Puschm. Ioann. Comm. in Gal. De sect.: I fol. 9v ed. Pav. 29–32] *cf.* Pall. Schol. in Gal. De sect.: p. 77,17–20 Baffioni

5 φλεγμός γ 6 *post* ἀλλὰ *add.* καὶ γ 9 ἀσύμμετρα γ 10 μέτρια *codd.*: *correxi* ὅπερ] ὢ τὸ *codd.*: *corr. Wk.* 14 τοιαῦτα] τρία L *post* οὖν *add.* ταῦτα τὰ L ξένα] ἕνα P: ἐ *ante spat. vac.* ζ 16 οὖν *om.* L 19 λέγει MP 23 γεγονότα *codd.*: *corr. Dietz* 24 τὸ ἐχρήσιμον, *ut vid.*, MP 26 ἡμᾶς ὁδὸν LM παιδεύων LPζ 29 περὶ MP 35 sq. τὰ – ἀναμνήσεως *add. Wk.* 36 εὔπορος L ὁ *om.* L εἰ *add. Wk.* προσηγορία *codd.*: *correxi*

the symptoms observed in diseases some are peculiar, well known and usual, while others are strange. In the case of pleurisy, for example, the peculiar symptoms are those (well known) four, coughing, difficult breathing, acute fever and throbbing pain. However, if coma, delirium, spitting blood or hiccups develop, these are strange symptoms for pleurisy. Now pleurisy is inflammation of the membrane lining the ribs, and since the inflammation is internal, the doctor diagnoses the disease from the four symptoms. The peculiar symptoms, then, show the type of disease, while the strange distinguish its character; and the character is of two kinds: for strange symptoms are either moderate or immoderate. If moderate, as for example mild bowel disturbance in pleurisy – this is a strange symptom, seeing that the matter is in another place –, they show that the disease is mild in character. But if they are immoderate like those we have mentioned for pleurisy, namely coma, delirium, spitting blood and spasm, they indicate that the disease is malignant in character. Strange symptoms such as these, then, always disturb nature and involve the art.

To put it briefly, then, Hippocrates has in mind to instruct us in the interpretation of symptoms of acute diseases, since these disturb nature and involve the art in the three ways we have described. But if someone should say, "As he goes on he deals with chronic diseases; for he discusses dropsy, diseased spleen and empyemas, which are chronic", our answer is that, although he does discuss those conditions, he devotes more attention to the acute; you see, he does not treat them as chronic (in themselves), but as conditions which have resulted from a change in acute diseases.

The usefulness (of the present book) is twofold; not only does it benefit the reader, but it is also a necessary work, setting us on the best road by its instruction, by which I mean the road to therapy, for, as the saying goes, "The one who prognoses best is also the best therapist." Note that there are three divisions of therapy: prevention, alleviation and cure, abnormal conditions also being three in number, namely diseases, symptoms and causes. When we fight against causes we are called preventors, against diseases healers, and against symptoms alleviators. Hence we have three forms also of symptom interpretation, prognosis, diagnosis and anamnesis. Using prognosis we take therapeutic precaution, through diagnosis we cure diseases, and through anamnesis we alleviate symptoms. But on this point of anamnesis we seem to run into a problem, if it is true that alleviation is concerned with present symptoms, while anamnesis has to do with past symptoms; anamnesis, then,

οὐδὲν οὖν συντελεῖ ἡ ἀνάμνησις πρὸς θεραπείαν, ἀλλὰ πρὸς τὰ συμπτώματα ἡ διάγνωσις μᾶλλον ἁρμόζει· ἢ ὅτι καὶ ἡ πρόγνωσις πρὸς θεραπείαν ἤτοι πρὸς παρηγορίαν. καὶ ἴσως ἀπορήσει τις ὅτι «Οὐδὲν ἡμῖν ὠφελεῖ ἡ ἀνάμνησις.» πρὸς ὃ λέγομεν ὅτι οὐδὲν ἡμῖν χρησιμεύει πρὸς θεραπείαν, πλὴν οὐ πάντη ἐστὶν ἄχρηστος, ἀλλὰ συμβάλλεται ἡμῖν καὶ αὕτη. διὰ γὰρ τῆς ἀναμνήσεως ἀναμιμνήσκομεν τὸν ἄρρωστον τὰ προγεγονότα ἀπό τινος μηδὲν ἀκούσαντες, καὶ λέγομεν αὐτῷ τῷ ἀρρώστῳ ὡς ἐν ὑποθέσει ὅτι «Ὑδροποσίᾳ ἐχρήσω ἢ ἀδηφαγίᾳ ἢ ὀπωροφαγίᾳ.» εἶτα ταῦτα τοῦ ἀρρώστου ἀναμιμνησκομένου μεγαλαυχεῖ τὸν τεχνίτην καὶ πειθήνιος γίνεται τῷ ἰατρῷ λέγων ὅτι «Οὗτος ἅπερ οὐκ εἶδεν οὐδὲ ἤκουσεν, ἀνέμνησέ με τῶν πραχθέντων παρ' ἐμοῦ.» καὶ τὸ τηνικαῦτα ῥᾴστη γενήσεται ἡ θεραπεία.

Ὅτι δὲ γνήσιόν ἐστι τὸ παρὸν σύγγραμμα τοῦ Ἱπποκράτους, πάντες ὡμοφώνησαν οἱ ἐξηγηταὶ ὅτι ἐκείνου τοῦ Ἱπποκράτους ἐστὶ τὸ παρὸν σύγγραμμα οὗτινος καὶ τὸ Περὶ διαίτης ὀξέων καὶ τὸ Περὶ τόπων ἀέρων ὑδάτων· ἐκεῖνα γὰρ κυρίως γνήσιά εἰσι τοῦ Ἱπποκράτους. ποίου δὲ Ἱπποκράτους εἰσὶν οὐκ ἴσμεν· τέσσαρες γὰρ Ἱπποκράται γεγόνασιν, ὁ Γνωσιδίκου, ὁ Ἡρακλείδα, ὁ Δράκοντος καὶ ὁ Θεσσαλοῦ. πλὴν ὑπολαμβάνομεν ὅτι τοῦ Ἡρακλείδα εἰσὶν Ἱπποκράτους τὰ συγγράμματα ταῦτα, ἐπειδὴ τοῦτον λέγουσιν εὐδοκιμήσαντα ἐν τοῖς ἔργοις τῆς τέχνης.

Ἐπιγέγραπται δὲ Προγνωστικὸν Ἱπποκράτους [καὶ] ἀπὸ σημειώσεως. καὶ μὴν τὴν σημείωσιν εἰς τρία διείλομεν, εἰς πρόγνωσιν καὶ
55 διάγνωσιν καὶ ἀνάμνησιν. | πῶς οὖν ἀπὸ ἑνὸς μέρους τὴν ἐπιγραφὴν ἐποιήσατο; καὶ λέγομεν ὅτι ἢ ὡς τιμιωτέραν ἢ ὡς καθολικωτέραν. τιμιωτέρα γάρ ἐστιν ἡ πρόγνωσις καὶ τῆς διαγνώσεως καὶ τῆς ἀναμνήσεως· μόνου γὰρ θεοῦ ἐστι τὸ προγινώσκειν. καὶ κατὰ τοῦτο οὖν ἐοίκαμεν θεῷ καὶ ἰσοθέους ἡμᾶς ἡγοῦνται, ἐκ τοῦ προγινώσκειν ἡμᾶς· ἡ γὰρ πρόγνωσις θείας τινὸς καὶ ὑπερτέρας ἐστὶ δυνάμεως. πάλιν δὲ καὶ ὡς καθολικωτέραν οὖσαν τὴν πρόγνωσιν, ἀπ' αὐτῆς ἐποιήσατο τὴν ἐπιγραφήν· ἐν γὰρ τῇ προγνώσει καὶ ἡ διάγνωσις καὶ ἡ ἀνάμνησις συνέ[ρ]χονται ὡς μερικώτερα.

Ἡ δὲ τάξις τῆς ἀναγνώσεως· δεῖ ἐν τοῖς Ἱπποκρατείοις συγγράμμασι πρότερον τὰ καθόλου ἀναγινώσκειν τῶν μερικῶν. διὸ δεῖ τοὺς Ἀφορισμοὺς ἀναγινώσκειν πρότερον, ἐπειδὴ πάντων τῶν μερῶν τῆς ἰατρικῆς διαλαμβάνουσιν, καὶ εἶθ' οὕτως ἐπὶ τὰ μερικὰ ἰέναι. ἀλλὰ ταῦτα διττά ἐστιν· ἢ

8 Ὑδροποσίᾳ – ὀπωροφαγίᾳ] *cf.* Schol. R *in* Gal. In Hipp. Progn. comm. I 2: CMG V 9,2 p. 198 *ad* lin. 19 16 sq.] *cf.* Pall. Schol. in Hipp. De fract.: XII p. 272 Chart. 22 sq.] *v. supra*, app. sim. *ad* p. 26,11–14 25 sq.] *cf.* Steph. Comm. in Hipp. Aph.: Ambros. S 19 sup. fol. 24ᵛ 26 sq.] *cf. infra*, p. 64,9 sq. Hipp. De decent. orn. 5: CMG I 1 p. 27 Pall. Schol. in Gal. De sect.: p. 71,13 Baffioni 31–32,25] *cf.* Pall. Schol. in Hipp. De fract.: XII pp. 271sq. Chart.

1 *ante* θεραπείαν *add.* τὴν L 10 οἶδε(ν) MP 11 γένηται L 12 Ὅτι] τί M: τι P 13 ὁμοφώνησαν Lζ 13 sq. σύγγραμμα τὸ παρὸν γ 17 ἡρακλειδᾶ L: ἡρακλείδας γ: *corr. Dietz* θεσσαλός *codd.*: *correxi* 18 ἡρακλειδᾶ L 21 καὶ *seclusi* ἀποσημείωσις *codd.*: *correxi* 23 τὴν ἐπιγραφὴν *post* οὖν *trsp.* γ 24 τιμιωτέρου ... καθολικωτέρου Pζ: *ambig.* M 25 μόνον L 26 καὶ[I] *om.* γ 28 οὖσαν *om.* γ 30 συνέρχονται *codd.*: *correxi* 34 ἐστιν] εἰσιν γ

contributes in no way towards the therapy of symptoms, rather diagnosis is more suited for this; or otherwise (we could say) that prognosis contributes to their therapy or alleviation. Perhaps someone will object that "Anamnesis is of no use to us at all." Our reply is that, even if it is of no help for therapy, it is not entirely useless and does make a contribution. For, using anamnesis, we can recall for the patient the things he has done, without being informed by anyone; we tell him, let us suppose, "You drank water or overate or took fruit." Then when this has been recalled to him he is all praise for the skilled man and puts his trust in the doctor; "This man", he says, "recalled to me the things I had done, without seeing or hearing about them." After this treatment will be simple.

As for the authenticity, all the commentators agree that the present work is by the same Hippocrates who wrote On Diet in Acute Diseases and On Places, Airs, Waters, these being above all authentic Hippocratic writings. But to which Hippocrates they belong we do not know; for there were four of them, the sons of Gnosidicus, Heracleides, Draco and Thessalus. However, it is our view that they were written by the son of Heracleides, since he is reputed to have distinguished himself in the practice of the art.

The title of the book, Prognosticon of Hippocrates, is taken from the sphere of symptom interpretation. We have already divided this into three, prognosis, diagnosis and anamnesis. Why, then, does he take the title from the one part? We say, either because prognosis is more important or because it is more comprehensive. For prognosis is more important than both diagnosis and anamnesis, since only God has the power of prognosis. And it is because of this, namely prognosing, that we (doctors) resemble God and are considered godlike; for foreknowledge belongs to a higher, divine power. Again, he takes the title from prognosis because it is more comprehensive; for both diagnosis and anamnesis are contained in prognosis as subdivisions.

As regards the reading order, among the writings of Hippocrates the comprehensive works should be read before those on particular subjects. This means that one ought to read first of all the Aphorisms, since these cover all the parts of medicine, then the writings concerned with particular topics. And here there are two kinds, those describing

γὰρ κατὰ φύσιν εἰσὶν ἢ παρὰ φύσιν. καὶ δεῖ πρότερον τὰ κατὰ φύσιν. ταῦτα δὲ τὰ κατὰ φύσιν τριττά εἰσιν· ἢ γὰρ πόρρω εἰσὶν ἢ προσεχῆ ἢ προσεχέστερα. καὶ δεῖ πρότερον τὰ πόρρω ἀναγινώσκειν, οἷον τὸ Περὶ ἀνθρώπου φύσεως, ἐπειδὴ ἐκεῖσε περὶ τῶν πορρωτάτω στοιχείων διαλέγεται. εἶτα δεῖ ἐπὶ τὰ προσεχῆ ἔρχεσθαι στοιχεῖα. διὸ δεῖ ἀναγινώσκειν τὸ Περὶ παιδίου φύσεως, τὸ Περὶ χυμῶν. ταῦτα γὰρ προσεχῆ εἰσιν στοιχεῖα, τὸ σπέρμα καὶ τὸ καταμήνιον, ἐξ οὗ τρέφεται τὸ ἔμβρυον, καὶ οἱ χυμοί. εἶτα μετὰ ταῦτα δεῖ ἐπὶ τὰ προσεχέστερα ἔρχεσθαι. διὸ δεῖ μετὰ ταῦτα τὸ Περὶ τροφῆς ἀναγινώσκειν· ταῦτα γὰρ προσεχέστερά εἰσι στοιχεῖα, λέγω δὴ αἱ τροφαί. εἶτα μετὰ τὰ κατὰ φύσιν δεῖ μετιέναι ἐπὶ τὰ παρὰ φύσιν. ἀλλὰ τῶν παρὰ φύσιν διττή ἐστιν ἡ διαφορά· ἢ γὰρ σποραδικά εἰσιν ἢ κοινά. καὶ δεῖ πρῶτον τὰ σποραδικὰ ἀναγινώσκειν. καὶ σποραδικὰ μέν ἐστι τὰ ἀλληνάλλως ἔχοντα περὶ τῶν
56 πα|θῶν. ταῦτα γὰρ τὰ σποραδικὰ διττά ἐστιν· ἢ γὰρ σημειωτικὰ ἢ θεραπευτικά. καὶ δεῖ πρότερον τὰ σημειωτικὰ ἀναγινώσκειν. διὸ δεῖ πρότερον τὸ παρὸν σύγγραμμα ἀναγινώσκειν καὶ τοῦ Περὶ διαίτης ὀξέων καὶ τοῦ Περὶ ἄρθρων καὶ τοῦ Περὶ ἀγμῶν, ἐπειδὴ ἐκεῖσε θεραπείας διδάσκει. καὶ μετὰ τὴν σημείωσιν δεῖ τὰς θεραπείας ἀναγινώσκειν, καὶ ἐν τῇ θεραπείᾳ τὰ ὁμοιομερῆ ἀναγινώσκειν ⟨πρότερον⟩ τῶν ὀργανικῶν. διὸ δεῖ πρότερον τὸ Περὶ διαίτης ὀξέων ἀναγινώσκειν, ἐπειδὴ ἐκεῖσε τὰ ὁμοιομερῆ θεραπεύει, καὶ εἶθ' οὕτως ἐπὶ τὰ ὀργανικὰ δεῖ ἔρχεσθαι. διὸ δεῖ τὸ Περὶ ἄρθρων καὶ ἀγμῶν ἀναγινώσκειν. τῶν δὲ κοινῶν τὰ μὲν ἔνδημά ἐστιν, τὰ δὲ ἐπίδημα. καὶ δεῖ πρῶτον τὰ ἔνδημα ἀναγινώσκειν. καὶ ἔνδημα μέν ἐστι τὰ ἐνυπάρχοντα, ἐπίδημα δὲ τὰ μὴ ὑπάρχοντα. διὸ δεῖ τὸ Περὶ τόπων ἀέρων ὑδάτων ἀναγινώσκειν, ἅπερ ἐστὶν ἔνδημα, καὶ εἶθ' οὕτως τὰ ἐπίδημα, τουτέστι τὰς 'Επιδημίας. καὶ τέλος πάντων δεῖ τὰ Γυναικεῖα ἀναγινώσκειν, διὰ τὸ περὶ γυναικείων παθῶν καὶ μόνον διαλέγεσθαι, ἄλλως τε δὲ ὅτι καὶ περὶ ἑνὸς μορίου πεπονθότος διαλέγεται, ἤγουν περὶ πεπονθυίας μήτρας.

Ἡ δὲ εἰς τὰ μόρια διαίρεσις· εἰς τρία τμήματα διαιρεῖται κατὰ τὸν Γαληνόν, κατὰ δὲ τὸν Ἱπποκράτην οὐκ ἔστι τμῆμα, ἀλλ' ὅσα θεωρήματα τοσαῦτα καὶ τμήματα.

Ἀνάγεται δὲ τὸ παρὸν σύγγραμμα ὑπὸ τὸ θεωρητικόν, καὶ τὸ θεωρητικὸν ὑπὸ τὸ σημειωτικόν.

Τρόπῳ δὲ διδασκαλικῷ οὐ κέχρηται ὁ Ἱπποκράτης ᾧτινι ὁ Γαληνὸς συνθετικῷ λόγῳ καὶ ἀναλυτικῷ ἐξ ὅρου διαλύσεως καὶ τοῖς τοιούτοις, ἀλλ'

29 κατὰ–30] *cf.* Pall. Comm. in Hipp. De morb. pop. VI: II p. 3,30–32 Dietz Ioann. Comm. in Hipp. De morb. pop. VI: 120b27–29 Pritchet Schol. in Hipp. De nat. pueri: II p. 207,26sq. Dietz 31sq.] *cf.* Steph. Comm. in Hipp. Aph.: Ambros. S 19 sup. fol. 2r 33–34,11 κέχρηται] *cf.* Steph. Comm. in Hipp. Aph.: II p. 240,1–13 Dietz Pall. Schol. in Hipp. De fract.: XII p. 272 Chart. Ioann. Comm. in Hipp. De morb. pop. VI: 120b30–36 Pritchet Γαληνὸς] Gal. Ars med., Prooem.: I p. 305 K.

1 τὰ *om.* L 1 sq. ταῦτα – φύσιν *om.* L 4 πορρωτάτων LM δεῖ] δὴ LPζ: *corr.* M 5 τὰ] τῶ L τὸ] τὰ *codd.*: *correxi* 8 δεῖ] δὴ LPζ: *corr.* M 14–23 *ubique* δὴ *pro* δεῖ L 15 καὶ^{I} *om.* γ 16 ἀκμῶν L: ἄκμων γ: *corr. Dietz* 17. 19 ὁμοιοτερῆ *bis* L 18 πρότερον^{I} *coni. Dietz* 20 ἀκμῶν *codd.*: *corr. Dietz* 26 μόνων PY 27 *verba* ἤγουν – 36,2 δυνήσηται *desunt in* L *(v. supra, p. 14)* 29 δὲ *om.* ζ 30 καὶ *om.* P 31 δὲ *supra lin. inser.* P: *om.* ζ τὸ^{II} *om.* M 31 sq. καὶ – σημειωτικόν *om.* ζ

normal conditions and those abnormal. The normal should come first; and they are of three kinds, remote, intermediate and immediate. One should first read the remote, namely On the Nature of Man, since he discusses there the most remote elements. Then one must proceed to the intermediate elements. So one should read On the Nature of the Child and On Humors, the intermediate elements being the sperm, the menses which nurture the embryo, and the humors. Next one should go on to the immediate. For which reason On Nutriment should then be read; for these, I mean foods, are immediate elements. After the normal we pass on to the writings on abnormal conditions, of which there are two kinds, sporadic and common. First one must read the sporadic, i.e., works which discuss diseases at random. And here we distinguish two groups, semeiotic and therapeutic. The semeiotic should come first, which means reading the present work before On Diet in Acute Diseases and before On Joints and On Fractures, because in those he gives instruction on therapy. After symptoms one should read about therapy, and within this class the works on homogeneous before those on organic parts. Hence one ought to begin with On Diet in Acute Diseases, since he gives there therapy for homogeneous parts. Next the works on organic parts, and so one should read On Joints and Fractures. Of the common works, on the other hand, some are endemic, others epidemic. The endemic are to be read first. Now endemic are inherent diseases, epidemic are non-inherent. Hence one should read On Places, Airs, Waters, which are endemic, after this the epidemic, which means the Epidemics. Last of all to be read is On the Diseases of Women, because it is devoted entirely to women's ailments, and the more so since only one affected part is discussed, viz. the diseased womb.

With regard to the division of the work, in Galen there are three sections, but Hippocrates has no divisions, sections corresponding to the number of topics discussed.

The present work belongs to the theoretical category and it is a theoretical treatise of the semeiotic class.

Hippocrates does not employ the same didactic method as Galen who uses synthesis, analysis, which is based on term resolution (?), and so

ἑτέροις τρόποις τρισὶ κέχρηται, ἀφοριστικῷ, ὑφηγηματικῷ καὶ μικτῷ. καὶ ἀφοριστικὸς μέν ἐστιν ὁ πενόμενος ταῖς λέξεσι, πλουτῶν δὲ τοῖς ἐνθυμήμασιν· ὑφηγηματικὸς δέ ἐστιν ὁ ἔχων προσδιορισμοὺς καὶ προθεωρήματα καὶ ἐπι-
57 λογισμοὺς καὶ παρεκβάσεις, καὶ ἁπλῶς εἰπεῖν | ἐξομοιούμενος καὶ ἐξ ἴσου ἔχων καὶ ἐξισάζων τοῖς ἐνθυμήμασι τὴν λέξιν. μικτὸς δέ ἐστιν ὁ μήτε οὕτως ὡς ὁ ἀφοριστικὸς μήτε ὡς ὁ ὑφηγηματικός, ἀλλὰ μέσως πως. ὁ δὲ ὑφηγηματικὸς εἰς τρία διαιρεῖται· ἢ γὰρ ὑψηλός ἐστι καὶ ἐπηρμένος ὁ χαρακτήρ, ὥσπερ τὸ Περὶ τόπων ἀέρων ὑδάτων, ἢ ταπεινὸς καὶ χθαμαλός, ὥσπερ τὰ Γυναικεῖα· περὶ γὰρ οὔρων, ὑποχωρημάτων καὶ τῶν τοιούτων ἐκεῖσε διαλέγεται· μέσος δὲ χαρακτήρ ἐστιν ᾧπερ ἐνταῦθα κέχρηται· οὔτε ὑψηλῷ καὶ ἐπηρμένῳ οὔτε ταπεινῷ, ἀλλὰ μέσῳ χαρακτῆρι κέχρηται. ἐν οἷς σὺν θεῷ ἡ πρᾶξις.

II

I 1 [1: 193,1 A. = II 110,2 L.] Τὸν ἰητρὸν δοκέει μοι ἄριστον εἶναι

Ἄξιον ἀπορίας ὅτι πῶς ὁ Ἱπποκράτης μὴ εἰωθὼς ἐν τοῖς οἰκείοις συγγράμμασι προοιμιάζεσθαι νῦν προοιμίῳ κέχρηται. καὶ λέγομεν ὅτι διὰ τοὺς μεθοδικοὺς τῷ προοιμίῳ ἠναγκάσθη χρήσασθαι, ἵνα ἀποδείξῃ ἀναγκαίαν τὴν πρόγνωσιν. ἐκεῖνοι γὰρ πάντῃ ἀνῄρουν τὴν πρόγνωσιν λέγοντες μηδὲν ὅλως λυσιτελοῦσαν τῷ ἰατρῷ. ἔφασκον γὰρ ὅτι ἰατροῦ ἐπιστήμονός ἐστι τὸ τὴν ὑγεῖαν φυλάττειν καὶ τὸ τὴν διαφθαρεῖσαν ὑγεῖαν ἀνακαλέσασθαι· τὸ δὲ προγινώσκειν μάντεώς ἐστιν ἢ προφητῶν τινων. ὁ οὖν Ἱπποκράτης θέλων ἐλέγξαι τοὺς μεθοδικοὺς καὶ ἀναγκαίαν ἀποδεῖξαι τὴν πρόγνωσιν τῷ προοιμίῳ ἐχρήσατο, ἐκ τριῶν συλλογιστικῶν ἀποδείξεων σκευάζων αὐτό.

Καὶ πρώτη ἐστὶν αὕτη· ὁ ἰατρὸς ἐξ ὧν προλέγει, πάντως γινώσκει τὴν φύσιν τοῦ ὑποκειμένου νοσήματος· ὁ δὲ γινώσκων τὴν φύσιν τοῦ ὑποκειμένου νοσήματος εὐπειθεῖς ἀπεργάζεται τοὺς νοσοῦντας· ὁ εὐπειθεῖς τοὺς νοσοῦντας ποιῶν εὐχερῶς καὶ ταχέως ἀπαλλάττει τὸν κάμνοντα τῆς νόσου· ὁ τοιοῦτος ἰατρὸς ἐξ ὧν προλέγει, εὐχερῶς καὶ ταχέως ἰᾶται τὸν κάμνοντα.

Δεύτερον συλλογισμὸν λέγει τοιοῦτον, ὅτι ὁ προγινώσκων ἰατρὸς προευτρεπίζεται· ὁ δὲ προπαρασκευαζόμενος οὐ ταράττεται· ὁ μὴ ταρατ-
58 τόμενος νικᾷ τὸν | ἀγῶνα· ὁ νικῶν τὸν ἀγῶνα τοῦ ἰδίου σκοποῦ περιγίνεται, ὅστις ἐστὶ τῆς ἰάσεως· οὗτος γὰρ ὁ σκοπὸς τῷ ἰατρῷ ἴασις. καὶ γὰρ ὁ προγινώσκων τὰς παρὰ φύσιν διαθέσεις τὰς μήπω γενομένας, μελλούσας δὲ

1sq.] *cf.* [Gal.] Def. med. V: XIX p. 349 K. 15–24] *cf.* Gal. In Hipp. Progn. comm. I 1: CMG V 9,2 p. 197,7–14 25–29] *cf.* Gal. In Hipp. Progn. comm. I 2: CMG V 9,2 p. 198,12–15 33–36,3] *cf.* Gal. In Hipp. Progn. comm. I 3: CMG V 9,2 p. 199,7–9

4 παρεμβάσεις Mζ: παραβάσεις P: *correxi* 10 ὅνπερ γ: *corr. Dietz* 13 *tit.* κείμενον *add.* Mζ τέλος τῆς προθεωρίας *et* ἀρχὴ τοῦ προγνωστικοῦ ἱπποκράτους *add.* V: τέλος τῶν προθεωριῶν *et* ἀρχὴ τοῦ προγνωστικοῦ τοῦ ἱπποκράτους ὑπὸ δαμασκίου φιλοσόφου *add.* Y ἰτρὸν M: ἰατρὸν P δοκέει μοι] δόκιμον P 15 *tit.* ἑρμηνεία *add.* ζ 16 προοιμιάζεται ζ 26 νοσώματος, *ut vid.*, P: σώματος Mζ: *corr. Dietz* 34 περὶ P *post* μήπω *add.* μὲν ζ

on. Hippocrates has three different styles, the aphoristic, the expository and the mixed. The aphoristic is poor in words but rich in meaning; the expository includes qualifying remarks, introductory discussions, further reflections and digressions, to put it simply, it assimilates, equalizes and evens expression to thought. The mixed is neither of these two but something intermediate. The expository is divided into three types: the character may be lofty and elevated as in On Places, Airs, Waters, or humble and down-to-earth as in On the Diseases of Women; for there he discusses urines and feces and the like; or in between, which is the character he uses here; he employs a style that is neither lofty and sublime nor humble, but intermediate. This, with God's help, is the lecture.

II

I 1 I think that the best thing for the doctor is

It is worth asking why Hippocrates, who usually does not have a preface in his works, now uses one. We say that he was forced to do so because of the Methodists, in order to show that prognosis is necessary. For those people did away with prognosis entirely, claiming that it was of no benefit whatsoever to the doctor. "The job of a skillful physician", they said, "is to preserve health and restore it when it has been lost; prognosis is for the seer or the prophets." Hippocrates, then, used the preface to refute the Methodists and to demonstrate the necessity of prediction, making it from three proofs in the form of syllogisms.

The first is as follows: judging from his prognosis the doctor must know the nature of the underlying disease; the one who understands the nature of the underlying disease makes the sick compliant; the one who makes the sick compliant effects in the patient an easy and swift cure from the disease; (therefore) such a doctor, from what he prognoses, easily and quickly cures the patient.

The second syllogism goes like this: the doctor who prognoses is well prepared; the one who is ready in advance is not thrown off balance; he who is not knocked off balance wins the struggle; the victor in the struggle is successful in his particular aim, which is healing, a doctor's objective being to heal. You see, the one who makes forecasts is able to eradicate and prevent diseased conditions while they are still threatening

ἔσεσθαι, ἐκκόπτει καὶ οὐκ ἐᾷ γενέσθαι. εἰ δὲ καὶ γένωνται, κἂν μὴ πάντῃ δυνήσηται αὐτὰς ἐκκόψαι, ἀλλ' ὅμως τὸ σφοδρὸν καὶ τὸ μέγεθος αὐτῶν καθαιρεῖ καὶ μετριάζει. οὕτως γοῦν πολλάκις προγινώσκοντες μέλλοντας παροξυσμοὺς εἰσβάλλειν μετὰ συγκοπῆς ἢ λιποθυμίας ἢ παραφορᾶς, παρέχοντες τροφὰς ἢ βοηθήμασιν ἐπιτηδείοις παρεσχηκότες, ἢ πάντῃ οὐ συνεχωρήσαμεν γενέσθαι ἤ, καὶ ἐὰν ἐγένοντο, ὑφειμένως καὶ μετρίως ἐγένοντο.

Τρίτον δὲ συλλογισμὸν οὐκέτι ἀπὸ τοῦ τέλους τῆς τέχνης λαμβανόμενον, ἀλλὰ ἀπὸ τοῦ ἀναίτιον καὶ ἀνεύθυνον αὐτόν τε καὶ τὴν τέχνην διατηρεῖν. φησὶ γὰρ ὅτι ὁ προγινώσκων ἰατρὸς προλέγει τοὺς σωθησομένους ἢ τεθνηξομένους· ὁ οὕτως προλέγων ἰατρὸς τὰ μέλλοντα ἔσεσθαι ἀναίτιον ἑαυτόν τε καὶ τὴν τέχνην καθίστησιν. ἐὰν γὰρ προγνῷ ὁ ἰατρὸς ὅτι περιεστηκός ἐστι τὸ νόσημα, πάντα τὰ δέοντα διαπράττεται καὶ κέχρηται ταχὺ καὶ φλεβοτομίᾳ καὶ καθάρσει καὶ ἑτέροις πλείστοις βοηθήμασιν. εἰ δὲ προγνῷ ὅτι ὀλέθριόν ἐστι τὸ νόσημα, οὐδ' ὅλως ἐγχειρεῖ τῷ νοσοῦντι παρατηρούμενος τὸ φάσκον ῥητὸν ὅτι «Τοῖς ὑπὸ τῶν νούσων κεκρατημένοις οὐ δεῖ ἐγχειρεῖν», καὶ τὸ «Φύσεως ἀντιπραττούσης πάντα κενεά». καὶ λοιπὸν οὐκ ἐφάπτεται, ἵνα μηδ' ὅλως οἱ λοιδορεῖν σπεύδοντες τῶν ἰδιωτῶν εἰς τὸ γινόμενον μέμψιν ἐπιθήσωσιν, ὅτι τυχὸν «Εἰ μὴ ἐφλεβοτομήθη[ν], οὐκ ἂν ἀπέθνῃσκεν».

I 2 [1: 193,1 A. = II 110,2 L.] ⟨Τὸν ἰητρὸν δοκέει μοι ἄριστον εἶναι⟩

Φησὶν ὁ Γαληνὸς ὅτι ἀσαφῶς πέφρασται τὸ ῥητόν, ἀλλὰ διὰ τὸ σαφὲς δεῖ ἡμᾶς ἐν ὑπερβατῷ οὕτως ἀναγνῶναι· «Δοκεῖ μοι ἄριστον εἶναι πρόνοιαν ἐπιτηδεύειν τὸν ἰατρόν.» φαμὲν οὖν ὅτι τὸ δοκεῖ κατὰ δύο σημαινομένων φέρεται· πρῶτον μὲν κατὰ τοῦ ἐνδοιαστικοῦ, ὥσπερ ἂν εἴπωμεν
59 «Δοκῶ τάδε βουλεύεσθαι ὑμᾶς». φέρεται | δὲ καὶ κατ' ἄλλου σημαινομένου, ὅταν μὴ ᾖ ἐνδοιαστικόν, οἷον ὡς ἂν εἴπωμεν ὅτι «Δοκεῖ τῷ θεῷ τόδε τι ποιῆσαι», «Δοκεῖ τῷ βασιλεῖ», καὶ τηνικαῦτα οὐ κατὰ τοῦ ἐνδοιαστικοῦ αὐτὸ λαμβάνομεν, ἀλλ' ὅτι δόγμα πεποίηται καὶ πάντως τοῦτο γενήσεται, ὃ ἔδοξεν αὐτῷ. οὕτως οὖν καὶ ἐνταῦθα ὁ Ἱπποκράτης τὸ δοκεῖ ἐξέλαβεν ἀντὶ τοῦ δόγμα τιθέναι.

Ἑτέρου. τὸν ἰητρὸν δοκέει μοι ἄριστον εἶναι· ἰστέον ὅτι τὸ δοκεῖ διάφορον ἔχει τὴν σημασίαν· σημαίνει γὰρ δισταγμὸν ἢ ἀξίωμα ἢ μέτριον ἦθος. καὶ διστακτικῶς μέν,

15 τὸ – ῥητὸν] Hipp. De arte 3: CMG I 1 p. 10,21sq. 16] Hipp. Lex 2: CMG I 1 p. 7,14 22–24] *nihil de hac re apud* Gal. In Hipp. Progn. comm. 33 μέτριον ἦθος] *cf.* Gal. In Hipp. Progn. comm. I 4: CMG V 9,2 p. 203,14–18

1 πάντ *(ambig.)* V: πάντα Y 3 καθαίρει *codd.*: *correxi* 5 παρεσχηκότες] χρώμενοι *exspectaveris* 7 οὐκέτι] οὐκ ἔστι L: *fort.* οὐ λέγει *scribendum est* 8 καὶ ἀνεύθυνον *om.* γ αὐτόν *codd.*: *correxi* 9 ὁ *post* προγινώσκων *trsp.* Pζ: *om.* M ἢ] καὶ γ 10 ἰατρὸς *post* ἔσεσθαι *trsp.* γ 11 τε *om.* γ 12 ταχὺ] τυχὸν L καὶ[II] *om.* L 13 καὶ[I]] ἢ L 15 νόσων L 16 κενά M: καινά L 17 μηδ'] μὴ L 18 ἐφλεβοτομήθην *codd.*: *corr. Dietz* 20 sq. Τὸν – εἶναι *addidi* 24 τὸ *om.* L σημαινομένω L 25 εἴπομεν γ 26 σημαινόμενον γ 27 εἴπομεν MPV τότε L 28 οὐ *om.* L 30 ὁ *om.* γ 32 ἕτερον Mζ(P?) 33 *ante* δισταγμὸν *add.* τὸν γ δικαστικῶς γ

and have not yet appeared. And even if they do develop and he does not manage to root them out entirely, all the same he can moderate their vehemence and lessen their seriousness. Thus, many times when we had predicted the onslaught of paroxysms in the form of syncope or fainting or delirium we were able, by administering nutriment or prescribing the proper remedies, either to completely prevent the attacks or, even if they did occur, to make them subdued and mild.

His third syllogism is based, not on the goal of the art, but on the idea that the one who prognoses keeps both himself and the art free from guilt and censure. For he says that the doctor who prognoses states in advance who will survive and who will die; the one who thus predicts the outcome leaves both himself and the art above reproach. For if his prognosis is that the disease can be cured, he does everything that should be done; he does not hesitate to open the veins or to purge or to employ many other remedies. However, if he predicts that the disease will prove fatal, he does not put a hand to the patient observing the prescriptions "Do not touch those already overcome by disease" and "When Nature is working against you everything is hopeless". Consequently he avoids the case so as to give no opportunity to those laymen who are just waiting to find fault in him; they would attach blame to the incident and say, for example, "If you hadn't cut his veins, he would not have died".

I 2 I think that the best thing for the doctor is

According to Galen the sentence as expressed is not clear and to make it so we must change the word order and read, "I think that the best thing for the doctor is to practice forecasting." We say, then, that (in Greek) the verb *dokein* (think) is used in two different senses. One is when there is doubt involved, as in the sentence, "It seems to me (*dokō*) that you are planning this". But it is used in another sense, when there is no uncertainty, as in "It pleases (*dokei*) God to do such and such" or "The Emperor sees fit (*dokei*)"; in these cases we do not take the word in the doubtful way, but (understand it to mean) that a decision has been made and what he has decided will certainly take place. Similarly here, then, Hippocrates employed the verb in the sense of making a judgement.

Another discussion of the text I think that the best thing for the doctor is: Note that the word *dokein* (think) is used in a variety of ways to convey doubt or self-evidence or moderation. In "The soul (appears to be?) immortal" it expresses

ὅτι «Ἡ ψυχὴ ἀθάνατος»· κατὰ γὰρ τοὺς ἔξω ἀμφιβάλλεται. ἀξιωματικῶς δὲ ὡς ἡνίκα ὑπὸ ἄλλου ἐρωτώμενος ὅτι «Ὁ ἄνθρωπος ζῷόν ἐστιν;» ἀποκρίνομαι λέγων «Οὕτως μοι δοκεῖ». μέτριον δὲ ἦθος καθάπερ οἱ φιλόσοφοι ποιοῦσιν ἐν τοῖς πράγμασιν ἐπὶ τῶν ἀληθῶν πραγμάτων, ἀποκρίνονται καὶ λέγουσιν ὅτι «Οὕτως μοι δοκεῖ», καίτοι γινώσκοντες ὅτι ἀληθῶς οὕτως ἔχει. ὁ οὖν Ἱπποκράτης ἀξιωματικῶς ἐχρήσατο τῷ δοκεῖ μοι ἢ ὡς διὰ μέτριον ἦθος.

Ἄλλη ἐξήγησις ἀνωνύμου τινὸς ἐξηγητοῦ σαφοῦς καὶ συντόμου καὶ θαυμαστοῦ. καθ' ὑπερβατὸν οὕτως ἀναγνωστέον· «Δοκέει μοι τὸν ἄριστον ἰατρὸν πρόνοιαν ἐπιτηδεύειν.» τὸ δοκέει μοί τινες ἐξηγήσαντο· φασὶ γὰρ ὅτι ὁ Ἱπποκράτης οὐκ ἐτόλμησεν οὕτως ἁπλῶς ἀποφήνασθαι διὰ τὸ μὴ παντελῶς θαρρεῖν· μετριάζων οὖν ἔφη δοκέει μοι ἀντὶ τοῦ νομίζω. οὐκ ἔστι δὲ ὡς ἐκεῖνοι ἐνόμισαν, ἀλλὰ δοκέει μοι ἀντὶ τοῦ «Δόγμα πεποίημαι καὶ δόγμα ἔχω τὸ τὸν ἰατρὸν τὸν ἄριστον πρόνοιαν ἐπιτηδεύειν.»

I 3 [1: **193,1 A.** = **II 110,2 L.**] Πρόνοιαν ἐπιτηδεύειν

Ἰστέον ὅτι ἡ πρόνοια τετραχῶς· δηλοῖ γὰρ τὴν φροντίδα καὶ τὴν προαίρεσιν καὶ τὴν κηδεμονικὴν τοῦ παντὸς δύναμιν καὶ τὴν πρόγνωσιν. καὶ ἐπὶ μὲν τῆς φροντίδος ἱστορεῖ ὁ Εὐριπίδης τὴν Πολυξένην φονευομένην ὑπὸ τοῦ Πύρρου ὅτι «Ἡ δὲ καὶ πίπτουσα ὅμως πολλὴν πρόνοιαν εἶχεν εὐσχήμως πεσεῖν καὶ κρύπτειν ἅπερ κρύπτεται ὄμματα ἀρρένων.» ἐπὶ
60 δὲ τῆς προ|αιρέσεως δηλοῖ τὸ παρὰ τῷ Σόλωνι τῷ νομοθέτῃ εἰρημένον, ὅτι «Δικάζειν δεῖ τὴν βουλὴν τὴν ἐν Ἀρείῳ πάγῳ φόνου καὶ τραύματος ἐκ προνοίας», τουτέστιν ὅτι οἱ κατὰ προαίρεσιν φονεῖς ἐν τῷ Ἀρείῳ πάγῳ εἶχον τὸ δικαστήριον, ὡς ἂν τῶν ἄλλων ἐγκλημάτων ἐν ἄλλοις τόποις ἐχόντων. ἐπὶ δὲ τῆς τοῦ παντὸς κηδεμονίας, ὡς ὅταν λέγωμεν ὅτι «Ὁ θεὸς προνοεῖται τοῦ τῇδε κόσμου.» ἐπὶ δὲ τῆς προγνώσεως αὐτὴ ἡ λέξις δηλοῖ ὅτι πρόνοια εἴρηται ἐκ τοῦ προνοεῖν τὸν νοῦν καὶ ἐκ τοῦ προλαμβάνειν τὸν νοῦν. ὁ οὖν Ἱπποκράτης τὴν πρόνοιαν κατὰ τῆς προγνώσεως ἔθηκεν ὡς ἰατρός.

Ἄλλως. τὸ δὲ τῆς προνοίας ὄνομα ἄλλοι ἄλλως ἐξηγήσαντο· οἱ μὲν γὰρ εἰρήκασιν πρόνοιαν αὐτὸν λέγειν τὴν φροντίδα, οἱ δὲ τὴν προπαρασκευήν. καὶ γὰρ πρόνοια καλεῖται ἡ φροντίς· ὅθεν λέγομεν ἐν τῇ κοινῇ συνηθείᾳ ὅτι «Ὁ δεῖνα τοῦδε προενοήσατο» ἀντὶ τοῦ φροντίζει. ἔχομεν δὲ τοῦτο καὶ παρὰ τῷ Εὐριπίδῃ τὸ ὄνομα εἰρημένον· βουλόμενος γὰρ σημᾶναι τὴν φροντίδα Πολυξένης ἐν τῇ Ἑκάβῃ ἔφησεν «Ἡ δὲ καὶ θνήσκουσα πολλὴν πρόνοιαν εἶχεν εὐσχήμως πεσεῖν.» λέγεται δὲ πρόνοια καὶ ἄλλως. οὕτως γὰρ λέγομεν πρόνοιαν τοῦ παντὸς διαιροῦντες ἀπὸ τοῦ αὐτομάτου καὶ τῆς τύχης· ἀντίκειται γὰρ τῷ

13–27] *cf.* Gal. In Hipp. Progn. comm. I 4: CMG V 9,2 p. 201,3–26 16 Εὐριπίδης] Eurip. Hecuba vv. 568–570 19 Σόλωνι] *v.* Gal. In Hipp. Progn. comm. I 4: CMG V 9,2 p. 201,4sq. 21 τουτέστιν – 23] *cf.* Schol. R *in* Gal. In Hipp. Progn. comm. I 4: CMG V 9,2 p. 201 *ad* lin. 24 28 sq.] *cf.* Gal. In Hipp. Progn. comm. I 4: CMG V 9,2 p. 201,11sq. 30–40,5] *cf.* Gal. In Hipp. Progn. comm. I 4: CMG V 9,2 pp. 201,3–203,10 32 ἐν τῇ Ἑκάβῃ] *v. supra*, linn. 16–18 33 sq.] *cf.* Gal. In Hipp. Progn. comm. I 4: CMG V 9,2 p. 202, 11–19

1 ὅτι – ἀθάνατος] *fort.* δοκεῖ *addendum est* 2 ὅτι *om.* γ 5 τὸ *codd.*: *correxi* ὡς *om.* L 9 φησὶ *codd.*: *corr. Dietz* ὁ *om.* γ 11 νομίζω – τοῦ^{II} *om.* L οὐκ ἔστι] οὐκέτι M ὡς – μοι *om.* M 13 *lemma om.* L 16 καὶ *om.* L 17 πίπτουσα] *v. l. apud Hermogenem, Περὶ εὑρέσεως δ' 12: p. 204 Rabe*: θνήσκουσ' *Eurip.* 18 καὶ – ἀρρένων] κρύπτουσ' ἃ κρύπτειν ὄμματ' ἀρσένων χρεών *Eurip.* κρύπτεσθαι *codd.*: *corr. Dietz* 19 περὶ MP 23 ὅταν] ὅτε L 25 ἐκ^{II}] ἐπὶ L 29 αὐτὸ γ 31 βούλομαι γ 32 θνήσκουσ' ὅμως *Eurip.*

uncertainty, the idea being disputed by unbelievers. It shows something as self-evident when, for example, in reply to the question "Is man an animal?", I say "I think so". (We have an example of its use) as a moderate expression when philosophers, in discussing truths, answer with the phrase "I believe so", knowing that it really is so. Hippocrates, then, used the word either to convey a principle or to express himself moderately.

Another explanation from an excellent unknown commentator who is clear and concise. One must change the order of the words and read "I think that the best doctor practices forecasting." Now some have commented on I think and assert that Hippocrates did not dare to state the matter without reserve because he was not entirely confident; hence he says I think in the moderate sense of "It is my opinion". But it is not as those people have thought; rather, I think means "I have made a judgement and hold it as a doctrine that the best doctor practices forecasting."

I 3 Practice forecasting

Note that *pronoia* (forecasting) is employed in four senses; for it means care, intent, the power that watches over the universe, and prognosis. The meaning "care" is in Euripides, where he describes Polyxena slain by Pyrrhus, "Even as she fell dying she took great care to fall gracefully and to cover that which is hidden from male eyes." "Intent" is illustrated by the quotation from Solon the Lawmaker, "The Boule on the Areopagus should judge cases of murder and injury with intent"; in other words, those who killed with premeditation had their court on the Areopagus, other charges being heard elsewhere. As to "the power that watches over the universe", (we use it) when we say, "God gives thought to the world here below." As for its meaning "prognosis", the word *pronoia* itself shows that it is formed from (elements which express) the mind's thinking beforehand and anticipating. Hippocrates, then, as a doctor used the term in the sense of prognosis.

From another commentary. Different people have explained the word *pronoia* in different ways, some maintaining that (Hippocrates) means by it care, others preparation. It can indeed be used to express care; hence the everyday expression "So and so has put his mind (*proenoēsato*) to this matter", meaning that he has taken care of it. We have an instance of the same use also in Euripides when he wishes to indicate the precaution of Polyxena in the "Hecuba", "Even as she was dying she took great care to fall gracefully." And the word is employed in other ways. For example, we use it to convey the power that watches over the universe as distinct from accident or

τῆς προνοίας ὀνόματι τὸ τῆς τύχης. λέγεται δὲ πρόνοια καὶ ἡ πρόγνωσις, ὡς ἡ ἐτυμολογία τοῦ ὀνόματος δείκνυσι· πρόνοια γὰρ τὸ πρῶτον ἐν νῷ ἔχειν ἤτοι γε τὸ ἐννοῆσαι πρὶν παρ' ἄλλου ἀκοῦσαι. ἐνταῦθα οὖν ὁ Ἱπποκράτης πρόνοιαν καλεῖ οὐ τὴν προπαρασκευήν, ἀλλὰ τὴν πρόγνωσιν. τὸ δὲ τῆς προγνώσεως ὄνομα λαμβάνεται παρ' αὐτοῦ κατὰ τῶν τριῶν χρόνων, παρεόντος τε καὶ μέλλοντος καὶ προγεγονότος.

I 4 [1: 193,2 A. = II 110,3 L.] Προγινώσκων γὰρ καὶ προλέγων παρὰ τοῖσιν νοσέουσιν

Ἰστέον ὅτι διαφέρουσι πρόγνωσις καὶ πρόρρησις, ὅτι ἡ μὲν πρόγνωσις
61 κατὰ ἐνδιάθετον λόγον γίνεται, ἡ δὲ πρόρ|ρησις κατὰ τὸν προφορικόν. καὶ
ἔστι προηγουμένη ἡ πρόγνωσις, ἑπομένη δὲ ἡ πρόρρησις.

Ἐντεῦθεν ἄρχεται τοῦ πρώτου συλλογισμοῦ. ὡς δὲ εἰρήκαμεν, ἔστιν οὕτως· ὁ ἄριστα προγινώσκων οἶδε τῶν νοσημάτων τὰς φύσεις· ὁ εἰδὼς τῶν νοσημάτων τὰς φύσεις προλέγει τοῖς κάμνουσιν· ὁ προλέγων τοῖς κάμνουσιν ἕξει πειθηνίους αὐτοὺς ἑαυτῷ· ὁ οὕτως ἄριστα προγινώσκων ἕξει πειθηνίους τοὺς κάμνοντας. καὶ οὕτως μὲν ὁ συλλογισμὸς οὗτος δεδόσθω ἀπὸ καθόλου καταφατικῆς τῆς μείζονος, καθόλου καταφατικῆς τῆς ἐλάττονος, καθόλου καταφατικὸν συνάγων συμπέρασμα.

⟨Ἄλλως.⟩ εἰδέναι δεῖ ὅτι ἄλλο ἐστὶ προγινώσκειν καὶ ἄλλο τὸ προλέγειν. καλῶς οὖν ὁ Ἱπποκράτης μηδὲ τοῦτο παραλιπὼν ἀλλὰ προτάξας τὰ ὀνόματα ὥσπερ ἔχει τὰ πράγματα. τὸ μὲν γὰρ προγινώσκειν αὐτὴν τὴν διάθεσιν τῆς ψυχῆς σημαίνει, τὸ δὲ προλέγειν τὴν προφορὰν αὐτὴν τῶν λεγομένων ἣν ποιούμεθα ἀλλήλοις ἀνακοινούμενοι τὰ πράγματα.

Ἑτέρα ἐξήγησις. Ἡρόφιλος ἐξηγήσατο ἄλλο εἶναι πρόγνωσιν καὶ ἄλλο πρόρρησιν. «Καὶ πρόγνωσις μέν», φησίν, «ὅταν προγνῶ, μὴ εἴπω δέ τινι· πρόρρησις δέ ἐστιν, ὅταν προεγνωκὼς εἴπω τὸ προεγνωσμένον.» καὶ αὕτη μὲν ἡ Ἡροφίλου ἐξήγησις, καταγέλαστος οὖσα. ἰστέον τοίνυν ὅτι πρόγνωσις καὶ πρόρρησις οὐδὲν διαφέρει πλὴν κατὰ τὴν ἕξιν τοῦ ἰατροῦ καὶ τοῦ νοσοῦντος. προγινώσκειν μὲν ἐκεῖνα λέγεται ἅτινα τῷ κάμνοντί ἐστιν ἀγνώριστα, οἷόν τί ἐστι τὸ λεγόμενον οἷον εἰσελθόντες πρὸς ἄρρωστον εὕρομεν αὐτὸν ὀδυνώμενον τὴν πλευρὰν καὶ ἔχοντα τὰ πολυθρύλλητα ἐκεῖνα τέσσαρα σημεῖα, βῆχα, πυρετὸν ὀξύν, δύσπνοιαν, νυγματῶδες ἄλγημα. αὐτὸς μὲν οὖν ἐπιδείκνυσι τὴν πλευράν, ἡμεῖς δὲ λέγομεν ὡς οὐκ ὀστέον ἐστὶ τὸ πεπονθός, οὐ μῦς, ἀλλ' ὁ ὑπεζωκὼς τὰς πλευρὰς ὑμήν· καὶ τοῦτο λέγεται πρόγνωσις. πρόρρησις δέ ἐστιν, ὅταν τὰ ἐγνωσμένα τῷ νοσοῦντι
62 εἴπωμεν, ὅτι καὶ βήξ ἐστι καὶ πυρετὸς | καὶ δύσπνοια καὶ νυγματῶδες ἄλγημα. καὶ οὕτως
λέγομεν πρόγνωσιν καὶ πρόρρησιν διαφέρειν, διότι ἡ μὲν πρόγνωσις ὡς πρὸς τὸν ἰατρὸν λέγεται, ἡ δὲ πρόρρησις ὡς πρὸς τὸν νοσοῦντα, ὅταν τὰ ἐγνωσμένα αὐτῷ προείπῃ.

I 5 [1: 193,2 A. = II 110,3 L.] Παρὰ τοῖσι νοσέουσι

1–5] *cf.* Gal. In Hipp. Progn. comm. I 4: CMG V 9,2 p. 202,20–26 8 sq.] *cf.* Gal. In Hipp. Prorrh. I comm., Prooem.: CMG V 9,2 p. 3 11 εἰρήκαμεν] *supra*, p. 34,25–29 23 Ἡρόφιλος] *cf.* Gal. In Hipp. Progn. comm. I 4: CMG V 9,2 pp. 203,19–204,18 28 εὕρομεν – 30] *cf. supra*, p. 28,2 sq.

8 πρόσρησις M P *(ante corr.)* 11 πρώτου *om.* γ εἰρήκαμεν *om.* γ 12 νόσων γ 14 sq. αὐτοὺς – πειθηνίους *om.* γ 16 *post* μείζονος *add.* καὶ Pζ 18 Ἄλλως *addidi* τὸ *om.* γ 21 ἀνακινούμενοι L 24 πρόγνωσιν *codd.*: *correxi* φασιν L 25 αὕτη – Ἡροφίλου] περὶ (παρὰ ζ) μὲν ἡροφίλῳ γ 28 τί *om.* γ 29 ὀδυρόμενον L 30 *post* δύσπνοιαν *add.* καὶ γ 32 τὸ ἐγνωσμένον γ 34 πρόρρησιν καὶ πρόγνωσιν Pζ διότι] ὅτι γ 36 τοῖσι] τοῖς LM νοσεύουσι L

chance, the words chance and *pronoia* being opposites. It is also employed with the meaning of prognosis, as the etymology of the word shows; for *pronoia* means having in mind first or thinking of before hearing from someone else. So Hippocrates means here by *pronoia* not preparation but prognosis. And he applies the word prognosis to the three tenses, present, future and past.

I 4 For if he prognoses and pronounces in the presence of the sick

It should be noted that prognosing and pronouncing are distinct processes in that the former is mental conception, while the latter is the expression of this. Prognosis precedes in time, pronouncing comes later.

At this point he begins the first syllogism. As we have said, it runs as follows: the one who prognoses best knows the natures of diseases; the one who knows the natures of diseases pronounces to the sick; the one who pronounces to the sick makes them compliant to himself; the one who thus prognoses best makes the sick compliant. This, then, is how the syllogism is composed: from a universal affirmative major premiss and a universal affirmative minor, a universal affirmative conclusion is drawn.

Someone else's comment. Note that there is a difference between prognosing and pronouncing. So Hippocrates is to be commended for not ignoring the distinction and for assigning the names to agree with the facts. For prognosis refers to the state of mind, while pronouncing means the actual verbal expression that we use in communicating with one another.

A different explanation. Herophilus in his comment distinguishes between prognosing and pronouncing. "Prognosis", he tells us, "is when I prognose something and do not reveal it to anyone; pronouncing is making known my prognosis." This is his explanation and a ridiculous one it is. Now, you should know that the only way in which prognosis and pronouncing differ is with respect to the dispositions (in knowledge) of doctor and patient. Prognosis, on the one hand, is used in reference to things not known to the patient; the following is an illustration: we come to a sick person and find him with a pain in the side and having those four well-known symptoms, coughing, acute fever, difficult breathing and a throbbing pain. He, for his part, points to the side, but we inform him that the part affected is not a bone nor a muscle, rather the membrane lining the ribs; this is what is called prognosis. Pronouncing, on the other hand, is when we tell the patient what he already knows, viz. that he has a cough, fever, difficult breathing and a throbbing pain. Thus we say prognosing and pronouncing differ, because the former is used with reference to the doctor, the latter from the patient's point of view, when the doctor tells him what he is already aware of.

I 5 In the presence of the sick

Δεῖ, φησίν, αὐτοῖς τοῖς νοσοῦσι προλέγειν· εἰ γὰρ τοῖς παρεοῦσιν εἴποις καὶ ὑπ' αὐτῶν μάθοι ὁ κάμνων, νομίζει αὐτοὺς ψεύδεσθαι· ἀλλὰ δεῖ αὐτῷ τῷ νοσοῦντι προλέγειν, ὅπως αὐτὸς πιστεύοι τῷ ἰατρῷ.

(III)

I 6 [1: 193,2 A. = II 110,3 L.] Τά τε παρεόντα καὶ τὰ προγεγονότα καὶ τὰ μέλλοντα ἔσεσθαι

Ἐντεῦθεν ἄρχεται ὁ πρῶτος συλλογισμός, ὅντινα ἐλέγομεν ἀπὸ τῶν τριῶν χρόνων τὴν πρότασιν ἔχειν. ἰστέον δὲ ὅτι ἐλέγετο ἐν τοῖς προλεγομένοις, ὅτι ὡς γενικωτέρᾳ ἐχρήσατο τῇ τοῦ Προγνωστικοῦ ἐπιγραφῇ φερομένου καὶ κατὰ διαγνώσεως καὶ ἀναμνήσεως καὶ ὅτι καὶ ἡ διάγνωσις ὑπὸ τὴν πρόγνωσιν ἀνάγεται. καὶ πάντων ῥίζα καὶ ἀρχή εἰσι τὰ ἐνιστάμενα καὶ τῶν φθασάντων καὶ τῶν μελλόντων. εἰ μὴ γάρ ἐστι τὸ ἐνεστός, ὃ νῦν διαγινώσκω, οὐ δύναμαι εἰπεῖν τὰ φθάσαντα ἢ τὰ μέλλοντα. καὶ ὅτι προφέρει πάντων ἡ διάγνωσις, ἐδήλωσε διὰ τούτων εἰρηκὼς καὶ καλῶς ἀπαριθμησάμενος πρώτην τὴν διάγνωσιν· ἡ γὰρ διάγνωσις ἐπὶ τῶν ἐνεστώτων λέγεται. φησὶν οὖν τὰ παρεόντα καὶ τὰ φθάσαντα καὶ τὰ μέλλοντα.

Ἀποροῦσι δὲ «Διὰ τί πρότερον τῶν παρεόντων ἐμνήσθη, εἴ γε πρότερον περὶ προγνώσεως προέθετο διαλεχθῆναι;» καὶ λέγομεν, ὅτι πᾶσα σημείωσις τῷ ἰατρῷ ἀπὸ τῶν παρόντων ἤτοι ἐνεστώτων ἀποδείκνυται. καὶ γὰρ καὶ τὴν ἀνάμνησιν ἀπὸ τῶν παρεόντων ποιούμεθα. ἐπεί τοι παρῆλθον ἐκεῖνα, ἀλλὰ λέγω τῷ ἀρρώστῳ ἀπὸ ὑδροποσίας ἢ ὀπωροφαγίας ἢ ἀδηφαγίας καὶ ἀπεψίας. καὶ ἰδοὺ ἀναμιμνῄσκω ἀπὸ τῶν παρεόντων τὸν ἄρρωστον, ὅτι
63 τοῦτο τὸ νόσημα ἢ | ὅτι αὕτη ἡ ψυχρὰ καὶ φλεγματικὴ ὕλη ἀπὸ τούτων ἠθροίσθη. καὶ ἰδοὺ ἀπὸ τῶν παρεόντων καὶ ἐνεστώτων τὰ παρελθόντα ἐνοήσαμεν.

Ἀλλὰ καὶ τὰ ἐσόμενα ἀπὸ τῶν παρόντων διαγινώσκομεν, ὥσπερ τὴν ἀρχὴν ἀπὸ σμικροσφυξίας καὶ συννεύσεως καὶ τῶν τοιούτων. ἀλλὰ καὶ τὴν ἀκμὴν ἀπὸ τῆς ἕξεως σημειούμεθα. καὶ πάλιν θεωροῦντες ἐν τῇ τετάρτῃ ἀμυδρᾶς πέψεως σημεῖα ἐν τοῖς οὔροις ἢ τοῖς ὑποχωρήμασιν προγινώσκομεν καὶ λέγομεν, ὅτι τῇ ἑβδόμῃ ἔχει κριθῆναι τὸ νόσημα. καὶ ἰδοὺ ἀπὸ τῶν παρόντων τὰ μέλλοντα προέγνωμεν, καὶ διὰ τοῦτο πρότερον τῶν παρεόντων ἐμνημονεύσαμεν.

I 7 [1: 193,3 A. = II 110,4 L.] Ὁκόσα τε παραλείπουσιν οἱ ἀσθενέοντες ἐκδιηγούμενοι

Δεῖ, φησί, τὸν ἰητρὸν προλέγειν μὴ μόνον ἅπερ παρὰ τῶν νοσούντων ἀκούει, ἀλλὰ καὶ τὰ παραλειπόμενα ὑπ' αὐτῶν προλέγειν. τίνα δέ εἰσιν ἅπερ

8 ἐν τοῖς προλεγομένοις] *v. supra*, p. 30,24–30

2 εἴπης L μάθη MP 5 τε *om.* L 9 ὡς *om.* L γενικωτέρω *codd.*: *corr. Dietz* *fort.* φερομένῃ *scribendum est* 14 καλῶς *om.* γ ἀπηριθμησάμενος MPV 18 γνώσεως γ προσέθετο L: διέθετο γ: *corr. Dietz* 24 *ante* ἐνεστώτων *add.* τῶν γ 27 καὶ[II] *om.* γ 32 *fort.* ἐμνημόνευσεν *scribendum est* 33 ὁπόσα L 34 διηγούμεθα γ 35 ἰατρὸν γ 36 δέ *om.* L

(Hippocrates) is saying that we must pronounce to the patients themselves; for if you tell something to those around the patient and he learns it from them, he will think that they lie; no, the doctor should inform the patient directly, in order to gain his trust.

(III)

I 6 The present, the past and the future

Here the first syllogism begins, the major premiss of which we have said comprises the three tenses. Note that in the introduction we said that (Hippocrates) uses the title Prognosticon as being the more comprehensive, prognosis covering both diagnosis and anamnesis, and that diagnosis is included under prognosis. Now present phenomena are the root and starting point for both past and future. For unless I first diagnose the present I cannot describe either the past or the future. And (Hippocrates) shows that diagnosis is superior to all by the words he uses and by rightly placing diagnosis in the first place; for diagnosis is used with reference to the present. Hence he writes the present, the past and the future.

And the problem is raised, "Why did he mention the present in the first place, if he proposed to discuss first prognosis?" We reply that it is on the present or existing (state of affairs) that the doctor bases all symptom interpretation. For even the past is recalled on the basis of the present. Even though the past is gone, I nevertheless tell the patient (that his trouble has come) from drinking water or eating fruit or overeating and indigestion. So you see, I remind the patient by means of the present that this illness or this cold, phlegmatic matter has accumulated from those actions. And thus we have apprehended the past from the present and existing (conditions).

But the future also we diagnose from the present; for example, the beginning from weak pulse or convergence (of innate heat to the interior) or the like. Similarly, we signal the acme from the (patient's present) state. So, too, when we observe on the fourth day signs of slight concoction in the urines or stools, we make a prognosis and declare that the disease will reach a crisis on the seventh. And so we have prognosed the future from the present, and this is why we have mentioned the present first.

I 7 And all the information left out from their accounts by the sick

(Hippocrates) says that the doctor must pronounce not only what he hears from the patients, but also what they omit. What do

παραλείπουσιν οἱ ἄρρωστοι; ἅπερ γινώσκοντες οὐκ ἐκφέρουσιν· οἷον πολλάκις ἀπὸ καταστήματος ψυχροτέρου ἢ ὑγροτέρου ἢ ἄλλως ὁπωσοῦν καταστήματος βλάπτεται, καὶ ἐπὶ τούτῳ κρύπτει τῷ ἰατρῷ καὶ οὐ λέγει. ἢ πολλάκις ἐν τῷ σώματι αὐτοῦ ὄγκος τις γίνεται, ἐρυσίπελας ἢ ἕρπης ἢ φλεγμονὴ ἢ βουβών, καὶ ἐγκρύπτεται ὁ νοσῶν. δι' ἣν δὲ αἰτίαν παραλιμπάνουσιν οἱ νοσοῦντες καὶ οὐ λέγουσι τῷ ἰατρῷ; ἢ διὰ βλακότητα ἢ διὰ δεινότητα ἢ κακοπραγίαν ἐκπειράζοντες τὸν ἰατρόν, ἐὰν δυνήσηται προγνῶναι καὶ εἰπεῖν τι ἐπιστημονικῶς· εἰ δὲ μή, ἵνα καταγελάσωσιν αὐτοῦ. ἢ δι' ὀλιγοψυχίαν, ὥσπερ πολλάκις ἐξησθένησαν καὶ κατέπεσον αἱ δυνάμεις τοῦ νοσοῦντος, καὶ οὐ δύναται εἰπεῖν τῷ ἰατρῷ. ὅθεν τινὲς τοὺς παρακολουθοῦντας αὐτοῖς ἐπιτρέπουσι λέγειν τὰ συμβάντα αὐτῷ τῇ νυκτὶ ἢ τῷ πρωΐ.

Ἄλλως. παραλείπουσί τινα οἱ νοσοῦντες τῶν συμβάντων ἐν τῷ διηγεῖσθαι τῷ
64 ἰατρῷ διὰ τρεῖς αἰτίας, ἢ δι' ἄγνοιαν ἢ | διὰ λήθην ἢ διὰ πανουργίαν. εἰσὶν οὖν πολλοὶ κρυψίνοοι καὶ ἀπατεῶνες καὶ βούλονται πειράζειν τοὺς ἰατρούς, ὡς καὶ ὁ συγγραφεὺς ἐν τῇ Σφυγμικῇ διέγνω τὸν λαβόντα τὸ φάρμακον ἐκ τοῦ σφυγμοῦ τὴν τούτου διάγνωσιν ποιησάμενος. περὶ ποίου οὖν λέγει παραλιμπανομένου; οὐχὶ περὶ τῶν δι' ἄγνοιαν· πῶς γὰρ δύναται ἀναμνῆσαι ἃ ἀγνοεῖ ὅλως ὅτι ἐγένετο; ἀλλὰ μᾶλλον περὶ τῶν κατὰ λήθην ἢ διὰ τὸ κρυψίνους εἶναι τοὺς τοιούτους.

Ἄλλη ἐξήγησις. τινὲς τῶν ἐξηγητῶν οὕτως εἰρήκασιν· «Φησὶ γὰρ ὅτι τὰ μὲν ἄλλα πάντα οἱ ἄρρωστοι ἴσασιν· εἰ ἔχουσι δὲ ἔμφραξιν ἐν ἥπατι ἢ ἐν σπληνὶ ἢ ἐν ἄλλῳ τινὶ τῶν μορίων, οὐκέτι, καὶ ταῦτά φησι παραλιμπάνουσι λέγειν. εἴ τις οὖν τῶν ἰατρῶν ταῦτα αὐτοῖς ἐκδιηγήσεται, θαυμάζεται παρ' αὐτοῖς.» ἐροῦμεν οὖν ἡμεῖς, ὅτι ἐψεύσαντο οἱ ταῦτα λέγειν ἐπιχειρήσαντες. οὐ γάρ, εἴ τις εἴπῃ τῷ ἀρρώστῳ τὸ ἀγνοούμενον αὐτῷ, ἤδη καὶ θαυμάσει· πῶς γὰρ ἔχει θαυμάσαι, ὃ οὐκ οἶδεν; ἀλλὰ θαυμάζοι τὸ ἤδη ἐγνωσμένον αὐτῷ ἀκούων. οἷον ἀνελθὼν ὁ ἰατρὸς πρὸς ἄρρωστον, ἁψάμενος αὐτοῦ τῆς ἀρτηρίας ἔγνω, ὅτι ἱδρῶτες αὐτῷ ἐγένοντο ἢ ἐθυμώθη, εἶτα εἴπῃ τῷ ἀρρώστῳ πρὶν ἀκούσῃ παρ' αὐτοῦ ἢ τῶν αὐτοῦ, θαυμάζεται παρὰ τῷ πάσχοντι. ὥστε οἱ ἄρρωστοι τὰ μὲν ἐναργῆ ἴσασιν, ἀγνοοῦσι δέ πως τὰ μὴ οὕτως ἔχοντα. εἴ τις οὖν τῶν ἐναργῶν τούτων προείπῃ τοῖς κάμνουσιν, εἰκότως θαυμασθήσεται.

I 8 [1: 193,4 A. = II 110,5 L.] Πιστεύοιτο ἂν μᾶλλον γινώσκειν τὰ τῶν νοσεόντων πρήγματα

Οὐκ εἶπεν ἁπλῶς τὰ τῶν ἀνθρώπων, ἀλλὰ τὰ τῶν νοσούντων, ἵνα μή τις ὑπολάβῃ, ὅτι περὶ χρυσοῦ καὶ ἀργύρου ἢ ἄλλου τινὸς τοιούτου πράγματος εἶπεν ὁ Ἱπποκράτης· ἀλλ' ἔφη τὰ τῶν νοσούντων εἰδέναι πράγματα. πράγματα δὲ ταῦτα, νοσήματα, αἴτια, συμπτώματα. |

65 I 9 [1: 193,5 A. = II 110,6 L.] Ὥστε τολμᾶν ἐπιτρέπειν τοὺς ἀνθρώπους σφᾶς ἑαυτοὺς τῷ ἰητρῷ

12–18] *cf.* Schol. R *in* Gal. In Hipp. Progn. comm. I 2: CMG V 9,2 p. 198 *ad* lin. 1   15 Σφυγμικῇ] Gal. De praesag. ex puls. I 1: IX pp. 218–220 K.

1 ἐκφέρονται γ   3 οὐ λέγει τῷ ἰατρῷ ἀλλὰ κρύπτει γ   4 ἐρυσίπελος L   ἕρπις *codd.*: *corr. Dietz*   7 δύναται γ   17 ἃ *ante* ἀναμνῆσαι *trsp.* L   18 κρυψίνοας γ   21 φησι *post* οὐκέτι *trsp.* γ   περιλιμπάνουσι MP   22 αὐτοῖς^{I}] αὐτῷ *codd.*: *correxi*   *ante* ἡμεῖς *add.* καὶ γ   23 αὐτὸς L   ἤδη] ἴδη *codd.*: *corr. Dietz*   24 θαυμάσει] θαυμάσῃ^{ει} Y: *ambig.* V: θαυμάσιον P   θαυμάζοι] θαυμάζει PV   25 ὁ *om.* γ   *fort.* εἰ γνῷ *scribendum est*   26 ἀκούσει Lζ: ἀκοῦσαι P   32 τὰ^{II} *om.* L

patients leave out? Things of which they are aware but do not express; for example, it often happens that a person is troubled by a rather cold or moist or some such condition, and he keeps this from the doctor and does not tell him. Or frequently a patient develops a swelling in his body, erysipelas or shingles or inflammation or groin swelling, and he conceals the fact. But why do the sick omit information and keep it from the doctor? They do it out of stupidity or cleverness or mischief, testing the doctor, to see if he can prognose and say something skillful, and if not, to ridicule him. Or because of weakness; often, for instance, the patient's faculties have become exhausted and collapsed, and he is unable to speak to the doctor. This is why some doctors instruct the patient's attendants to report what he experienced in the night or in the morning.

Someone else's explanation. There are three reasons why the sick leave certain things out of the account of their experiences to the doctor; they do it through ignorance or forgetfulness or deception. For there are lots of dissemblers and cheats who want to put doctors to the test, just as the writer (Galen) in Pulses recognized the one who had taken the drug by making the diagnosis from his pulse. Which type of omission, then, is (Hippocrates) speaking about? Surely not those caused by ignorance; for how can a person recall events the occurrence of which is entirely unknown to him? No, he is referring rather to omissions stemming from either poor memory or deception by such people.

Another explanation. Some commentators have explained the matter as follows: "(Hippocrates) is saying that the sick know more or less everything; if, however, there is obstruction in the liver or spleen or any other part, they are not aware of it, and this, according to him, is what they leave out. When a doctor, then, explains such things to them, he wins their admiration." We say that this attempted explanation is false. For, telling the patient something that he was not aware of is no guarantee of his admiration; how can he admire (being told) something of which he had no knowledge? On the contrary he will be impressed to hear what he knows already. For example, if a doctor visiting a patient and feeling his artery finds out that he has been sweating or in a passion, and he announces this before being informed by the patient or those attending him, he gains the patient's admiration. The fact is that the sick know what is visible, but what is not visible they do not know. So if a doctor pronounces to his patients any of these visible symptoms, he will be justly admired.

I 8 He will be more easily credited with understanding the affairs of the sick

Hippocrates says the affairs of the sick and not just "the affairs of men", in order that no one take him to be speaking about gold or silver or any such thing; no, he says understanding the affairs of the sick, and affairs are these: diseases, causes and symptoms.

I 9 So that men will have the confidence to entrust themselves to the doctor

Ἰδοὺ ἐνταῦθα κατασκευάζει τὴν συλλογιστικὴν ἀπόδειξιν, ἣν ἀνωτέρω προεῖπεν.

Ἄλλως. ἀντὶ τοῦ πείθεσθαι τοὺς ἀρρώστους τῷ ἰητρῷ καὶ πειθηνίους αὐτοὺς ἔχειν, καὶ τοῦτό ἐστι τὸ ἐπιτρέπειν αὐτοὺς ἑαυτοὺς τῷ ἰητρῷ.

I 10 [1: 193,6 A. = II 110,7 L.] Τήν τε θεραπείαν ἄριστα ἂν ποιέοιτο προειδὼς τὰ ἐσόμενα ἐκ τῶν παρεόντων παθημάτων.

Ἐνταῦθα τὸν δεύτερον συλλογισμὸν ἐκτιθέμεθα, ὅνπερ ἀνωτέρω προείπομεν. καλῶς δὲ καὶ θαυμασίως ἔφη προγινώσκειν τὰ μέλλοντα ἐκ τῶν παρεόντων παθημάτων ὡς πρὸς ἀντιδιαστολὴν τῆς τοῦ θεοῦ προγνώσεως. οἱ μὲν γὰρ ἄνθρωποι ἐκ τῶν παρεόντων τὰ μέλλοντα γινώσκουσιν, οἷον οἰωνοσκόπος θεωρῶν τὴν πτῆσιν τῶν πτηνῶν εἴτε πρὸς βορρᾶν πέτονται εἴτε πρὸς νότον, εἴτε εἰς ὕψος εἴτε χθαμαλῶς, εἴτε κράζοντα, οὕτως προγινώσκει. ἀλλὰ καὶ αἱ λοιπαὶ τέχναι ἀπό τινων σημείων προγινώσκουσι. δηλονότι καὶ ὁ ἰατρὸς ἀπό τινων σημείων προγινώσκει καὶ ἐν χρόνῳ καὶ διαμεμερισμένως. ὁ θεὸς δὲ οὐ δεῖται χρόνου πρὸς τὸ προγνῶναι, ἀλλ' ἀχρόνως καὶ ἀδιασπάστως πάντα προγινώσκει, ἐπειδὴ τὰ πάντα αὐτὸς ἐποίησεν.

Ἄλλως. τοῦτό ἐστι τοῦ πρώτου συλλογισμοῦ τὸ συμπέρασμα ὡς εἴρηται, ὅτι ὁ ἄριστα εἰδὼς τοὺς τρεῖς χρόνους, θεραπεύει. ἀλλὰ μὴν καὶ ἀρχὴ[ν] τοῦ δευτέρου συλλογισμοῦ. εἴρηται γὰρ ὁ δεύτερος συλλογισμὸς ἀπὸ μόνου τοῦ τρίτου χρόνου λαμβάνεσθαι οὕτως· ὁ προειδὼς τὰ μέλλοντα προευτρεπίζεται κατὰ τοῦ νοσήματος· ὁ προευτρεπιζόμενος ἄριστα θεραπεύει. ἐντεῦθεν οὖν ἤρξατο τοῦ δευτέρου συλλογισμοῦ. ἀλλ' ἰστέον
66 ὅτι πολλάκις οἱ ἀρχαῖοι προτάσεις ἔλεγον μόνον, κελεύ|οντες ἡμᾶς τῶν συμπερασμάτων ὑπακούειν. ὥσπερ καὶ ὁ Γαληνὸς ἐν τῷ προοιμίῳ τοῦ Περὶ στοιχείων εἰρηκὼς μόνας τὰς προτάσεις τὰ συμπεράσματα ἡμᾶς ἐκέλευσε προσυπακούειν. οὕτως οὖν κἀντεῦθεν δείκνυται, ὅτι πρὸ Ἀριστοτέλους ὁ Ἱπποκράτης διαλεκτικὴν μέθοδον ἤσκησεν· εἰρηκὼς γὰρ συμπέρασμα ἐκέλευσεν ἡμᾶς προτάσεων προσυπακούειν.

Ἄλλη ἐξήγησις. Ἱπποκράτης ἐνταῦθα τοῦ δευτέρου συλλογισμοῦ ποιεῖται τὴν ἀρχήν. ὡς βραχυλόγος δὲ καταλείψας τὰς προτάσεις τὸ συμπέρασμα ἐπήγαγεν· ἴσμεν δὲ ποῖος οὗτος, ὅτι ὁ προγινώσκων οἶδε τὸ μέλλον· ὁ εἰδὼς τὸ μέλλον προπαρασκευάζεται· ὁ προπαρασκευαζόμενος ἄριστα θεραπεύει.

I 11 [1: 193,6 A. = II 110,8 L.] Προειδὼς τὰ ἐσόμενα ἐκ τῶν παρεόντων παθημάτων

Καὶ πάλιν διὰ τούτων βεβαιοῦται, ὅτι ῥίζα πάντων ἐστὶν ἡ διάγνωσις, ὡς καὶ ἀνωτέρω ἐλέγετο. οὐδὲ γὰρ δυνάμεθα προγνῶναι ἢ μεμνηκέναι τῶν φθασάντων, εἰ μὴ διαγνῶμεν τὰ παρεόντα. διὰ τοῦτο πρῶτον εἶπεν

1 ἀνωτέρω] *v. supra*, p. 34,25–29, 7 ἀνωτέρω] *v. supra*, p. 34,30–33, 24 ἐν — στοιχείων] Gal. De elem. sec. Hipp. I 1: pp. 1sq. Helmr. = I pp. 413–415 K., *ubi de hac re nihil cerno* 26] *cf.* Ioann. Comm. in Hipp. De morb. pop. VI: 134a5; 146c11; 149b57 Pritchet 35 ἀνωτέρω] *v. supra*, p. 42,11

2 *fort.* προείπομεν *scribendum est* 4 ἰατρῷ γ 7 τῶν δύο συλλογισμῶν γ ὧνπερ γ 11 οἰωνοσκοπίας γ 12 *post* κράζοντα *fort. exciderunt* εἴτε μὴ κράζοντα 15 ἀναγνῶναι γ 19 ἀρχὴν *codd.*: *correxi* 21 ὁ^{I} *om.* L κατὰ] ἐκ γ 24 τοῦ *om.* L 27 προϋπακούειν γ 35 μεμνημένα L 36 πρῶτον *om.* γ

Here we see him setting out the proof by syllogism mentioned earlier.

From another commentary. By entrust themselves to the doctor he means that the sick will believe in him and he will have their confidence.

I 10 And he will give the best treatment by prognosing the future from present conditions.

Here we set out the second syllogism described above. Prognosing the future from present conditions – this he rightly and admirably expressed in distinction to the foreknowledge of God, since men use the present to get to know the future. For example, an augur observing the flight of birds makes his predictions according to whether they fly northwards or southwards, whether they fly high or low, or whether they emit a cry. The other arts, too, prognose from certain signs. Obviously the doctor, too, prognoses from certain signs, through time and step by step. God, on the other hand, does not need time to prognose; he foresees everything independent of time and dimension, being himself the creator of all things.

Someone else's explanation. This is the conclusion of the first syllogism, as stated above: that the one who best knows the three times, cures. But it is also the beginning of the second. For this one, as we noted, is based entirely on the third tense, as follows: he who prognoses the future is prepared for the disease; the one who is prepared gives the best treatment. This, then, is his starting point for the second syllogism. But we should be aware that it is a common practice of the ancients to express only the premisses, telling us to understand the conclusions. Galen, for example, does this in his introduction to On the Elements; he gives just the premisses and tells us to understand the conclusions. The present instance, then, proves that Hippocrates used the dialectic method before Aristotle, because he provides us with the conclusion and instructs us to supply the premisses.

From a different commentator. Here Hippocrates begins the second syllogism. But in his fondness for brevity he gives just the conclusion omitting the premisses; we know, however, what the syllogism is, viz. that the one who prognoses knows what is going to happen; he who knows what is going to happen is prepared; the one who is prepared gives the best treatment.

I 11 Prognosing the future from present conditions

These words are a further confirmation of our earlier statement, that diagnosis is the basis of all. For we cannot prognose (the future) or recall the past, if we do not diagnose the present. This is why he said in

προειδὼς τὰ ἐσόμενα ἐκ τῶν παρεόντων παθημάτων.

Ἰστέον ὅτι τὰ παλαιὰ τῶν ἀντιγράφων νοσήματα ἔχει. καὶ καλῶς ἔχει· εἴρηται γὰρ ὡς τῶν Ἱπποκρατείων οὐκ ἦν διῃρημένα τὰ νοσήματα καὶ τὰ συμπτώματα καὶ τὰ αἴτια, ἀλλὰ πάντα κοινῷ ὀνόματι ἐκαλοῦντο νοσήματα. διὰ τοῦτό φησι προειδὼς τὰ ἐσόμενα ἐκ τῶν παρεόντων νοσημάτων, συμπτωμάτων, αἰτίων.

I 12 [1: 193,7 A. = II 110,9 L.] Ὑγιέας μὲν γὰρ ποιέειν ἅπαντας τοὺς ἀσθενέοντας ἀδύνατον

Ἰδοὺ εἰς τὸν τρίτον λόγον εἰσέβαλεν ἑαυτὸν ἐν ᾧ φησιν ὅτι ὁ προγινώσκων ἰατρὸς προλέγει τούς τε σωθησομένους καὶ ἀπολλυμένους. καλῶς δὲ καὶ θαυμασίως ἔφη ὁ Ἱπποκράτης· ὑγιάζειν ἅπαντας τοὺς ἀσθενοῦντας ἀδύνατον· τοῦτο γὰρ καὶ τοῦ προγινώσκειν τὰ μέλλοντα
67 ἀπο|βήσεσθαι κρεῖσσον ἂν εἴη. τουτέστιν ὅτι ἀδύνατόν ἐστι πάντας τοὺς ἀσθενοῦντας ὑγιάζειν. εἰ γὰρ τοῦτο ἠδυνάμεθα ποιεῖν, ἀναγκαιότερον ἂν ἦν καὶ τῆς προγνώσεως καὶ οὐκ εἴχομεν τοιαύτην μέριμναν θέσθαι περὶ τὴν πρόγνωσιν. καὶ ἄνευ γὰρ τοῦ προγνῶναι ἐπὰν εἶχεν ὑγιασθῆναι, οὐκ ἔμελ[λ]ε τὸ προγνῶναι. ἀλλ' ἐπειδὴ ἀδύνατόν ἐστιν ἅπαντας ὑγιάζειν, διὰ τοῦτο ἀναγκαῖον ἡμῖν ἐστι πολλὴν σπουδὴν καὶ ἐπιμέλειαν θέσθαι περὶ τὴν πρόγνωσιν, ὥστε ἐπίστασθαι αὐτὴν καὶ προγινώσκειν τὰ μέλλοντα ἔσεσθαι. τῷ προγινώσκειν γὰρ καὶ προλέγειν ἀναίτιον ἑαυτόν τε καὶ τὴν τέχνην καθίστησιν.

Ἄλλη ἐξήγησις. ἐνταῦθα συμπεπλήρωνται οἱ δύο συλλογισμοί, ὁ πρῶτος καὶ ὁ δεύτερος. λοιπὸν ἡ ἀκοὴ ἀναμένει τὸν τρίτον ῥηθῆναι. ὁ δὲ οὐ παραδίδωσιν εὐθέως τὸν τρίτον, ἀλλ', εἰ καὶ βραχυλόγος ἐστὶν ὁ Ἱπποκράτης, ἠκολούθησε τοῖς πλατικώτερον ἐκδιδοῦσι τὰ συγγράμματα καὶ διὰ τοῦτο ἀσάφειαν ἐποίησεν ἐν τῷ ῥητῷ. παραδίδωσι μὲν γὰρ προτέλειά τινα συμβαλλόμενα ἡμῖν πρὸς τὸν τρίτον συλλογισμὸν καὶ προαναμιμνῄσκει τῶν φθασάντων· καὶ εἶθ' οὕτως τὸν τρίτον συλλογισμὸν ἐκτίθεται. εἰσὶ δὲ ταῦτα τὰ προτέλεια· ἰστέον ὅτι ἡ ἰατρικὴ αὐτὴ καθ' ἑαυτὴν θεωρουμένη ἄπταιστός ἐστιν ἐπιστήμη. διὰ δὲ τὸ ῥευστὸν τῆς ὕλης καὶ εὐμετάβλητον καὶ ἄλλοτε ἄλλως ἔχον — καλῶς γὰρ ὁ Πλάτων ποταμῷ ῥέοντι ἀπείκασε τὰ ἡμέτερα σώματα —, καὶ διὰ τοῦτο οὐκ ἔχει τὸ βέβαιον ἡ τέχνη. εἰ μὲν πάντες οἱ νοσοῦντες ἀπέθνησκον, οὐκ ἦν ἔγκλημα τῷ ἰατρῷ, εἰ καὶ μὴ προλέγοι. εἰ δὲ πάντες ὑγίαινον, οὐδὲν ἐδεῖτο τῆς προρρήσεως.

I 13 [1: 193,7 A. = II 110,9 L.] Ὑγιέας μὲν γὰρ ἅπαντας ποιέειν

Τίνος αὐτῷ προκειμένου τὸν λόγον ἐπήγαγε τοῦτον τὸν λέγοντα ὑγιέας μὲν γὰρ ἅπαντας ποιέειν τοὺς ἀσθενέοντας ἀδύνατον

28–31] *cf. infra,* pp. 50,4–11; 52,3sq. Prolog. R *ad* Gal. In Hipp. Progn. comm.: CMG V 9,2 p. XXX,25–31 Olymp. In Plat. Gorg. comm.: pp. 18,23–19,6 Westerink Ps.-Eliae Lect. in Porph. Isag.: p. 16,19 Westerink Dav. Proleg.: CAG XVIII 2 pp. 44,23–45,11 30 ὁ Πλάτων] Plat. Crat. 402a?

2 παλαιὰ] πολλὰ M: παρὰ Pζ 5 *ante* νοσήματα *add.* τὰ γ 13 ἀποβήσεσθαι *om.* γ 15 ἂν *om.* L 17 ἔμελλε *codd.*: *correxi* 20 τῷ] τὸ *codd.*: *corr. Wk.* γὰρ *om.* L τε *om.* γ 23 ἡ ἀκοὴ] ἀκοὴ P: ἡ κοὴ M 26 παντέλεια L τὸν *om.* γ 27 τὸν] πρὸς γ 28 τὰ *om.* Pζ αὐτὴ] αὕτη L 31 *post* μὲν *add.* γὰρ γ 32 μὴ *om.* L 33–50,16 *fort. alia explicatio distinguenda est* 33 *et* 35 ποιέειν ἅπαντας *Hipp. (cf. lin. 7)* 34 τινὸς γ

the first place prognosing the future from present conditions.

It should be noted that the old copies have diseases (instead of conditions). And they are correct, for, as has been observed, in the Hippocratic writings there is no division into diseases, symptoms and causes, all being called by the common term "diseases". For this reason he says prognosing the future from present diseases, symptoms and causes.

I 12 Now it is not possible to restore all sick people to health

(Hippocrates) begins the third argument at the point where he says that the doctor who prognoses tells in advance who will survive and who will die. But how right and admirable Hippocrates is to state that it is not possible to restore all sick people to health; for this would be even better than prognosing how the future will turn out, implying that it is impossible to cure every patient. If this were within our power, it would be more important than even prognosis, and we would not have to worry so much about forecasting. If cures could be effected without the aid of prognosis, prognosis would not count. However, since it is not possible to cure all, we are forced to take great pains and care with prognosis, so as to understand it and predict what is going to happen. For it is by prognosing and predicting that the doctor keeps both himself and the art free from blame.

Another explanation. At this point the first two syllogisms have been completed. Then we expect to hear the third mentioned. But Hippocrates does not give it straightaway; despite his preference for brevity, he follows those who write with more detail and, as a result, has obscured his narrative. He gives some preliminaries to help our understanding of the third syllogism and repeats beforehand things already mentioned; after this he sets out the third syllogism. These are the preliminaries: we must understand that medicine considered in itself is an infallible science. But since the matter (it deals with) is fluid, changeable and unpredictable – Plato rightly compared our bodies to a flowing river –, for this reason the art does not possess certainty. If every patient died, the doctor would not be held responsible, even if he failed to forecast (death). And, on the other hand, if all sick people were restored to health, there would be no need to predict.

I 13 To restore all sick people to health

What does (Hippocrates) have in mind when he states, Now it is not possible to restore all sick people to health etc.? We say that

68 καὶ τὰ ἑξῆς; καὶ λέγομεν ὅτι | ὡς συμβαλλόμενον τοῦτο κατὰ τὸν τρίτον συλλογισμὸν προέφη καὶ εἶπε. τοῦτο γάρ φησιν ὅτι εἰ ἐνεδέχετο πάντας ὑγιάζειν, περιττὴ ἂν εἴη ἡ πρόγνωσις· ἐπειδὴ δὲ οὐ δυνατὸν πάντας ὑγιάζειν, οὐχ ὅτι περιττὴ ἡ πρόγνωσις. τί οὖν; ὅτι πταιστὴ ἡ τέχνη. αὕτη μὲν καθ' ἑαυτὴν ἄπταιστός τε καὶ ἀναμάρτητος· εἰ δὲ πολλάκις οἷα εἰκὸς ἁμαρτάνει, οὐ δι' ἑαυτήν, ἀλλὰ διὰ τὴν ὑποκειμένην ὕλην ῥευστήν τε καὶ εὐμετάβλητον οὖσαν. οὕτω καὶ τεκτονική τε καὶ οἰκοδομικὴ ἁμαρτάνουσιν, οὐ δι' ἑαυτάς, ἀλλὰ διὰ τὰς ὑποκειμένας ὕλας αὐταῖς. ὅσαι δ' ἔχουσι τὴν ὑποκειμένην ὕλην ἀμετάβλητον, αὗται καὶ τὸ ἄπταιστον ηὐτύχησαν, καθάπερ ἀστρονομία τε καὶ γεωμετρία. ἐπεὶ οὖν ῥευστὴ ὕλη ὑπόκειται τῇ ἰατρικῇ – σώματα γάρ εἰσιν ἀνθρώπεια –, διὰ ταύτην τὴν αἰτίαν πταίει. δεῖ οὖν πάντα τρόπον ποιεῖν ἄμεμπτον φυλάττεσθαι τὴν τέχνην. πῶς δὲ αὐτὴν ἄμεμπτον φυλάξωμεν, εἰ μὴ ὅτι τῷ προγνῶναι τὸ μέλλον; κἄν τε σωτήριον ᾖ τὸ νόσημα κἄν τε ὀλέθριον, ἀναγκαία ἡ τούτου πρόγνωσις ὥστε, κἂν ἀποτυχία τις ἔσται, διὰ τοῦ προλέγειν ἄμεμπτος ἡ τέχνη διαμενεῖ.

I 14 [1: 193,9 A. = II 110,11 L.] Ἐπειδὴ δὲ οἱ ἄνθρωποι ἀποθνήσκουσιν οἱ μὲν πρὶν ἢ καλέσαι τὸν ἰατρὸν ὑπὸ τῆς ἰσχύος τῆς νόσου, οἱ δὲ καὶ ἐκκαλεσάμενοι παραχρῆμα ἐτελεύτησαν, οἱ μὲν ἡμέραν μίαν ζήσαντες

Ἀποροῦσί τινες ὅτι «Τούτου ἀκαίρως ἐμνημόνευσεν ὁ Ἱπποκράτης· ἐὰν γὰρ πρὸ τοῦ καλέσαι τὸν ἰατρὸν ἀποθάνῃ ὁ ἄρρωστος, τότε ἀναίτιός ἐστιν· οὐδὲ γὰρ ἐθεώρησε τὸ πρόσωπον τοῦ θνήξαντος ἐν τῷ ζῆν αὐτόν.» πρὸς ὃ λέγομεν ὅτι καὶ ἀναγκαίως αὐτοῦ ἐμνημόνευσε κατὰ δύο αἰτίας· ἢ γὰρ διὰ τὸ τέλειον τῆς διαιρέσεως ἐμνημόνευσε τὸ πρὶν ἢ καλέσαι τὸν ἰατρὸν
69 ἀποθνήσκουσιν, ἢ | διὰ τὸ διδάξαι ἡμᾶς τὴν παρὰ φύσιν διάθεσιν τῶν ὀξέων νοσημάτων ἐμνημόνευσε τούτου τοῦ ῥησειδίου. καὶ διὰ μὲν τὸ τέλειον τῆς διαιρέσεως οὕτως· οἷον ὁ νοσῶν ἢ περισῴζεται ἢ ἀπόλλυται, καὶ ὁ ἀπολλύμενος ἢ πρὸ τοῦ κληθῆναι τὸν ἰατρὸν ἀποθνήσκει ἢ μετὰ τὸ καλέσαι τὸν ἰατρὸν καὶ ἀπελθεῖν, καὶ μετὰ τὸ ἀπελθεῖν τὸν ἰατρὸν καὶ ἐπισκέψασθαι ἢ ἐν τῇ αὐτῇ ἡμέρᾳ ἀπόλλυται ἢ μετὰ μίαν ἢ μετὰ δύο ἢ τρεῖς καὶ ἐπέκεινα. διὰ δὲ τὸ διδάξαι ἡμᾶς τὰ ὀξέα νοσήματα· πολλάκις γὰρ κάτοξύ ἐστι νόσημα, καὶ πρὶν καλέσαι τὸν ἰατρὸν ἀποθνήσκει ὁ νοσῶν καὶ οὐκ ἀναμένει τὴν παρουσίαν τοῦ ἰατροῦ· πολλάκις δὲ ὀξύ ἐστι τὸ νόσημα καὶ οὐ κάτοξυ, καὶ ἀναμένει τὴν παρουσίαν τοῦ ἰατροῦ, καὶ μετὰ τὸ καλέσαι τὸν ἰατρὸν ἢ ἐν τῇ αὐτῇ ἡμέρᾳ ἀποθνήσκει ἢ μετὰ μίαν ἢ μετὰ δύο ἢ μετὰ τρεῖς καὶ ἐπέκεινα. διὰ ταύτας οὖν τὰς δύο αἰτίας ἀναγκαίως τοῦ ῥησειδίου τούτου ἐμνημόνευσεν.

4–11] *v. supra*, app. sim. *ad* p. 48,28–31

1 καὶ^{II} *om.* L *ante* τοῦτο *add.* αὐτῇ L 2 εἰ *om.* L 4 οὐχ ὅτι] οὐκέτι γ *post* περιττὴ *add.* ἦν γ 10 ἐπεὶ οὖν] ἐπειδὴ ἂν γ 11 ἀνθρώπινα γ 13 τῷ] τοῦ *codd.*: *correxi* 14 *verba* τὸ νόσημα – 52,18 τοιούτῳ *desunt in* L *(v. supra, p. 14)* 19 ἐσκαλεσάμενοι *Hipp.* 21 τοῦτο P 23 οὐ MY ἐθεώρησας, *ut vid.*, ζ 25 τέλει M 26 περὶ MP 33 *ante* νόσημα *add.* τὸ M 36 ἀποθνήσκουσιν Pζ: *corr.* M

he states it beforehand as a contribution to the third syllogism. What he means is that, if it were possible to cure everyone, prognosis would be redundant; but since it is not possible to cure all, prognosis is not superfluous. Why? Because the art is liable to error. Now, considered in itself it is infallible and unerring; but if obviously it makes frequent mistakes this happens not because of itself, but because of the unstable and changeable nature of the matter it deals with. In this way both carpentry and building make mistakes, not from themselves, but from the nature of their subject matter. On the other hand, arts such as astronomy and geometry, whose subject matter is unchangeable, have attained to infallibility. Medicine, then, since it deals with unstable matter, bodies being mortal, for this reason makes blunders. Consequently, we must do everything to keep the art free from censure. And how else can we preserve it blameless if not by prognosing the future? Whether the disease be curable or fatal it is necessary to prognose it, so that, even if some failure should occur, the art will remain blameless by having made the prognosis.

I 14 But since men do die, some before they summon the doctor owing to the severity of the disease, others just after they have called him living one day

Some raise the difficulty, "Hippocrates has said this unadvisedly; for if the patient dies before the doctor is called, the doctor is free from responsibility, since he did not even get to examine the dead man's face while still alive." Our answer is that (Hippocrates) has been obliged to include this phrase for two reasons; he says they die before they summon the doctor either to complete the division or to instruct us on the abnormal condition of acute diseases. To complete the division, as follows: a patient either recovers or dies; one dies either before the summons of the doctor or after he has been called and has departed; the one who dies following the doctor's visit and departure succumbs either on the same day or after one or two or three or more days. To inform us about acute diseases: many times a disease is extremely acute and the patient does not last until the doctor comes, but dies before he is called; on the other hand, a disease is often acute without being extremely so; the patient survives until the doctor has arrived, then passes away on the day of the summons or after one or two or three or more days. These are the two reasons, then, that have compelled him to include this phrase.

Ἄλλως. «Ἐπειδὴ δέ τινες», φησίν, «ἀποθνήσκουσι μετὰ τὸ καλέσαι τὸν ἰατρὸν παραχρῆμα, οἱ δὲ μετὰ ὀλίγας ἡμέρας, οἱ δὲ πρὶν ἢ ἐκκαλέσαι τὸν ἰατρὸν ἐτελεύτησαν, διὰ τοῦτο», φησί, «βούλομαί σε εἰδότα τὸ ῥευστὸν τῆς ὕλης καὶ τὸ ἄλλοτε ἄλλως ἔχον προγινώσκειν καὶ προλέγειν.» ἀλλ' ἴσως τις ἀπορήσοι ὅτι «Καὶ ποίαν μέμψιν ἔχει ὁ ἰατρός, ἐὰν πρὶν ἐκκαλέσασθαι ἐτελεύτησε;» καὶ νόμιζε λέγειν τὸν Ἱπποκράτην ὅτι «Οὐκ ἔχει ἐπὶ τούτῳ ὁ ἰατρὸς μέμψιν· ἀλλὰ βούλομαί σε εἰδέναι τὸ ῥευστὸν τῆς ὕλης καὶ διὰ τοῦτο προλέγειν, ἵνα μὴ μεμπτέος ἔσῃ.»

Ἄλλη ἐξήγησις. ἐνταῦθα ἄρχεται τοῦ τρίτου συλλογισμοῦ. ἴσμεν δὲ ὅτι ἐστὶν οὕτως· ὁ προγινώσκων οἶδε τὴν ἔκβασιν· ὁ εἰδὼς τὴν ἔκβασιν προλέγει τὸ μέλλον· ὁ προ-
70 λέγων τὸ μέλλον ἀνέγκλητον φυλάξει τὴν τέχνην. οὕτως ὅτι | ἀναγκαία ἡ πρόγνωσις διὰ τὸ εἰδέναι τὴν ἔκβασιν τοῦ μέλλοντος. ἰατρός τις ἰδιώτης μὴ προγνοὺς τὸ μέλλον ἀνελθὼν πρὸς ἄρρωστον καὶ ὁρῶν τοῦτον ἱδροῦντα συγκοπτικῶς, εἶτα νομίσας ἐλλιπῶς γίνεσθαι τοὺς ἱδρῶτας, μὴ γνοὺς ὅτι κατὰ συγκοπὴν ἐγένοντο οὗτοι οἱ ἱδρῶτες, ἐνόμισε δεῖν ἐπὶ πλέον ἐκφορῆσαι τὴν ὕλην. ἀπήγαγεν οὖν τὸν ἄρρωστον εἰς λουτρὸν καὶ τοῦτο⟨ν⟩ ἐποίησεν ἐπὶ πλέον διαφορηθῆναι, καὶ ἅμα τῷ διαφορηθῆναι τετελεύτηκεν ὁ ἄνθρωπος, καὶ τὴν πᾶσαν ἀπηνέγκατο μέμψιν ὁ ἰατρός, αἴτιος αὐτῷ τοῦ θανάτου γενόμενος. οὐχ ὅτι δὲ αὐτὸς αἴτιος τοῦ θανάτου· ἔμελλεν γὰρ θνήσκειν ὅσον ἐκ τοῦ προηγησαμένου συμπτώματος· ἀλλ' ἐπειδὴ οὐ προέγνω τὸ μέλλον ὥστε μὴ ἐγχειρῆσαι τοιούτῳ τολμήματι, ἐγχειρήσας οὖν, τὴν πᾶσαν αἰτίαν ἐκληρονόμησεν. ὥστε οὖν ἵνα μὴ τὸ αὐτὸ πάθωμεν ἐκείνῳ τῷ ἰδιώτῃ, ἀναγκαῖον ἀσκεῖν τὴν πρόγνωσιν.

I 15 [1: 194,2 A. = II 112,2 L.] Πρὶν ἢ τὸν ἰατρὸν τῇ τέχνῃ πρὸς ἕκαστον νόσημα ἀνταγωνίσασθαι

Θαυμασίως πάνυ τῇ πληθυντικῇ φωνῇ ἐχρήσατο εἰπὼν πρὸς ἕκαστον νόσημα· ἐνδέχεται γὰρ μὴ ὑπὸ ἑνὸς νοσήματος ἔχεσθαι τὸν κάμνοντα, ἀλλ' ὑπὸ δύο νοσημάτων καὶ ἔστιν ὅτε καὶ τριῶν, καὶ διὰ τοῦτο ἔφη πρὸς ἕκαστον νόσημα.

Ἄλλως. τὸ πρὸς ἕκαστον νόσημα· εἰ μὲν κατὰ πολλῶν νοσημάτων εἴπωμεν, ἐπὶ διαφόρων λαμβάνομεν ἀνθρώπων, ἐπειδὴ πληθυντική ἐστιν ἡ φωνή. εἰ δὲ ἐπὶ ἑνὸς ἀνθρώπου τὸ τῶν νοσημάτων λαμβάνομεν, ἀντὶ τοῦ περὶ αἰτιῶν, συμπτωμάτων, νοσημάτων. καὶ καλῶς πάνυ προῆλθεν ἡ ἐξήγησις.

Ἄλλη ἐξήγησις. ἕκαστον λέγει ἢ πρὸς τὴν αἰτίαν ἢ πρὸς τὸ νόσημα ἢ πρὸς τὸ σύμπτωμα· ὁ γὰρ ἰατρὸς πρὸς ἕκαστον ἀγωνίζεται τούτων. ἐὰν οὖν βίαιον ᾖ τὸ νόσημα
71 ὡς εἶναι τοῦτο ὑπὲρ τὴν δύναμιν, οὐδενὶ τῶν εἰρημένων ἐλπὶς ἀν|τιστῆναι τοῦτον. εἰ γὰρ καὶ πρὸς τὴν αἰτίαν σταίη, εἰκότως ἕτερον αἴτιον ἰσχυρότερον εὑρεθήσεσθαι τούτου, ὃ φθάσει περιγινόμενον καὶ τῆς δυνάμεως, ὡς καὶ ταύτην καταλῦσαι. πολλάκις δὲ ἕτερον μὲν αἴτιον οὐκ ἀντιπράττει, τὸ δὲ νόσημα αὐτὸ ὀχληρότερον καθίσταται. ἔστι δ' ὅτε τὸ μὲν νόσημα κατεπείγει οὐδέν, ἀλλὰ τὰ συμπτώματα. πολλάκις γοῦν ἐν ᾧ χρόνῳ πρὸς ἕν τι διαμάχεται, φθάνει ἕτερον ἰσχυρότερον εὑρεθὲν ἀνελεῖν τὴν δύναμιν. διὰ οὖν τὴν βίαν τῶν τοιούτων ὀλεθρίων ὄντων ἀναγκαῖον κατορθοῦν τὴν πρόγνωσιν.

3sq.] *v. supra*, app. sim. *ad* p. 48,28–31 11–16] *cf.* Gal. In Hipp. Progn. comm. I 4: CMG V 9,2 p. 200,9–13

1 Ἄλλως] ⟨κ⟩είμενον M 2 καλέσαι P 3 *fort.* ἔχειν *scribendum est* 4 ἔχῃ MPY 6 τοῦτο γ: *correxi* 7 μεμπτὸς M: μεμπτοὶ ζ 8 Ἄλλη] ἑτέρα ζ 10 οὕτως] ὄντως γ: *corr. Wk.* ὅτι] ἐστὶν P 11 μὴ] μὲν P 13 οἱ *om.* M 14 τοῦτο γ: *correxi* 16 γινόμενος ζ 17 αὐτὸ M ἔμελε M θνήσκειν] ὁ θνήσκων M 18 ἐγχειρίσαι Mζ: *corr.* P ἐγχειρίσας Lζ: ἐγχειρίσαι M: *corr.* P 19 μὴ *om.* L τῶ αὐτῶ L 23 πρὸς] καθ' γ 25 καὶ[I] *om.* γ 27 εἴπομεν *codd.*: *correxi* 28 sq. ἐπὶ . . . λαμβάνομεν] ἐστιν . . . λαμβανόμενον *codd.*: *corr. Wk.* 30 καὶ καλῶς καὶ πάνυ καλῶς γ 32 ἢ *om.* L 33 τοῦτον] τούτων L 34 ἰσχυρότερον *om.* γ 35 προγενόμενον L

From another commentary. (Hippocrates) is saying, "Since some die just after calling the doctor, others a few days later, and some before he has been summoned, for this reason I want you to prognose and forecast, being aware of the unstable and changing nature of the subject matter." Here perhaps the objection will be raised, "What blame can be laid to the doctor if the patient dies before he has been called?" You may imagine this to be Hippocrates' reply: "He is not responsible in such a case; but I want you to be conscious of the unstable nature of the matter and, for this reason, to predict so as to avoid reproach."

From a different commentator. Here he begins the third syllogism which, as we know, runs as follows: the one who prognoses knows the outcome; he who knows the outcome forecasts the future; the one who forecasts the future will keep the art free from blame. Thus we see that prognosis is necessary for discovering how the future will turn out. A certain amateur, who did not practice prognosis, came to a patient and found him sweating like one with syncope; then, failing to recognize it as sweat from syncope, he decided that he was not sweating sufficiently and that the matter must be cleared out further. So he brought him to the bath and had him dissipate more; but as soon as this was accomplished the patient died and the entire blame was placed on the doctor, because (it was claimed) he had caused the man's death. The fact is, however, that he was not the cause; the man was going to die from the antecedent symptom. However, since he did not prognose what was going to happen, (which would have told him) not to attempt such a risk, he tried it and got all the blame. The conclusion is that, in order to avoid what happened to that amateur, we must practice prognosis.

I 15 Before the doctor has been able to combat each disease with the art

When he uses the plural phrase each disease it is a very good choice of words; for a patient can be suffering from not just a single disease but from two and sometimes even three; this explains his saying each disease.

A different explanation of the phrase each disease: When we speak in terms of many diseases, we understand them to refer to different people, "diseases" being plural. On the other hand, when we use "diseases" of one person, we mean causes, symptoms and diseases. And thus the explanation is quite successful.

From another commentator. Each refers to the cause or to the disease or to the symptom; for the doctor struggles against each of these. Now if the disease is violent enough to exceed the body's power, the doctor has no hope of withstanding any of the three. For if he takes his stand against the cause, he may reasonably expect another, more powerful one to show up, one that will manage to surpass and break down the power of the body. On the other hand, it often is the case that he is not confronted by another cause, but the disease itself becomes more troublesome. Again, sometimes the disease is not at all urgent, but the symptoms are. So in many instances while he has been engaged against one, another and stronger one has developed to destroy the body's power. It is necessary, then, because of the force of such deadly conditions, to practice prognosis successfully.

I 16 [1: 194,4 A. = II 112,4 L.] Ὁκόσον ὑπὲρ τὴν δύναμίν εἰσι τῶν σωμάτων

Δεῖ εἰδέναι ὅτι αἱ τοῦ σώματος δυνάμεις εἰσὶ τρεῖς, φυσική, ζωτική, ψυχική. δεῖ τοίνυν, φησί, τὰς τοῦ σώματος δυνάμεις παραβαλεῖν πρὸς τὴν τοῦ νοσήματος καὶ εἰδέναι, εἰ οὐκ ἐξισχύουσι κατ' αὐτοῦ, καὶ ποῖαι, ὅτι ἀπεῖπον. εἰ μὲν γὰρ αἱ κρείττονες ἀπεῖπον, οἷον ἡ ζωτική, ἥτις ἀπὸ καρδίας ὁρμᾶται, ἢ ἡ ψυχικὴ ἡ ἐκ τοῦ ἐγκεφάλου, μένει δὲ ἡ φυσική, τηνικαῦτα ὁ θάνατος ὑπόγυιος γίνεται ὡς τῆς ἐλάττονος ἐρρωμένης, τῶν κρειττόνων καταβεβλημένων. ὡς δήπου κἀμοὶ ὤπται τοῦ ἀρρώστου ἄριστον †ὕδωρ εἰς† ἐκκρίνοντος· καὶ ἐντεῦθεν εἴχαμεν ἐρρῶσθαι τὴν φυσικὴν δύναμιν, καταβεβλῆσθαι δὲ τὴν ζωτικήν, διότι συγκοπτικὸν εἶχεν ἱδρῶτα, καὶ ὁ τοιοῦτος ἐτελεύτα.

(IV)

I 17 [1: 194,4 A. = II 112,5 L.] Ἅμα δὲ καὶ εἴ τι θεῖον ἔνεστιν ἐν τῇσι νούσοισιν

Λέγει ὁ συγγραφεὺς ὅτι δεῖ, φησί, μὴ μόνον τὰ κατὰ ἁπλούστερον τρόπον περὶ τοὺς ἀρρώστους συμβαίνοντα προγινώσκειν καὶ ἅπερ οἱ κάμνοντες παραλιμπάνουσι προλέγειν, ἀλλὰ καὶ εἴ τι θεῖον ἔνεστιν ἐν ταῖς νόσοις,
72 καὶ τούτου δεῖ τὴν πρόνοιαν ποιεῖσθαι, ἤτοι πρό|γνωσιν ἐκμελετᾶν.
Καὶ οἱ μέν φασι θεῖον εἰρηκέναι τὸν Ἱπποκράτην τὴν θεομηνίαν, καθὸ νοσήματα διάφορα τοῖς ἀνθρώποις εἴωθε γίνεσθαι, ἅπερ πιστούμενοι εἰς μαρτυρίαν παράγουσι τοὺς λεγομένους βλητοὺς καὶ τοὺς ἐπιλήπτους. ὁ μέντοι Γαληνὸς οὐ δέχεται τὴν τοιαύτην γνώμην τῶν ἐξηγητῶν λέγων ὅτι οὐδέποτε ἐν τοῖς ἑαυτοῦ συγγράμμασι φαίνεται ὁ Ἱπποκράτης οὑτινοσοῦν νοσήματος τὴν αἰτίαν εἰς τὸ θεῖον ἀναφέρων. ἄλλως τε δὲ ἐν τῷ Περὶ διαίτης ὀξέων βιβλίῳ μνημονεύσας τὸ πάθος τῶν βλητῶν τὴν αἰτίαν ἐδίδαξε, καθ' ἣν τὸ τοιοῦτον πάθος τοῖς ἀνθρώποις συμβαίνει. ἀλλὰ καὶ ἐν τῷ Περὶ τῆς ἱερῆς νόσου συγγράμματι ἀντιρρητικῶς ἔχει ⟨πρὸς⟩ τοὺς λέγοντας αὐτὸ κατὰ θεομηνίαν γίνεσθαι.

20–29] *cf.* Gal. In Hipp. Progn. comm. I 4: CMG V 9,2 p. 206,9–15 23 Γαληνὸς] Gal. In Hipp. Progn. comm. I 4: CMG V 9,2 pp. 206,9–208,21 26 Περὶ διαίτης ὀξέων] Hipp. De diaeta acut. 17 (5): I p. 117,7–22 Kw. = II pp. 260,7–262,13 L. 28 Περὶ – νόσου] Hipp. De morb. sacr.: Ars Medica II 1 pp. 60–90 = VI pp. 352–396 L.

1 ὁκόσιν L: ὁκόσοισιν γ: *sec. Hipp. corr. Dietz* εἰσι] ἐς τὸ L 4 παραβάλλειν ζ: περιβάλλειν P: περιβάλον *(sic)* M 5 εἰ *om.* γ οὐ κατισχύουσι γ 7 ὁ *om.* L 8 ὑπόγυος γ 9 ἀρρώστου – 10 δύναμιν] οὕτως δεῖ γρ(άφειν) ἄρρ(ωστον) καὶ οὖν ὥρων *(sic)* εἰσεκκρίνοντα καὶ ἐνταῦθα ἔγνων ἐρρῶσαι τὴν φυσικὴν δύναμιν καὶ τὰ ἑξῆς *in mg.* L 9 sq. ὕδωρ εἰς] οὐ δῶρον L: οὖρον *coni. Dietz* 10 ἐκκρίνοντα L 15 τοῖσι *codd.*: *corr. Dietz* 16 συγγραφεὺς] ποιητὴς γ 19 ποιεῖσθαι *om.* γ 20 θεῖον *om.* L 22 τοὺς[II] *om.* γ 23 ὁ *om.* L γνώμην *post* ἐξηγητῶν *trsp.* γ τῶν *om.* L 25 ἀναφέρειν L 28 ἱερᾶς L πρὸς *coni. Dietz* 29 αὐτῶ γ

I 16 How far they exceed the power of the body

Note that the faculties of the body are three in number, the natural, vital and psychic. So we must, (Hippocrates) says, compare the body's faculties with the strength of the disease, and we should know whether they do not match up to the disease, and which do not, because they are exhausted. For if the more important give out, namely the vital whose source is the heart or the psychic which originates in the brain, and the natural is left, then death becomes imminent, the lesser being intact and the more important having failed. I personally have seen this happen; the patient was passing (?) very well; so it meant that the natural faculty was strong, but the vital was exhausted, since he had a syncoptic sweat, and he died.

(IV)

I 17 And at the same time if there is anything divine in the diseases

Our author says that we ought to prognose not only the straightforward things that happen to the sick and tell in advance what they leave out, but if there is anything divine in the diseases, we must make the prognosis or prediction of this as well.

Some (commentators) maintain that Hippocrates means by divine the wrath of God which is commonly held to cause various diseases in man; those who believe in such diseases cite as evidence the so-called stricken (or palsies) and epileptics. Galen, however, does not accept this view of the commentators; Hippocrates, he says, in his writings never attributes to the divine the cause of any disease. Moreover, in On Diet in Acute Diseases, when discussing palsy, he gives the reason why this condition occurs in man. And in the treatise On the Sacred Disease he criticizes those who claim that it is brought about by divine wrath.

Αὐτίκα γοῦν τὸ τῶν λεγομένων βλητῶν πάθος τοιῷδέ τι⟨νι⟩ τρόπῳ συμβαίνει συνίστασθαι· ἐπειδὴ ὡς μάλιστα ἐν τοῖς λοιμοῖς τὸ τοιοῦτον συμβαίνει τοῖς κάμνουσιν – ἴσμεν γὰρ ὅτι τὰ λοιμικὰ πάθη τὴν σηπεδονώδη τοῦ ἀέρος κατάστασιν αἰτίαν τῆς οἰκείας γενέσεως εὐπόρησεν σηπομένων καὶ διαφθειρομένων δηλονότι τῶν ἐν τοῖς σώμασι χυμῶν –, ἐκ τῆς τοιαύτης τοίνυν σηπεδόνος καὶ ὀξείας καὶ ἀλλοκότου καὶ ταραχώδους τῶν χυμῶν κινήσεως ἀγομένη ἡ φύσις ἐπείγεται πρὸς ἀπώθησιν καὶ ἔκκρισιν καὶ διαφόρησιν τῶν ἀνιόντων. τούτου δὲ τυχεῖν μὴ δυναμένη δι' οἰκείαν ἀσθένειαν, προκαταλαμβάνοντος τὸ ἔργον τοῦ θανάτου, μέχρι μέν τινος ὠθήσασα τὴν ὕλην, τὸ ἐντεῦθεν ἐκλείπει. εἶτα αὐτὴ ἡ ἐκριφεῖσα ὕλη ὡς ἐπὶ τὰ ὑπὸ τὸ δέρμα χωρία ἐκεῖσε ἐνεχθεῖσα καὶ σφηνωθεῖσα τῷ πλήθει καὶ τῇ ὑπερπληρώσει ῥήγνυσι τὰ λεπτὰ τῶν ἀγγείων καὶ ἐκχεῖται τὸ τηνικαῦτα εἰς τὰς παρακειμένας κενὰς χώρας. οὗτινος γενομένου πελιδνοῦνται καὶ μελαίνονται οἱ τοῦτο πάσχοντες τόποι δίκην τῶν ἐκχυμωμάτων, ὡς αἴσθησιν αἰκισμῶν τινων καὶ μαστίγων τοῖς ἀγυμνάστοις τῶν ὁρώντων ἐμποιεῖν.
73 ὅθεν οἱ ἰδιῶται ὁρῶντες τοὺς τοῦτο παθόντας κατά τινα | θείαν ὀργὴν ὑπὸ ἐναντίας δυνάμεως μαστιγωθῆναι λέγουσιν ἐκείνους. ὅθεν καὶ βλητοὺς αὐτοὺς ὀνομάζουσι παρὰ τὸ κατὰ θείαν μῆνιν ὑπὸ ἐναντίας βεβλῆσθαι δυνάμεως.

Καὶ τὸ τῶν ἐπιλήπτων δὲ πάθος οὐκ ἔχει θείαν ὀργὴν αἰτίαν τῆς γενέσεως, ἀλλὰ γίνεται ἡ ἐπιληψία κατά τινα σεληνιακὴν περίοδον, οὐ τοῦτο λέγοντός μου, ὅτι ἡ τοῦ θεοῦ ὀργὴ διὰ τῆς τῶν οὐρανίων κινήσεως ἐπιπέμπει τοῖς ἀνθρώποις τὸ πάθος. ἀλλ' ἰστέον ὅτι ἡ σελήνη, ἡνίκα πλησιφαὴς γένηται καὶ αὔξῃ αὐτῆς τὸ φῶς, χλιαρᾶς τινος θερμασίας καὶ συμμέτρου αἰτία τοῖς σώμασι γίνεται, ὑφ' ἧς θερμασίας διαχεῖσθαι συμβαίνει τοὺς χυμοὺς καὶ πληροῦν μάλιστα τὰς κεφαλάς, διὰ τὸ γυμνὰς ταύτας καὶ πρώτας σχεδὸν τοῦ λοιποῦ σώματος τῷ περιέχοντι ὁμιλεῖν ἀέρι. ὑπὸ οὖν τῆς αὐτῆς χύσεως ἀνάγκη παροξύνεσθαι τὸ πάθος τῶν ἐπιτηδείως οὕτως διακειμένων πρὸς τὸ πάθος τῆς ἐπιληψίας. ἔνθεν αὐξούσης τῆς σελήνης παροξύνονται οἱ ἐπιληπτικοὶ καὶ πάλιν ληγούσης παρακμάζουσιν. ἔστι δὲ τεκμήρασθαι τὸ αὐτὸ τοῦτο, φημὶ ὅτι ἡ σελήνη ἐξάρχει χλιαρᾶς τινος θερμασίας, καὶ ἐξ ἑτέρων πλείστων. οἵ τε γὰρ ἐγκέφαλοι τῶν ζῴων αὐξάνοντος τοῦ σεληνιακοῦ φωτὸς μείζονες ἑαυτῶν γίνονται, καὶ τὰ ὀστρακόδερμα δὲ λεγόμενα αἰσθητὴν ἔχουσι τὴν κατ' οὐσίαν ἐπίδοσιν τὸ τηνικαῦτα, ὅπερ ἐν αὐτοῖς μάλιστα διαφαίνεται τῶν ἄλλων διὰ τὸ ὑγρὸν τῆς οὐσίας. ἐπεί τοί γε ἡ τοιαύτη ἀναλογία διὰ πάντων διήκει τῶν σωμάτων, λέγω δὴ αὐξανόντων κατ' οὐσίαν πλησιφαοῦς γινομένης τῆς σελήνης, μειουμένης δὲ συγκαθαιρο⟨υ⟩μένων. τοῦ δὲ τοιούτου πάθους ὁ ἥλιος τὴν πρώτην ἔχει αἰτίαν· αὐτὸς γὰρ

1–30] *cf.* Schol. R *in* Gal. In Hipp. Progn. comm. I 4: CMG V 9,2 p. 206 *ad* lin. 11   21–58,3] *cf.* Ioann. Comm. in Hipp. De morb. pop. VI: 143d19–34 Pritchet

1 τινι] τι *codd.*: *suppl. Dietz*   4 εὐπόρησιν V: ἀπόρη *(ambig.)* MP   6 ὀξέως *codd.*: *correxi*   7 ἀγομένη] εὐομένη L   διαφύρησιν L   8 *fort.* τούτον *(sic)* L   μὴ *om.* L   9 ὠθήσασα] ἀνατρέψασα *in mg.* L   11 τὸ *om.* MP   13 παρακειμένας *om.* γ   21 ἐπίληψις γ   22 κινήσεων *codd.*: *corr. Dietz*   24 αὔξει γ   28 τῶν *om.* γ   29 ἐπιλήψεως γ   30 ἐπίληπτοι γ   31 ὅτι *om.* γ   37 πλησιοφαοῦς γ   συγκαθαιρομένων *codd.*: *corr. Dietz*

Here, then, is a description of how the condition of palsy develops: Since the disease happens to patients for the most part in plagues – for we know that plague diseases have, as the cause of their own origin, the putrid state of the atmosphere, namely when the body humors have become corrupted and rotten – nature, then, roused by this putrefaction and by the vehement, abnormal and confused movement of the humors, is eager to eject, excrete and dissipate the matter which comes up (for elimination). But it is unable to accomplish this due to its own weakness, seeing that death is already anticipating the work of nature; and having forced the matter to a certain point it then fails. After this the matter expelled as far as the subcutaneous areas, having reached there and being impacted by the great quantity and excess, ruptures the small vessels and spills over then into the surrounding vacant areas. When this happens the affected areas turn livid and black as in ecchymosis, so as to create for the untrained eye the impression of torture and scourging. Consequently laymen, upon seeing victims of this condition, say that they have been scourged by an adverse power in accordance with some divine wrath. And this is why they call them the "stricken", from their having been struck by an adverse power as a result of divine wrath.

Neither does the condition of epileptics have divine wrath as a cause of its generation; rather, epilepsy develops according to a particular phase of the moon, by which I do not mean that the wrath of God sends the disease to men through the movement of the heavenly bodies. But note that the moon, when it is full and has increased light, becomes the cause of a warm and moderate heat in the body; this heat makes the humors spread around and fill the head especially, this part being exposed and usually the first in the body to be in contact with the surrounding air. Then the same flow (of humors) necessarily produces a heightening of the condition in those who are disposed in the right way for epilepsy. This is why, as the moon becomes fuller, epileptics experience paroxysms, but as it disappears, their condition abates. It is possible to prove this particular point, namely that the moon sets off a certain moderate heat, from many other examples as well. For animal brains grow larger than normal with increasing moonlight, and in the case of the so-called testaceans there is during this period a noticeable increase in substance, which is much more visible in them than in other creatures because of their moist nature. As a matter of fact the same kind of change extends to all bodies, namely that they increase in substance as the moon gets larger and subside as it decreases. But it is the sun which is the principal

πάντα ἀλλοιοῖ τὰ τῇδε σώματα τῷ δραστηρίῳ τῆς θερμότητος. ἐπὶ μέντοι τὴν σελήνην ἀναφέρομεν τὸ τοιοῦτον ἔργον, διὰ τὸ περίγειον αὐτῆς καὶ προσεχὲς μᾶλλον ἡμῖν.

Ἕτεροι δὲ λέγουσι θεῖον εἰρηκέναι τὸν Ἱπποκράτην τὰς κρισίμους ἡμέρας· ὅτι δεῖ προγινώσκειν τὰς κρισίμους ἡμέρας, διὰ τί ἡ μὲν τετάρτη
74 κρίνει, ἡ δὲ πέμπτη οὐ κρίνει, ἡ δὲ ἕκτη κρίνει | μέν, ἐπὶ κακῷ δέ, καὶ ἡ ἑβδόμη κρίνει, ἀλλ' ἐπ' ἀγαθῷ· ταῦτα δὲ οὐκ ἄλλῳ τινὶ γίνονται ἀλλ' ἢ θείᾳ τινὶ ἐπιφοιτήσει. ὁ δὲ Γαληνὸς ἐκβάλλει καὶ ταύτην τὴν αἰτίαν λέγων ὅτι πῶς ὁ Ἱπποκράτης ἐν ἄλλοις συγγράμμασι πλατικῶς περὶ τῶν κρισίμων ἡμερῶν διαλεχθείς — ἐν Ἀφορισμοῖς φησι —, παρακεκαλυμμένως εἶχε περὶ τῶν κρισίμων εἰπεῖν καὶ συλλογιστικῶς εἶχε τοῦτο ποιῆσαι ἀπὸ τῆς θείας φωνῆς, τουτέστι διὰ τοῦ θείου;

Ἕτεροι δὲ λέγουσι τὸν ἔρωτα θεῖον καλεῖν τὸν Ἱπποκράτην ἐνταῦθα· καὶ γὰρ θεῖόν τι χρῆμά ἐστιν ὁ ἔρως, ὡς δηλοῦσι τὰ σύμβολα, ἃ οἱ γραφεῖς γράφουσι περὶ αὐτοῦ· γράφουσι γὰρ αὐτὸν παιδίον πτερὰ ἔχοντα καὶ λαμπάδα κατέχοντα· καὶ παιδίον μὲν ὡς νέον καὶ ἀγήρατον καὶ ὡς ἄφθαρτον αὐτὸν ὄντα, πτερωτὸν δὲ διὰ τὸ ὑψιπετὲς καὶ ἐπάρσιον αὐτὸν παραπέτασθαι, λαμπάδα δὲ κατέχειν ὡς φωτίζοντα καὶ ζωοποιοῦντα· ταῦτα δὲ πάντα θείας τινός εἰσι δυνάμεως. ὁ οὖν Ἱπποκράτης θεῖον ἐνταῦθα τὸν ἔρωτα καλεῖ, ἐπειδὴ ἔστι τι πάθος ἐρωτικὸν γινόμενον ἐν τοῖς ἀνθρώποις ἐγκεκρυμμένον· καὶ τοῦτό φησι δεῖ προγινώσκειν. οὕτως γοῦν φασιν Ἀντίοχον τὸν υἱὸν Σελεύκου τοῦ Μακεδόνων βασιλέως, καθ' ὧν καὶ αἱ πόλεις Ἀντιόχεια καὶ Σελεύκεια ὠνομάσθησαν, τοῦτον οὖν τὸν Ἀντίοχόν φασιν ἑαλωκέναι ἔρωτι πρὸς Εὐρυδίκην τὴν μητρυιὰν αὐτοῦ, καὶ εἶχε τοῦτο τὸ ἐρωτικὸν πάθος ἐγκεκαλυμμένον, καὶ ἐν μέσῳ ζωῆς καὶ θανάτου αὐτὸν τετυχηκέναι, καὶ πολλὴν ἐπιμέλειαν οἱ ἐν τῷ παλατίῳ ἰατροὶ πρὸς τὰ νομισθέντα αὐτοῖς ἐποίησαν. ἀλλὰ καὶ ἄλλους πλείστους ἰατροὺς ἀπὸ τῶν πόλεων μεταχειρισάμενοι καὶ ἀπὸ τῶν κωμῶν καὶ ἀπὸ τῶν ἀγρῶν καὶ μηδὲν ἰσχύσαντες ποιῆσαι διὰ τὸ ἐγκατακεκρυμμένον ἔχειν τὸ πάθος, ἐγνώσθη τῷ βασιλεῖ Σελεύκῳ περὶ Ἐρασιστράτου τοῦ Σαμίου ὅτι ἄριστός ἐστιν ἰατρός. καὶ δὴ παραγενομένου τοῦ Ἐρασιστράτου πρὸς τὸν Σέλευκον διελέχθησαν περὶ τοῦ υἱοῦ. καὶ εἰσελθόντος τοῦ Ἐρασιστράτου πρὸς τὸν Ἀντίοχον ἐπέβαλε τὴν χεῖρα ἐπὶ τῷ καρπῷ τοῦ Ἀντιόχου, καὶ δὴ σφυγμολογοῦντος τοῦ Ἐρασιστράτου
75 κατά τινα τύχην | τις ἐκ τῶν ἐκεῖσε ἑστώτων ἐμνημόνευσεν Εὐρυδίκης, καὶ εὐθέως γεγόνασιν οἱ σφυγμοὶ ἄτακτοι, καὶ διέγνω ἐν ἑαυτῷ ὁ Ἐρασίστρατος ὅτι ἐρωτικῶς διάκειται πρὸς Εὐρυδίκην ὁ νεανίας. καὶ παρασιωπήσας

8 Γαληνὸς] Gal. In Hipp. Progn. comm. I 4: CMG V 9,2 p. 207,15–20 15–18] *cf.* Gal. In Hipp. Progn. comm. I 4: CMG V 9,2 p. 207,13sq. 21–62,4] *cf.* Gal. In Hipp. Progn. comm. I 4; I 8: CMG V 9,2 pp. 206,16–207,14; 218,17–219,5 De praecognit. 6: CMG V 8,1 p. 100,7–14 Appian. Syr. 59–61 Plut. Demetr. 38 Iulian. Misopog.: II pp. 446–448 Wright Lucian. De dea Syr. 17–18

2 τῆς σελήνης L 11 εἶχε^{I} – συλλογιστικῶς *om.* L 17 περιπέτασθαι MP 19 τινός *om.* γ 22 ὧν *cod. Cyriaci Anconitani (v. supra, p. 19)*: ὃν *cett.* 23 γοῦν γ 29 ἐγκεκρυμένον γ 35 ἐμνημόνευσεν Εὐρυδίκης *ante* τις *trsp.* γ 36 διέγνων L αὐτῷ γ ὁ *om.* γ

cause of this condition; for it affects all earthly bodies by the activity of its heat. However, we attribute this effect to the moon, because it is close to earth and nearer to us (than the sun).

Others, however, say that what Hippocrates means by divine are the critical days; (and so) we must have previous knowledge of them, why the fourth is critical and the fifth not, why the sixth is critical and for the worse, the seventh critical but for the better; these things happen in this way only by divine direction. But Galen rejects this explanation also; why should Hippocrates, he asks, who in other works discusses the critical days at length – he means in the Aphorisms –, have to mention them here in a cryptic manner and in such a way that they have to be inferred from a sacred word, namely divine?

Others maintain that by divine Hippocrates means love in this instance; and love (they argue) is something divine, as is shown by the symbolism adopted by writers to depict it; for they represent it as a boy with wings and carrying a torch – a boy, love being young, unaging and immortal; winged, because it soars aloft to greater heights; and holding a torch, since it brings light and imparts life. All these are characteristics of a divine power. Hippocrates, then, means love here by divine, since there occurs in men a certain love sickness which is concealed; and this, he says, we must prognose. In this connection they relate the story about Antiochus the son of King Seleucus of Macedonia, who have given their names to the cities of Antioch and Seleucia; this Antiochus, they say, fell in love with Eurydice, his stepmother, and kept his passion concealed, and was between life and death; the court physicians took great care with him and tried everything they knew. Even when many other doctors were summoned from city, town and country, they had no success, because (Antiochus) kept his condition hidden; then King Seleucus heard about Erasistratus of Samos, that he was the best doctor. So when Erasistratus came to Seleucus they discussed the son. Erasistratus went to Antiochus and placed his hand on Antiochus' wrist; and as Erasistratus was taking his pulses one of those present happened to mention Eurydice's name and straightaway the pulses became irregular; so Erasistratus diagnosed to himself that the young man was in love with Eurydice. But he kept the discovery

ἐπυνθάνετο λέγων ὅτι «Δεῖ καὶ δεύτερον καὶ τρίτον ἐπιστῆναι τῇ σημειώσει πρὸς ἀσφαλῆ διάγνωσιν τοῦ πάθους», καὶ εἰπὼν ἀπηλλάγη. εἶτα ἐλθὼν τῇ ἐπαύριον λέγει τινὶ τῶν μετ' αὐτοῦ ὅτι «Ἡνίκα νεύσω σοι, μνημόνευσον Εὐρυδίκης.» καὶ ἐπέβαλε τὴν χεῖρα ἐπὶ τῷ καρπῷ τοῦ Ἀντιόχου καὶ εὗρε τοὺς σφυγμοὺς οἷοί περ καὶ ἐν τῷ κατὰ φύσιν· καὶ δὴ σημειουμένου αὐτοῦ ἔνευσε τῷ μετ' αὐτοῦ, καὶ ἐμνημόνευσεν Εὐρυδίκης. καὶ εὐθὺς γέγονεν ἡ ἀρτηρία ἐν ταράχῳ πολλῷ καὶ ἀτάκτῳ κινήσει, καὶ διέγνω ὁ Ἐρασίστρατος ἀσφαλῶς ὅτι ἔρωτα εἶχε πρὸς Εὐρυδίκην· τίς δ' ἦν ἡ Εὐρυδίκη οὐκ ἐγίνωσκε. καὶ δὴ πάλιν εἰρηκὼς ὅτι «Ἔτι δεόμεθα τῆς σημειώσεως» ἀνεχώρησεν. εἶτα εἰς ὕστερον ἐλθὼν ὁ Ἐρασίστρατος ἔφη πρὸς τὸν Σέλευκον ὅτι «Θέλω πάσας τὰς θεραπαίνας τὰς ἐν τῷ παλατίῳ οὔσας διελθεῖν ἔμπροσθεν ἡμῶν, ἵνα τὴν ἐπιτηδειοτάτην ἐκλεξώμεθα πρὸς ὑπουργίαν τοῦ νεανίσκου, ἵνα τὰ ὑφ' ἡμῶν ἐπιτασσόμενα βοηθήματα ποιῇ.» καὶ δὴ τοῦτο ἐποίησεν ὁ βασιλεὺς καὶ ἐκέλευσε πάσας διέρχεσθαι ἔμπροσθεν τοῦ Ἀντιόχου. ὁ δὲ Ἐρασίστρατος ἐσφυγμολόγει αὐτόν, καὶ παρῆλθον αἱ θεράπαιναι, καὶ οὐδεμία ἀνωμαλία γέγονεν ἐν τῇ ἀρτηρίᾳ. καὶ δὴ ἐν ἀμηχανίᾳ γεγονὼς ὁ Ἐρασίστρατος ἔφη πρὸς τὸν Σέλευκον ὅτι «Οὐκ ἀπολέλειπται ἄλλη θεραπαινίς, ἥτις γνωρίμη ἐστὶ τῷ νεανίσκῳ;» καί φησιν ὁ βασιλεὺς ὅτι «Οὐκ ἀπολέλειπται ἄλλη κορασίς, εἰ μὴ τὸ γύναιόν μου.» καί φησιν ὁ Ἐρασίστρατος ὅτι «Ἐλθέτω καὶ αὕτη.» καὶ δὴ ἐρχομένης τῆς Εὐρυδίκης, ἅμα ἐθεώρησεν ὁ Ἀντίοχος, γέγονεν ἡ ἀρτηρία αὐτοῦ ἐν ἀνωμαλίᾳ· ὁ γὰρ Ἐρασίστρατος ἔμεινε σφυγμολογῶν αὐτὸν ἀπ' ἀρχῆς μέχρι τέλους. καὶ δῆθεν ἐπιστώσατο καὶ διέγνω ὅτι πρὸς τὴν Εὐρυδίκην τὴν μητρυιὰν αὐτοῦ ἔρωτι ἑαλωκέναι· καὶ δή, φασί, πρὸς τὸν πατέρα τοῦ Ἀντιόχου ἀπεφήνατο λέγων ὅτι «Οἶδα τὸ νόσημα καὶ
76 διέγνων αὐτό, ὅπερ νοσεῖ ὁ υἱός σου, καὶ δύναμαι αὐτὸν | θεραπεῦσαι, οὐ βούλομαι δέ.» καὶ δὴ εὐθὺς ὁ βασιλεὺς πολλὰς ὑπέσχετο καὶ τιμὰς καὶ ἀξίας δοῦναι τῷ Ἐρασιστράτῳ, ἵνα ἰάσηται τὸν υἱὸν αὐτοῦ ἐκ τῆς νόσου. ὁ δὲ Ἐρασίστρατος εἶπε πάλιν τὰ αὐτά, ὅτι «Διέγνων μὲν τὸ νόσημα καὶ δύναμαι αὐτὸν θεραπεῦσαι, οὐ βούλομαι δέ.» καὶ δὴ τοῦτο ἐπὶ πολὺ τοῦ Ἐρασιστράτου λέγοντος ἐθυμώθη ὁ βασιλεὺς καὶ ἀπειλὰς καὶ ἐμβριμήσεις τύραννος ὢν ἀπένεμε τῷ Ἐρασιστράτῳ, ὅτι τυχὸν «Εἰ μὴ θέλεις αὐτὸν θεραπεῦσαι, φονεύω σε.» καί φησιν ὁ Ἐρασίστρατος· «Τί ἐθυμώθης, ὦ βασιλεῦ; ὅτι τῆς γυναικός μου ἐρᾷ καὶ θέλεις δίδωμι τὴν ἐμὴν γυναῖκα, ἵνα συνδιαφθαρῇ αὐτῷ· ἄκαιρον τοῦτό ἐστιν.» καὶ δή φησιν ὁ βασιλεὺς ὅτι «Ἐὰν τοῦτο ποιήσῃς καὶ δώσεις τὴν γυναῖκά σου καὶ ἰαθῇ ὁ υἱός μου, πολλὰ χρήματα δώσω σοι καὶ συγκοινωνὸς τῆς βασιλείας μου ἔσῃ.» καί φησιν ὁ Ἐρασίστρατος ὅτι «Εἰ τῆς γυναικός σου ἤρα, παρεῖχες ἂν τῷ νεανίσκῳ ὥστε ὑγιασθῆναι αὐτόν;» ὁ δὲ βασιλεὺς μετὰ πολλοῦ ὅρκου ἐξομνύμενος ὅτι «Ἐὰν τῆς γυναικός μου ἤρα, ἐδίδουν ἂν αὐτῷ, ἵνα ὑγιασθῇ», καὶ τοῦτο κατασφαλισάμενος ὁ Ἐρασίστρατος, λέγει πρὸς τὸν βασιλέα ὅτι «Ἵνα γινώσκῃς, ὦ βασιλεῦ, τῆς γυναικός σου ἐρᾷ.» καὶ

4 τὸν καρπὸν L, *sed cf. p. 58,34* 9 Ἔτι] ἔδει L 16 ἐν[I] *om.* L 20 ὅτι *om.* L 21 ἐχώρησεν γ *ante* γέγονεν *add.* καὶ γ 24 φησί(ν) *codd.*: *corr. Dietz* 26 δύναμαι] βούλομαι γ (ἴσως δύναμαι *in mg.* V) 27 εὐθέως γ 29 διέγνω μὲν P: διέγνομεν M 40 ἂν *om.* L 42 βασιλεῦ V: βασιλεῦς Y: -εὺς M(P?)

to himself; he remarked that he would need to observe the symptoms a second and a third time in order to ensure correct diagnosis of the condition, and having said this he left. On his return the following day he gave instructions to one of those with him, "When I nod, mention Eurydice's name." Then he put his hand on Antiochus' wrist and found his pulses normal; this observation made he nodded to the one with him, and he mentioned Eurydice. Immediately the young man's artery became very disturbed and irregular, and Erasistratus knew for certain that he was in love with Eurydice; but who Eurydice was he did not know. So once again saying "Further observation is necessary", he left. Later on Erasistratus came to Seleucus and said, "I would like all the female servants at the palace to come before us, so that we may choose the most suitable one for helping the young man to take the remedies we have prescribed." The king agreed and ordered all the servants to go before Antiochus. Erasistratus kept taking the pulses, the servants came, and nothing unusual happened to the artery. So Erasistratus was at a loss and he asked Seleucus, "(Are you sure that) there is no other female left that the young man knows?" To which the king replied, "There is no other woman left apart from my wife." And Erasistratus said, "Have her come too." So Eurydice came and as soon as Antiochus laid eyes on her his artery became abnormal; for Erasistratus was taking his pulses from start to finish. He had now confirmed and diagnosed that (Antiochus) was in love with Eurydice his stepmother; whereupon, the story goes, he addressed Antiochus' father as follows, "I have diagnosed your son's illness", he said, "and know what is ailing him; I can cure him, but I do not want to." The king immediately promised Erasistratus many honors and titles (to persuade him) to cure his son's illness. But Erasistratus repeated the same thing, "I have diagnosed the illness and can cure him, but I am not willing to." The king became angry when Erasistratus kept repeating this and, being a tyrant, he grew indignant and threatened him, saying for example, "If you do not agree to cure him, I will have you executed." To which Erasistratus replied, "Why are you angry Your Majesty? The question is that he is in love with my wife, and you want me to submit her to be corrupted with him; this is improper." But the king said, "If you do this, if you give your wife and my son is cured, I will pay you a large sum of money and share my kingdom with you." Erasistratus then said, "Suppose it were your wife that he loved; would you offer her to have the young man cured?" The king swore to the high heavens that "If he were in love with my wife, I would give her to him so that he might be cured"; so Erasistratus, now that he was assured of this, said to the king, "Your Majesty, I want you to know that it is your wife whom

δὴ εὐθέως ἐκέλευσεν ὁ βασιλεὺς τὴν Εὐρυδίκην εἰσελθεῖν πρὸς τὸν Ἀντίοχον. καί τινες μέν φασιν ὅτι συνεφθάρη αὐτῇ καὶ οὕτως ἀπηλλάγη τοῦ πάθους ὁ Ἀντίοχος. ἕτεροι δὲ εἶπον ὅτι ἐν ἐξουσίᾳ αὐτὴν λαβὼν καὶ περιβαλὼν καὶ καταφιλήσας ἀπηλλάγη· οἶδε γὰρ ἡ ἐξουσία καὶ τὸ αὐτεξούσιον ἀπαλλάξαι τοιούτου πάθους καὶ πόθου. ἀλλὰ καὶ ὁ Ἱπποκράτης διέγνω τοιοῦτον πάθος ἔρωτος τοῦ Περδίκκου. ἀλλὰ καὶ αὐτὸς ὁ Γαληνός φησιν ὅτι διέγνω τοιοῦτον πάθος θυγάτριον ἔχον ἔρωτος πρὸς Πυλάδην ὀρχηστὴν ἐν τοῖς τότε καιροῖς γενόμενον. ὁ οὖν Ἱπποκράτης θεῖον ἐνταῦθα τὸν ἔρωτα, ὥς τινες ὑπενόησαν, καλεῖ· ὅτι δεῖ καὶ τοῦτο προγινώσκειν, μή τι πάθος τοιοῦτον ἐγκατακέκρυπται ἐν τοῖς ἀνθρώποις.

Ὁ δὲ Γαληνὸς οὐδὲ ταύτην τὴν αἰτίαν ἐδέξατο, ἀλλ' ἐλέγχει αὐτοὺς ὡς κακῶς τοῦτο ἐννοήσαντας λέγων ὅτι αἰσχρόν ἐστιν ὁ ἔρως· καὶ ὅτι |
77 τοῦτο ἀληθές, δηλοῦσι τὰ σύμβολα, ἃ οἱ γραφεῖς γράφουσι. παιδίον μὲν αὐτὸν γράφουσιν οὐ διὰ τὸ νέον, ἀλλὰ διὰ τὸ ἐλλιπές, πτερωτὸν δὲ οὐ διὰ τὸ ὑψιπετῆ αὐτὸν εἶναι, ἀλλὰ διὰ τὸ ἄστατον τῇδε κἀκεῖσε περιφερόμενον, λαμπάδα δὲ κρατοῦντα οὐ διὰ τὸ φωτίζειν, ἀλλὰ πῦρ κρατοῦντα καὶ καπνίζοντα, ἅπερ αἰσχρὰ καὶ κίβδηλά εἰσιν. οὕτως διελέγξας αὐτοὺς λέγει αἰτίαν τοιαύτην, ὅτι θεῖον ἐνταῦθα ὁ Ἱπποκράτης τὰ προκαταρκτικὰ αἴτια λέγει καὶ τὴν κατάστασιν τοῦ περιέχοντος ἡμᾶς ἀέρος ὑποτίθεται. οὕτως γὰρ καὶ ἐν Ἐπιδημίοις ὑποτίθεται καὶ ἐν Ἀφορισμοῖς, ὡς δηλοῖ ἡ ῥῆσις λέγουσα οὕτως· «ἢν ὁ χειμὼν αὐχμηρὸς καὶ βόρειος γένηται, τὸ δὲ ἔαρ ἔπομβρον καὶ νότιον, ἀνάγκη τοῦ θέρεος πυρετοὺς ὀξεῖς καὶ ὀφθαλμίας καὶ δυσεντερίας γενέσθαι, μάλιστα τῇσι γυναιξὶ καὶ τοῖσιν ὑγρὰς ἔχουσι τὰς φύσιας.» καὶ ἄλλα πολλὰ εὑρήσεις εἰπόντα τὸν Ἱπποκράτην. ταῦτα οὖν δεῖ προγινώσκειν. καὶ [ὅτι] θεῖον ἐκάλεσεν ἐνταῦθα τὸ προγινώσκειν τὸν ἰατρὸν τὴν κατάστασιν τοῦ περιέχοντος ἡμᾶς ἀέρος, ἐπειδὴ ἀφανῶς καὶ ἀνεπαισθήτως ποιεῖ ἡμῖν, ὡς δηλοῦσιν αἱ λοιμικαὶ διαθέσεις ἀπὸ τῆς σηπεδόνος τοῦ περιέχοντος ἡμᾶς ἀέρος γινόμεναι. καὶ δεῖ, φησί, παρὰ πάντα τὰ νοσήματα τὰ ἐπιδήμια γινώσκειν τὰ ἀπὸ τοῦ περιέχοντος ἡμᾶς ἀέρος γινόμενα, εἴτε σωτήριά εἰσιν εἴτε ὀλέθρια.

Καὶ ἀποροῦσί τινες ὅτι «⟨Τί⟩ δήποτε μὴ ἐσαφήνισεν ἡμῖν ὁ Ἱπποκράτης καὶ σαφῶς ἀπεκρίνατο ὅτι δεῖ προγινώσκειν τὴν κατάστασιν τοῦ ἀέρος τοῦ ἡμᾶς περιέχοντος, ἀλλὰ θεῖον αὐτὸ ἔφη καὶ ἀσαφῶς;» καὶ

5sq. Ἱπποκράτης – Περδίκκου] *cf.* Sor. Vita Hipp. 5: CMG IV p. 176,4–11   7 ὁ Γαληνός] Gal. De praecognit. 6: CMG V 8,1 pp. 100,15–102,27 *cf.* Gal. In Hipp. Progn. comm. I 8: CMG V 9,2 pp. 218,20–219,5   12 Γαληνὸς] Gal. In Hipp. Progn. comm. I 4: CMG V 9,2 p. 207,10–14   18sq. αἰτίαν τοιαύτην] *cf.* Gal. In Hipp. Progn. comm. I 4: CMG V 9,2 pp. 208,10–25 *et* 207,5   21 ἐν Ἐπιδημίοις] Hipp. Epid. III 15: I pp. 231,19–232,6 Kw. = III pp. 98,6–100,6 L.   ἐν Ἀφορισμοῖς] Hipp. Aph. III 11: IV p. 490,2–5 L.

4 περιλαβὼν *codd.*: *corr. Wk.*   5 ὁ *om.* γ   6 τοιούτου πάθους *codd.*: *correxi*   7 αὐτὸν τὸν γαληνόν *codd.*: *correxi*   ἔρωτα γ   8 πυλάδου *codd.*: *corr. Dietz*   9 καλεῖ *post* ἐνταῦθα *trsp.* γ   13 αἰσχρὸς γ   16 εἶναι] ὄντα L   20 ἡμᾶς *om.* γ   21 καὶ[II] *om.* L   23 ἦρ γ   26 ὅτι *seclusi*   ἐκέλευσεν L   29 γινομένων *codd.*: *corr. Dietz*   παρὰ *om.* γ   32 Τί *addidi*   ἡμῖν *om.* L   33 *post* προγινώσκειν *add.* καὶ L   34 *post* ἀλλὰ *add.* καὶ L   αὐτῷ L   καὶ[II] *om.* γ

he loves." At this the king straightaway ordered Eurydice to go to Antiochus. According to some Antiochus had illicit intercourse with her and in this way was cured of the condition. But others maintain that he was cured by taking her in his arms and embracing and kissing her with her consent; for permission and freedom can rid a person of this kind of passion and desire. Hippocrates, too, diagnosed this love sickness in Perdiccas. And Galen himself tells us that he diagnosed such a sickness in a young woman who had fallen in love with a certain dancer of those times called Pylades. Hippocrates, then, according to the supposition of some, means love by divine in this instance, (and he says) that we must employ prognosis to see if such a condition is being kept hidden in men.

Galen, however, did not accept this explanation either and criticizes its proponents for misunderstanding the matter; he says that love is something base; and that this is true is borne out by the symbols used by writers to describe it. They portray love as a boy not for its youthfulness, but for its immaturity; with wings, not for its loftiness but for its fickle shifting from place to place; holding a torch, not because it gives light but because it brings fire and smoke, and these are base and dishonorable. Having thus thoroughly refuted them he gives this explanation: Hippocrates here means by divine the predisposing causes, by which he understands the state of the air surrounding us. For such is his assumption in both the Epidemics and Aphorisms, as we see from the following passage: "If the winter is dry and northerly, the spring very wet and southerly, then summer must bring acute fevers, eye diseases and dysentery, especially in women and those with moist constitutions." And you will find Hippocrates saying many other things (of this sort). These are the things, then, that we must prognose. So in the present instance (Hippocrates) uses divine in the sense of the doctor's prognosing the state of the air surrounding us, since it works on us unnoticed and imperceptively, as is shown by the plague conditions which develop from putrefaction of the surrounding atmosphere. And we must, he says, get to know above all diseases the epidemics which are produced by the atmosphere surrounding us, (to see) whether they are curable or fatal.

Some raise the question, "Why does Hippocrates not make things clear for us? Why does he not simply say that we must prognose the state of the air surrounding us, but calls it divine ambiguously?" We answer

ἀπολογούμεθα ὅτι διὰ τοῦτο οὐκ ἐμνημόνευσεν ὡς ὑμεῖς εἴπατε, ἐπειδὴ κατεσκεύασται αὐτῷ ἡ τοιαύτη πραγματεία ἐν πολλοῖς, καὶ ἐν Ἐπιδημίοις γὰρ καὶ ἐν Ἀφορισμοῖς καὶ ἐν ἄλλοις πλείστοις. ἐνταῦθα μέντοι πλατικῶς οὐκ ἠθέλησε τοῦτο ποιῆσαι.

I 18 [1: 194,5 A. = II 112,6 L.] Οὕτω γὰρ ἄν τις θαυμάζοιτό τε δικαίως καὶ ἰητρὸς ἀγαθὸς ἂν εἴη.

Φησὶν ὅτι ὁ προγινώσκων ἰατρὸς καὶ εἴ τι θεῖον ἔνεστιν ἐν ταῖς
78 νόσοις, τὴν ἴασιν εὐχερῶς περιτυγχάνει. | καὶ δεῖ θαυμάζειν τὸν τοιοῦτον δικαίως καὶ θαυμασίως, ὅτι ὁμοίωται τῷ θεῷ ὁ ἰατρὸς κατὰ τὸ δυνατὸν ἀνθρώποις κατὰ τὴν πρόγνωσιν.

I 19 [1: 194,6 A. = II 112,7 L.] Καὶ γὰρ οὓς οἷόν τε περιγενέσθαι ἔτι μᾶλλον δύναιτο διαφυλάττειν ἐκ πλείονος χρόνου προβουλευόμενος πρὸς ἕκαστα

Ἰδοὺ ἐκ τούτου τοῦ ῥησειδίου δυνατόν ἐστι βεβαιῶσαι τὴν τοῦ Γαληνοῦ ἐξήγησιν, ὅτι θεῖον ἐνταῦθα ὁ Ἱπποκράτης λέγει τὰ προκαταρκτικὰ αἴτια ἤτοι τὴν κατάστασιν τοῦ περιέχοντος ἡμᾶς ἀέρος, ἐκ τοῦ εἰπεῖν αὐτὸν ἐκ πλείονος χρόνου προβουλευόμενος πρὸς ἕκαστα.
Προγινώσκων γὰρ οὓς οἷόν τε περιγενέσθαι, τουτέστιν ὁ προγινώσκων ἰατρὸς ἅπερ σῴζονται νοσήματα καὶ περιγενέσθαι ἐκ πλείονος χρόνου προβουλευόμενος πρὸς ἕκαστον νόσημα, οὗτος δύναται εὐχερῶς ἰᾶσθαι τὰς νόσους· ὥσπερ ἐκ τοῦ χειμῶνος δύναται ὁ ἰατρὸς προγνῶναι τὰ ἐν τῷ θέρει μέλλοντα συμβῆναι καὶ εἰπεῖν νοσήματα· καὶ δύναται πρὸ πολλοῦ ἔτι περιεστηκῶς αὐτῶν ἐχόντων, λέγω δὴ τῶν νοσημάτων, προπαρασκευασθῆναι καὶ ἰάσασθαι τὰ τοιαῦτα νοσήματα· καὶ οὕτως ἀπαλλάττεται τοῦ κινδύνου.

V

I 20 [2: 194,10 A. = II 112,12 L.] Σκέπτεσθαι δὲ χρὴ ὧδε ἐν τοῖσιν ὀξέσι νοσήμασι, πρῶτον μὲν τὸ πρόσωπον τοῦ νοσέοντος

2 ἐν πολλοῖς] *cf.* Gal. In Hipp. Progn. comm. I 4: CMG V 9,2 p. 208,17–19 7sq. καὶ – νόσοις] Hipp. Progn. 1: p. 194,4sq. A. = II p. 112,5sq. L. 9 ὁμοίωται τῷ θεῷ] *cf. supra*, p. 30,26 Ioann. Comm. in Gal. De sect.: I fol. 6ᵛ ed. Pav. Ps.-Eliae Lect. in Porph. Isag.: p. 18,9sq. Westerink Dav. Proleg.: CAG XVIII 2 pp. 20,29; 55,35sq. Eliae Proleg.: CAG XVIII 1 pp. 16,10–16; 27,9–13 Plat. Theaet. 176a/b

2 αὐτῶν γ 3 γὰρ *om.* γ 6 ἰατρὸς γ 8 παρατυγχάνει *codd.*: *correxi* 9 ὡμοίωται γ τῷ *om.* γ 12 δύναιτο *om.* γ διαφυλάττει L 18 Προγινώσκων] γινώσκω *post spat. vac.* L *post* τουτέστιν *add.* ὅτι γ 20 οὕτως L 21 ἰάσασθαι γ ἐκ] ἀπὸ γ 23 περιεστηκὼς *codd.*: *correxi; cf. infra, pp. 266,23; 282,5*

that he does not express himself in the way you put it, because he has treated the matter fully in several works including the Epidemics and Aphorisms and many others. Here, however, he has no wish to go into detail.

I 18 For in this way he will be justly admired and be a good doctor.

He is saying that the doctor who prognoses to see if there is anything divine in the diseases effects cures easily. Such a person fully and justly deserves our admiration, because the doctor, by using prognosis, is assimilated to God to the greatest degree possible for man.

I 19 For he will be even more capable of saving those who can survive by taking precautions far in advance against each disorder

This statement, viz. taking precautions far in advance against each disorder, can be used to confirm Galen's explanation that by divine Hippocrates means here the predisposing causes or the state of the air surrounding us.

Prognosing who can survive: he means that the doctor who prognoses those diseases that are curable and takes precautions long beforehand against each disorder to save the patient is able to cure diseases easily; for example, the doctor can prognose and predict from winter the diseases that will develop in the summer; and he is able far ahead of time, when they, I mean the diseases, can still be survived, to take measures against and cure such diseases; in this way (the patient) is freed from danger.

V

I 20 In acute diseases the doctor must investigate as follows: first (he should examine) the patient's face

Ἰστέον ὅτι ἡ σημείωσις τριττή ἐστιν, ἐπιστημονική, τεχνική, ἰδιωτική. κέχρηται δὲ τῇ τεχνικῇ σημειώσει. καὶ σημειοῦται οὐκ ἀπὸ τοῦ γένους· οὔτε γὰρ περὶ ὀργανικῶν διαλέγεται οὔτε περὶ ὁμοιομερῶν· ἀλλ' οὐδὲ ἀπὸ τοῦ εἴδους, εἴτε καῦσος εἶεν εἴτε σύνοχος καὶ τὰ τοιαῦτα· ἀλλὰ σημειοῦται, εἴτε σωτήριόν ἐστι τὸ νόσημα εἴτε ὀλέθριον, τουτέστιν ἀπὸ τοῦ ἤθους, ὅπερ ἀπὸ τῶν ἑπομένων καὶ ἐπιγενομένων συμπτωμάτων χαρακτηρίζεται.

Σημειοῦται δὲ τὸ ὀξὺ νόσημα ἀπὸ τοῦ προσώπου διὰ τὸ φανερὸν καὶ
79 ἑτοίμως αὐτὸ ὁρᾶσθαι ὑπὸ τοῦ ἰατροῦ. καὶ λέγει | πρῶτον μὲν τὸ πρόσωπον τοῦ νοσέοντος, εἰ ὅμοιόν ἐστι τοῖσι τῶν ὑγιαινόντων, μάλιστα δὲ εἰ αὐτὸ ἑαυτῷ, τουτέστιν ὅτι δεῖ ἀντεξετάζειν τὸ πρόσωπον τοῦ νοσοῦντος, εἰ ὅμοιόν ἐστι τοῖσι τῶν ὑγιαινόντων ἢ ἀνόμοιον, μάλιστα δὲ τὴν παραβολὴν ποιεῖσθαι, εἰ αὐτὸ πρὸς ἑαυτό ἐστιν ὅμοιον ἢ ἀνόμοιον. καὶ αὕτη μᾶλλον ἡ ἀρίστη σημείωσις. πολλοὶ γὰρ ἐν τῷ κατὰ φύσιν ἔχουσιν ἰσχνὸν τὸ πρόσωπον ἢ μολιβδῶδες ἢ ἰκτερῶδες ἢ ὠχρόν, καὶ ἐὰν πρὸς τοὺς ὑγιαίνοντας ποιήσῃς τὴν παραβολήν, εἰς πολλοὺς παραλογισμοὺς ἐμπέσεις. καὶ τοῦ μὲν ὁμοίου καὶ κατὰ φύσιν ὁ συγγραφεὺς οὐκ εἶπε διαφοράν, ἀλλ' εἴασεν αὐτὸ οὕτως ἀδιαίρετον. τὸ δὲ ἀνόμοιον διαιρεῖ καὶ λέγει αὐτοῦ διαφοράς· φησὶ γὰρ ὅτι τὸ ἀνόμοιον ἢ πλεῖστον ἀφέστηκε τοῦ κατὰ φύσιν καὶ ἐν ἀκροτάτῳ τοῦ παρὰ φύσιν γέγονεν, ὅπερ κινδυνότατόν ἐστιν, ἢ μέσως πως ἀφέστηκεν. καὶ τοῦτο πάλιν πολλὰς ἔχει διαφορὰς παρὰ τὸ μᾶλλόν τε καὶ ἧττον· ἢ γὰρ τῷ κατὰ φύσιν πλησιάζει ἢ τῷ πάντῃ ἀφεστηκὸς ἀνομοίῳ. καὶ ἐφ' ὅσον μὲν τῷ κατὰ φύσιν πλησιάζει, ἧττόν ἐστι κινδυνῶδες, ἐφ' ὅσον δὲ τῷ παρὰ φύσιν, κινδυνῶδές ἐστιν.

Ἔστι δὲ καὶ ἄλλην αἰτίαν θαυμαστοτάτην ἀποδοῦναι. διὰ τοῦτο τὴν σημείωσιν ἀπὸ τοῦ προσώπου ποιεῖται, τὸ πρόσωπον ἐξ ἀνομοιομεροῦς οὐσίας σύγκειται· τὸ γὰρ πλεῖστον μέρος αὐτοῦ ὀστῶδές ἐστι, τὸ δὲ λοιπὸν σάρκες καὶ ὑγρὰ καὶ πνεύματα ἀναπληροῦσιν. ἐπειδὴ οὖν τὰ ὀξέα νοσήματα συντηκτικὰ καὶ δαπανητικά εἰσι τῶν σαρκῶν καὶ ὑγρῶν καὶ πνευμάτων, τὰ δ' ὀστᾶ δυσπαθῆ ὄντα τῇ δαπάνῃ τῶν σαρκῶν καὶ τῶν ὑγρῶν καὶ πνευμάτων, μένει ἡ ὀστώδης φύσις ὡς δυσπαθής. καὶ δυνατόν ἐστιν ἐκ τούτου ἐπιστῆναι τῇ σημειώσει ὅτι ὀλέθριόν ἐστι τὸ νόσημα.

Οὕτως ἡ τῶν ῥηΐστων σημείωσις ἀπὸ τοῦ προσώπου ὑφέστηκεν. ἀλλὰ καὶ ἡ τῶν μεγίστων σημείωσις ἐν τῷ προσώπῳ συνίσταται. μέγιστα δὲ σημεῖά ἐστιν ὅτι τὰς τρεῖς ἀρχὰς σημαίνει τὸ πρόσωπον τὸ πῶς διάκεινται,
80 ἐγκέφαλον λέγω καὶ καρδίαν καὶ ἧπαρ. καὶ αὕτη λέγεται | μεγίστη σημείωσις. καὶ τὸν μὲν ἐγκέφαλον δηλοῖ τὸ πρόσωπον τὸ πῶς διάκειται ἀπὸ τῶν αἰσθήσεων· αἱ γὰρ αἰσθήσεις ὡς δορυφόροι τινὲς κάθηνται περὶ τὸ πρόσω-

1] *cf.* [Gal.] De aff. ren. ins. dign. et cur. 3: XIX p. 653 K. 16–23] *cf.* Gal. In Hipp. Progn. comm. I 5: CMG V 9,2 p. 210,16–25 32–68,19] *cf.* Schol. R *in* Gal. In Hipp. Progn. comm. I 5: CMG V 9,2 p. 209 *ad* lin. 15 32 Οὕτως – 33] *cf.* Gal. In Hipp. Progn. comm. I 5: CMG V 9,2 p. 210,1

1 ἰδιωτική] ἰατρική L, *sed cf. [Gal.] XIX 653,7 K.* 4 εἶεν] *sic codd.* 6 ἐπιγινομένων MZ 8 αὐτῷ L 10 ἑαυτῷ] ἑαυτό γ 11 τοῖς γ 16 ἐμπέσῃς P: *ambig.* ζ 17 αὐτῷ γ 19 τοῦ] τοῦτο L 20 ἔχει πολλὰς γ 21 τῷ[I]] τὸ *codd. (et ubique linn. 21–23)*: *corr. Dietz* 29 καὶ[I] *om.* LM συμπαθῆ γ 33 δὲ *om.* L

It should be noted that there are three kinds of symptom interpretation, scientific, technical and specific. (Hippocrates) uses the technical (here). For he bases it neither on genus, since he does not discuss either organic diseases or those of homogeneous parts; nor on species, (not being concerned with) whether the fever be a causus or an unremittent or the like; rather, he interprets whether the disease will prove curable or fatal; that is, his basis is the character of the disease, and this is shaped by the symptoms which follow and develop (after it has struck).

He interprets acute disease from the face, because it is clearly and easily seen by the doctor. He says, first the patient's face, if it is like those of healthy people and above all if it is like its usual self, this means that we must examine the patient's face by comparison to see if it resembles those of the healthy or not; but above all we must compare to see if it is like itself or not. And this is by far the best kind of interpretation. For there are many whose faces are naturally lean or whose normal complexions are like lead or jaundiced or pale; so if you make the comparison with the healthy, you will draw many false conclusions. Now within the class of the like or normal face our author does not distinguish differences but leaves it as it is, undivided. The unlike, on the other hand, he divides into different degrees; he tells us that it either diverges from the normal to the greatest extent and is extremely abnormal, which is very dangerous, or it is moderately distant from it. This again admits of many degrees more or less; for either it approaches the normal or it is separated from it by total dissimilarity. The closer it comes to normal the less dangerous it is, while the nearer it approaches the abnormal it is (that much more) serious.

One can give another and very admirable explanation. Interpretation is made from the face because the face is composed of matter which is not homogeneous; for the greater part of it consists of bone, while the rest is filled out by flesh, fluids and pneumas. And since acute diseases dissolve and consume flesh, fluids and pneumas, but bones are not affected by the destruction of flesh, fluids and pneumas, the bones remain intact. It is possible, then, on the basis of the face to establish the interpretation that the disease is fatal.

Thus interpretation of the simplest symptoms is made from the face. But the face provides also the most important signs. They are the most important, because the face tells us the condition of the body's three principal parts, namely the brain, the heart and the liver. This is called the most important interpretation. As regards the brain, the face reveals its condition through the senses; for the senses, like bodyguards

πον ὡς βασιλέα δορυφοροῦσαι τὸν ἐγκέφαλον, καὶ εὖ ἐνεργουσῶν τῶν αἰσθήσεων δηλοῦσι τὸν ἐγκέφαλον καλῶς διακεῖσθαι· εἰ δὲ βεβλαμμένως ἐνεργοῦσι, δηλοῦσι κακῶς διακεῖσθαι. ἀλλὰ καὶ τὴν καρδίαν σημειούμεθα ἀπὸ τοῦ προσώπου· εἰ μὲν γὰρ εὔχρουν ἐστὶ τὸ πρόσωπον, δηλοῖ τὴν καρδίαν καλῶς διακεῖσθαι, ἐπειδὴ ἡ εὐχροια ἀπὸ τοῦ ἐμφύτου θερμοῦ γίνεται ἀπὸ τῆς καρδίας καὶ διὰ τῶν ἀρτηριῶν ἐπινάεται τὸ πρόσωπον καὶ γίνεται εὔχρουν. εἰ δὲ κακόχρουν ἐστὶ τὸ πρόσωπον, δηλοῖ τὴν καρδίαν κακῶς διακειμένην· ἡ γὰρ κακόχροια γίνεται ἢ κακοχυμίας τινὸς πλεοναζούσης ἐν τῇ καρδίᾳ ἢ φερομένης ἀπό τινος μορίου, καὶ τὸ τηνικαῦτα μολύνεται τὸ ἔμφυτον θερμὸν καὶ ὁ ζωτικὸς τόνος, καὶ ἐντεῦθεν κακόχρουν γίνεται τὸ πρόσωπον, ἢ δι' ἀσθένειαν ἐνδεὴς γίνεται ἡ τοῦ ἐμφύτου θερμοῦ ἀνάδοσις, καὶ διὰ τοῦτο κακόχρουν γίνεται τὸ πρόσωπον. ἀλλὰ καὶ τὸ ἧπαρ σημαίνει εἴτε καλῶς διάκειται εἴτε κακῶς· εἰ μὲν γὰρ εὔτροφόν ἐστι τὸ πρόσωπον, δηλοῖ ὅτι καλῶς διάκειται τὸ ἧπαρ καὶ ἀμέμπτως ἐνεργεῖ. εἰ δὲ ἰσχνόν ἐστι τὸ πρόσωπον, δηλοῖ κακῶς διακεῖσθαι τὸ ἧπαρ· ἢ γὰρ κακοχυμία τις πλεονάζει ἐν τῷ ἥπατι καὶ συναναδίδοται τῷ λόγῳ τροφῆς ἐν τῷ προσώπῳ φερομένῳ, καὶ διὰ τὸ κακόχυμον αὐτὸ εἶναι καὶ ἀκάθαρτον οὐ τρέφεται, ἀλλ' ἰσχναίνεται, ἢ ἐνδεὴς γίνεται ἡ ἀνάδοσις διά τινα ἀσθένειαν, καὶ τὸ τηνικαῦτα ἰσχναίνεται τὸ πρόσωπον.

Ἀλλὰ καὶ εὐσχημός ἐστιν ἡ ἀπὸ τοῦ προσώπου σημείωσις· οὐδὲ γὰρ δεῖται ἀνακαλύψεως τὸ πρόσωπον, ὡς εἰώθαμεν ἀνακαλύπτειν ἐπὶ τῶν σπλάγχνων κακῶς διακειμένου στομάχου ἢ γαστρὸς ἢ ἥπατος ἢ σπληνὸς καὶ τῶν τοιούτων· ἐπὶ τούτων γὰρ ἀνακαλύπτομεν. ἐπὶ δὲ τῇ σημειώσει τοῦ προσώπου οὐκ ἀνακαλύπτομεν· αὐτόθεν γὰρ γυμνὸν ὑποπίπτει. καὶ εὐσχημός ἐστιν ἡ τοιαύτη σημείωσις μάλιστα ἐπὶ τῶν παρθενευουσῶν ἢ
81 τῶν | ὁπωσοῦν κόσμιον καὶ σεμνὸν βίον διαγόντων γυναικῶν. ⟨ἀλλὰ καὶ⟩ εὐσχημός ἐστιν ἡ ἀπὸ τοῦ προσώπου σημείωσις διὰ τὸ πάντα ⟨τὰ⟩ ὁπωσοῦν νενομοθετημένα σημεῖα ἐν τῷ Κατ' ἰητρεῖον συγγράμματι ἐν τῷ προσώπῳ συνίστασθαι.

I 21 [2: 194,13 A. = II 114,2 L.] Ῥὶς ὀξεῖα, ὀφθαλμοὶ κοῖλοι, κρόταφοι συμπεπτωκότες, ὦτα ψυχρὰ καὶ συνεσταλμένα καὶ οἱ λοβοὶ τῶν ὤτων ἀπεστραμμένοι

Ὅτι κακά εἰσι καὶ ὀλέθρια τὰ ἓξ ταῦτα συμπτώματα καὶ χαρακτηριστικὰ νεκρώδους προσώπου, πιστοῦται ὁ Γαληνὸς διά τε τοῦ ἐπιλογισμοῦ καὶ τοῦ ἀναλογισμοῦ, τουτέστιν ἀπὸ τῆς πείρας καὶ ἀπὸ τοῦ λόγου. καὶ ἀπὸ μὲν τῆς πείρας οὕτως, ὅτι ἐφ' ὧν νοσημάτων συνέβη ταῦτα, ἔφησεν ὅτι

28 ἐν – ἰητρεῖον] Hipp. De off. med. 1: II p. 30,2–7 Kw. = III p. 272,1–5 L. *cf.* Gal. In Hipp. Progn. comm. I 5: CMG V 9,2 pp. 209,17–210,15 34 ὁ Γαληνὸς] Gal. In Hipp. Progn. comm. I 6: CMG V 9,2 p. 211,11–17

1 *post* βασιλέα *add.* καὶ L 4 γὰρ *om.* L 6 καὶ^{I} *om.* L ἐπινεύεται P*(-ευ- ex -α-, ut vid., mut.)* ζ 16 τῷ^{II}] τὸ Μζ 17 φερόμενον *codd.*: *correxi* 19 τὸ *om.* L 25 εὔχυμος L 26 διαγόντων] *sic codd.; cf. infra, p. 284,10* ἀλλὰ καὶ *add. Wk.* 27 εὔχημος, *ut vid.*, L: εὔσημός *coni. Wk.* τὸ *om.* L τὰ *add. Wk.* 28 κατιητρίω *codd.*: *corr. Dietz* 33 τὰ] τάδε L 35 ἀπὸ^{II} *om.* γ

are placed about the face watching over the brain like over an emperor; when the senses are working well they show that the brain is in good condition; if their functions are impaired, it means that the brain is out of order. The state of the heart also we interpret from facial symptoms; if the complexion is good, it shows that the heart is functioning well; for the healthy color develops when the innate heat, which originates in the heart, travels through the arteries and the face receives an influx and becomes healthy looking. But if the face has a bad complexion it indicates a malfunctioning heart; for the color turns bad either because an excess of bad humor develops in the heart or comes (to it) from some other part, and this corrupts the innate heat and vital tone, leaving the face's color bad; or, the complexion becomes bad due to deficient distribution of innate heat caused by weakness. In the case of the liver, too, (the face) reveals whether it is in a good or bad state; if the face looks well-nourished, it means that the liver is in fine condition and is functioning perfectly. A lean face, on the other hand, indicates trouble in the liver; for either the organ contains an excess of bad humor which is distributed with the matter conveyed to the face in the form of nutriment; whereupon the face, because polluted by the bad humor, is not nourished but becomes emaciated; or, distribution becomes defective because of some weakness and then the face becomes emaciated.

Interpretation made from the face is dignified as well, since the face does not need to be uncovered, as we are wont to do in the case of the inner parts, when there is a disorder in the orifice (of the stomach) or stomach or liver or spleen or the like; for in these cases we uncover. But for interpretation of the face we do not uncover, since it is naturally exposed. And this type of symptom interpretation is particularly becoming when dealing with nuns or women who lead any kind of disciplined and chaste lives. And interpretation from the face is also dignified because all the symptoms laid down by the work In the Surgery are found in the face.

I 21 Sharp nose, sunken eyes, collapsed temples, cold and contracted ears and turned-back lobes

That these six symptoms are dangerous, fatal and characteristic of the mortified face is confirmed by Galen both empirically and logically, that is, by experience and reasoning. By experience, in this way: he says that whenever those symptoms appear in a disease it always

ὀλέθριόν ἐστι τὸ νόσημα ἐκεῖνο. ἀπὸ δὲ τοῦ λόγου, ὅτι ἐν τῷ καθόλου κατὰ δύο αἰτίας γίνεται τὸ τοιοῦτον πάθος ἐν τῷ προσώπῳ· ἢ γὰρ διὰ δριμύτητα ὕλης φερομένης καὶ δαπανώσης καὶ διαφθειρούσης τὰ εὐπαθῆ, ἅπερ ἐστὶ σάρκες καὶ ὑγρὰ καὶ πνεύματα, ὡς ἐν τῇ θεωρίᾳ εἰρήκαμεν, καὶ οὕτως γίνεται τὸ πάθος τοῦτο. ἢ δι' ἀσθένειαν τοῦ ἐμφύτου θερμοῦ τοῦτο γίνεται· ἀσθενοῦντος γὰρ τοῦ ἐμφύτου θερμοῦ οὐ δύναται ἐπεκτανθῆναι ἐπὶ τὰ πόρρω καὶ ἄκρα μόρια, ἀλλ' ἐμφωλεύει περὶ τὰ σπλάγχνα καὶ ἐκεῖσε ἐνειλίσσεται, καὶ τὸ τηνικαῦτα λειφαιμοῦντα καὶ ἀμοιροῦντα τοῦ ἐμφύτου θερμοῦ καὶ ζωτικοῦ τόνου ψύχονται τὰ ἄκρα καὶ ἀπομαραίνονται καὶ οὕτως ἀπονεκροῦνται. καὶ γὰρ τὸ πρόσωπον ἄκρον ἐστὶ μόριον, ἀλλὰ καὶ ἄσκεπον ἀείσε ἐστί. διὰ τοῦτο καὶ ἡ παραλλαγὴ τοῦ κατὰ φύσιν τῷ προσώπῳ μάλιστα γίνεται. ἐντεῦθεν καὶ τὰ ἓξ ἐκεῖνα συμπτώματα ἐν τῷ προσώπῳ συνίστανται διὰ τὰς αὐτὰς δύο αἰτίας.

Καὶ τέως, ῥὶς ὀξεῖα· ἡ ῥὶς ὀξεῖα γίνεται τρόπῳ τοιούτῳ· ἡ ῥὶς 82 ὀστοῦν χονδρῶδές ἐστι· τὸ μὲν ἐντὸς ὀστῶδές ἐστι, τὸ δὲ ἔμπρο|σθεν χόνδρος· μόνα δὲ τὰ πτερύγια σαρκώδη εἰσὶ καὶ ὑγρά· ταῦτα οὖν τὰ πτερύγια ὡς ὑγρὰ ὄντα καὶ εὐπαθῆ συμβαίνει διὰ μίαν τῶν αἰτιῶν δαπανᾶσθαι καὶ φθείρεσθαι. ἢ γὰρ διὰ δριμύτητα τῆς ὕλης δαπανῶνται καὶ ἐξαναλίσκονται, ἢ δι' ἀσθένειαν τοῦ ἐμφύτου θερμοῦ τῆς ψύξεως τὸ τηνικαῦτα πιλούσης καὶ ἐκπυρηνιζούσης καὶ δι' ἀτροφίαν φθείρει τὰ πτερύγια. τούτων δὲ μειουμένων καὶ τῶν παρ' ἑκάτερα μερῶν δαπανωμένων ἐξ ἀνάγκης ὀξεῖα γίνεται ἡ ῥίς. καὶ ἐπὶ σιμῆς δὲ ῥινὸς τὸ ἀνάλογον γίνεται, καὶ ὀξύνεται καὶ ἡ σιμὴ ῥίς. ἀλλὰ καὶ ἡ γρυπὴ καὶ ἡ ὁπωσοῦν ῥὶς ὀξύνεται, καὶ δεῖ αὐτὴν πρὸς ἑαυτὴν τὴν ῥῖνα ἀντεξετάζειν.

᾿Οφθαλμοὶ κοῖλοι· καὶ οἱ ὀφθαλμοὶ κοῖλοι γίνονται διὰ μίαν τῶν αἰτιῶν· ἢ γὰρ διὰ κακοχυμίαν καὶ δριμεῖαν ὕλην ἐξαναλίσκουσαν καὶ ἐκδαπανῶσαν τὰ ἐν τοῖς ὀφθαλμοῖς, λοιπὸν δὲ καὶ τὰ πνεύματα· πλείστη γὰρ μοῖρα πνεύματος ὀπτικοῦ πέμπεται εἰς τοὺς ὀφθαλμούς· τούτων δὲ δαπανωμένων ὡς εὐπαθῶν ἐξ ἀνάγκης οἱ ὀφθαλμοὶ κοῖλοι γίνονται. διὰ δὲ ἄκραν ψῦξιν κοῖλοι γίνονται οἱ ὀφθαλμοί, ἐπειδὴ ἡ ἄκρα ψῦξις πύκνωσιν καὶ πίλησιν καὶ συνίζησιν καὶ ἐκπυρηνισμὸν ἀπεργάζεται· λοιπὸν καὶ ἀτροφία ἐν αὐτοῖς γίνεται, καὶ τῷ λόγῳ τούτῳ ἐξ ἀνάγκης κοῖλοι γίνονται οἱ ὀφθαλμοί.

Κρόταφοι ξυμπεπτωκότες· πρὸ πάντων τῶν ἐν τῇ κεφαλῇ μορίων οἱ κροταφῖται μύες δαπανῶνται διὰ τὰς αὐτὰς αἰτίας· ἢ γὰρ τῇ δριμύτητι τῆς ὕλης δαπανώμενοι συμπίπτουσιν οἱ κρόταφοι ἢ διὰ τὴν ἄκραν ψῦξιν.

1–13] *cf.* Gal. In Hipp. Progn. comm. I 7: CMG V 9,2 p. 212,7–19 4 ἐν τῇ θεωρίᾳ] *v. supra*, p. 66,28–30 14–24] *cf.* Gal. In Hipp. Progn. comm. I 7: CMG V 9,2 p. 212,19–25 25–33] *cf.* Gal. In Hipp. Progn. comm. I 7: CMG V 9,2 p. 212,27–30 34 sq.] *cf.* Gal. In Hipp. Progn. comm. I 7: CMG V 9,2 p. 213,1sq.

1 ἐστι *om.* γ 8 λειφαιμοῦνται γ ἀμοιροῦνται γ: ἀλροῦντα L: *corr. Dietz* 14 Καὶ τέως *om.* γ 15 ἐστι^{II} *om.* γ 20 ἐμπυρηνιζούσης γ 21 καὶ — δαπανωμένων *om.* L 29 *post* γίνονται *add.* διὰ μίαν τῶν αἰτιῶν γ 30sq. πύκνωσις καὶ πίλησις γ 31 συνίζησις V: συνίζησι MP 34 *post* μορίων *add.* μόνοι L

proves fatal. By reasoning: in general the condition develops in the face for two reasons; either from the acridness of matter borne (there) which consumes and destroys the easily affected parts, namely, as we have said in the general discussion, flesh, fluids and pneumas, and the condition arises in this way. Or it arises from weakness of the innate heat; for in this state the heat cannot reach the distant parts at the extremities, but lurks in and wraps itself around the viscera; whereupon the extremities, deprived of blood, innate heat and vital tone, grow cold, wither and thus mortify. The fact is that the face is an extremity and it is always exposed. This explains why it in particular is the scene of abnormal change. Then those six symptoms, too, appear in the face for the same two reasons.

First, sharp nose: The nose becomes sharp in this way; the nose is composed of bone and cartilage, bone on the inside, cartilage in front and only the alae are fleshy and moist; the alae, then, being moist and easily affected are consumed and perish for one of the (two) reasons. They either are consumed and waste away because of the acridness of the matter; or, due to weakness of the innate heat they are compressed and squeezed out by the cold and perish from lack of nourishment. When these parts diminish and both sides are consumed, the nose necessarily sharpens. Even the snub nose is subject to the same kind of change and becomes pointed. The aquiline, too, and any other type of nose sharpens, and the nose should be compared to its normal self.

Sunken eyes: The eyes, too, sink for one of the (two) reasons; either because of unwholesome humor and acrid matter which destroys and consumes the substance of the eyes, including the pneumas; for a very great quantity of optic pneuma is sent to the eyes; and when these substances, being vulnerable, are destroyed, the eyes of necessity become sunken. Again, the eyes become sunken due to extreme cold, since extreme cold condenses, compresses, squeezes and forces out (the substance); then atrophy develops in them, and for this reason the eyes of necessity become sunken.

Collapsed temples: More than any of the parts of the head the temporal muscles are consumed by these same causes; the temples collapse either because they have been corroded by the acridness of the matter or because of extreme cold.

῏Ωτα ψυχρὰ καὶ συνεσταλμένα· τὰ ὦτα ἐπειδὴ χονδρώδη εἰσί, φύσει ψυχρά εἰσι. καὶ εἰκότως ὑπὸ τῆς ἄκρας ψύξεως ψυχρὰ γίνονται. ἀλλὰ καὶ διὰ τοῦτο συνεσταλμένα γίνονται, διὰ τὴν ψῦξιν· ἡ γὰρ ἄκρα ψῦξις συν⟨αι⟩ρεῖ αὐτὰ καὶ οἷον συσπᾷ αὐτά, καὶ γίνονται συνεσταλμένα. |

83 Καὶ οἱ λοβοὶ τῶν ὤτων ἀπεστραμμένοι· εἰκότως, ἐπειδὴ παρὰ πάντα τὰ μόρια τῶν ὤτων σαρκωδέστεροι καὶ ὑγρότεροι οἱ λοβοί εἰσι· δαπανώμενοι οὖν καὶ ἰσχναινόμενοι ἀποστρέφονται ἐπὶ τὰ ὀπίσω. καὶ διὰ ποίαν αἰτίαν ἐπὶ τὰ ὀπίσω ἀποστρέφονται οἱ λοβοὶ καὶ μὴ πρὸς τὰ ἔμπροσθεν μέρη; καὶ λέγομεν ὅτι διὰ τοῦτο, ἐπὶ τὰ ὀπίσω ἀποστρέφονται ὡς ἐπὶ τὴν οἰκείαν ἀρχήν, ἐπειδὴ ἀπὸ τῶν ὀπίσω δέχονται τὰ ὦτα αἰσθητικὰ νεῦρα. τῇ οὖν ἄκρᾳ ψύξει σπώμενα τὰ αἰσθητικὰ νεῦρα πρὸς ἑαυτὰ ἐφέλκονται τοὺς λοβοὺς τῶν ὤτων· καὶ διὰ τοῦτο ἐπὶ τὰ ὀπίσω ἀποστρέφονται.

Ἐντεῦθεν καὶ ἡ δόξα ἐκείνη ἐκβάλλεται τῶν ὁρισαμένων τὸν σπασμὸν κίνησιν ἀπροαίρετον ἐν κινητικοῖς μορίοις συνισταμένην, οὐ μὴν ἐν τοῖς αἰσθητικοῖς καὶ ἀκινήτοις. ἰδοὺ γὰρ ἀποδέδεικται ἐνταῦθα ὅτι οὐ μόνον ἐν τοῖς κινητικοῖς μορίοις συνίσταται ὁ σπασμός, ἀλλὰ καὶ ἐν τοῖς αἰσθητικοῖς ἤτοι τοῖς ἀκινήτοις νεύροις. καλῶς δὲ λοιπὸν ὡρίσαντο οἱ εἰπόντες τὸν σπασμὸν κίνησιν ἀπροαίρετον ἐν προαιρετικοῖς μορίοις συνισταμένην· ἀμφότερα γὰρ περιλαμβάνει ὁ ὁρισμὸς οὗτος. καὶ οἱ λοβοὶ τῶν ὤτων ἀπεστραμμένοι.

I 22 [2: 194,15 A. = II 114,4 L.] Καὶ τὸ δέρμα τὸ περὶ τὸ μέτωπον σκληρόν τε καὶ περιτεταμένον καὶ καρφαλέον ἐόν

Εἰκότως τοῦτο γενήσεται, ἐπειδὴ σχεδὸν ἄσαρκόν ἐστι τὸ μέτωπον ὀστῶδες τυγχάνον, εἰ μή τι δ' ἂν ἐλαχίστη μοῖρα ἀπὸ τοῦ μυώδους πλατύσματος φέρεται παρὰ τὸ μέτωπον καὶ κινεῖ αὐτό. καὶ διὰ μίαν τῶν εἰρημένων αἰτιῶν συμβαίνει καὶ τοῦτο δαπανᾶσθαι καὶ φθείρεσθαι καὶ σκληρὸν γίνεσθαι καὶ περιτεταμένον καὶ καρφαλέον τὸ δέρμα τοῦ μετώπου. ταῦτα γὰρ πάντα ἐπιτεταμένην ξηρότητα δηλοῦσιν.

I 23 [2: 195,1 A. = II 114,5 L.] Καὶ τὸ χρῶμα τοῦ ξύμπαντος προσώπου χλωρόν τε ἢ πελιὸν ἢ καὶ μέλαν ἐόν

Ταῦτα πάντα τὰ χρώματα ὑπὸ ψύξεως γίνονται. καὶ τὸ μὲν μέλαν κατὰ
84 ἐπίτασιν γίνεται ψύξεως· οὕτως | γὰρ καὶ τὸ αἷμα ἐν ταῖς φλεβοτομίαις ἢ ὁπωσοῦν κενούμενον θρομβοῦται, εἶτα πήγνυται, καὶ οὕτως τῷ χρόνῳ μελαίνεται. τὸ δὲ χλωρόν τινες καὶ τὸ ὠχρὸν ταὐτὸν ἐνόμισαν εἶναι· διαφέρουσι δὲ ἀλλήλων ταῦτα. πρῶτον μὲν γὰρ τὸ ὠχρὸν γίνεται χρῶμα ὑπὸ τῆς

1–2 γίνονται] *cf.* Gal. In Hipp. Progn. comm. I 7: CMG V 9,2 p. 213,4sq. 9–20] *cf.* Gal. In Hipp. Progn. comm. I 7: CMG V 9,2 p. 213,10–17 24sq.] *cf.* Gal. In Hipp. Progn. comm. I 7: CMG V 9,2 p. 213,20sq. 32–74,4] *cf.* Gal. In Hipp. Progn. comm. I 7: CMG V 9,2 p. 213,23–30

4 συνρεῖ *codd.*: *corr. Wk.* καὶ[I] – αὐτά *om.* γ 5 παρὰ] περὶ ζ: *om.* P 8 τὰ[II] *om.* L 10 *post* ὦτα *fort. excidit* τὰ 11 τῇ – νεῦρα *om.* γ 19 οὕτω γ 24 μή τι δ' ἂν] μὴ *coni. Dietz* 29 Καὶ *om.* γ 30 χλωρόν – ἐόν] *sic nullus test. Hipp.* 31 *post* Ταῦτα *add.* γὰρ γ 35 γὰρ *om.* γ

Cold and contracted ears: The ears being composed of cartilage are cold by nature. So it is no wonder that they become so when subjected to extreme cold. Contraction also has the same cause, namely the cold; for extreme cold shortens and, as it were, draws them together and they become contracted.

And turned-back lobes: This is not surprising since, compared to all the other parts of the ears, the lobes contain more flesh and fluid; so when they are consumed and become emaciated, they turn backwards. But why are the lobes turned towards the back and not towards the front parts? We say that it is for this reason: they turn back to their own source, since the ears receive the sensory nerves from behind. When the sensory nerves, then, are contracted by extreme cold, they draw the lobes towards themselves; and this explains why they are turned backwards.

On this basis also we are able to refute the opinion of those who define spasm as an involuntary movement in the motor parts, but not in the sensory or immobile parts. For, here we have proof that the spasm occurs not only in the motor parts, but also in the sensory or immobile nerves. Hence those who have characterized the spasm as an involuntary movement in the voluntary parts have produced a good definition; for it includes both (the motor and the sensory). (So much for) and turned-back lobes.

I 22 And the skin around the forehead hard, taut and dry

This is only to be expected; for the forehead has practically no flesh, being (all) bone except for the very small piece of the broad muscle which stretches along the brow and moves it. This part, too, is liable to consumption and destruction by one of the (two) causes which have been mentioned, and the skin becomes hard, taut and dry. For all these conditions point to intense dryness.

I 23 And the color of the whole face yellow or livid or black

All these colors result from cold. Black for its part is produced by extreme cold; thus we see blood shed by venesection or in any other way (first) clotting, then hardening and eventually turning black. Some have considered yellow and pale to be the same; but there is a difference. For pale is the first color to be produced by cold, next livid

ψύξεως, εἶτα τὸ πελιδνόν, καὶ εἶθ' οὕτως τὸ μέλαν. καὶ τὸ μὲν ὠχρὸν χρῶμα τοῦ προσώπου ὑπὸ τῆς ἀρχῆς τῆς ψύξεως γίνεται· τὸ δὲ χλωρὸν ἔτι ἐπιτεινομένης τῆς ψύξεως· τὸ δὲ πελιδνὸν ἔτι πλεῖον ἐπιτεινομένης· τὸ δὲ μέλαν ἐπὶ μεγίστῃ καὶ ἀκροτάτῃ ψύξει γίνεται, ὅπερ νέκρωσίς ἐστιν.

Οὕτως οὖν τὴν αἰτίαν ἑκάστου συμπτώματος ἀποδέδωκεν ὁ Γαληνός. πλὴν δεῖ εἰδέναι οὐ πάντοτε ταῦτα τὰ συμπτώματα θανατώδη εἰσίν. ἐὰν γὰρ ἐπὶ χρονίῳ νοσήματι γίνωνται, τῷ μήκει καὶ τῇ ἐκτάσει τοῦ χρόνου ἐκτήκονται, καὶ οὐ πάντως θάνατος ἐπακολουθεῖ· ἀλλ' ὑγιαίνουσιν οἱ οὕτως πάσχοντες καὶ ἐξειλοῦσι τοῦ κινδύνου διά τε ἡλικίαν ἀκμαστικοῦ ὄντος τοῦ νοσοῦντος καὶ κρᾶσιν θερμὴν καὶ ὥραν θερινὴν καὶ τὰ τοιαῦτα. ἐὰν οὖν συνέλθωσιν, ἐκφεύγει τὸν κίνδυνον. ἀλλ' ἐπὶ τῶν ὀξέων νοσημάτων ταῦτα γινόμενα ὀλέθριά εἰσι, καὶ μάλιστα ἐὰν ἐν τῇ ἀρχῇ τῆς νόσου γένωνται, πλὴν εἰ μή τι δι' ἑτέραν αἰτίαν ἐγγίνονται, καὶ τότε οὔκ εἰσι θανατώδη. ποία δέ ἐστιν ἡ αἰτία ἐκείνη, ἡ ἐφεξῆς θεωρία δηλώσει.

VI

I 24 [2: 195,2 A. = II 114,6 L.] Εἰ μὲν οὖν ἐν ἀρχῇ τῆς νόσου τὸ πρόσωπον χλωρὸν ᾖ καὶ μέλαν ἐὸν καὶ μήπω οἷόν τε

Φησὶν ὅτι, ἐὰν ἐν ἀρχῇ τοῦ νοσήματος τὸ νεκρῶδες γένηται πρόσωπον, γίνωσκε ὅτι διὰ κακοήθειαν ὀξέου νοσήματος ἐγένετο ἢ διά τινα προκαταρκτικὴν αἰτίαν. καὶ διὰ μὲν κακοήθειαν νοσήματος οὕτως· ἵνα ὑποστῇ ἡ κακοήθεια τοῦ νοσήματος, τριῶν δεῖται συνδρομῆς, ἵνα ἡ καθεκτικὴ δύναμις τοῦ παντὸς σώματος ἀσθενὴς ᾖ καὶ ἵνα λεπτοί εἰσιν οἱ χυμοὶ καὶ πυρετὸς διακαὴς καὶ ζέων. τί γάρ; ὅτι τῆς καθεκτικῆς δυνάμεως ἀσθενούσης πολλὴ
85 γίνεται διαφόρησις τῆς ἀδήλου διαπνοῆς ἀνεπαισθήτως, | καὶ μάλιστα λεπτῶν ὄντων τῶν χυμῶν πολλὴ γενήσεται ἡ διαφόρησις. λοιπὸν δὲ καὶ ὅτι συνεργεῖ τῇ διαφορήσει ὁ διακαὴς πυρετός. τούτων οὖν τῶν τριῶν συντρεχόντων ἰσχναίνεται τὸ σῶμα καὶ νεκρῶδες γίνεται τὸ πρόσωπον. καὶ ἀναλογεῖ αὕτη ἡ διαφόρησις, ἡ ἀενάως γινομένη καὶ ἀνεπαισθήτως, ταῖς μεγίσταις κινήσεσι ταῖς διὰ τῶν φυσικῶν ὑπονόμων γινομέναις, ἐκταράξει γαστρὸς ἢ ἐμέτῳ ἢ αἱμορραγίᾳ.

Διὰ δὲ χρόνιον νόσημα νεκρῶδες γίνεται πρόσωπον οὕτως· τῷ γὰρ μήκει τῆς νόσου διαφοροῦνται οἱ χυμοὶ καὶ τὰ ὑγρὰ καὶ τὰ πνεύματα· λοιπὸν δὲ καὶ αἱ δυνάμεις κακῶς διατίθενται. καὶ ἐνταῦθα ἀτροφοῦνται τὰ μόρια, ἰσχναίνεται τὸ σῶμα καὶ νεκρῶδες γίνεται τὸ πρόσωπον.

6–13] *cf.* Gal. In Hipp. Progn. comm. I 7: CMG V 9,2 p. 214,2–11 14 ἡ[II] – δηλώσει] *infra*, pp. 76,28–78,1, *ut vid.* 20–30] *cf.* Gal. In Hipp. Progn. comm. I 7: CMG V 9,2 p. 215,3–12

1 *post* ψύξεως *fort. exciderunt* εἶτα τὸ χλωρόν 2 τῆς[I] *om.* γ 7 ἐκστάσει γ 9 ἐξηλοῦσι *codd.*: *correxi* 9sq. τοῦ νοσοῦντος *om.* γ 11 συνέλθῃ γ 12 ἐν *om.* L τοῦ νοσήματος γ 16 οὖν *om.* γ 17 χλωρὸν – ἐὸν] τοιοῦτον ᾖ *Hipp.* (*cf. supra, p. 72,30; infra, p. 76,14*) 19 ἐγένετο *om.* γ ἢ διά τινα] ἅτινα L 26 συνερχόντων L; *sed cf. lin. 21* 28 αὐτ' L: αὐτῷ γ: *corr. Wk.* ἀννάως L 33 ἀτροφοῦντα L

and finally black. The face turns pale from beginning cold, yellow from intensified, livid from further intensified, and black from the most intense and extreme state of cold, which is mortification.

This is how Galen, then, explained the cause of each symptom. However, it should be realized that these symptoms are not always fatal. For if they develop in a chronic disease, they disappear with the long and extended period of time and death does not necessarily result; rather, those affected in this way recover their health and escape the danger, whether because of youth if the patient is in his prime, or from a warm temperament or summer weather and so on. If these factors prevail at the same time, (the patient) escapes the danger. In acute diseases, on the other hand, these symptoms are deadly, especially when they show up at the beginning of the disease, unless they occur for some other reason, and then they are not fatal. What this reason is, the next general discussion will show.

VI

I 24 If at the beginning of the disease the face is yellow or black and it is not yet possible

He is saying that if at the start of the disease the face takes on a deadly appearance, understand that it has been produced by malignancy of an acute disease or by some predisposing cause. By malignancy of a disease, as follows: in order to develop in a disease, malignancy requires the concurrence of three factors, namely a weak retentive faculty throughout the body, thin humors and a burning and seething fever. Why? Because when the retentive faculty is weak there occurs a great imperceptible dissipation of invisible transpiration, and the dissipation is great especially when the humors are thin. Burning fever also contributes to dissipation. When these three factors, then, coincide, the body wastes away and the face becomes mortified. And this constant imperceptible dissipation is analogous to the major movements which take place in the natural channels (of the body), namely bowel disturbance, vomiting and haemorrhage.

The face assumes the appearance of death from chronic illness in this way: the humors, fluids and pneumas are dissipated due to the length of the disease and, besides, the faculties are in poor condition. Hence the parts are left without nourishment, the body withers and the face becomes mortified.

Διὰ δὲ προκαταρκτικὴν αἰτίαν οὕτως, ἀλλὰ τοῦτο τριχῶς· ἢ γὰρ δι' ἀγρυπνίαν ἄμετρον ἢ διὰ πολλὴν ἐκτάραξιν τῆς γαστρὸς ἢ διὰ λιμὸν ἐπιτεταμένον· ἕκαστον γὰρ τούτων δύναται νεκρῶδες ποιῆσαι πρόσωπον. ἡ μὲν κένωσις τῆς γαστρὸς ἡ ἐπιτεταμένη δηλονότι ἰσχναίνει τὸ σῶμα καὶ νεκρῶδες ποιεῖ τὸ πρόσωπον. ἀλλὰ καὶ ἡ ἀγρυπνία ἡ ἐπιτεταμένη οἶδε διαφόρησιν ποιεῖν καὶ νεκρῶδες ἀπεργάζεσθαι τὸ πρόσωπον. καὶ ὁ λιμὸς οὖν, εἴτε ἑκούσιός ἐστιν εἴτε ἀκούσιος, τῷ λόγῳ τῆς ἐνδείας καὶ τῆς ἀσιτίας δύναται νεκρῶδες ποιῆσαι τὸ πρόσωπον. μνημονεύσας δὲ τὴν κένωσιν πᾶσαν κένωσιν ἀμέτρως γινομένην ἐδήλωσεν εἴτε δι' ἐμέτων εἴτε δι' αἱμορραγίας εἴτε δι' οὔρων εἴτε δι' ἱδρώτων. διὰ δὲ τοῦ μνημονεῦσαι ὕπνου πάντα τὰ ψυχικὰ πάθη τὰ δυνάμενα συγκοπὰς καὶ λιποθυμίας ποιῆσαι ἐδήλωσεν, ὥσπερ φροντὶς καὶ θυμὸς καὶ τὰ τοιαῦτα.

Τί οὖν φησιν ὁ Ἱπποκράτης; ἢν μὲν οὖν ἐν ἀρχῇ τῆς νόσου τὸ πρόσωπον χλωρὸν ἢ μέλαν ἐόν. ἰστέον ὅτι ἡ ἀρχὴ τριχῶς διαιρεῖται· ἢ γὰρ ἄχρονος καὶ ἀκαρής ἐστιν, ἥτις ἐν αὐτῷ τῷ ἄρχεσθαι ἀλλοιοῦσθαι ἐπὶ τὸ παρὰ φύσιν τὸν ἄνθρωπον περιγράφεται, ἥτις ἀχρόνως γίνεται. ἔστιν
86 ἀρχὴ καὶ ἡ ἐν πλάτει θεωρουμένη. αὕτη δὲ διχῶς | διαιρεῖται· ἢ γὰρ τεχνική ἐστιν ἢ ἁπλῶς πλατικὴ καὶ ἄτεχνος, ἥτις ἐν τρισὶν ἡμέραις θεωρεῖται. ἔγνωσται γὰρ καὶ αὕτη τοῖς ἰατροῖς, καὶ εἰώθασιν ἀρχὴν τὰς τρεῖς ἡμέρας καλεῖν ἐπὶ παντὸς νοσήματος. ἡ δὲ τεχνική ἐστιν ἥτις ἀντιδιαστέλλεται τοῖς λοιποῖς καιροῖς, ἀναβάσει λέγω καὶ ἀκμῇ καὶ παρακμῇ. τοσαυταχῶς τῆς ἀρχῆς λαμβανομένης ὁ Ἱπποκράτης ἐνταῦθα περὶ τοῦ δευτέρου σημαινομένου λέγει, λέγω δὴ τῆς πλατικῆς ἀρχῆς ἤτοι τῆς ἀτέχνου τῆς ἐν τρισὶν ἡμέραις θεωρουμένης, ὡς δηλοῖ τὸ ἐπαγόμενον, ἢν δὲ καὶ παλαιοτέρου ἐόντος τοῦ νοσήματος ἢ τριταίου, ὡς ἂν ὅτι τῆς ἀρχῆς ἐν τρισὶν ἡμέραις θεωρουμένης, ἐὰν νεκρῶδες γένηται τὸ πρόσωπον. εἶτα καὶ ἀρχῆς μνημονεύσας ἐξέβαλε τὸ ἓν σημαινόμενον τοῦ νεκρώδους προσώπου, λέγω δὴ τοῦ ἐπὶ χρονίῳ νοσήματι γινομένου. διὰ δὲ τοῦ εἰπεῖν ἐπανερέσθαι μὴ ἠγρύπνησεν ὁ ἄρρωστος ἢ τὰ τῆς κοιλίης ἐξυγρασμένα ἢ λιμῶδές τι εἶχεν αὐτὸν ἐδήλωσε τὰ προκαταρκτικὰ αἴτια τὰ ποιοῦντα τὸ πρόσωπον νεκρῶδες. φησὶ γὰρ ὅτι, ἐπειδὴ οὐκ ἐπὶ πάντων φαντὰ καὶ γνώριμα καὶ ὁμολογούμενά εἰσιν ἡμῖν τὰ σημεῖα, δεῖ τῇ ἀνακρίσει χρήσασθαι καὶ ἐρωτῆσαι τὸν ἄρρωστον· «Μὴ ἐκτάραξις γαστρὸς ἄμετρος γέγονέν σοι ἢ ἠγρύπνησας ἐπιτεταμένως ἢ ἠσίτησας;» καὶ εἰ μὲν φαίη τι τούτων, ἰδοὺ γινώσκεις ὅτι ἐπὶ προκαταρκτικῇ αἰτίᾳ γέγονε νεκρῶδες τὸ πρόσωπον. καὶ ἔστι μὲν κακόν, πλὴν ἧττον κακόν ἐστιν ὡς πρὸς κακοήθειαν νοσήματος. εἰ δὲ μηδὲν τούτων συνθῆταί σοι γεγονέναι, γίνωσκε ὅτι ἐπὶ κακοηθείᾳ ὀξέου νοσήματος γέγονε

1–3] *cf.* Gal. In Hipp. Progn. comm. I 8: CMG V 9,2 p. 215,28sq. 6sq.] *cf.* Steph. Comm. in Hipp. Aph.: Ambros. S 19 sup. fol. 36[v] 14 ἡ — διαιρεῖται] *cf.* Gal. In Hipp. Progn. comm. I 9: CMG V 9,2 p. 220,16–26 Steph. Comm. in Hipp. Aph.: Ambros. S 19 sup. fol. 17[v]; 26[v] 24sq. ἢν — τριταίου] Hipp. Progn. 2: p. 195,9 A. = II p. 114,15 L. 28 ἐπανερέσθαι — 30 αὐτὸν] Hipp. Progn. 2: p. 195,4sq. A. = II p. 114,8–10 L.

7 ἀκούσιος . . . ἑκούσιος γ 8 τὴν *coni. Wk.*: τρίτην *codd.* 10 δὲ *in* καὶ *mut.* L 12 ὥσπερ — 14 ἰστέον *om.* γ 18 ἡμέραισιν LP: ἡμέρησιν Mζ: *corr. Dietz* 29 ἢ τὰ] εἶτα γ 33 σοι γέγονεν γ

When a predisposing cause is responsible (the condition develops) in one of these three ways: from immoderate insomnia or severe bowel disturbance or prolonged hunger, each of these being capable of producing a mortified face. Extensive evacuation of the bowels obviously emaciates the body and gives the face a look of death. Severe insomnia as well can cause dissipation and produce a corpse-like face. Again, hunger, whether it be voluntary or involuntary, is capable of leaving the face mortified from neglect and lack of food. When (Hippocrates) speaks here of evacuation he means all forms of excessive evacuation whether by vomiting, bleeding, passing urine or sweating. By his mention of sleep he means all the psychic conditions capable of producing syncope and fainting, such as worry, anger and the like.

What, then, does Hippocrates say? If in the beginning of the disease the face is yellow or black. You should know that beginning is divided into three kinds: One is timeless or momentary; it is limited to the moment in which a person's condition begins to turn abnormal and it takes place instantaneously. There is a beginning in an extensive sense. And here there are two types; for it is either technical or simply extensive and non-technical, which is counted as three days. And this, too, is known among doctors; for they usually call the (first) three days of any disease the beginning. The technical beginning is the one distinguished from the other periods (of a disease), namely the heightening, crisis and abatement. These, then, are the number of beginnings and in the present instance Hippocrates is referring to the second, that is, to the extensive or non-technical beginning which is considered as three days; this is shown by what he goes on to say, If in a disease that lasts longer than three days – implying that the beginning is considered as three days –, the face becomes mortified. Now, by his mention of beginning he precluded one type of corpse-like face, namely that caused by a chronic disease. On the other hand, by saying, One must go on to ask whether the patient has been sleepless or has had loose bowels or felt some hunger he referred to the predisposing causes that produce mortification of the face. For he is saying that since we do not in all cases see, recognize and agree upon the symptoms, it is necessary to interrogate the patient and ask him if his bowels have been very loose or he could not sleep for a long time or went without food. If he answers affirmatively to one of these, it will tell you that the face has been left corpse-like by a predisposing cause, which is bad, though not as serious as the malignancy of a disease. But if he acknowledges to you that none of these things has happened, you will know that the face has been mortified by malignancy

νεκρῶδες τὸ πρόσωπον, ὅπερ ὀλέθριόν ἐστι καὶ κινδυνῶδες.

Πλὴν καὶ τοῦτο δεῖ σε γινώσκειν, ὅτι πολλάκις ἡ ἀγρυπνία καὶ ἡ ἐκτάραξις τῆς γαστρὸς οὐχ ὡς προκαταρκτικὰ αἴτια ὑπάρχοντα νεκρῶδες ποιοῦσι τὸ πρόσωπον, ἀλλ' ἔστιν ὅτε καὶ διὰ κακοήθειαν ὀξέου νοσήματος ἀμφότερα γίνεσθαι, καὶ τὴν ἀγρυπνίαν καὶ τὴν ἐκτάραξιν τῆς γαστρὸς καὶ τὸ νεκρῶδες πρόσωπον. καὶ πόθεν τοῦτο ὀφείλομεν γνῶναι, εἴτε ἡ κακοήθεια
87 τοῦ νοσήματος ταῦτα | ἐποίησε εἴτε ὡς προκαταρκτικὰ ὄντα ἐποίησαν νεκρῶδες τὸ πρόσωπον, τυχὸν ἡ ἀγρυπνία καὶ ἡ ἐκτάραξις τῆς γαστρός; ἔσο γινώσκων ὅτι τοῦτο διαγινώσκεις εἰς τὸ ἡμερονύκτιόν σου προσφόρως καὶ ἁρμοδίως διαιτῶντος. εἰ μὲν γαστρόρροιά ἐστιν, χρῆσαι τῇ σταλτικῇ τροφῇ, τυχὸν ψιχίοις ἀφράτου εἰς ὑδροροσᾶτον. εἰ δὲ ἀγρυπνία ἐστί, δεῖ σε ὑγροτέρᾳ τροφῇ χρήσασθαι, τυχὸν χυλῷ πτισάνης ἢ λαχάνων καὶ τοῖς τοιούτοις. εἰ δὲ ἀσιτία ἐστὶ καὶ ἔνδεια, καὶ ἐνταῦθα ταῖς δυναμέναις ἀνακαλέσασθαι καὶ τονῶσαι τροφαῖς χρήσασθαι. καὶ ἐὰν ταῦτά σου ποιήσαντος καταστῇ ἡμερονύκτιον, γίνωσκε ὅτι ἐπὶ προκαταρκτικῇ αἰτίᾳ γέγονε νεκρῶδες τὸ πρόσωπον. εἰ δὲ μείνῃ ὡσαύτως ἔχον, ἥ τε ἀγρυπνία καὶ ἡ γαστρόρροια, τότε γίνωσκε ὅτι διὰ κακοήθειαν νοσήματος πάντα γεγόνασι, καὶ ἡ ἀγρυπνία καὶ ἡ γαστρόρροια καὶ τὸ νεκρῶδες πρόσωπον. πλὴν ἐπειδὴ οὐκ ἐπὶ πάντων τῶν παθῶν ἡ αὐτὴ ἀκολουθία ἐστί, δεῖ σε καὶ εἰς τὰ σύστοιχα ἀποβλέπειν. ἐὰν ἀκμαστική ἐστιν ἡ ἡλικία καὶ θερινὴ ὥρα καὶ ἡ κρᾶσις καὶ τὸ χωρίον θερμόν, καὶ ἐὰν ἐνδεής ἐστι περὶ τὴν τροφὴν καὶ βίον ἄγρυπνον καὶ ἐπίπονον καὶ φροντιστικὸν καὶ φιλοταλαίπωρον ζῇ, γίνωσκε ἐπὶ κακοηθείᾳ τοῦ νοσήματος νεκρῶδες τὸ πρόσωπον γέγονε καὶ κινδυνῶδές ἐστι.

Καὶ ταῦτα μὲν ἐντὸς τῶν τριῶν ἡμερῶν. εἰ δέ γε ὑπερπέσῃ τὴν τρίτην ἡμέραν, ὡς δηλοῖ τὸ εἰπεῖν αὐτὸν ἢν δὲ καὶ παλαιοτέρου ἐόντος τοῦ νοσήματος ἢ τριταίου, τουτέστιν ἐπὶ πλέον τῶν τριῶν ἡμερῶν ἐάν τε γένηται νεκρῶδες τὸ πρόσωπον, πρὸς τούτοις πᾶσι τοῖς εἰρημένοις — τὰ ἓξ ἐκεῖνα ὀλέθρια συμπτώματα καὶ ἀνιχνεύοντός σου καὶ τὰ προκαταρκτικὰ αἴτια —, χρὴ δὲ πρὸς τούτοις ἐπιβλέπειν καὶ ἕτερα πλεῖστα σημεῖα ἐν ὀφθαλμοῖς θεωρούμενα. καὶ οἷον ἐπιβεβαιοῖ τὴν σημείωσιν τοῦ ὀλέθριον εἶναι τὸ νόσημα ἀπὸ ἐννέα τινῶν ἐν τοῖς ὀφθαλμοῖς συνισταμένων. καὶ λέγει ὅτι οἱ τοιοῦτοι τὴν αὐγὴν ἀποφεύγουσιν, οἱ τοιοῦτοι ἀπροαιρέτως δα-
88 κρύουσι, ἐπὶ τῶν τοιούτων ὁ | ἕτερος τοῦ ἑτέρου ὀφθαλμοῦ ἐλάσσων γίνεται, τὰ φλέβια τὰ ἐπὶ τῶν ἐπιπεφυκότων τῶν ὀφθαλμῶν ἐρυθρὰ γίνονται ἢ πελιὰ ἢ μέλανα, ἢ λήμας ἔχουσι περὶ τὰς ὄψεις, ἐπὶ τούτων ἐξίστανται οἱ ὀφθαλμοὶ καὶ ἀπαιώρηνται, καὶ προπετεῖς

26sq. ἢν – τριταίου] Hipp. Progn. 2: p. 195,9 A. = II p. 114,15 L. 33 τὴν – 80,3 ἠλλοιωμένον] Hipp. Progn. 2: pp. 195,12–196,5 A. = II p. 116,4–10 L.

1 νεκρῶδες – κινδυνῶδες *om.* M ὅπερ – 96,6 περιπνευμονία *om.* L ὅπερ] καὶ ζ 6 καὶ – 8 πρόσωπον *om.* M 11 ψιχία ἀφράτα ὑδροροσάτον *scripserit Wk.* ψιχία γ: *corr. Kollesch* ἀφράτα γ: *correxi* *ante* εἰς *add.* καὶ P ὑδρο-ῆς-ροσατον *(sic)* P 12 τρυφῇ P λαχάνοις ζ: λαχάνης M 14 τροφαῖς V: τροφᾶς M: τροφῆς Y 17 *ante* νοσήματος *add.* ὀξέου M 19 ἀκολουθία] ἀκολασία ζ 20 θερινὴ] ἡμερινὴ ζ 22 ζῆν γ: *corr. Dietz* 33 τὴν *om.* M 36 ἔχουσαι ζ 37 οἱ *om.* ζ

of an acute disease; and this is deadly and dangerous.

You should also be aware, however, that often insomnia and bowel disturbance do not act as predisposing causes to bring about mortification of the face, but there are times when all, namely insomnia, bowel disturbance and a corpse-like face, are caused by malignancy of an acute disease. How are we to find out whether these symptoms result from the malignancy of the disease or are in fact predisposing causes that have produced mortification, i.e. insomnia and bowel disturbance? This you will discover by administering the correct diet in proper amounts for a period of twenty-four hours. If it is diarrhoea, employ an astringent diet, e.g., crumbs of fine bread in rose-water. But if it is insomnia you should use food which is more on the fluid side, like a decoction of barley or vegetables, etc. In the case of hunger or diet deficiency give food capable of restoring and building up strength. If the patient recovers within twenty-four hours after this treatment, it means that a predisposing cause was responsible for the face being corpse-like. But if it remains the same and the insomnia and diarrhoea (continue), then you will know that all – insomnia, diarrhoea and the mortified face – are the results of the malignancy of a disease. However, since not all conditions develop in the same way, you must consider the concomitant circumstances as well. If the (patient's) age is prime, the weather summer-like, the temperament and locality hot, and if he is deficient in nourishment, lives a hard life full of work, worry and little sleep, conclude that his face has become mortified from a malignancy of the disease and is dangerous.

This (holds good) within the three day period. However, when the condition continues beyond that, as is shown by his saying If the disease lasts longer than the third day, in other words, if the corpse-like face persists more than three days, in addition to looking for all the signs we have mentioned – namely those six deadly symptoms and the predisposing causes – one must also consider many other symptoms besides which are to be observed in the eyes. And there are nine eye conditions from which he confirms, so to say, the interpretation that the disease is fatal. He says that people affected in this way avoid the light, weep involuntarily, have one eye smaller than the other, the blood vessels in the conjunctivae of their eyes become red or livid or black, or they have rheum around the eyeballs, in these cases the eyes are restless and move about, and

αὐτοὺς ἴσχουσιν ἢ κοίλους, ἐπὶ τούτων ἀστήρικτοί εἰσιν οἱ ὀφθαλμοί, ἢ τὸ σύμπαν χρῶμα τοῦ σύμπαντος προσώπου καὶ αὐτῶν τῶν ὀφθαλμῶν ἠλλοιωμένον ἔχουσιν. ἐὰν οὖν πρὸς τοῖς εἰρημένοις καὶ ταῦτα συνέλθωσιν, ὀλέθριόν ἐστι καὶ δεῖ προλέγειν τὸν θάνατον.

I 25 [2: 195,2 A. = II 114,6 L.] Ἢν μὲν οὖν ἐν ἀρχῇ τῆς νόσου τὸ πρόσωπον χλωρὸν ᾖ καὶ μέλαν ἐόν, τοιοῦτον ᾖ καὶ μήπω οἷόν τε ᾖ τοῖσιν ἄλλοισι σημείοισι ξυντεκμαίρεσθαι, ἐπανερέσθαι χρὴ μὴ ἠγρύπνηκεν ὁ ἄνθρωπος

Φησὶν ἐνταῦθα ὁ Ἱπποκράτης ὅτι, ἐὰν ἐν τῇ ἀρχῇ τοῦ νοσήματος, τουτέστιν ἐν τῇ πρώτῃ ἡμέρᾳ ἢ τῇ δευτέρᾳ, νεκρῶδες γένηται τὸ πρόσωπον μήπω ἔχον ἐγνωσμένα τὰ συμπτώματα — ἐγνωσμένα δὲ συμπτώματα ἀκουστέον τὴν αἰτίαν, ὑφ' ἧς γέγονε τὸ νεκρῶδες πρόσωπον —, ἐπερωτᾶν δεῖ τὸν ἄρρωστον μὴ ἠγρύπνησεν ἢ ἐκτάραξις τῆς γαστρὸς γέγονεν αὐτῷ μεγίστη ἢ ἐλιμαγχονήθη ἤγουν ἐν ἀσιτίᾳ διέμεινεν. πλὴν οὐ μόνον ἐπὶ τούτοις τοῖς σημείοις γίνεται νεκρῶδες πρόσωπον, ἀλλὰ καὶ ἐπὶ ἀκροτάτῃ ψύξει δι' ὥραν χειμερινὴν ἢ διὰ κατάστημα ψυχρότατον ἢ καὶ δι' ἔσχατον γῆρας. ἀλλ' οὔκ εἰσιν οὕτως κινδυνώδη.

Καὶ ταῦτα μὲν ὁ Ἱπποκράτης. ὁ δὲ Γαληνὸς μείζονι τέχνῃ νῦν ἑαυτὸν ἐπιτρέψας λέγει ὅτι δυνατόν ἐστιν ἡμᾶς προγνῶναι πᾶσαν αἰτίαν νεκρῶδες ἐργασαμένην τὸ πρόσωπον μηδεμιᾶς ἐρωτήσεως δεηθέντας. τί γάρ; ὅτι δεῖ σε ἀναδραμεῖν καὶ ἀποβλέψαι εἰς τὰ σύστοιχα· ἐὰν ἡ ὥρα θερινὴ ἐστιν καὶ τὸ κατάστημα θερμὸν καὶ ξηρόν, καὶ ἡ κρᾶσις τοῦ κάμνοντος θερμὴ καὶ ἡλικία ἀκμαστική, ἡ δίαιτα ἐνδεής, βίον διάγων φροντιστικὸν καὶ
89 ἐπίπονον, | καὶ οἱ σφυγμοὶ ἠτονημένοι καὶ βραδεῖς καὶ μικροὶ καὶ ἀμυδροί, καὶ ἁπτομένου σου τῇ ἁφῇ καυσώδης καὶ διακαὴς ὑποπίπτει ἡ θερμασία, καὶ ἐπὶ τούτῳ ἐν τῇ πρώτῃ ἢ ἐν τῇ δευτέρᾳ ἡμέρᾳ νεκρῶδες γέγονε τὸ πρόσωπον, γίνωσκε ὅτι διὰ κακοήθειαν νοσήματος γέγονεν. ἐὰν δὲ ἐπὶ γαστρορροίᾳ γέγονε νεκρῶδες τὸ πρόσωπον, ἔχεις ἀσφαλέστατον σημεῖον τῶν ὀφθαλμῶν· ἐπὶ γὰρ τῆς γαστρορροίας ἔγκοιλοι γίνονται οἱ ὀφθαλμοὶ αὐτῶν, καὶ ἐξηραμμένους αὐτοὺς ἔχουσιν ὡς μὴ δύνασθαι τὰ βλέφαρα ἀνατείνειν. ἐπὶ δὲ τῆς ἀγρυπνίας ἀσφαλέστατον σημεῖον εὑρήσεις ἐπὶ τῶν σφυγμῶν τὸ δίκην χορδῆς τεταμένην εὑρίσκεσθαι τὴν ἀρτηρίαν. τοὺς δὲ διὰ κακοήθειαν νοσήματος ἀπὸ τῆς ἁφῆς σημειώσῃ· ἐπιβαλὼν γὰρ τὴν ἁφὴν ⟨οὐ⟩ μόνον κατὰ τὸν καρπὸν ἀλλὰ καὶ παράνω, τυχὸν κατὰ τὸν βραχίονα, εὑρήσεις καυσωδεστάτην καὶ ζέουσαν τὴν ἀναφερομένην θερμασίαν καὶ δριμεῖαν καὶ καπνώδεις ἀναθυμιάσεις ἀνεῖσθαι πρὸς τὴν ἁφήν· καὶ γινώσκεις ὅτι ὀξύς ἐστιν ὁ πυρετὸς καὶ διαφορητικώτατος ὁ τὸ νεκρῶδες ποιήσας πρόσωπον.

18 Γαληνὸς] *cf.* Gal. In Hipp. Progn. comm. I 8: CMG V 9,2 pp. 216,9–218,13

2 αὐτοὶ ζ 3 ἠλλοιωμένων Μζ: ἠλλοιωμένη P: *corr. Dietz* 6 χλωρὸν — ἐόν] *hic nullus test. Hipp.* 6 sq. ᾖ^{II} ... ᾖ] ἢ ... ἢ γ: *sec. Hipp. correxi* 11 ἔχωσι Y: ἔχορι V 20 δεηθέντος MP: *ambig.* ζ: *corr. Dietz* 28 *post* σημεῖον *fort. excidit* ἐπὶ *(cf. infra, linn. 31 sq.)* 33 σημειώσεις M: *ambig.* ζ 34 οὐ *addidi* ὑπεράνω *coni. Dietz*

they are either prominent or sunken, further, their eyes are unstable and their color as well as that of the entire face is changed. If, then, these symptoms develop in addition to those already discussed, (the disease) is fatal and we must forecast death.

> I 25 If at the beginning of the disease the face is yellow or black, if it is in such a condition, then, and it is not yet possible with the help of the other symptoms to make a conjecture, one must go on to ask whether the patient has been sleepless

Hippocrates says here that if in the beginning of the disease, i.e., on the first or second day, the face becomes corpse-like but the symptoms have not yet been recognized – by recognized symptoms we understand the reason why the face has become corpse-like – it is necessary to ask the patient whether he has been sleepless or his bowels have been very disturbed or he has been weakened by hunger, i.e., has been without food for a long time. However, these are not the only symptoms that produce mortification of the face, it is also caused by extreme cold resulting from winter season or very cold weather or even advanced old-age. But these are not so dangerous.

This is what Hippocrates says. Galen, on the other hand, relying here on greater skill, states that we can prognose every cause which has made the face corpse-like without having to ask a question. How? You must go back and examine the circumstances; if it is summer, the weather hot and dry, the patient's temperament warm and he is in his prime, if his diet is deficient and he leads a life full of worries and work, if his pulses are weak, slow, shallow and faint and on touching him you find the heat (of his body) feverish and burning, and if in these circumstances the face assumes a deadly aspect on the first or second day, you may conclude that the cause is the malignancy of the disease. On the other hand, if the face has become mortified due to diarrhoea, the eyes will provide you with the surest sign; for with diarrhoea their eyes become hollow and dried up, so that the eyelids cannot be opened. For sleeplessness you have the surest sign in the pulses, when you find the artery stretched like a string. But when the condition is caused by the malignancy of the disease you will interpret it by means of touch; by placing your hand not only on the wrist but further up also, i.e., along the arm, you will find the heat coming up there burning, seething and stinging, and the touch of your hand will set off steaming vapor; this will tell you that the fever which has left the face corpse-like is acute and is causing very severe dissipation.

I 26 [2: 195,5 A. = II 114,10 L.] Καὶ ἢν μέν τι τουτέων ὁμολογέει, ἧσσον νομίζειν δεινὸν εἶναι.

Φησὶν ὅτι τὸ νεκρῶδες πρόσωπον, ἐὰν διά τινα προκαταρκτικὴν γένη⟨ται⟩ αἰτίαν, τυχὸν εἴτε διὰ γαστρόρροιαν εἴτε διὰ λιμὸν εἴτε δι' ἀγρυπνίαν, κακὸν μέν ἐστιν, ἀλλ' ἧττον ὡς τὸ διὰ κακοήθειαν γινόμενον.

I 27 [2: 195,12 A. = II 116,4 L.] Ἢν γὰρ τὴν αὐγὴν φεύγωσιν

Ἰστέον ὅτι τὰ τρία ταῦτα ἀντιπαράκεινται ἀλλήλοις, φῶς, ἀκτὶς καὶ αὐγή. καὶ τὸ φῶς συνουσίωται τῷ ἡλίῳ, ἡ δὲ ἀκτίς ἐστιν ἡ ἐκ τοῦ φωτὸς πεμπομένη, αὐγὴ δέ ἐστιν ἡ ἐκ τῆς ἀκτῖνος πεμπομένη, περὶ ἧς καὶ ἔστι νῦν ὁ λόγος· ἐν γὰρ τῇ αὐγῇ ἀείσε ἐσμὲν καὶ ἄνευ αὐτῆς εἶναι οὐ δυνάμεθα. πῶς οὖν οὐ κακὸν τοῦτο ἐπὶ ὀξεῖ νοσήματι; δηλοῖ γὰρ ἄκραν καταβολὴν τῶν ὀπτικῶν δυνάμεων. πλὴν φεύγουσι πολλοὶ τὴν αὐγὴν καὶ δι' ἄλλην αἰτίαν, ὥσπερ οἱ ὀφθαλμιῶντες καὶ οἱ †τεζηβοί†. ταῦτα δὲ οὔκ εἰσιν ἐνδεικτικὰ κινδύνων. |

90 **I 28** [2: 196,1 A. = II 116,4 L.] Ἢν δακρύωσιν ἀπροαιρέτως

Ἐὰν ἐν τοῖς ὀξέσι νοσήμασιν ἀπροαιρέτως δακρύωσιν οἱ νοσοῦντες, γίνωσκε ὅτι δι' ἄκραν ἀσθένειαν τῆς καθεκτικῆς δυνάμεως ἀπροαιρέτως δακρύουσιν, ὅπερ κακόν ἐστι σημεῖον, ἐπειδὴ αὐτὸ τὸ ὀλίγον ⟨ὑγρὸν⟩ τὸ λόγῳ τροφῆς φερόμενον ἐν τοῖς ὀφθαλμοῖς οὐ κατέχεται, ἀλλ' ὥσπερ ἀπὸ ἀψύχου ἀπορρεῖ καὶ κενοῦται.

I 29 [2: 196,1 A. = II 116,5 L.] Ἢ διαστρέφονται

Ἢ γὰρ διὰ παράλυσιν τῶν ἐν τοῖς ὀφθαλμοῖς μυῶν παραλυομένων ἢ διὰ σπασμόν. εἰ μὲν διὰ παράλυσιν, εἰς τὸ ἐναντίον διαστρέφονται τὰ παραλυόμενα μόρια· εἰ δὲ διὰ σπασμόν, ἐφ' ἑαυτὸ σπᾶται καὶ διαστρέφεται, καθ' ἣν οἱ στραβισμοὶ γίνονται. καὶ τοῦτο διαγινώσκεις ἐκ τῆς ὀδύνης καὶ τῆς ἀτροφίας· ἐπὶ γὰρ τοῦ σπασμοῦ ὀδυνῶνται, ἀλλὰ καὶ ἀτροφία ἕπεται.

Ταῦτα δὲ τὰ πάθη, ὁ σπασμὸς λέγω καὶ ἡ παράλυσις, ἢ δι' αὐτοὺς τοὺς ὀφθαλμοὺς γίνονται ἢ διὰ τὸν ἐγκέφαλον. καὶ εἰ μὲν διὰ τὸν ἐγκέφαλον διαστραφῶσιν οἱ ὀφθαλμοί, εἴτε παραλυομένων αὐτῶν εἴτε σπωμένων, ὀδυνῶνται τὸ μέτωπον, τὸ νωτιαῖον, τοὺς ὀφθαλμοὺς καὶ τοὺς κροτάφους, καὶ μάλιστα πρότερον ἐκεῖνα ἅπερ καὶ προσεγγίζουσι τῷ ἐγκεφάλῳ μόρια. καὶ κακόν ἐστιν, ἡνίκα μὴ διὰ τοὺς ὀφθαλμοὺς ἡ διαστροφὴ γένηται, ἀλλὰ διὰ τὸν ἐγκέφαλον· δηλοῖ γὰρ καὶ αὐτὴν τὴν πρώτην ἀρχὴν κακῶς διακεῖσθαι, ὅπερ κάκιστόν ἐστι σημεῖον ἐπὶ ὀξέου νοσήματος.

12sq.] *cf.* Gal. In Hipp. Progn. comm. I 10: CMG V 9,2 p. 221,18–20 17sq. δι' — σημεῖον] *cf.* Gal. In Hipp. Progn. comm. I 10: CMG V 9,2 p. 222,1sq.

2 νομίζει MP 4 γένη γ: *suppl. Dietz* 5 *post* ὡς *fort.* πρὸς *addendum est* 8 συνουσιοῦται M: συνουσῖται P 13 τεζηκοί *(?)* P: τζιμβλοί *(i. q.* lippi*) coni. Dietz* 15 Ἢν] ἢ *Hipp.* δακρύουσιν Mζ: δακρύσουσιν P: *corr. Dietz* 16 δακρύουσιν γ: *corr. Dietz* 18 τὸ ὀλίγον *om.* M 19 ὑγρὸν *addidi (cf. infra, p. 84,30)* 20 ἀποψύχου P: ἀπὸ ἀψύχρου M 22 ὀφθαλμοῖς *om.* M 27sq. αὐτοῦ τοῦ ὀφθαλμοῦ γ: *correxi*

I 26 And if he confirms one of these you may consider it less dangerous.

He means that if mortification of the face is due to a predisposing cause, i.e. whether due to diarrhoea or hunger or insomnia, it is bad, but less so than the one caused by malignancy.

I 27 For if they avoid the light

Note that these three, illumination, ray and light, are correlatives. Illumination is essentially connected with the sun, the ray is that which comes from illumination and light is the product of the ray. Here we are dealing with the third; for we are always in the light and cannot exist without it. It is surely a bad sign, then, in acute illness (if the eyes shun the light), because it indicates serious failure of the optical faculties. However, many avoid the light for another reason too, such as those suffering from ophthalmia and the .... But these conditions do not signal danger.

I 28 If they weep involuntarily

If patients with acute diseases cry against their will, conclude that they are shedding tears involuntarily because the retentive faculty is extremely weak; this is a bad sign, because even the small amount of fluid conveyed in the eyes in the form of nutriment is not retained, but runs off and is evacuated as from a lifeless body.

I 29 Or are distorted

(The eyes are distorted) either by paralysis, the muscles in the eyes becoming paralyzed, or by spasm. If by paralysis the affected parts are twisted in opposite directions; but if by spasm (the part) is drawn together and contorted towards itself, which is the cause of people becoming squint-eyed. This condition is diagnosed from the pain and atrophy; for with spasm they suffer pain, and atrophy follows.

These affections, spasm and paralysis, are caused either by the eyes themselves or by the brain. If the brain is responsible for distorted eyes, whether by paralysis or spasm, pains are experienced in the brow, at the back (of the head), in the eyes and temples and before all in those parts which are near the brain. It is a bad sign when distortion is produced not by the eyes but by the brain; for it means that the first principle itself is in poor condition, which is a very dangerous sign in acute illness.

I 30 [2: 196,1 A. = II 116,5 L.] Ἢ ὁ ἕτερος τοῦ ἑτέρου ἐλάσσων γίνεται

Διὰ τί ὁ ἕτερος ὀφθαλμὸς τοῦ ἑτέρου ἐλάσσων γίνεται; ἐπὶ ἐνδείᾳ καὶ ἐπὶ ἀτροφίᾳ καὶ ἐπὶ ἄκρᾳ ξηρότητι καὶ ἐπὶ καταβολῇ τῶν ἐν αὐτῷ φυσικῶν δυνάμεων, ὅπερ καὶ τοῦτο ἐπὶ ὀξεῖ νοσήματι κάκιστόν ἐστι σημεῖον.

I 31 [2: 196,2 A. = II 116,6 L.] Ἢ τὰ λευκὰ ἐρυθρὰ ἴσχωσιν

Ὅτι τὰ φλέβια τὰ ἐν τῷ ἐπιπεφυκότι – λευκὸν γὰρ αὐτὸν τὸν ἐπι-
91 πεφυκότα καλεῖ νῦν – ἐρυθρὰ ἴσχουσι. διὰ | πλείονας αἰτίας τοῦτο γίνεται· ἢ γὰρ δι' ὀφθαλμίαν, ὥσπερ ἐπὶ τῶν ⟨ἐκ⟩χυμωμάτων, ἢ διὰ μέθην τὰ λευκὰ ἐρυθραίνονται ἢ διὰ ἔμετον ἢ διὰ πληθώραν αἱματικὴν ἢ διὰ φλεγμονὴν τῶν μηνίγγων. καὶ διὰ μὲν πληθώραν ἐρυθρὰ γίνονται τὰ φλέβια τοῦ ἐπιπεφυκότος τρόπῳ τοιούτῳ· τῷ πλήθει ἀπελαύνεται ἐπὶ τοὺς ὀφθαλμοὺς τὸ αἷμα καὶ τείνει τὰ φλέβια τὰ ἐν τῷ ἐπιπεφυκότι, ἐπειδὴ στενὰ καὶ λεπτά εἰσι· μὴ φέροντα οὖν τὴν τάσιν ῥήγνυνται καὶ ἐκχεῖται τὸ αἷμα καὶ ἐρυθρὰ γίνονται. ἐὰν οὖν ὀξέου νοσήματος ὑποκειμένου καὶ καυσώδους πυρετοῦ ἔ[σ]τι καὶ ἢ φλεγμονὴ ἐν ταῖς μήνιγξιν ἢ πληθώρα ὑπόκειται, παγκάκιστόν ἐστι καὶ τοῦτο σημεῖον.

I 32 [2: 196,2 A. = II 116,6 L.] Ἢ πελιὰ ἢ μέλανα

Ταῦτα τὰ χρώματα, τὸ πελιὸν καὶ τὸ μέλαν, ἐπὶ ἄκρᾳ καταψύξει γίνονται. ἐὰν οὖν πελιὰ γίνωνται ἢ μέλανα τὰ ἐν τοῖς ὀφθαλμοῖς λευκά, τουτέστιν ὁ ἐπιπεφυκώς, παγχάλεπόν ἐστι σημεῖον ἐπὶ ὀξέου νοσήματος.

I 33 [2: 196,3 A. = II 116,7 L.] Ἢ λῆμαι φαίνονται περὶ τὰς ὄψιας

Λῆμαι γίνονται ἐπὶ τοὺς ὀφθαλμοὺς ἢ διά τι πάθος περὶ αὐτοὺς συνιστάμενον, ὥσπερ ἐπὶ τῶν ὀφθαλμιώντων, ἢ ὑγρότητός τινος φερομένης καὶ ποιούσης λήμας. δεῖ γὰρ εἰδέναι ὅτι ἡ λήμη γίνεται ἐν τοῖς ὀφθαλμοῖς ἐπὶ ἀπεψίᾳ τοῦ λόγῳ τροφῆς ἐν τοῖς ὀφθαλμοῖς φερομένου. ἐὰν οὖν ὀξέος ὑποκειμένου νοσήματος καὶ διακαοῦς πυρετοῦ καὶ ἀτροφίας καὶ ξηρότητος λῆμαι γίνωνται περὶ τοὺς ὀφθαλμούς, παγκάκιστόν ἐστι καὶ τοῦτο σημεῖον· δηλοῖ γὰρ ὅτι καὶ αὐτὸ τὸ ἐλάχιστον ὑγρὸν τὸ λόγῳ τροφῆς φερόμενον ἐκεῖσε οὐκ ἰσχύει ἡ ἀλλοιωτικὴ δύναμις πέψαι καὶ ἀλλοιῶσαι, ἀλλ' ἀπεπτούμενον τὰς λήμας ποιεῖ.

I 34 [2: 196,3 A. = II 116,8 L.] Ἢ ἐναιωρούμενοι

9 δι' – 15] *cf.* Gal. In Hipp. Progn. comm. I 10: CMG V 9,2 p. 222,12–15   19 καταψύξει] *cf.* Gal. In Hipp. Progn. comm. I 10: CMG V 9,2 p. 222,24sq.   24–32] *cf.* Gal. In Hipp. Progn. comm. I 10: CMG V 9,2 p. 223,1–11

9 χυμωμάτων γ: *supplevi*   16 ἔστι *codd.*: *corr. Dietz*   ἢ[I]] ἡ γ: *corr. Dietz*   20 γίνονται P: γένωνται M   23 ὄψεις M   27 τοῦ] τῶ γ: *correxi*   φερόμενον γ: *correxi*   28 ὀξέου *codd.*: *correxi*   29 γίνονται P   παρὰ M   30 τὸ[II]] τῶ MV: *corr.* PY   32 ἀπεπτούμενα γ: *correxi*

I 30 Or one becomes smaller than the other

Why does one eye become smaller than the other? From deficiency in nutriment, atrophy, intense dryness or through collapse of its natural faculties; this also is a very bad symptom in acute disease.

I 31 Or the white parts are red

(He is saying) that the blood vessels in the conjunctiva – for he calls the conjunctiva itself the white part here – have turned red. This takes place for a number of reasons; the white parts become red either from ophthalmia, as in cases of ecchymosis, or from being drunk, or from vomiting, or from a plethora of blood or from inflammation of the membranes. The blood vessels of the conjunctiva become red from a plethora in the following way: due to the surplus the blood is driven to the eyes where it puts a strain on the conjunctiva's vessels, these being narrow and thin; then, not being able to bear the strain they rupture, whereupon the blood spills all around and they turn red. If, then, in a case of acute disease accompanied by burning fever there is also either inflammation in the membranes or a plethora (of blood), it is an extremely dangerous sign.

I 32 Or livid or black

These colors, livid and black, are produced by extreme cold. If, then, the white part in the eyes, or conjunctiva, becomes livid or black, it is a most serious symptom in an acute disease.

I 33 Or rheum appears around the eye-balls

Rheum develops in the eyes either from a local affection, as in the case of ophthalmia, or when a certain fluid is conveyed to them and produces the rheum. For it should be noted that the rheum in the eyes results when the matter conveyed in the form of nutriment to the eyes is not digested. If, then, rheum shows up around the eyes in a case of acute disease accompanied by burning fever, atrophy and dryness, this also is an extremely bad sign; for it means that the converting faculty is not strong enough to digest and convert even the very small quantity of fluid brought there in the form of nutriment, but it is undigested and creates the rheum.

I 34 Or (the eyes) move about

Ἐναιωρούμενοί εἰσιν οἱ ὀφθαλμοὶ οἱ ἀστήρικτοι οἱ τῇδε κἀκεῖσε περιφερόμενοι ἀτάκτως καὶ ἀρρύθμως ἐν τῷ μὴ ἑδράζεσθαι μηδὲ στηρίζεσθαι ὑπὸ τῶν μυῶν. ἀστήρικτοι δὲ καὶ ἐναιωρούμενοι γίνονται οἱ ὀφθαλμοὶ ἢ
92 διὰ τρομώδη διάθεσιν ἐν αὐτοῖς τοῖς μυσὶ τῶν ὀφθαλμῶν συνισ|ταμένην ἢ διὰ παραφροσύνην. ὀξέος οὖν ὑποκειμένου νοσήματος καὶ διακαοῦς πυρετοῦ εἴτε διὰ τρόμον γένωνται οἱ ὀφθαλμοὶ ἀστήρικτοι εἴτε διὰ παραφροσύνην, παγχάλεπόν ἐστι καὶ τοῦτο σημεῖον.

I 35 [2: 196,3 A. = II 116,8 L.] Ἢ ἐξίσχοντες ἢ ἔγκοιλοι ἰσχυρῶς γιγνόμενοι

Καὶ ἔγκοιλοι μὲν γίγνονται οἱ ὀφθαλμοὶ δι' ἔνδειαν καὶ ἀτροφίαν καὶ ἄγαν ξηρότητα· ἐξίσχοντες δὲ τῷ λόγῳ τῆς ἀκρατείας τῶν μυῶν, διὰ τοῦτο προκύπτουσι.

Καὶ τὸ χρῶμα τοῦ ξύμπαντος προσώπου ἠλλοιωμένον γίνεται τῷ λόγῳ τῆς νεκρώσεως, τοῦ κακῶς διακεῖσθαι τὸν ζωτικὸν τόνον.

VII

I 36 [2: 196,5 A. = II 116,11 L.] Σκοπεῖν δὲ καὶ τὰς ὑποφάσεις τῶν ὀφθαλμῶν ἐν τοῖσιν ὕπνοισιν. ἢν γάρ τι ὑποφαίνηται ξυμβαλλομένων τῶν βλεφάρων τοῦ λευκοῦ

Τὸ λεγόμενον τοιοῦτόν ἐστιν, ὅτι, ἐὰν ἐν τοῖς ὕπνοις μὴ συμβάλλωνται μηδὲ ἀσφαλίζωνται τὰ βλέφαρα, ἀλλ' ὑποφαίνηταί τι μέρος τοῦ ἐπιπεφυκότος – λευκὸν γὰρ τὸν ἐπιπεφυκότα ἐκάλεσε –, κάκιστόν ἐστι καὶ τοῦτο σημεῖον ἐν ὀξεῖ νοσήματι γινόμενον· δηλοῖ γὰρ ἢ σπασμὸν ἢ παράλυσιν τῶν ἀνοιγόντων καὶ κλειόντων τὰ βλέφαρα. ἑκάτερον δὲ κάκιστόν ἐστιν· ἡ μὲν γὰρ παράλυσις ἀσθένειαν καὶ ἀκράτειαν δηλοῖ τῶν ψυχικῶν δυνάμεων, ὁ δὲ σπασμὸς ἄκραν ξηρότητα, ὅστις καὶ ἀνίατός ἐστιν ἐν ὀξεῖ νοσήματι.

Καὶ ἐπεὶ τῶν ἐν τοῖς βλεφάροις μυῶν ἐμνημονεύσαμεν, φέρε εἴπωμεν καὶ περὶ αὐτῶν. ἰστέον ὅτι τρεῖς εἰσι μύες οἱ ἀνοίγοντες καὶ κλείοντες τὰ ἄνω βλέφαρα· τὰ γὰρ κάτω ἀκίνητά εἰσι. καὶ εἷς μέν ἐστιν ὁ ἀνοίγων μῦς, δύο δὲ οἱ ἀσφαλίζοντες τὸ βλέφαρον. καὶ ὁ μὲν ἀνοίγων μῦς κατὰ τοῦ μεσαιτάτου βλεφάρου τέτακται πανσόφως ὑπὸ τῆς φύσεως τοῦτο μηχανευσαμένης. τὰ γὰρ βαρέα τῶν σωμάτων κατὰ τοῦ μεσαιτάτου ἑλκόμενα εἴκει ἑτοίμως καὶ ἀνέλκεται. οὕτως οὖν καὶ ὁ ἀνοίγων μῦς κατὰ τοῦ μέσου βλεφάρου τέτακται, ἵνα πρὸς ἑαυτὸν ἐπισπώμενος ἀνοίγῃ καὶ ἕλκῃ αὐτό.
93 οἱ δὲ | ἀσφαλίζοντες δύο μύες καθ' ἑκάτερον μέρος τῶν βλεφάρων εἰσὶ τεταγμένοι, εἷς μὲν πρὸς τὸν μέγαν κανθὸν καὶ ὁ εἷς πρὸς τὸν μικρόν. οὗτοι

1–7] *cf.* Gal. In Hipp. Progn. comm. I 10: CMG V 9,2 p. 223,12–15 35–88,6] *cf.* Gal. De usu part. X 9: II pp. 87sq. Helmr. = III pp. 805sq. K.

5 ὀξέως γ: *corr. Dietz* 16 *post* δὲ *praeb.* χρὴ *Hipp.* ὑποφάσιας M 20 ὑποφαίνεται MP: ὑποφαίνει ζ: *corr. Dietz* 25 ξηρότητος γ: *corr. Dietz* 27 ἐπὶ MP: *corr.* ζ εἴπομεν γ: *corr. Dietz* 29 μῦς *om.* M 31 τούτου P μηχανευσάμενος γ: *correxi* 33 ἥκει γ: *correxi* 34 ἑσπόμενος M

Moving eyes are those which are unstable and shift in every direction without order or rhythm, not being fixed or secured by the muscles. Unstable and moving eyes are caused either by a trembling condition in the eye muscles themselves or by delirium. In an acute disease, then, with burning fever, if the eyes become unstable, whether from trembling or delirium, this, too, is a very unfavorable symptom.

I 35 And they are either prominent or véry sunken

The eyes are sunken from deficiency in nutriment, atrophy and extreme dryness; they become prominent from loss of power in the muscles, and so they protrude.

The complexion of the whole face is changed by the mortification and by the poor condition of the vital tone.

VII

I 36 One must examine the partial openings of the eyes during sleep. For if a part of the white shows through when the eyelids are drawn together

What he is saying is this: if during sleep the eyelids do not come into contact and are not closed, but a part of the conjunctiva is visible – the white is his expression for the conjunctiva –, this also is a very bad sign in acute disease; for it means either spasm or paralysis of the eyelid's opening and closing (muscles). And each is very bad; for paralysis indicates weakness and powerlessness of the psychic faculties; spasm means extreme dryness and is also incurable in acute disease.

Since we have mentioned eyelid muscles we will discuss them (at this point). Note that there are three muscles which open and close the upper lids; the bottom ones do not move. One muscle is for opening and the other two for closing the lid. The opening muscle is situated at the exact center of the lid, having been very cleverly placed there by the contrivance of nature. For heavy objects move readily and can be drawn up when pulled at the very center. In the same way, then, the opening muscle has been placed in the middle, in order to draw the lid towards itself and open it. The two closing muscles, on the other hand, are situated on either side of the eyelids, one at the large corner and the

οὖν οἱ μύες, καὶ οὗτοι ὡς πρὸς ἑαυτοὺς καὶ ἐπὶ τὰ ἔσω ἕλκοντες τὰ βλέφαρα κλείουσιν αὐτά. συμβαίνει οὖν τὸ τηνικαῦτα ὁ μὲν σπασμὸς ἐν τῷ ἄνω μυΐ, λέγω δὴ τὸν ἀνοίγοντα, συνίστασθαι, ἡ δὲ παράλυσις ἐν τοῖς κλείουσι. σπωμένου οὖν τοῦ ἄνω μυὸς τοῦ ἀνοίγοντος, ὡς πρὸς ἑαυτὸν ἐφέλκεται τὸ ἄνω βλέφαρον, καὶ ἐπιφαίνεται μέρος τοῦ ἐπιπεφυκότος· ὁ γὰρ σπασμὸς πρὸς τὴν οἰκείαν ἀρχὴν ἕλκει τὸ μόριον. ἀλλὰ καὶ ἐπὶ τῶν ἀσφαλιζόντων τοῦτο γίνεται, τὸ ὑποφαίνεσθαί τι μέρος τοῦ ἐπιπεφυκότος, ἀλλὰ τούτων οὐ σπωμένων, ἀλλὰ παραλυομένων· ἡ γὰρ παράλυσις ἐπὶ τὸ ἐναντίον τοῦ κατὰ φύσιν ποιεῖται τὴν κίνησιν. παραλυομένων οὖν τῶν κλειόντων μυῶν οὐ συμβάλλονται τὰ βλέφαρα, ἀλλ' ἀνεῳγότας αὐτοὺς ἔχουσι. καὶ πάλιν φαίνεται ὁ ἐπιπεφυκώς, ὡς δοκεῖν κλειστανοίκτους εἶναι τοὺς ὀφθαλμούς. καὶ ταῦτα μὲν ἐπὶ ἀνθρώπων. ἐπὶ δέ τινων ζῴων οὔκ εἰσιν οἱ ἀσφαλίζοντες μύες τὰ βλέφαρα, ἀλλὰ μόνον τοὺς ἀνοίγοντας ἔχουσιν. ὅθεν ἐν τῷ ὑπνοῦν τὰ τοιαῦτα τῶν ζῴων ἐπὶ τὴν θαλάμην ἀντιστρέφειν τοὺς βολβοὺς καὶ αὐτὴν τὴν κόρην ἐντὸς εἶναι τῆς θαλάμης, ἵνα μὴ λυμαίνωνται ὑπὸ τῶν προσπιπτόντων. οὕτως ἐπὶ δορκάδων καὶ λαγωῶν καὶ ἐπί τινων ἰχθύων ἐστίν. εἶτα καὶ διὰ τοῦτο εἷς μὲν ἔστι μῦς ὁ ἀνοίγων, ἐπειδὴ ὀλίγου καιροῦ δέεται ἀναβαστάζειν τὸ βλέφαρον, καὶ παραυτίκα διαδέχονται αὐτὸν οἱ κλείοντες. δύο δὲ μύες γεγόνασιν οἱ κλείοντες διὰ δύο
94 αἰτίας, διά τε τὸ ταχέως ἀσφαλίζεσθαι τὰ βλέφαρα, ἐπειδὴ ὁ ὀφθαλ|μὸς εὐπαθής ἐστιν· εὐπαθὴς δὲ καθέστηκεν, ἵνα ἑτοίμως ἀντιλαμβάνωνται τά τε χρώματα καὶ τῶν μικρῶν καὶ τῶν μεγάλων σωμάτων· ἐν γὰρ τῷ πάσχειν ἀντιλαμβάνονται οἱ ὀφθαλμοί. διὰ οὖν τὴν εὐπάθειαν ἐδεήθη ἡ φύσις ⟨εἰς⟩ τὸ τάχος τῶν ἀσφαλιζόντων δύο μυῶν τοῦ πλείονας εἶναι, ἵνα τάχιστα ποιῶνται τὴν μύσιν καὶ ἐκφύγωσι τὴν βλάβην ἀπὸ τῶν προσπι⟨πτόντων⟩, κάρφου⟨ς⟩ λέγω καὶ κονιορτοῦ ἢ σμηγμάτων τινῶν ἢ ζῳυφίων καὶ τῶν τοιούτων. καὶ διὰ τὸ μόνιμον· κατά τινα γὰρ καιρὸν καὶ μονῆς δεῖται πρὸς τὸ εἶναι ἠσφαλισμένα τὰ βλέφαρα. καὶ ἀναγκαίως τοῦτο κατεσκευάσθη, ὥσπερ ἐν τοῖς ὕπνοις πᾶσα ἀνακωχὴ καὶ ἀνάπαυλα τῆς τε φύσεως καὶ τῶν ψυχικῶν δυνάμεων γίνεται διὰ τὸ ἐν τῷ ἐγρηγορέναι κάμνειν αὐτὰς καὶ κοπιᾶν. καὶ ταῦτα μὲν οὕτως.

Εἶτα καὶ ἀποροῦσί τινες ὅτι «Διὰ τί μὴ ἐν τῷ ἐγρηγορέναι ἐμνημόνευσε τοῦ τοιούτου σημείου, ἀλλ' ἐν τῷ καθεύδειν;» καὶ λέγομεν ὅτι ἐν τῷ ἐγρηγορέναι οὐ διαφαίνεται τοῦτο τὸ σημεῖον, διὰ τὸ πλεῖστον φέρεσθαι εἰς τοὺς ὀφθαλμοὺς τὸ ὀπτικὸν πνεῦμα. εἰ δὲ καὶ ἴδωμεν ὅτι ὑποφαίνεται, ὑπόγυον δηλοῖ τὸν θάνατον, ὅπερ καὶ οἱ ἰδιῶται διαγινώσκουσι τοῦτο. καὶ ἡμᾶς οὖν ὁ Ἱπποκράτης οὐ περὶ ὄντος καὶ ἤδη ἐνισταμένου θανάτου βούλεται διδάξαι, ἀλλὰ περὶ μέλλοντος, ἵνα προγινώσκοντες πρὸ πολλοῦ χρόνου ἀνεγκλήτους καὶ ἑαυτοὺς καὶ τὴν τέχνην φυλάξωμεν.

Εἶτα καὶ προσδιορισμοῖς κέχρηται, καὶ λέγει ὅτι ἐὰν μὴ ἐκ διαρροίας

3 συνίσταται ζ 4 αὐτὸν ζ 11 κλειστανοίκτους *coni. Wk.*: κλεῖς ἀνοικτοὺς γ 14 ἀντιστρέφον P: ἀντιστρέφει Y: ἀντιστρέφουσιν V 20 σφαλίζεσθαι P *post* βλέφαρα *iter.* κλείουσιν – σπασμὸς *(v. supra, linn. 2–5)* M 21 δὲ *om.* M 22 *post* χρώματα *fort. exciderunt* καὶ τὰ μεγέθη καὶ τὰ σχήματα *vel sim.* τῶν^{II} *om.* ζ 23 ἀναλαμβάνονται γ: *correxi* 24 εἰς *addidi* τῶν *om.* M τοῦ] τοὺς *codd.*: *corr. Wk.* 25 ποιοῦνται γ: *corr. Dietz* 25 sq. προσπικάρφου γ: *suppl. Dietz* 32 μὴ] μὲν M 40 προδιορισμὸν M

other at the small. These, then, are the (closing) muscles and they shut the lids by drawing them towards themselves and to the inside. It so happens, then, in that situation, that spasm occurs in the upper muscle, I mean the opener, and paralysis in the closers. When the upper muscle or the opener is convulsed, then, it draws the upper lid towards itself and part of the conjunctiva appears; for spasm pulls the part in the direction of its own source. In the case of the closers, too, the same happens and a portion of the conjunctiva shows through; here, however, the muscles are not convulsed but paralysed; for paralysis produces movement in the direction opposite of normal. When the closers, then, are paralysed the lids do not shut, but (the eyes) are kept open. Here again the conjunctiva can be seen, so that the eyes look half open and half shut. This is the situation in humans. Certain animals, on the other hand, do not possess the muscles which close the eyelids, but only have the openers. Whence it happens that when such animals sleep they turn the eyeballs into the sockets and the pupil itself is within the socket, to prevent injury from colliding objects. This is the case with antelopes, hares and certain types of fish. Another reason why there is one opening muscle is because it requires little time to open the lid, whereupon the closers immediately take over. But there are two closers and this for two reasons; first, to enable the lids to close quickly, because the eye is a sensitive part; it is sensitive in order to perceive easily the colors of small and large objects; for the eyes perceive by being acted upon. Because of this vulnerability, then, nature needed in the interest of speed more than one closer, i.e., two, so that they might make the closing in the shortest time and prevent injury from colliding objects, such as chaff, dust, soap, insects and so on. The second reason is stability; in order to remain closed for a certain length of time the eyelids need staying power. And this is a necessary provision; for example, after being worn out from activity during waking hours it is during sleep that nature and the psychic faculties get all their rest and relief. This is how these things are.

At this point the question is raised: "Why did he not give this symptom for the waking state, but (only) for sleep?" We reply that this symptom does not show in waking because of the great quantity of optic pneuma conveyed to the eyes. However, if we do see it appear it means imminent death, and this is something even laymen can diagnose. It is not Hippocrates' intention, then, to instruct us on death that has set in and is already taking place, but on death that is threatening, in order that by making the prognosis far ahead of time, we may keep both ourselves and the art free from blame.

Next he adds some qualifying remarks saying, unless the conjunctiva is visible because of diarrhoea or (the patient)

τινὸς ὑποφαίνηται ὁ ἐπιπεφυκὼς ἢ καὶ εἴθιστο οὕτως καθεύδειν· ἐὰν γὰρ διά τι τούτων ὑποφαίνηται ὁ ἐπιπεφυκώς, οὐκ ἔστι τοῦτο κινδυνῶδες, ἐπειδὴ ἀνακτώμεθα τὴν τοιαύτην διάθεσιν. ἔστι δ' ὅτε ὑπὸ γαστρορροίας φαίνεται τῇ κενώσει ξηρανθέντα τὰ βλέφαρα καὶ οὐ συμβάλλονται· καὶ τοῦτο ἀνακτώμεθα. πολλάκις δὲ εἴθιστο οὕτως καθεύδειν ὁ ἄνθρωπος, καὶ πολλοί εἰσιν ἐν τῷ κατὰ φύσιν οὕτως ἐξ ἔθους κοιμώμενοι ἀνεῳγότας ἔχοντες τοὺς ὀφθαλμούς, οὕστινας οἱ ἰδιῶται λέγουσι τὸ λαγωδάτον κοιμᾶσθαι. ἐὰν οὖν μὴ διὰ ταύτας τὰς αἰτίας φαίνηταί τι τοῦ ἐπιπεφυκότος ἐν τῷ καθεύδειν,
95 θα|νατῶδές ἐστι τὸ σημεῖον.

Εἶτα ἐπιβεβαιῶν τὴν τοιαύτην σημείωσιν τοῦ ὀλέθρου καὶ ἕτερα σημεῖα ἡμῖν παραδίδωσιν λέγων οὕτως· ἢν δὲ ῥικνὸν ἢ καμπύλον γένηται ἢ πελιὸν βλέφαρον ἢ χεῖλος ἢ ῥὶς μετά τινος τῶν ἄλλων σημείων. καὶ τὸ μὲν ῥικνόν ἐστιν ἔνδεια καὶ ἀτροφία μετὰ [ἐρ]ῥυτίδος, τουτέστι τὸ ἐρρυτιδωμένον μετὰ ἄκρας ξηρότητος· ἔστι γὰρ καὶ μετὰ ὑγρότητος [ἐρ]ῥυτίδωσις. ἐνταῦθα οὖν τὸ μετὰ ξηρότητος ἐρρυτιδωμένον ἐκάλεσε ῥικνόν.

Ἢ καμπύλον· καμπύλον λέγει τὸ ἑτερόρροπον· καὶ τοῦτο ὑπὸ ξηρότητος γίνεται ὡς ἐπίπαν. τὴν γὰρ διαστροφὴν λέγει τὸ καμπύλον, τυχὸν ἐὰν διαστραφῇ ἓν τούτων, ἢ ῥὶς τυχὸν ἢ χεῖλος ἢ βλέφαρα. διαστρέφονται δὲ εἴτε ἐπὶ σπασμῷ, τοῦ σπασμοῦ ἐπὶ ξηρότητι γινομένου, εἴτε διὰ παράλυσιν, ἥτις ἐπὶ ἄκρᾳ ψύξει γίνεται, καθ' ἣν καὶ τὸ πελιὸν γίνεται χρῶμα· ἐπὶ γὰρ ἄκρᾳ ψύξει καὶ τοῦτο γίνεται. ἐὰν οὖν καὶ ταῦτα γίνωνται τὰ σημεῖα μετὰ τῶν ἤδη προειρημένων συνερχόμενα, ὑπόγυον δηλοῦσι τὸν θάνατον. εἰ δὲ μόνα ταῦτα γένωνται, κακὰ μέν εἰσι, πλὴν οὐχ οὕτως κινδυνώδη.

VIII

I 37 [3: 197,4 A. = II 118,7 L.] Κεκλιμένον δὲ χρὴ καταλαμβάνεσθαι τὸν νοσέοντα ὑπὸ τοῦ ἰατροῦ ἐπὶ τὸ πλευρὸν τὸ δεξιὸν ἢ τὸ ἀριστερόν

Ἐνταῦθα σημειοῦται τὴν κατὰ φύσιν ἀνάκλισιν καὶ λέγει τρία σημεῖα, ἤγουν τρία σχήματα, τῆς κατὰ φύσιν κλίσεως. φησὶ γὰρ ὅτι ⟨πρῶτον⟩ σχῆμα κατακλίσεώς ἐστι τὸ ἐπὶ τὸ δεξιὸν ἢ τὸ ἀριστερὸν πλευρὸν κατακεκλίσθαι. δεύτερον σχῆμά ἐστιν, ὅτι δεῖ ἐπικεκαμμένα ἔχειν ὀλίγον τὰ σκέλη καὶ τὰς χεῖρας καὶ τὸν τράχηλον· ὅθεν καὶ τὸ ἐγγώνιον σχῆμα τῆς χειρὸς ἀποδεχόμεθα παρὰ τὸ ἄγαν ἐκτεταμένον ἢ συγκεκαμμένον,

7 τὸ – κοιμᾶσθαι] *cf.* Steph. Comm. in Hipp. Aph.: Escor. Σ. II. 10 fol. 268^{v} 18–20] *cf.* Gal. In Hipp. Progn. comm. I 12: CMG V 9,2 p. 226,18

1 ὑποφαίνεται ζ   ὁ] καὶ P   6 οὕτως *post* εἰσιν *trsp.* M   7 λεγωδάτον ζ   11 ἡμῖν *post* παραδίδωσιν *trsp.* M   δὲ] μὲν M   ῥικνὸν ἢ καμπύλον] *sic nullus test. Hipp.*   13 ἐρρυτίδος γ: *corr. Dietz*   14 γὰρ] δὲ P   ἐρρυτίδωσις γ: *correxi*   18 ἢ[I]] ἡ Pζ: *corr.* M   27 ἰητροῦ ζ   30 πρῶτον *addidi*   32 δεῖ] δὴ γ: *correxi*   ἐπικεκαυμένα γ: *corr. Dietz*   34 περὶ MP: *corr.* ζ   τεταμένων M   συγκεκαυμένον γ: *corr. Dietz*

usually sleeps in this way; for if the conjunctiva shows for one of these reasons it is not dangerous, since one can recover from such a condition. Sometimes in diarrhoea it shows, when the eyelids become dry due to the evacuation and do not close; but from this we recover. Again, it often happens that the patient is accustomed to sleeping in this manner and many healthy people have a habit of sleeping thus, keeping the eyes open; these are the ones who, in the layman's expression, sleep like the hare. If part of the conjunctiva, then, can be seen during sleep and not for one of these reasons, the symptom is fatal.

After this he gives us other signs to confirm the prognosis of death, saying, if, in addition to one of the other symptoms, eyelid, lip or nose becomes shrivelled, bent or livid. Shrivelled means wrinkled by deficiency and atrophy, in other words wrinkled with intense desiccation, there being also a wrinkling with moistness. So in this case by shrivelled he means wrinkled with dryness.

Or bent: By bent he means turned to one side, a condition brought about for the most part by desiccation. For he is using the word bent in the sense of distorted and is saying, if one of these, nose or lip or eyelid, is distorted. And they are distorted either by spasm, the spasm being produced by dryness, or by paralysis, which is caused by intense cold; paralysis is also responsible for the livid color; for this too occurs with extreme cold. If these symptoms, then, develop in conjunction with the ones already mentioned, they indicate that death is imminent. However, if they appear on their own, they are bad, but not so dangerous.

VIII

I 37 The doctor should come upon the patient reclining on his right or left side

Here he discusses the symptoms for the normal bed position and he gives us three signs, or three forms, of normal reclining. The first, he says, is that the patient should be lying on his right or left side. The second form is that in which the legs, arms and neck should be slightly bent; hence we find the angular form of the arm preferable to the overly stretched or folded, because in this posture the muscles

ἐπειδὴ ἐν τῷ ἐγγωνίῳ σχήματι ἐν ἀνέσει τυγχάνουσιν οἱ μύες. λέγει καὶ τρίτον σχῆμα κατὰ φύσιν, ὅτι δεῖ ἀντιπροσώπως ἀνακεκλίσθαι, καθ' ἣν
96 ποι|εῖται τὰς εἰσόδους ὁ ἰατρός. τί γάρ; ὅτι δύναται καὶ πρὸς τὰ ἐρωτώμενα ὑπὸ τοῦ ἰατροῦ πρὸς ἔπος ἀποκρίνασθαι καὶ δεόντως ἀπολογεῖσθαι.

Ἐφ' οἷς καὶ τὴν αἰτίαν τῶν τοιούτων κατακλίσεων, ὅτι κατὰ φύσιν εἰσί, λέγει ὁ Ἱπποκράτης τῷ ἐπιλογισμῷ χρώμενος ἐκ τοῦ φαινομένου. φησὶν οὕτως γὰρ καὶ οἱ πλεῖστοι τῶν ὑγιαινόντων κατακλίνονται. ἄρισται δέ εἰσι τῶν κατακλίσεων αἱ ὅμοιαι τῇσι τῶν ὑγιαινόντων. ὁ δὲ Γαληνὸς τῷ λογισμῷ κεχρημένος καὶ ἐξ αὐτῆς τῆς φύσεως τῶν πραγμάτων ὁρμώμενος λέγει ὅτι ταῦτα τὰ σχήματα τῆς κατακλίσεως κατὰ φύσιν εἰσί, καί φησιν ὅτι τὸ ἀντιπροσώπως τῷ ἰατρῷ κατακεκλίσθαι τὸν κάμνοντα, καθ' ἣν ποιεῖται τὰς εἰσόδους, καὶ ἐκεῖσε ἀποβλέπειν καὶ ἀναμένειν τὴν παρουσίαν τοῦ ἰατροῦ ἀγαθόν ἐστιν, ἐπειδὴ δηλοῖ ὅτι καλῶς διάκειται τὸν λογισμόν. καὶ ἀγαθόν ἐστιν, ὡς δηλοῖ τὸ τοῦ Ἱπποκράτους ἐν Ἀφορισμοῖς εἰρημένον· «Ἐν πάσῃ νούσῳ τὸ ἐρρῶσθαι τὴν διάνοιαν καὶ εὖ ἔχειν πρὸς τὰ πρόσφορα ἀγαθόν, τὸ δὲ ἐναντίον κακόν.» ἀλλὰ καὶ τὸ ἐπικεκαμμένας ἔχειν ἐπ' ὀλίγον τὰς χεῖρας καὶ τὸν τράχηλον καὶ τὰ σκέλη κατὰ φύσιν ἐστίν, ἐπειδὴ δηλοῖ ἐρρωμένην καὶ ἰσχυρὰν τὴν συνέχουσαν καὶ στηρίζουσαν καὶ συνδεσμοῦσαν τὴν συνεκτικὴν δύναμιν τοῦ ὅλου σώματος. τὸ δὲ τοιοῦτον σχῆμα καὶ μεταξύ ἐστι τῶν ὑπερβολικῶν σχημάτων καὶ δηλοῖ ἐν ἀνέσει τυγχάνοντας τοὺς μύας καὶ τὰ νεῦρα. ὑπερβολικὰ δὲ σχήματά εἰσι τὸ ἄγαν ἐκτεταμένας ἔχειν τὰς χεῖρας καὶ τὰ σκέλη καὶ οἷον ἐξεωσμένα⟨ς⟩ καὶ ⟨ἐκ⟩κεκαλυμμένα⟨ς⟩· δηλοῖ γὰρ παράλυσιν καὶ ἀκράτειαν τῶν μυῶν καὶ τῶν νεύρων. ἀλλὰ καὶ τὸ ἄγαν συγκεκαμμένας ἔχειν τὰς χεῖρας καὶ τὰ σκέλη ὑπερβολικὸν σχῆμά ἐστι καὶ κακόν· δηλοῖ γὰρ τάσιν τῶν νεύρων καὶ μυῶν, ὅθεν καὶ ὑγρὸν ἐκάλεσε τὸ μεταξὺ σχῆμα· ἔφη γὰρ καὶ τὸ σύμπαν σῶμα ὑγρὸν ἔχοντα κείμενον. ὑγρὸν δὲ ἐκάλεσε τὸ σχῆμα τοῦτο διὰ τὸ ὥσπερ τὰ ὑγρὰ οὐκ ἐκτείνονται καθάπερ τὸ ὕδωρ, οὕτως καὶ τὸ ἐπ' ὀλίγον ἐπικεκαμμένον σχῆμα οὐκ ἔχει ἐκτεταμένα τὰ νεῦρα ἢ τοὺς μύας, ἀλλ' ἐν ἀνέσει τυγχάνοντας.

97 Οὕτως σημειωσάμενος τὴν κατὰ φύσιν | κατάκλισιν τρέπεται καὶ ἐπὶ τὴν σημείωσιν τῆς παρὰ φύσιν κατακλίσεως καὶ λέγει ἑπτὰ σχήματα. καὶ πρῶτον σχῆμα λέγει τοιοῦτον, ὅτι ἐὰν ὕπτιος κεῖται ὁ ἄρρωστος ἐκτεταμένας ἔχων τὰς χεῖρας καὶ τὰ σκέλη, κακόν ἐστι· δηλοῖ γὰρ ἀκράτειαν καὶ ἀσθένειαν τῆς στηριζούσης καὶ κρατυνούσης τὸ σῶμα συνεκτικῆς δυνάμεως καὶ βλάβην τοῦ λογισμοῦ, εἰ μήτι ὅτι διὰ κακότητα ἢ τῦφον ἢ ὑπερηφάνειαν τυραννικῶς φερόμενος καὶ μηδ' ὅλως προσποιούμενος τὴν παρουσίαν τοῦ ἰατροῦ.

1 λέγει] *immo Galenus, v.* In Hipp. Progn. comm. I 13: CMG V 9,2 p. 227,16sq. 9–30] *cf.* Gal. In Hipp. Progn. comm. I 13: CMG V 9,2 pp. 227,13–228,20 15 ἐν Ἀφορισμοῖς] Hipp. Aph. II 33: IV p. 480,5sq. L.

1 *post* σχήματι *add.* τῆς χειρὸς M καὶ] δὲ P 6 τῶν ἐπιλογισμῶν γ: *corr. Dietz* 8 ἄριστα ζ τῇσι] τοῖς γ: *correxi* 12 ἀποβλέπων ... ἀναμένων γ: *corr. Dietz* 16 τὰς προσφορὰς *Hipp.* 22 ἐκτεταμμένον γ: *corr. Dietz* 23 καὶ[I] – 25 σκέλη *om.* M ἐξεασμένα καὶ κεκαλυμμένα Pζ: *correxi* 24 συγκεκαμμένον Pζ: *correxi* 34 ἔχειν MP: *corr.* ζ 35 κρατούσης ζ

are relaxed. For the third normal form he says that (the patient) should be facing the direction from which the doctor enters. Why? Because (this way) he can answer the doctor's questions directly and speak properly for himself.

Next, proceeding by inference from observation, Hippocrates gives the reason why these positions are normal. He says, *For this is how the majority of the healthy recline. And the best reclining postures are most like the positions of the healthy.* Galen, on the other hand, arguing from reason and basing himself on the very nature of things states that these reclining positions are normal and he says that it is a good sign when the patient lies facing the direction of the doctor's entrance, watching and waiting like that for the doctor's arrival, since it indicates that his mind is working well. And it is good, as is shown by what Hippocrates says in the Aphorisms, "In any disease it is a good sign if (the patient's) mind is sound and he likes what is given to him, the opposite is bad." It is normal for the arms, neck and legs to be slightly bent, for it means that the sustaining faculty of the whole body, which maintains, supports and holds it together, is healthy and strong. Such a posture is intermediate between the exaggerated positions and shows that the muscles and nerves are relaxed. The exaggerated are the positions where the arms and legs are excessively stretched and, so to say, extruded and uncovered; (which is bad,) since it means paralysis and loss of power in the muscles and nerves. To have the arms and legs extremely bent is also an exaggerated position and bad, indicating tension in the nerves and muscles; this is why he called the intermediate position *fluid*, saying *and the entire body in a fluid state*. He called this position *fluid* because, just as fluids, e.g. water, are not in a state of tension, likewise in the slightly bent position the nerves or muscles are not tensed but relaxed.

Having thus given the symptoms of the normal reclining position, he turns to the symptoms for the abnormal position and gives seven forms. The first form he gives is this, if the *patient lies supine with outstretched arms and legs*, it is bad; for it shows loss of power and weakness of the sustaining faculty which supports and controls the body, and impaired reasoning, unless (the patient) is acting contemptuously out of badness or conceit or arrogance, pretending that the doctor is not present at all.

Δεύτερον δὲ τὸ προπετῶς καταρρεῖν ἀπὸ τῆς κλίνης τὸν ἄρρωστον ἐπὶ πόδας. κακόν ἐστι καὶ τοῦτο σημεῖον· δηλοῖ γὰρ καὶ ἐνταῦθα ἀκράτειαν καὶ ἀσθένειαν τῆς κρατυνούσης καὶ στηριζούσης τὸ σῶμα συνεκτικῆς δυνάμεως καὶ ὑπ' αὐτῆς μηδ' ὅλως κατέχεσθαι, ἀλλὰ τῷ οἰκείῳ βάρει τῷ φυσικῷ ἐπὶ πόδας ἀντικαταρρεῖν, ὅπερ μέγιστον κακὸν σημεῖόν ἐστι.

Τρίτον σχῆμα τῆς παρὰ φύσιν κατακλίσεώς ἐστι τὸ ἀπογυμνοῦν τοὺς πόδας καὶ ἀσκεπάστους ἔχειν καὶ τὰς χεῖρας καὶ τὸν τράχηλον καὶ περιερριμμένους καὶ ἐκλελυμένους καὶ περιφερομένους τῆδε κἀκεῖσε. καὶ τοῦτο κακόν ἐστι τὸ σημεῖον ἐν ὀξεῖ νοσήματι· δηλοῖ γὰρ ἀλυσμόν, τουτέστι δυσφορίαν ἄκραν ἐν τῷ στομάχῳ, καὶ δακνομένου τοῦ στομάχου καὶ ἀνιωμένου ὑπὸ τῆς κακοχυμίας οὕτως κατακέκλιται, εἰ μήτι ὅτι διὰ βλακείαν τινὰ ἢ δι' ὀξὺν καὶ διακαῆ πυρετὸν ταῦτα ποιεῖ· τότε γὰρ δήλη ἐστὶν ἡ αἰτία, καθ' ἣν τοῦτο ποιεῖ, τοῦ καταψυχθῆναι καὶ παραμυθίαν καὶ παρηγορίαν ἀναλαβεῖν διὰ τὴν ζέσιν τοῦ πυρετοῦ. καὶ τοῦτο οὐκ ἔστι τοιοῦτον κακόν. εἰ δὲ μήτε διὰ τὸν πυρετὸν γυμνοῖ τοὺς πόδας μήτε μὴν διὰ βλακότητα καὶ ἦθος τοιοῦτον, τότε κάκιστόν ἐστι καὶ τοῦτο σημεῖον· δηλοῖ γὰρ ἢ παραφροσύνην ἢ μεγίστην δυσκρασίαν ἐν τῷ στομάχῳ.

Τέταρτον σχῆμα τῆς παρὰ φύσιν κατακλίσεως τὸ κεχηνότως καθεύδειν, ὅπερ δηλοῖ ἢ παράλυσιν τῶν κλειόντων μυῶν τὸ στόμα ἢ σπασμὸν τῶν ἀνοιγόντων, ὥσπερ καὶ ἐπὶ τῶν βλεφάρων ἐλέγομεν. ἀλλ' ἐπὶ τοῦ
98 ὀφθαλμοῦ ἧττον ἦν κακόν, ἐπειδὴ ἐν τοῖς | ὕπνοις αὐτὸ παρελάβομεν. ἐνταῦθα δὲ ἐν τῷ ἐγρηγορέναι αὐτὸ παραλαμβάνομεν· τὸ γὰρ καθεύδειν ἐνταῦθα τὸ ἀνακεκλίσθαι λέγει, οὐ τὸ ὑπνοῦν, ὅπερ κακόν ἐστι σημεῖον καὶ τοῦτο ἐν ὀξεῖ νοσήματι, εἴτε διὰ σπασμὸν γένηται εἴτε διὰ παράλυσιν εἴτε διὰ τὰ συναμφότερα.

Πέμπτον δέ, ἐὰν ὕπτιος ἀνακέκλιται καὶ κεκαμμένα ἔχει τὰ γόνατα καὶ ἀπερριμμένα ἀπ' ἀλλήλων ἤγουν συμπεπλεγμένα καὶ ἄγαν συγκεκαμμένα, τουτέστι τοὺς μηροὺς καὶ τὰ γόνατα ἐναλλὰξ παραπεπλεγμένα ἔχει καὶ ἐπὶ γαστέρα συγκεκαμμένα· κακόν ἐστι καὶ τοῦτο σημεῖον διὰ τὸ μὴ πάντῃ οὕτως εἰθίσθαι ἀνακεκλίσθαι τοὺς ἀνθρώπους ἐν τῷ ὑγιαίνειν· δηλοῖ γὰρ ἢ παραφροσύνην ἢ μεγίστην ὀδύνην τῶν περὶ τὴν γαστέρα χωρίων, φυσικῶς τοῦτο ποιοῦντες· συγκάμπτοντες γὰρ ἐπὶ τὴν γαστέρα τοὺς μηροὺς καὶ τὰ γόνατα τῇ προσψαύσει τοῦ ὁμοίου σώματος παρηγοροῦνται. οὕτως γὰρ καὶ ἡμεῖς ποιοῦμεν στροφούμενοι ἢ ὀδυνώμενοι πρός τι μόριον· τὰς χεῖρας ἐπιτιθέμενοι καὶ προσψαύοντες παρηγορούμεθα τῷ ὀδυνωμένῳ μορίῳ.

Ἕκτον δὲ τὸ ἐπὶ γαστέρα κεῖσθαι ἐν τῇ κλίνῃ· δηλοῖ γὰρ μεγάλην διάθεσιν τῶν περὶ τὴν γαστέρα χωρίων, ἐὰν μὴ οὕτως εἴθιστο κοιμᾶσθαι,

18–20] *cf.* Gal. In Hipp. Progn. comm. I 17: CMG V 9,2 p. 230,26sq. 18 κεχηνότως καθεύδειν] Hipp. Progn. 3: p. 197,14 A. = II p. 120,2sq. L. 20 ἐλέγομεν] *supra*, p. 88,2–10 37–96,3] *cf.* Gal. In Hipp. Progn. comm. I 19: CMG V 9,2 p. 232,1–5 37 ἐπὶ – κεῖσθαι] Hipp. Progn. 3: p. 198,1 A. = II p. 120,4 L.

5 καταρρεῖν M 6 περὶ P 18 *post* σχῆμα *add.* σημεῖον M κεχηνότας *coni. Dietz*: κεχηνότα *Hipp.* 21 περιελάβομεν γ: *correxi* 26 κεκαυμένα ζ: καυμένα M 27 ἀπ' – συμπεπλεγμένα *om.* M συγκεκαυμένα ζ 28 περιπεπλεγμένα P 30 ἔθιστο M 32 τὴν *om.* ζ 33 προψαύσει P

Second, if the patient sinks away without control from the bed towards his feet. This is also a dangerous symptom, pointing in this case as well to loss of power and weakness of the sustaining faculty which controls and supports the body; (it means that the body) is not controlled by it at all, but slips down to the feet under its own natural weight, which is an extremely dangerous sign.

The third form of abnormal position is to have the feet bared and the arms and neck uncovered, tossed about, scattered and flung around in disarray. And this is a bad symptom in acute disease; for it points to distress, i.e., severe distress in the stomach; (the patient) assumes this posture when his stomach is irritated and stung by the bad humor, provided he is not doing it as a stupid trick or because of acute burning fever; for then the reason is clear why he does it: to cool himself and get relief and alleviation on account of the seething heat of the fever. This is not so serious. However, if it is not due to fever or stupidity or some such disposition that he leaves his feet bare, then the symptom is very bad. For it betokens either delirium or very severe stomach distemper.

The fourth form of abnormal position is to rest with the mouth open; it indicates either paralysis of the mouth's closing muscles or spasm in the openers, just as we described in the case of the eyelids. But the symptom in the eye was not as serious, since we encountered it during sleep. Here, however, we find it in the waking state; for by to rest in the present instance he means to lie back (in the bed), not, to sleep; and this too is a bad sign in acute disease, whether the cause be spasm or paralysis or both together.

The fifth is if (the patient) lies on his back with the knees bent and thrown apart from one another or locked together and overly bent, that is, when his thighs and knees are interlocked and twisted up into the belly; it is an unfavorable sign, since healthy persons are never in the habit of lying thus; it indicates either delirium or severe pain in the areas around the belly, and they do this as a natural reaction; for by bending the thighs and knees towards the belly they get relief through rubbing against a similar body. We too do the same thing when suffering from colic or from pain in some part; we place our hands on the sore spot and ease the pain by rubbing.

The sixth is to lie in bed on the belly; (this is abnormal) for it means a severe condition in the parts around the belly, unless (the individual) is accustomed to sleeping thus, especially in digestion, since

καὶ μάλιστα εἰς τὰς πέψεις διὰ τὸ συνεργεῖσθαι πρὸς τὴν πέψιν. εἰ δὲ μὴ ὦσιν εἰθισμένοι οὕτως καθεύδειν, κάκιστόν ἐστι· δηλοῖ γὰρ οὐ μόνον μεγίστην ὀδύνην τῶν περὶ τὴν γαστέρα χωρίων, ἀλλὰ καὶ παραφροσύνην.

Ἕβδομον δέ ἐστι τὸ ἄφνω ἀνακαθέζεσθαι καὶ ἐξανίστασθαι καὶ ζητεῖν ἀπὸ τόπου ἐπὶ τόπον μετελθεῖν· κάκιστον σημεῖον ἐν ὀξεῖ πυρετῷ καὶ μάλιστα ἐπὶ τῶν περιπνευμονικῶν. ἡ γὰρ περιπνευμονία φλεγμονή ἐστι τοῦ πνεύμονος· ἐν οὖν τῇ τοιαύτῃ φλεγμονῇ δηλονότι καὶ πυρετὸς διακαὴς σύνεστιν. ἐν οὖν τῇ κατακλίσει οὐκ ἀντεισάγεται ὁ ἀρκῶν ἀὴρ καὶ πνεῦμα πρὸς τὸ ἐμψῦξαι, ἐπειδὴ συμπίπτει ὁ θώραξ ὡς ἐπὶ τὴν ῥάχιν καὶ ἀποστενοῦται·
99 καὶ ἐκβιαζόμενοι ἀνακαθέζονται, ἵνα τῇ εὐρυχωρίᾳ καὶ τῷ τοιούτῳ | σχήματι δαψιλέστερον πνεῦμα εἰσπνέωσιν, καὶ παραμυθοῦνται. ἐὰν οὖν ἐν ὀξεῖ νοσήματι αἰφνίδιον ἀνακαθέζωνται καὶ ἐξανίστανται, καὶ μάλιστα ἐν τῇ ἀκμῇ, ὅτε ὤφειλεν ἐν ἀνέσει τυγχάνειν — ἐν γὰρ τῇ ἀκμῇ ἀναπαύεται ἡ φύσις καὶ αἱ δυνάμεις, ἐπειδὴ κάμνουσιν ἐν τῇ ἀρχῇ καὶ ἐν τῇ ἀναβάσει —, ἐν τῇ ἀκμῇ ἐν ἀνέσει ὀφείλουσαι τυγχάνειν, ἐὰν ἐξανίστανται ἀθρόως, κάκιστόν ἐστι καὶ τοῦτο τὸ σημεῖον· δηλοῖ γὰρ μεγίστην φλόγωσιν καὶ ζέσιν καὶ σηπεδόνα ἐν τοῖς ἀναπνευστικοῖς μορίοις συνισταμένην.

Πρὸς τούτοις δὲ καὶ ἕτερον σημεῖον προστίθησι λέγων ὅτι κάκιστόν ἐστι σημεῖον ἐν ὀξεῖ νοσήματι τὸ τρίζειν τοὺς ὀδόντας· δηλοῖ γὰρ σπασμώδη διάθεσιν τῶν κροταφιτῶν καὶ σιαγονιτῶν μυῶν καὶ παραφροσύνην μεγίστην ἐν ὀξεῖ νοσήματι, χωρὶς εἰ μὴ εἴθιστο ἐκ παιδόθεν τρίζειν τοὺς ὀδόντας. πολλοὶ γὰρ οὕτως εἰσὶν εἰθισμένοι τρίζειν τοὺς ὀδόντας διὰ φυσικὴν ἀσθένειαν οὕτως κατασκευασθέντων τῶν σιαγονιτῶν μυῶν, καὶ λοιπὸν διὰ τὴν ἀκράτειαν τρίζουσι τοὺς ὀδόντας. ὥσπερ οὖν καὶ τοὺς ὀφθαλμοὺς ὁρῶμεν τρομωδῶς καὶ ἀτάκτως τῇδε κἀκεῖσε περιφερομένους ἐπί τινων ἐξ ἀρχῆς τοῦτο πάσχοντας, ὅπερ καὶ τοῦτο διὰ φυσικὴν ἀσθένειαν τῶν στηριζόντων μυῶν οὕτως κατασκευασθέντων γίνεται.

Εἶτα παρακατιὼν λέγει ὅτι ἀλλὰ προλέγειν ἐπ' ἀμφοῖν τὸν κίνδυνον. ποῖον λέγει ὅτι δεῖ προλέγειν ἐπ' ἀμφοτέρων τὸν κίνδυνον — ἰδοὺ γὰρ εἴρηκεν ὅτι θανατῶδες — ὡς ἂν τοῦ κινδύνου πλέον θανατωδεστάτου ὄντος; καὶ λέγομεν ὅτι δυνατόν ἐστι καὶ πρὸς τὰ ἄνω αὐτὸν ἐξηγήσασθαι καὶ πρὸς τὰ κάτω. καὶ πρὸς μὲν τὰ ἄνω οὕτως· ὅτι ἀμφοῖν ἔφη ὅτι, ἐὰν τρίζῃ τοὺς ὀδόντας καὶ ἀπειλῇ καὶ μελετᾶται γενέσθαι μανία, ἐπὶ ἀμφοτέρων δεῖ προλέγειν τὸν κίνδυνον· τὸ γὰρ τοῦ θανάτου παρεκτείνεται καὶ ἐπὶ τοῦ κινδύνου. καὶ ἵνα μὴ ταὐτολογήσῃ ἐν βραχεῖ χωρίῳ, διὰ τὸ θανατῶδες εἰπεῖν ἐπήγαγε τὸν κίνδυνον· καὶ ἐπὶ
100 ἀμφοτέρων παρεκτείνεται τὸ θανατῶδες. πρὸς δὲ τὰ | κάτω οὕτως δεῖ

4–17] *cf.* Gal. In Hipp. Progn. comm. I 20: CMG V 9,2 p. 232,10–21 18–27] *cf.* Gal. In Hipp. Progn. comm. I 21: CMG V 9,2 p. 233,3–25 28sq. ἀλλὰ – κίνδυνον] Hipp. Progn. 3: p. 198,7 A. = II p. 120,10sq. L. 30 θανατῶδες] Hipp. Progn. 3: 198,7 A. = II p. 120,10 L.

1 διὰ τὸ] δι' ἃς γ: *corr. Wk.* 5 *post* κάκιστον *add.* ἐστι P 6 περιπνευμονία] περιπνεύμονος γ: *corr. Dietz* 7 *post* σύνεστιν *add.* ἐν οὖν τῇ τοιαύτῃ κατακλίσει δηλονότι καὶ πυρετὸς διακαὴς σύνεστιν L 14 κάμνωσιν LPζ: *corr.* M 16 φλόγωσιν] φλεγμονὴν L 19 σημεῖον *om.* γ 20 μεγίστην *om.* γ 28 *post* Εἶτα *add.* καὶ γ 29 ὅτι – κίνδυνον *om.* L 30 θανατωδέστατον L 33 γενέσθαι *om.* L 36 εἰπὼν *codd.*: *correxi*

(those parts) contribute to coction. But if this is not the usual way of sleeping, it is a very bad sign, signalling not only severe pain in the parts around the belly, but delirium as well.

The seventh is sudden rising and sitting up (in the bed) and wanting to change from place to place; this is a very bad sign when there is acute fever and especially in cases of pneumonia. For pneumonia is inflammation of the lungs and the inflammation is obviously accompanied by burning fever. In lying down, then, sufficient air and pneuma for cooling are not introduced, since the chest sinks towards the spine and is restricted; so in their plight they sit up in order to inhale a larger supply of air with the help of the wider space which this position affords, and they are alleviated. In an acute disease, then, if they suddenly raise themselves and sit up (in the bed), especially at the crisis, when (the body) ought to be relaxed – for during crisis nature and the faculties take a rest, being hard pressed in the beginning and during the heightening –, if during crisis they raise themselves suddenly, when nature and the faculties should be relaxing, it is a very dangerous symptom; for it means serious inflammation, seething heat and putrefaction in the respiratory parts.

To these he adds yet another symptom stating that in acute disease to grind the teeth is a very serious sign; for it shows a convulsive condition in the temporal and jawbone muscles and severe delirium in acute disease, provided that (the patient) has not had the habit of grinding the teeth from childhood. For there are many who in this way habitually grate their teeth, the jawbone muscles being thus disposed by an innate weakness, and so they grate the teeth due to the debility. In the same way we see some people who are born with eyes that tremble and move about without control; this, too, is caused by a natural weakness, the stabilizing muscles having been made thus.

Then he goes on to say, *But we must forecast danger from both.* Why does he say *we must forecast danger from both* – for he already said that it is *deadly* – as if danger were more than very deadly? We say that it is possible to explain him in relation to both his preceding and succeeding statements. In terms of what precedes: he says *both* in the sense that if (the patient) grinds his teeth and madness threatens and prepares to develop, we must forecast danger from both, the idea of death going hand in hand with that of danger. But seeing that he has already used the word *deadly*, he says *danger* here in order to avoid repetition within a short space; and the notion of deadliness extends to both. We should relate (the sentence) to what

συνάψαι, ἐπειδὴ γὰρ παρακατιὼν λέγει ἢν δὲ καὶ παραφρονέων τοῦτο ποιέῃ, ὀλέθριον κάρτα ἤδη γίνεται, τουτέστι τὸ τρίζειν τοὺς ὀδόντας.

Καὶ ἴσως ἐρεῖ τις ὅτι «Τί δήποτε καὶ ἄνω μανίαν εἶπε καὶ πάλιν ἐνταῦθα παραφρονέων τοῦτο ποιέει ὡς ἂν τῆς μανίας οὐκ οὔσης παραφορᾶς, καίτοι ἐπιτεταμένη παραφορά ἐστιν ἡ μανία; ταὐτολογεῖ οὖν.» καὶ λέγομεν ὅτι οὐ ταὐτολογεῖ· ἀνωτέρω μὲν γὰρ μελετωμένην ὑπέθετο τὴν μανίαν, οὔπω δὲ γενομένην. καὶ ἔλεγεν ὅτι, ἐὰν τρίζῃ τοὺς ὀδόντας καὶ μανία μελετᾶται γενέσθαι, ἐπ' ἀμφοτέρων δεῖ προλέγειν τὸν κίνδυνον· ἐνταῦθα οὖν λέγει ὅτι, ἐὰν τρίζῃ τοὺς ὀδόντας καὶ παραφρονῇ, ⟨ὀλέθριον⟩ κάρτα ἤδη γίνεται, τουτέστιν ὅτι πλησίον ἐστὶν ὁ θάνατος.

I 38 [3: 197,4 A. = II 118,7 L.] Κεκλιμένον δὲ χρὴ καταλαμβάνεσθαι τὸν νοσέοντα καὶ τὰ ἑξῆς

Τινὲς λέγουσι νομοθετεῖν ἐνταῦθα τὸν Ἱπποκράτην τὸ ἀμηνυτὶ καὶ ἀπροόπτως καὶ ἀπὸ ταὐτομάτου εἰσιέναι τὸν ἰατρὸν εἰς τοὺς κάμνοντας, ὥστε μὴ γινώσκοντας ποιεῖσθαι τὰς ἐπισκέψεις, ὡς δηλοῖ τὸ εἰπεῖν αὐτὸν κεκλιμένον δὲ χρὴ καταλαμβάνεσθαι τὸν νοσέοντα ὑπὸ τοῦ ἰητροῦ, ὅτι τυχὸν ἀμηνυτὶ καὶ μὴ γινώσκοντος τοῦ ἀρρώστου δεῖ ποιεῖσθαι τὴν ἐπίσκεψιν καὶ οἷον καταλαμβάνειν αὐτὸν μὴ γινώσκοντα μήτε μεταχειρισάμενον αὐτόν· οὕτως γὰρ ἀμηνυτὶ εἰσερχομένου τοῦ ἰατροῦ, μεγάλην τιμὴν καὶ δόξαν ἑαυτῷ καὶ τῇ τέχνῃ χαρίζεται. κακῶς δὲ λέγουσιν οὗτοι· τοὐναντίον γάρ· ὁ γὰρ Ἱπποκράτης οὐ παρακελεύεται τὸν ἰατρόν, ἵνα ἀμηνυτὶ ποιῆται τὴν ἐπίσκεψιν. τί γάρ; ὅτι πολλάκις πράγματά τινα μυστηριώδη ἔχουσι καὶ διαπράττονται καὶ οὐ θέλουσιν, ἵνα γνῷ ὁ ἰατρός. καὶ τί λέγω ὁ ἰατρός; ἀλλ' οὐδὲ ἀναγκαῖον αὐτοῦ συγγενῆ ἢ φίλον θέλει ἵνα γνῶσι τὰ μυστήρια ἅπερ διαπράττεται ὁ νοσῶν. ἀμηνυτὶ γὰρ εἰσερχομένου τοῦ ἰατροῦ, ὡς οὗτοι ὑπέθεντο, ἀτιμίαν προσάγομεν καὶ τῇ τέχνῃ καὶ ἑαυτοῖς
101 καὶ φορτικοὶ γινόμεθα | τοῖς ἀρρώστοις καὶ μισούμεθα ὑπ' αὐτῶν. ἀλλὰ τοὐναντίον δεῖ ποιεῖν. λέγει ὁ Ἱπποκράτης ὅτι μετὰ εἰδήσεως καὶ γνώσεως τοῦ ἀρρώστου εἰσιέναι δεῖ τὸν ἰατρὸν καὶ ποιῆσαι τὴν ἐπίσκεψιν, ἐπειδὴ οὕτως ποιούντων ἡμῶν καὶ εἰσιόντων, μεγάλην τιμὴν καὶ ἑαυτοῖς καὶ τῇ τέχνῃ προσάγομεν, ὅτι προευτρεπίζεται δεόντως ὁ νοσῶν καὶ ἐκδέχεται μετὰ μεγάλης τιμῆς τὴν παρουσίαν τοῦ ἰατροῦ, ὅπερ ὡς εἴρηται μεγάλην τιμὴν προσάγει τῇ τέχνῃ, τὸ μετὰ εἰδήσεως καὶ γνώσεως τῶν καμνόντων εἰσιέναι τὸν ἰατρὸν καὶ ποιεῖσθαι τὴν ἐπίσκεψιν. ἀλλὰ καὶ σημεῖον ἡμῖν

1sq. ἢν – γίνεται] Hipp. Progn. 3: p. 198,7sq. A. = II pp. 120,11–122,1 L. 4–11] *cf.* Gal. In Hipp. Progn. comm. I 21: CMG V 9,2 p. 234,8–27

2 ποιέει γ 2 sq. τουτέστι – ὀδόντας] τυχὸν τὸ τρίζειν τοὺς ὀδόντας *ante* ὀλέθριον *(lin. 2) trsp.* γ 4 τίς ἐρεῖ γ 5 οὐκ οὔσης] ἀκούσης γ 6 μανία] παραφροσύνη L 7 λέγομεν *scripsi*: ἔλεγεν *codd.* ὅτι *om.* L ὑπέσχετο γ 8 ἔλεγεν *scripsi*: λέγομεν *codd.* 9 ἀμφότερα γ 10 παραφρονεῖ Mζ: *corr.* P: *ambig.* L 11 ὀλέθριον *addidi* 12 χρὴ καταλαμβάνεσθαι *om.* L 17 κεκλιμένον δὲ *om.* γ 18 ἰατροῦ γ 21 ἑαυτὸν καὶ τὴν τέχνην L 23 ποιῆται *ex* -ῆσαι, *ut vid.*, *corr.* L: ποιεῖται MV: ποιῆσαι P 24 sq. ἵνα – θέλει *om.* γ 27 καὶ[I] *om.* γ καὶ ἑαυτοῖς *om.* γ 30 καὶ ποιῆσαι] πρὸς γ 33 sq. ὅπερ ... τὸ] ᾧπερ ... τῷ *coni. Dietz* 34 προσάγομεν *codd.*: *correxi*

comes afterwards because he goes on to say, And if he does this, i.e., grinds his teeth, after delirium has developed, it is an extremely deadly sign.

But someone may say, "Why did he say mania above and here again if he does this after delirium has developed, as if mania were not delirium, when in fact mania is an intense form of delirium. He is repeating himself then." But we say no; for in the first instance he is speaking of the mania as threatening but not yet developed. And he said that if (the patient) grinds his teeth and mania threatens, we must forecast danger from both; here, on the other hand, he tells us that if (the patient) grinds his teeth and he is delirious, it is very deadly, in other words, death is imminent.

I 38 (The doctor) should come upon the patient reclining etc.

Some claim that Hippocrates is laying down a rule here that the visits of the doctor to his patients should be unannounced, unexpected and impromptu, so that he can see them without their knowing it, as is shown by his saying, The doctor should come upon the patient reclining, that is, he must make his inspection sudden and without the patient's knowledge, and, as it were, catch him unawares and unprepared; for, by entering thus without warning, the doctor will gain great honor and reputation for himself and the art. But these people are wrong; Hippocrates means the opposite, for he is not advising the doctor to make the inspection unannounced. Why? Because (patients) often have private matters to see to and they do not want the doctor to know. But why do I say the doctor? A sick person does not wish even a relative or friend to be aware of his personal affairs. By coming without warning, as these people suggest, we doctors give the art and ourselves a bad reputation, we make nuisances of ourselves to the patients and are hated by them. The opposite is the proper procedure. Hippocrates says that the doctor should enter and make inspection with the patient's knowledge and awareness, since by acting and entering in this way we bring great honor on both ourselves and the art, because the patient is properly prepared in advance and receives the doctor with much respect; and this, as we have remarked, brings great honor on the art, namely entering and inspecting with the awareness and knowledge of the patients. As well, it gives us an indication of how the patient's

καθίσταται τὸ πῶς διάκειται ὁ κάμνων περὶ τὴν ἔννοιαν καὶ τὸν λογισμόν· ἐὰν γὰρ μετὰ εἰδήσεως αὐτοῦ ποιήσηται ὁ ἰατρὸς τὴν ἐπίσκεψιν, σχηματίζει ἑαυτὸν δεόντως καὶ κατὰ φύσιν, ὅπερ σημεῖόν ἐστι τοῦ καλῶς ἐνεργεῖν τὸν λογισμόν.

Τὸ δὲ καταλαμβάνεσθαι ἀντὶ τοῦ εὑρίσκεσθαι ἐν τῷ κατὰ φύσιν σχήματι τὸν κάμνοντα ὑπὸ τοῦ ἰατροῦ ἔφη ὁ Ἱπποκράτης. διὰ τί δὲ ἔφη ἐπὶ τὸ πλευρὸν τὸ δεξιὸν ἢ τὸ ἀριστερὸν καὶ μόνου τοῦ ἑνὸς πλευροῦ οὐκ ἐμνημόνευσεν, ἀλλὰ τῶν δύο; καὶ λέγομεν τούτου δύο αἰτίας. πρῶτον μὲν τοιαύτην, ὅτι ἐπειδὴ κοπιῶδές ἐστι καὶ μοχθηρὸν τὸ ἐπὶ τὸ ἓν πλευρὸν ἀείσε καὶ ἐπιμόνως ἀνακεκλίσθαι οὐ μόνον ἐπὶ τῶν νοσούντων, ἀλλὰ καὶ ἐπὶ τῶν ὑγιαινόντων, ἀλλὰ ποτὲ μὲν ἐπὶ τὸ δεξιόν, ποτὲ δὲ ἐπὶ τὸ ἀριστερὸν ἀνακεκλίσθαι, ἄλλοτε ὕπτιοι, καὶ διὰ τοῦτο τῶν δύο σχημάτων ἐμνημόνευσε, λέγω δὴ τῶν δύο πλευρῶν. αὕτη πρώτη αἰτία. δευτέρα δὲ αἰτία ἐστίν, ὅτι οὐ πάντες ἐπὶ τῷ δεξιῷ πλευρῷ ἀείσε ἀνακεκλιμένοι οἱ κάμνοντες εὐαρμόστως ἔχουσιν, ὥστε ἀντιπροσώπως κεῖσθαι ἐν ᾧ τὴν ἐπίσκεψιν ποιεῖται ὁ ἰατρός, ἀλλὰ ποτὲ μὲν ἐπὶ τὸ δεξιὸν κείμενοι πλευρὸν ἀντιπροσώπως εὑρίσκονται ⟨ὑπὸ⟩ τοῦ ἰατροῦ, ποτὲ δὲ ἐπὶ τὸ ἀριστερόν, ἄλλοτε δὲ ὕπτιοι. πολλάκις οὖν ἀπέστραπται καὶ γινώσκων, ὅτι ἐμήνυσεν ὁ ἰατρός, σχηματίζει ἑαυτὸν
102 ἀντιπροσώπως ὥστε δεόντως τὰς ἐντεύ|ξεις καὶ ἀνταποκρίσεις ποιήσασθαι ὡς πρὸς τὰ ἐπερωτώμενα ὑπὸ τοῦ ἰατροῦ. καὶ διὰ τοῦτο τῶν δύο ἐμνημόνευσε πλευρῶν.

IX

I 39 [3: 198,9 A. = II 122,1 L.] Ἕλκος δέ, ἤν τε καὶ προγεγονὸς τύχῃ ἔχων ἤν τε καὶ ἐν τῇ νούσῳ γίνοιτο, καταμανθάνειν χρή. ἢν γὰρ μέλλῃ ἀπολεῖσθαι ὁ ἄνθρωπος, πρὸ τοῦ θανάτου ἢ πελιδνὸν καὶ ξηρὸν ἔσται ἢ ὠχρόν τε καὶ ξηρόν.

Φησὶν ὅτι δεῖ σκοπεῖν, ἐὰν ἕλκος προγεγονὸς εἶχεν ὁ ἄρρωστος ἢ ἐν αὐτῇ τῇ νούσῳ οὐ πρὸ πολλοῦ γέγονε. καὶ εἰ μὲν ἄνικμον πάντῃ ἐστὶ καὶ κατάξηρον τὸ ἕλκος, γίνωσκε ὅτι ὅσον οὔπω θνήσκει ὁ ἄνθρωπος. καὶ λέγουσί τινες ὅτι «Τί φής, ὦ Ἱππόκρατες; οὐκ αὐτὸς εἶπας· 'Ἕλκεα ξύμπαντα οὐ δεῖ ἐπιτέγγειν πλὴν οἴνῳ', τουτέστιν ὅτι δεῖ ξηρότερα εἶναι τὰ ἕλκη ὥστε ἀπουλωθῆναι αὐτά; πῶς οὖν ἐνταῦθα διαβάλλεις λέγων ὅτι, ἐὰν ἄνικμα καὶ ξηρά εἰσι τὰ ἕλκη, ἐγγὺς ὁ θάνατος;» καὶ λέγομεν ὅτι ἐκεῖσε ξηρὰ ἔλεγεν, ἵνα ἄνευ περιττωματικῆς τινος ὑγρότητος καὶ ἐπιρροῆς ἔσωνται, ἐπειδὴ ἡ πλαδαρὰ σὰρξ ἑτοιμόφθαρτός ἐστι. καὶ οὐκ ἄγονται εἰς οὐλὴν τὰ ἕλκη. ἐπεί τοί γε οὐ πάντῃ λέγει ἄνικμα εἶναι τὰ ἕλκη — ἐπεὶ πῶς ἔχουσι

30 αὐτὸς εἶπας] Hipp. De ulc. 1: VI p. 400,1 L.

5 ἐν] ἂν L   6 ἰατροῦ *om.* γ   9 ὅτι *om.* L   τὸ[II] *om.* L   10 καὶ ἐπιμόνως *om.* L   κατακεκλίσθαι L   οὐ μόνον — 11 ὑγιαινόντων *om.* L   12 ἀνακεκλίσθαι *post* δεξιόν *(lin. 11) trsp.* γ   13 δὲ *om.* Μζ   16 κείμενον γ   πλευρὸν *post* δεξιὸν *trsp.* γ   17 ὑπὸ *addidi*   δὲ[II] *om.* L   18 οὖν] δὲ γ   19 ἀποκρίσεις L   ποιήσηται γ   20 ὡς *om.* γ   23 προσεγόνει L   24 ἤν τε — 26 ξηρόν *om.* γ   γένηται *aut* γίνηται *codd. Hipp.*   28 νόσω γ   29 ὅτι *om.* L; *cf. supra, p. 14*   30 ὅτι *om.* L   31 οἴνου *codd.*: *sec. Hipp. correxi*   33 ἐκεῖ γ   34 ἵνα] ὅτι γ

mind and reason are working; for if the doctor makes the inspection with his knowledge, he arranges himself in a proper and normal position, which means that his faculty of reason is functioning well.

When he said come upon Hippocrates meant that the doctor should find the patient in the normal position. But why did he say on the right or left side, mentioning both instead of one? We give two reasons for this. First, since to lie on one side all the time and continuously is tiring and distressing not only for the sick but for the healthy as well, they lie sometimes on the right, sometimes on the left and at other times in a supine position; and this is why he mentioned the two forms, that is to say, the two sides. This is the first reason. The other is that not all those patients who always recline on the right side are in the correct position to be facing the doctor when he makes his inspection; no, sometimes they will be found to face the doctor when reclining on the right, sometimes when on the left and sometimes when they are on their backs. It often happens, then, that (the patient) is turned the other way, and learning that the doctor has announced his arrival he arranges himself to be facing him, in order to respond properly and answer the doctor's questions. This explains why he speaks of both sides.

IX

I 39 If (the patient) had a sore beforehand or if one develops during the disease, you must observe it closely. For if the patient is going to die, before death it will be either livid and dry or greenish and dry.

He says that if the patient had a sore beforehand or if one recently developed during the disease itself, you must examine this. If the sore has no moisture at all and is completely dry, you may conclude that the person will die very soon. Here some say, "What do you mean Hippocrates? Have you yourself not said, 'No sore should be moistened except with wine', in other words, that sores have to be on the dry side in order to heal? So why do you consider it a bad sign here, saying that if sores are dry and without moisture, death is at hand?" We say that he said dry there to mean that they should be free of all superfluous moisture and flux, since damp flesh decomposes easily and sores fail to cicatrize. However, he does not state that sores must be absolutely

σαρκωθῆναι καὶ ἀφουλωθῆναι; –, ἀλλὰ δεῖ χρηστὴν ὑγρότητα ἔχειν τὰ ἕλκη. ἐνταῦθα δὲ τὰ ἄνικμα πάνυ καὶ κατάξηρα διαβάλλει, ἅτινα δηλοῦσι μεγίστην καταβολὴν καὶ ἀσθένειαν τῶν φυσικῶν δυνάμεων καὶ μεγάλην ἔνδειαν καὶ ἀτροφίαν, ὅπερ χαλεπόν ἐστιν ἐν ὀξεῖ νοσήματι καὶ θανατῶδες. ἀλλὰ δεῖ, φησί, καὶ τὸ χρῶμα τοῦ ἕλκους σκοπεῖν· δυνατὸν γὰρ ἐκ τοῦ χρώματος τοῦ ἐν τῷ ἕλκει διαγνῶναι τὸν πλεονάζοντα χυμόν, ἐν ᾧ ὁ κίνδυνος ἐπακολουθεῖ. εἰ μὲν γὰρ χολή ἐστιν ἡ πλεονάζουσα, ὠχρὸν γίνεται τὸ ἕλκος, τουτέστιν ἰῶδες· τὸ δὲ πελιδνὸν καὶ μέλαν χρῶμα νεκρώσεώς εἰσι δηλωτικά. καὶ λέγουσί τινες ὅτι «Τί δήποτε ἀπὸ τοῦ ἐν ὅλῳ τῷ σώματι χρώματος οὐκ ἐσημειώσατο, ἀλλ' ἀπὸ τοῦ ἐν τῷ ἕλκει;» καὶ λέγομεν τούτου
103 δύο αἰτίας, μίαν μὲν τοιαύτην, ὅτι αἱ | σάρκες ἐρυθραί εἰσιν, ἐπὶ δὲ τοῦ ἕλκους γυμναὶ οὖσαι, ἑτοίμως διαφαίνεται τὸ χρῶμα. δευτέρα δὲ αἰτία, ὅτι, ἔνθα τὸ ἕλκος ἐστί, πάντως ἀσθενέστερόν ἐστιν ἐκεῖνο τὸ μόριον· ἐν οὖν τῷ ἀσθενεστέρῳ μορίῳ μᾶλλον γίνεται ἐπιρροὴ τοῦ πλεονάζοντος χυμοῦ· καὶ ἐντεῦθεν ἐν τῷ ἕλκει σαφῶς διαφαίνεται καὶ τὸ χρῶμα, ὅπερ θανατῶδές ἐστι σημεῖον. καὶ διὰ τοῦτο ἀπὸ τοῦ ἐν τῷ ἕλκει χρώματος τὴν σημείωσιν ἐποιήσατο.

Δεύτερόν ἐστι κεφάλαιον, ἐν ᾧ περὶ χειρῶν φορᾶς καὶ κινήσεως διαλέγεται. καί φησιν ὅτι, ἐὰν τὰς χεῖρας περιφέρωσιν ὡς ἐπὶ τὸν ἀέρα ἢ καὶ παρὰ τὸ πρόσωπον καὶ δοκοῦσι ζῳύφιά τινα θηρᾶν ἢ καρφολογεῖν ἢ κροκύδας ἀνασπᾶν ἀπὸ τῶν ἱματίων ἢ ἄχυρα ἐκ τοῦ τοίχου δοκοῦσιν ἀφαιρεῖν, κάκιστόν ἐστιν ἐν ὀξεῖ πυρετῷ καὶ ἐν περιπνευμονίᾳ καὶ ἐν φρενίτιδι καὶ ἐν κεφαλαλγίᾳ· δηλοῖ γὰρ τὴν ὁρατικὴν αἴσθησιν ἀπατωμένην περὶ αἰσθητά τινα νομιζόμενα εἶναι, οὐκ ὄντα δέ. τὴν δὲ αἰτίαν, καθ' ἣν ἀπατᾶται ἡ ὁρατικὴ δύναμις εἰς τὰ τοιαῦτα φαντάσματα, λέγει ὁ Γαληνός, ὅτι ἡ ἀπάτη γίνεται διὰ δύο αἰτίας· ἢ γὰρ κατὰ πρωτοπάθειαν ἢ ἰδιοπάθειαν αὐτῶν τῶν ὀφθαλμῶν οὕτως ὡς ἐπὶ τῶν ὑποχεομένων· ἐπὶ γὰρ τῶν ὑποχυμάτων πολλάκις δι' ἀτονίαν τῆς ὁρατικῆς δυνάμεως ὑγρόν τι ἀθροίζεται μεταξὺ τῆς κόρης καὶ τοῦ ᾠοειδοῦς ὑγροῦ· τὸ δὲ κρυσταλλοειδὲς οὐκέτι λαμπρὰν καὶ ἀκραιφνῆ ποιεῖται τὴν ἐνέργειαν, ἀλλ' ἀμαυροῖ αὐτοῦ τὴν ἐνέργειαν καὶ τὴν ὁρατικὴν δύναμιν μολύνει. καὶ τούτων οὕτως γινομένων ἀπατῶνται περὶ τὴν ὅρασιν καὶ ὅπερ ἐντός ἐστι πάθος, δοκοῦσι κατὰ ἀπάτην ἔξω ὁρᾶν αὐτό· τῆς γὰρ ὁρατικῆς δυνάμεως προσπιπτούσης τῷ ὑγρῷ ἐκείνῳ, ἔνθα τὸ μὲν ᾠοειδὲς ὡς εἴρηται ἐπαχύνθη, τὸ δὲ κρυσταλλοειδὲς ἠμαυρώθη, λοιπὸν δὲ καὶ ἡ ὁρατικὴ δύναμις ἐμολύνθη προσπίπτουσα ἐντὸς καὶ παρ' αὐτῷ τῷ ὑγρῷ, καὶ τῷ πάθει τῷ ἐντὸς ἐνεργοῦσα, ἀπατω-
104 μένη δοκεῖ ἔξω ὁρᾶν αὐτό, καὶ διὰ τοῦτο δοκοῦσι | ζῳύφιά τινα θηρᾶν ἢ

7–9] *cf.* Gal. In Hipp. Progn. comm. I 22: CMG V 9,2 p. 235,8–12   18 περὶ – 23 κεφαλαλγίᾳ] Hipp. Progn. 4: p. 199,1–5 A. = II p. 122,5–9 L.   25 ὁ Γαληνός] Gal. In Hipp. Progn. comm. I 23: CMG V 9,2 p. 236,1–17

2 ἄνικμα πάνυ] ἄγαν ἄνικμα γ   8 πέλιον γ   13 ἐστιν *om.* γ   15 καὶ *scripsi*: κατὰ *codd.*   16 τοῦτο ἀπὸ *bis scr.* L   ἐν τῷ *om.* L   18 ἐστι *om.* L   19 περιφέρουσι(ν) Pζ   22 περιπνεύμονι γ   24 νομιζομένην γ   26 sq. ἰδιοπάθειαν ἢ πρωτοπάθειαν γ   29 ὠειδοῦς γ: ἀειδοῦς L: *corr. Dietz*   33 *ante* τῷ *add.* ἐν γ   34 ὠειδὲς γ   35 δύναμις αὕτη P: αὕτη δύναμις ζ

dry – (otherwise) how could they receive flesh to heal over?–, but sores should contain useful moisture. In the present case, on the other hand, he considers it an unfavorable symptom for sores to be extremely dry and lacking moisture; they indicate severe collapse and weakness of the natural faculties as well as serious lack of nutriment and atrophy, which is dangerous and deadly in acute disease. We must, he tells us, examine also the sore's color; for it is possible from the color of the sore to identify the superfluous humor responsible for the danger. If the superfluity is bile, the sore turns greenish, that is to say, verdigris; livid and black colors, on the other hand, point to mortification. Here the question is posed, "Why did he make the observations, not from the color of the whole body, but from that of the sore?" We give two reasons for this; first, flesh is red and, since it is exposed during ulceration, the color readily shows through. The second reason is that, where the sore is located, that part is necessarily weaker; the weaker part, then, is more subject to an influx of superfluous humor; hence the color shows through clearly in the sore, which is a deadly symptom. This is why he based the observation on the color in the sore.

In a second chapter he discusses the behavior and movement of the hands. If (the patients), he tells us, wave their hands in the air or around the face and think that they are chasing insects or picking up bits and pieces (from the bed) or plucking nap from the blankets or chips from the wall, it is very dangerous in acute fever, pneumonia, phrenitis and headache; it shows that the optic faculty has been deceived about perceiving certain objects which it thinks exist, but which in fact do not. Galen gives the reason why the faculty of sight is deluded by visions of this sort and the deception has two causes: it may be due to a primary or peculiar affection of the eyes themselves, as in cataracts; for frequently in cataracts a fluid accumulates between the pupil and the ovoid humor because the optic faculty has lost its tone; (as a result) the crystalline humor no longer functions clearly and purely, but (the fluid) obscures its action and taints the optic faculty. When this happens they are deluded in their vision, and whatever affection occurs inside, they are misled to believe that they see it outside; for when the optic faculty comes into contact with that fluid, in which the ovoid humor, as we noted, is thickened and the crystalline is obscured, then the optic faculty, too, is tainted when it encounters the fluid itself internally and, functioning on the internal sensation, it is deceived and imagines that it is seeing it outside; so this explains why (the patients) believe that they are chasing insects or

καρφολογεῖν καὶ τὰ λοιπά. καὶ οὕτως μὲν κατὰ πρωτοπάθειαν. ἀλλὰ καὶ κατὰ συμπάθειαν τοῦτο γίνεται, ἀλλὰ διχῶς· ἢ γὰρ ἐν ὅλῳ τῷ σώματι οὔσης τῆς κακοχυμίας τοῦτο γίνεται ἢ ἐν αὐτῷ τῷ ἐγκεφάλῳ. καὶ εἰ μὲν ἐν ὅλῳ τῷ σώματί ἐστιν ἡ κακοχυμία, ἀναπέμπονται παχέα πνεύματα ἀπὸ τῆς κακοχυμίας ἐπὶ τὴν κεφαλήν· εἶτα φέρονται ἐπὶ τὰ ὀπτικὰ νεῦρα καὶ ἐπὶ αὐτοὺς τοὺς ὀφθαλμούς· εἶτα ταῦτα τὰ παχέα φερόμενα προσαναλύουσι, καὶ ἐντεῦθεν ὑγρά τινα ἐρχόμενα προστίθενται τῷ ᾠοειδεῖ καὶ ἀμαυροῦσι τὸ κρυσταλλοειδὲς καὶ τὴν ὁρατικὴν καὶ ὀπτικὴν δύναμιν μολύνουσι, καὶ γίνεται ταῦτα, ἅπερ εἰρήκαμεν, τὸ τόδε ὁρᾶν ἢ τὸ τόδε κατὰ ἀπάτην, καθάπερ ἐπὶ τῶν περιπνευμονικῶν καὶ τοῦ ὀξέος πυρετοῦ. εἰ δὲ ἐν αὐτῇ τῇ κεφαλῇ ἐστιν ἡ κακοχυμία, πέμπεται εἰς τοὺς ὀφθαλμοὺς καὶ ταῦτα ποιεῖ, ἅπερ εἰρήκαμεν· παχύνεται τὸ ᾠοειδές, ἀμαυροῦται τὸ κρυσταλλοειδές, μολύνεται ἡ ὁρατικὴ δύναμις, καὶ πάλιν κατὰ ἀπάτην ὁρῶσιν, ἅπερ εἰρήκαμεν, καθάπερ ἐπὶ τῶν φρενιτικῶν.

Καὶ λέγουσί τινες ὅτι «Καὶ πόθεν τὰ διάφορα εἴδη ταῦτα τῶν συμπτωμάτων ὁρῶσι;» καὶ λέγομεν ὅτι διὰ τρεῖς αἰτίας ταῦτα ὁρῶσι, διά τε τὸ ποσὸν τῆς ὕλης καὶ τὴν σύστασιν καὶ τὸ χρῶμα· ἢ γὰρ ὀλίγη ἐστὶν ἡ ὕλη ἢ πολλή, καὶ ὁρῶσιν ἢ μικρὰ ἢ μεγάλα. ἀλλὰ καὶ κατὰ τὴν σύστασιν· εἰ μὲν γὰρ ἐπιμήκης ἐστὶν ἡ ὕλη, ὁρῶσι τριχοειδῆ καὶ κάρφη καὶ ἄχυρα καὶ τὰ τοιαῦτα· εἰ δὲ στρογγυλώδης ἐστίν, ὁρῶσι κροκύδας καὶ κέγχρους καὶ τὰ τοιαῦτα. ἀλλὰ καὶ κατὰ τὸ χρῶμα τῆς ὕλης ἢ ἐρυθρὰ ὁρῶσιν ἢ ὠχρὰ ἢ χλωρὰ ἢ πελιδνὰ ἢ μέλανα καὶ τὰ τοιαῦτα. πλὴν καὶ τοῦτο δεῖ εἰδέναι, ὅτι τὰ πάθη ταῦτα τὰ κατὰ ἀπάτην γινόμενα πολλάκις ἐπὶ βλάβῃ μόνῃ τῆς ὁρατικῆς δυνάμεως γίνονται, καθ' ἃς εἰρήκαμεν αἰτίας, τοῦ λογισμοῦ ὑγιῶς ἔχοντος. καὶ τοῦτο ἧττόν ἐστι κακόν, πλὴν οὐκ ἀκίνδυνον οὐδὲ τοῦτο. |

X

105 **I 40** [5: 199,6 A. = II 122,11 L.] Πνεῦμα δὲ πυκνὸν μὲν ἐὸν πόνον σημαίνει ἢ φλεγμονὴν ἐν τοῖς

Ἰστέον ὅτι τὰ συμπτώματα τριττά εἰσιν· ἢ γὰρ ἐν διαθέσει θεωροῦνται ἢ ἐν βλάβαις ἐνεργειῶν ἢ ἐν κενουμένοις καὶ ἐπεχομένοις. λοιπὸν σημειωσάμενος τὸ ὀξὺ νόσημα ἀπὸ τῶν ἐν διαθέσει λέγει νῦν περὶ τῶν ἐν βλάβαις ἐνεργειῶν. καὶ λέγει περὶ βλάβης ἐνεργείας, οὐ τῆς τυχούσης δέ· περὶ γὰρ βλαβείσης ἀναπνοῆς περὶ τὴν ἐνέργειαν διαλέγεται, ἥτις ἐστὶν ἀξιολογω-

1–14] *cf.* Gal. In Hipp. Progn. comm. I 23: CMG V 9,2 pp. 237,8–238,2 29sq.] *cf.* [Gal.] De urinis ex Hipp. Gal. aliisque quibusdam 1: IX p. 612 K. Gal. De sympt. diff. 2: VII p. 53 K. Steph. Comm. in Gal. Ad Glauc. de med. meth.: I p. 243 Dietz

1 sq. ἀλλὰ – συμπάθειαν *om.* L 3 ἢ *om.* γ 7 ἐρχόμενα *om.* γ τὸ ὠ(ο)ειδὲς *codd.*: *correxi* 8 δύναμιν *post* ὁρατικὴν *trsp.* γ μολύνουσι] ἀμβλύνουσι L, *sed cf. supra, p. 102,31; infra, lin. 12* 10 ὀξέου γ τῇ *om.* L 11 ταῦτα] τὰ αὐτὰ γ ἅπερ] ὥσπερ γ 12 ὠειδές γ 13 ὁρῶν γ 15 ὅτι *om.* L Καὶ[II] *om.* γ 21 ὁρῶσιν] ὦσιν γ 22 πέλια γ 23 τὰ *om.* L 25 ἐστὶν ἧττον γ 28 ἢ – τοῖς *om.* γ 29 ἐστιν γ 30 ἐνεργεῖ γ κενουμένω καὶ ἐπεχομένω γ 33 βλαβείσης] βλάβης καὶ γ

picking up bits of material and so on. This is how the condition results from a primary affection. But it can also be produced by a sympathetic affection, and in two ways: it happens either when the unwholesome humor is in the whole body or when it is in the brain itself. If the unwholesome humor is throughout the body, dense gases from the unwholesome humor are transmitted to the head; then they are carried to the optic nerves and to the eyes themselves; next these dense (gases) break up and certain fluids issue which combine with the ovoid humor, darken the crystalline and taint the optic and seeing faculty, and those things happen which we have described: (the victims) are deluded by visions of one or other of those objects, just as in cases of pneumonia and acute fever. But if the unwholesome humor is in the head itself, it is conveyed to the eyes and produces what we have said: the ovoid humor thickens, the crystalline is obscured, the optic faculty is tainted and again they are deceived by those visions which we have described, as in cases of phrenitis.

And some say, "How do you explain their seeing these different kinds of object?" We reply that they see these things for three reasons: the quantity, composition and color of the matter; for either there is little or much matter, and so they see small or large objects. And according to the composition: for if the matter is oblong they see hair-like objects, twigs, chaff and so on; but if it is round, they see pieces of wool and grain and the like. Depending on the color of the matter, they see red, yellowish, green, livid, black objects and so on. However, it should also be noted that these deceptive visual sensations often result solely from a defect in the optic faculty, for the reasons we have given, while the faculty of reason remains sound. This is less serious, though even this is not without danger.

X

I 40 When the breath is frequent it means pain or inflammation in the

Note that there are three kinds of symptoms: for they are observed in the (body's) condition, or in impaired functions, or in evacuations and retentions. Having interpreted acute disease from the symptoms of the (body's) condition, he now discusses those appearing with impaired functions. But the impaired function he speaks of is not just any one; for he is discussing the impaired function of respiration, which is extre-

τάτη, ἐπειδὴ ζωογονεῖ καὶ ἀνακτᾶται τὸ ἔμφυτον θερμόν, καὶ ὑγιῶς αὐτῆς ἐχούσης, εἰς τὸ ζῆν συμβάλλεται τοῖς ζῴοις, βεβλαμμένως δὲ ἐχούσης, σφάλλει τὰ ζῷα καὶ φθείρει αὐτά.

Ἀλλ' ὥσπερ μέλλοντες εἰπεῖν περὶ σφυγμοῦ ἐζητήσαμεν, τίνα καὶ πόσα εἰσὶ τὰ συνεκτικὰ αἴτια, καὶ εὕρομεν ὅτι τρία εἰσί, χρεία, δύναμις καὶ ὄργανον — ἄνευ γὰρ τούτων οὐ δύναται εἶναι σφυγμός —, οὕτως οὖν καὶ ἐνταῦθα δεῖ ἡμᾶς ζητῆσαι τὰ γενεσιουργὰ αἴτια τῆς ἀναπνοῆς. καὶ χρή σε εἰδέναι ὅτι εἰσὶ τέσσαρα, ποιητικόν, ὀργανικόν, ὑλικόν, τελικόν. καὶ ποιητικὸν μὲν αἴτιόν ἐστι τῆς ἀναπνοῆς αὐτὴ ἡ δύναμις ἡ κινοῦσα τοὺς μύας τοῦ θώρακος. ὑλικὸν δὲ αἴτιόν ἐστιν αὐτὸ τὸ εἰσπνεόμενον καὶ ἐκπνεόμενον πνεῦμα. τελικὸν δὲ αἴτιόν ἐστιν ἡ χρεία· διττὴ δὲ αὕτη· διὰ μὲν τῆς εἰσπνοῆς εἰσάγει καθαρὸν ἀέρα καὶ ἐμψύχει τὸ ἔμφυτον θερμόν, διὰ δὲ τῆς ἐκπνοῆς ἐξάγει τὰ λιγνυώδη περιττώματα. ὀργανικὸν δὲ αἴτιόν ἐστι τὸ διάφραγμα· τὸ γὰρ διάφραγμα τὴν κατὰ φύσιν καὶ ἀβίαστον ἀναπνοὴν ἀπεργάζεται. εἰ δὲ συντεταμένη ἐστὶν ἡ ἀναπνοή, τότε καὶ οἱ μεσοπλεύριοι μύες ἐνεργοῦσιν. εἰ δὲ ἔτι πλέον ἐστὶν ἐπιτεταμένη ἡ ἀναπνοή, τότε καὶ οἱ ὑψηλοὶ λεγόμενοι μύες ἐνεργοῦσι. καὶ ὥσπερ ἐν τῷ ἠρέμα ἡμᾶς βαδίζειν ἐνεργεῖ τὸ διάφραγμα τὴν κατὰ φύσιν ἀναπνοήν, οὕτως τὴν ἐπιτεταμένην ἀναπνοήν, ἐπειδὴ οὐκ ἐξαρκεῖ μόνον τὸ
106 διάφραγμα ἀναπληρῶσαι τὴν χρείαν, ἐνεργοῦσι καὶ οἱ μεσο|πλεύριοι μύες, ὥσπερ ἐπὶ τῶν ὀξέως βαδιζόντων. εἰ δὲ ἔτι πλέον ἐστὶν ἐπιτεταμένη καὶ βεβιασμένη ἡ ἀναπνοή, ἐπειδὴ οὐκ ἐξαρκοῦσι τότε τὸ διάφραγμα καὶ οἱ μεσοπλεύριοι μύες ἀναπληρῶσαι τὴν χρείαν, τότε καὶ οἱ ὑψηλοὶ λεγόμενοι μύες ἐνεργοῦσιν, ὥσπερ ἐπὶ τῶν τρεχόντων καὶ ἐντεταμένως γυμναζομένων.

Δεύτερον δὲ ἔστιν εἰπεῖν, κατὰ πόσους τρόπους βλάπτεται ἡ ἀναπνοή. καὶ ἰστέον ὅτι κατὰ τρεῖς, κατὰ μέγεθος, κατὰ ποιότητα καὶ κατὰ τὸν χρόνον τῶν διαλειμμάτων. ⟨καὶ κατὰ μὲν τὸν χρόνον τῶν διαλειμμάτων,⟩ καθὸ ἀραιὰ ἢ πυκνὴ γίνεται ἡ ἀναπνοή· καὶ εἰ μὲν πολὺν χρόνον κρατεῖ τὸ διάλειμμα, γίνεται ἀραιά· εἰ δὲ ὀλίγον, πυκνή. κατὰ δὲ τὸ μέγεθος, καθὸ μεγάλη ἢ μικρὰ γίνεται ἡ ἀναπνοή· αὕτη δὲ ἡ μεγάλη ἀναπνοὴ ἢ φαίνεται καὶ ἔστι μεγάλη κατὰ ἀλήθειαν ἢ φαίνεται μέν, οὐκ ἔστι δέ. καὶ φαίνεται μὲν μεγάλη καὶ ἔστι τοιαύτη κατὰ ἀλήθειαν, ὥσπερ ἐπὶ τῆς ἐπιτεταμένης ἀναπνοῆς, καθάπερ ἐπὶ τῶν κατὰ ἔντασιν γυμναζομένων ἢ τρεχόντων. καὶ φαίνεται μὲν μεγάλη ἡ ἀναπνοή, ἐπειδὴ τὸ τρίτον γένος τῶν μυῶν ἐνήργησεν, ἀλλὰ καὶ ἔστι κατὰ ἀλήθειαν, ἐπειδὴ ἡ χρεία ἀνεπληρώθη· τὸ γὰρ φαίνεσθαι καὶ μὴ φαίνεσθαι κατὰ τὴν συστολὴν καὶ τὴν διαστολὴν τοῦ θώρακος φέρεται, τὸ δὲ ἔστι καὶ μὴ ἔστι κατὰ τὴν ἐνέργειαν νοεῖται. φαινομένη δὲ μεγάλη ἀναπνοή,

4 ἐζητήσαμεν] *v. supra*, p. 13 5 χρεία – ὄργανον] *cf.* Gal. De caus. puls. I 1: IX p. 1 K. De caus. respir.: IV pp. 465sq. K. 25–27] *cf.* Gal. De diff. respir. III 3: VII p. 897 K.

1 ζωοποιεῖ γ 4 τίνα καὶ *om.* γ 8 ὑλικὸν ὀργανικὸν γ 11 ἐστιν αἴτιον γ 13 ἐστιν αἴτιον γ 14 ἀναπνοὴν *post* φύσιν *trsp.* γ 18 οὕτως – ἀναπνοήν *om.* γ 21 τὸ *om.* γ 22 ψηλοὶ MP 27 καὶ – διαλειμμάτων *addidi* 28 διάφραγμα L 29 δὲ[II]] μὲν L τὸ *om.* γ 30 ἢ μικρὰ *om.* γ αὕτη – ἀναπνοὴ *om.* L 34 *post* ἐπειδὴ *add.* καὶ γ 36 τὴν[II] *om.* γ φέρεται – 108,1 ἔμφραξιν *om.* L

mely important, being that which creates the innate heat and keeps it alive, and when respiration is working properly it contributes to the life of living creatures, but when damaged it causes their downfall and destruction.

But just as at the beginning of our discussion on the pulse we investigated how many and which are the essential causes and found them to be three, function, faculty and organ – for without these there can be no pulse –, in the same way here we must ask what the generative causes of respiration are. You should know that they are four, the efficient, organic, material and final. The efficient cause of respiration is the very faculty that moves the thorax muscles. The material cause is the inhaled and exhaled breath itself. The final cause is the function, which is twofold; for through inspiration it draws in clean air and cools the innate heat, while by expiration it expels the sooty residues. The organic cause is the diaphragm; for the diaphragm produces normal, unforced breathing. However, if respiration is put under pressure, then the intercostal muscles also go to work. And if there is further strain on respiration, then the so-called elevated muscles go into action as well. And just as the diaphragm produces normal breathing when we walk slowly, so the intercostal muscles create the more intense respiration when we walk fast, the diaphragm being unable on its own to fulfil the function. But if respiration is under even more pressure and strain, e.g. in running or performing strenuous exercises, the so-called elevated muscles are activated, seeing that neither the diaphragm nor the intercostal muscles are capable of doing the job.

The second point for discussion is the number of ways in which respiration is impaired. Note that ⟨it can be affected⟩ in three ways: in quantity, quality and pause duration. First, in the duration of the pauses, which makes breathing either intermittent or frequent: if the interval lasts a long time, ⟨breathing⟩ becomes intermittent; but if it is short, ⟨breathing⟩ is frequent. And in quantity, which determines whether respiration is deep or shallow: deep breathing either appears to be and is really deep or it seems to be but is not so. It appears deep and really is such in pressured breathing, for example in those who run or do strenuous exercises. On the one hand breathing appears to be deep, since the third class of muscles has been activated, but it is in truth deep, because the function has been fulfilled; for appearance and non-appearance refer to the contraction and expansion of the thorax, while real and unreal ⟨deepness⟩ are considered in terms of function. On the other hand,

οὐκ οὖσα δέ, αὕτη διττή ἐστιν· ἢ γὰρ κατὰ ἔμφραξιν φαίνεται καὶ οὐκ ἔστι, καθάπερ ἐπὶ τῶν περιπνευμονικῶν. τί γάρ; ὅτι κινεῖται τὸ διάφραγμα ὥστε τὴν ἀναπνοὴν ποιῆσαι, οὐκ ἐξαρκεῖ δὲ ὥστε τὴν χρείαν ἀναπληρωθῆναι· εἶτα κινοῦνται καὶ οἱ μεσοπλεύριοι μύες, οὐκ ἐξαρκοῦσιν οὐδ' οὕτως ἀναπληρῶσαι τὴν χρείαν· τότε δὲ κινοῦνται καὶ οἱ ὑψηλοὶ μύες, καὶ οὐδ' οὕτως ἀναπληροῦται ἡ χρεία. καὶ φαινομένη λέγεται μεγάλη ἀναπνοή, ἐπειδὴ τὸ τρίτον γένος τῶν μυῶν ἐκινήθη, οὐκ οὖσα δὲ κατὰ ἀλήθειαν, ἐπειδὴ ἡ χρεία οὐκ ἀνεπληρώθη. τί γάρ; ὅτι ἔμφραξις ὑπόκειται τῶν βρογχίων τοῦ
107 πνεύμονος, ἔνθα ἡ πάροδος τοῦ πνεύματος γίνεται, | καθ' ἣν ἐπὶ τὴν καρδίαν φέρεται. τούτων οὖν ἐμφραττομένων οὐ γίνεται εἰσαγωγὴ τοῦ πνεύματος ἐπὶ τὴν καρδίαν, καὶ οὕτως γίνονται λιγνυώδη περιττώματα, ἐπειδὴ ἐναπειλημμέναι εἰσὶ καὶ ἐμπεφραγμέναι ⟨αἱ⟩ ὁδοὶ τοῦ πνεύματος, καὶ ἡ χρεία οὐκ ἀναπληροῦται. καὶ οὕτως διὰ τὴν ἔμφραξιν. ἢ διὰ τὴν ἀσθένειαν τῶν μυῶν καὶ ἀτονίαν τῶν κινούντων τὸν θώρακα φαίνεται μεγάλη ἡ ἀναπνοή, οὐκ οὖσα δέ, τρόπῳ τοιούτῳ. τί γάρ; ὅτι ἐνεργεῖ τὸ διάφραγμα, ἀλλ' ἀτόνως ἐνεργεῖ καὶ οὐκ ἀναπληροῦται ἡ χρεία· εἶτα κινοῦνται καὶ οἱ μεσοπλεύριοι μύες καὶ αὐτοὶ ἀτόνως, καὶ οὐδ' οὕτως ἀναπληροῦται ἡ χρεία· εἶτα ἐξ ἀνάγκης τῆς χρείας κατεπειγούσης κινοῦνται καὶ οἱ ὑψηλοὶ μύες καὶ αὐτοὶ ἀτόνως, καὶ οὐδ' οὕτως ἀναπληροῦται ἡ χρεία. καὶ ἐπειδὴ τὸ τρίτον γένος τῶν μυῶν ἐκινήθη, φαίνεται μὲν μεγάλη ἡ ἀναπνοή, οὐκ οὖσα δέ, ἐπειδὴ οὐκ ἀνεπληρώθη ἡ χρεία διὰ τὸ ἀτόνως καὶ ἀσθενῶς ἐνεργῆσαι τοὺς μύας. ὁ οὖν Ἱπποκράτης περὶ τῶν κατὰ τὸ μέγεθος καὶ περὶ τῶν κατὰ τὸν χρόνον ⟨τῶν⟩ διαλειμμάτων διαλέγεται, τουτέστι περὶ τῆς μεγάλης καὶ μικρᾶς ἀναπνοῆς καὶ ἀραιᾶς καὶ πυκνῆς, παρῆκε δὲ τὴν κατὰ ποιότητα. τοῦτο δὲ ἐποίησε διὰ δύο αἰτίας, ἢ ὅτι συνεισάγεται ἡ κατὰ ποιότητα καὶ συνδιαφαίνεται τούτοις, λέγω δὴ τῇ μεγάλῃ καὶ τῇ πυκνῇ συνεισάγεται δὲ καὶ τὸ τάχος, τῇ δὲ μικρᾷ καὶ τῇ ἀραιᾷ συνεισάγεται καὶ ἡ βραδύτης. ἢ τὸ ἄλλο εἰπέ, ὅτι ἡ κατὰ ποιότητα διαφορὰ ποικιλωτέρα ἐστί, καὶ ὡς ἂν οὔσης αὐτῆς ποικιλωτέρας, παρῆκεν αὐτὴν ἐνταῦθα, ὡς δεομένης αὐτῆς ἰδίας ἐπεξεργασίας διὰ τὸ ποικίλον.

Καὶ ἐπειδὴ δ' συμπλοκαὶ τῆς ἀναπνοῆς συνίστανται, ἥ τε μεγάλη καὶ πυκνή, καὶ ἡ μεγάλη καὶ ἀραιά, καὶ ἡ μικρὰ καὶ πυκνή, καὶ ἡ μικρὰ καὶ ἀραιά — αἱ γὰρ δύο οὐ συνίστανται, ἥ τε μεγάλη καὶ μικρά, καὶ ἡ πυκνὴ καὶ ἀραιά —, δεῖ οὖν ἡμᾶς εἰπεῖν, πῶς γίνονται καὶ τί σημαίνουσι. καὶ πρότερον εἴπωμεν περὶ τῆς μικρᾶς καὶ πυκνῆς, ἐπειδὴ ταύτην καὶ Ἱπποκράτης πρότερον
108 μεταχειρίζεται. | αὕτη οὖν ἡ μικρὰ καὶ πυκνὴ δύσπνοια ὀδύνην σημαίνει ἐν

31–32 ἀραιά] *cf.* Gal. De diff. respir. III 2: VII pp. 892sq. K. 33] *cf.* Ioann. Comm. in Hipp. De morb. pop. VI: 124d51–53 Pritchet 36–110,1] *cf.* Gal. In Hipp. Epid. III comm. III 78: CMG V 10,2,1 p. 170,17–19 De diff. respir. I 12: VII p. 788 K.

2 πνευμονικῶν γ 8 βραχίων, *ut vid.*, L 10 ἡ ἀγωγὴ γ 11 οὕτως] ἐντεῦθεν γ 12 αἱ *addidi* ὁδοὶ *om.* L πνεύμονος γ 14 ἡ *om.* γ 17 οὐδ' οὕτως] οὐδόλως L 21 ἀπόνως L 22 τῶν[I]] τοῦ *codd.*: *correxi* τὸ *om.* γ 23 τῶν *add.* *Kollesch* 26 *fort.* δὲ *delendum est* 27 τῇ δὲ] τῇδε τῇ L 32 καὶ[I] — πυκνή *om.* γ 33 *ante* μικρά *add.* ἡ Μζ *post* ἀραιά *habet ex lin. 32* καὶ[III] — ἀραιά γ 34 εἰπεῖν ἡμᾶς L; *cf. supra, p. 14* γίνεται γ σημειοῦμεθα γ εἴπομεν γ 36 ὀδύνην] λοιπὸν γ

breathing which appears deep but is not, is of two types; for it appears to be, but is not so, due to a stoppage, as in cases of pneumonia. Why? Because the diaphragm moves to produce respiration, but is unable to fulfil the function; then the intercostal muscles go into action as well, but even this is not enough to do the needed; next the elevated muscles, too, are activated and still the function is not fulfilled. And since it appears so, the third muscle class having been activated, this breathing is called deep; but in fact it is not, because the function has not been performed. Why? Because there is an obstruction in the lung's bronchial tubes, which constitute the passage of the breath, along which it is carried to the heart. Once these are blocked, then, breath is not introduced to the heart, and thus sooty residues develop, the air passages having been stopped and clogged, and the function is not carried out. This is how it is caused by a stoppage. Or, breathing that seems to be deep, but is not (really), is caused by weakness and lack of tone in the muscles that move the thorax, in the following way. Why? Because the diaphragm functions, but without power, so the function is not carried out; next the intercostals are set in motion, but these also lack strength and the job is not completed; then the need inevitably becomes urgent and the elevated muscles are activated, but they are weak as well and the function is not fulfilled. And since the third class of muscles has gone into action, the breathing appears to be deep, but is not, seeing that the need has not been satisfied due to the toneless and weak state of the muscles. Hippocrates, then, discusses the types of respiration based on quantity and pause duration, in other words, deep and shallow, intermittent and frequent, but he left out the quality (distinction). He did so for (one of) two reasons, either because the qualitative difference is included in and represented by the others, i.e., fastness is included in deep and frequent, slowness in shallow and intermittent. For the other reason you may say that the difference based on quality is rather complicated and as such he passed it over here, because it would require separate treatment in view of its complexity.

Since there are four combinations of breathing, deep and frequent, deep and intermittent, shallow and frequent, shallow and intermittent – for the (other) two, deep and shallow, frequent and intermittent, do not exist –, we should, then, discuss how they arise and what they signify. Let us speak first about shallow and frequent, this being the first (combination) that Hippocrates deals with. This shallow and frequent dyspnoea, then, shows pain in the respiratory parts brought about by

τοῖς ἀναπνευστικοῖς μορίοις συνισταμένην διά τινα φλεγμονὴν ἢ δι' ἕλκωσιν ἢ διὰ ῥευματικὴν διάθεσιν. ἔγνωμεν οὖν τὸ τί σημαίνει ἡ μικρὰ καὶ πυκνὴ δύσπνοια· λοιπὸν δεῖ ἡμᾶς εἰπεῖν τὸ πῶς γίνεται. καὶ ὅσον μὲν ἐπὶ τῇ ὑποκειμένῃ διαθέσει ὤφειλε μεγάλη γίνεσθαι ἡ ἀναπνοή· ἡ δὲ μεγάλη ἀναπνοὴ ἐπὶ μεγίστῃ κινήσει τοῦ θώρακος γίνεται· ἡ δὲ μεγίστη κίνησις τοῦ θώρακος χύσιν ποιεῖται τῶν ὑλῶν· ἐπὶ δὲ τῇ χύσει ἐπιτείνονται οἱ ῥευματισμοί· ἐπιτεινομένων δὲ τῶν ῥευματισμῶν ἐξ ἀνάγκης ἐπιτείνονται τὰ τῆς ὀδύνης. φειδόμενοι οὖν ἑαυτῶν οἱ οὕτως πάσχοντες οὐκ ἀναπνέουσι μέγα διὰ τὸ μὴ ἐπιταθῆναι αὐτοῖς τὰ τῆς ὀδύνης· ἀλλὰ μικρὰν ποιοῦνται τὴν ἀναπνοήν, τῇ δὲ πυκνότητι κατεπείγουσι, καὶ ὅπερ τῇ μικρότητι πλημμελοῦσι τῇ ἀναπνοῇ, τῇ πυκνότητι ἀναπληροῦσι τὴν χρείαν. καὶ προηγεῖται μὲν ἡ μικρὰ ἀναπνοή, ἕπεται δὲ ἡ πυκνή. καὶ ταῦτα μὲν περὶ τῆς πρώτης διαφορᾶς τῆς δυσπνοίας.

Δευτέρα δέ ἐστι διαφορὰ δυσπνοίας μεγάλη καὶ πυκνή, ἥτις γίνεται ἐπὶ τῶν τρεχόντων καὶ κατὰ ἔντασιν γυμναζομένων καὶ ἐπὶ τῶν ὀξέως πυρεττόντων. τί γάρ; ὅτι ἡ μεγάλη ἀναπνοὴ οὐκ ἐξαρκεῖ τὴν χρείαν ἀναπληρῶσαι καὶ λοιπὸν γίνεται καὶ πυκνὴ καὶ κατεπείγει τῇ πυκνότητι καὶ οὕτως ἀναπληροῦται ἡ χρεία. καὶ προηγεῖται ἡ μεγάλη ἀναπνοή, ἕπεται δὲ ἡ πυκνή.

Τρίτη διαφορὰ δυσπνοίας μεγάλη καὶ ἀραιά, ἥτις γίνεται ἐπὶ τῶν φρενιτικῶν, ὅτι τοῦ λογισμοῦ περί τινα φαντάσματα ἀπησχολημένου ἐπὶ τῶν φρενιτικῶν, ἐπιλανθάνεται τῶν οἰκείων ἔργων καὶ οὐ κινεῖ τὸν θώρακα, ἵνα ἡ ἀναπνοὴ γίνηται, ἀλλὰ παρέρχεται καὶ μία καὶ δευτέρα καὶ τρίτη κίνησις καὶ ἐν τῷ διαλείμματι τοῦ χρόνου ἐμβραδύνει, καθ' ἣν καὶ ἀραιὰ γίνεται ἡ ἀναπνοή. ἐπειδὴ δὲ περὶ τὸ εἶναι συμβάλλεται ἡμῖν ἡ ἀναπνοή, ἵνα μὴ
109 ἐν ἡμῖν εἴη τὸ ζῆν, ἀναμνημονεύει τῶν οἰκείων | ἔργων ἡ ψυχή, καὶ ὅπερ ἐν τῷ διαλείμματι ἐπλημμελήθη, ὑφ' ἓν θέλουσα ἀναπληρῶσαι τὸ πλημμεληθέν, μεγάλην ποιεῖται τὴν ἀναπνοήν. οὕτως γίνεται καὶ ἐπὶ τῶν λυπουμένων διὰ τὰς αὐτὰς αἰτίας. τί γάρ; ὅτι καὶ ἐνταῦθα τοῦ λογισμοῦ ἀπασχολουμένου περὶ τῶν λυπηρῶν, ἐπιλανθάνεται τῶν οἰκείων ἔργων καὶ παρέρχεται καὶ μιᾶς καὶ δύο, ἔστι δ' ὅτε καὶ τριῶν κινήσεων ἀναπνοῆς χρόνος· εἶτα ὀψέ ποτε ἀναμνημονεύουσα ἡ ψυχὴ τῶν οἰκείων ἔργων, θέλουσα ἐφάπαξ τὸ πλημμεληθὲν ἀναπληρῶσαι μεγάλην ποιεῖται τὴν ἀναπνοήν, ὅπερ καὶ στεναγμὸς καλεῖται. ἐνταῦθα δὲ ἐπὶ τῶν λυπουμένων ἡ μεγάλη ἀναπνοὴ καὶ ἀραιὰ μετὰ στεναγμοῦ γίνεται. εἰκότως, διά τε τὸ τὸ πλημμεληθὲν ἀναπληρῶσαι καὶ διὰ τὸ πολλὰ λιγνυώδη περιττώματα γεννᾶσθαι ἐπ' αὐτῶν καὶ χρεία ἐστὶν ἐξαγωγῆς, ὅπερ διὰ τοῦ ἀναστεναγμοῦ ἐξωθοῦσι,

14–16] *cf.* Gal. De diff. respir. III 5: VII p. 911 K. 20–23] *cf.* Gal. De diff. respir. II 3: VII p. 830 K.

2 *ante* πυκνὴ *add.* ἡ L 4 ἡ^{I} *om.* L 6 ἐπὶ] ἐπεὶ L 12 πυκνή] πυκνότης γ 14 δύσπνοια γ 18 προηγεῖται] πληροῦται γ μεγάλη *om.* L 21 ἀπησχολησμένου L 21sq. ἐπὶ τῶν φρενιτικῶν *om.* γ 23 γένηται γ περιέρχεται γ 25 δὲ *om.* γ παρὰ L 28 μεγάλως γ γίνεται] γὰρ γ 31 ἔστιν ὅτε γ κινήσεως MPV 33 ὑφάπαξ γ μεγάλως γ 35 τὸ^{II} *supra lin. inser.* L: *om.* γ 36 τὸ πολλὰ] τοῦτο τὰ γ 37 *ante* ἐξαγωγῆς *add.* καὶ γ στεναγμοῦ γ

some inflammation or ulceration or a flux condition. Now that we know what the shallow and frequent dyspnoea means, we should next describe how it develops. In view of the underlying condition the breathing ought to be deep; but deep breathing is produced by very great movement of the thorax; and very great movement of the thorax creates a flow of the matters; the flow intensifies the fluxes and, when this occurs, the pain is bound to heighten. So the victims of this condition spare themselves by not breathing deeply, in order to avoid aggravating the pain; instead they make their breathing shallow and speed it up by (increasing) the frequency, and whatever error they make in respiration by shallowness, they (compensate and) fulfil the need by frequency. The shallow respiration comes first and the frequent follows. So much for the first variety of dyspnoea.

The second variety of dyspnoea is deep and frequent, which occurs in those who run or perform strenuous exercises or in cases of acute fever. Why? Because deep breathing is not capable of satisfying the need, and so it becomes frequent as well and forces itself by frequency, and thus the need is fulfilled. Deep breathing precedes, frequent comes later.

The third variety of dyspnoea, deep and intermittent, develops in cases of phrenitis, because in these cases the mind is absorbed in fantasies, forgets its own work and fails to create the thorax movement necessary for respiration; the movement skips once, twice, three times and lags behind because of the interval of time, which causes intermittent breathing. However, since respiration contributes to our existence, in order that life should not depend on us, the soul remembers its own functions and, because it wants to supply at once whatever was lost in the pause, it makes the breathing deep. The same thing happens also to the grief-stricken and for the same reasons. Why? Because here, too, the mind is preoccupied by the distress, neglects its own functions and the respiratory movements skip once, twice and occasionally even three times; then at the last the soul recalls its duties and wishing to make up the loss in one effort produces the deep breathing which is also known as groaning. Here in the case of the grief-stricken the deep and intermittent respiration is accompanied by groaning. And this is reasonable, both because the loss is made good and because a large quantity of superfluities develops in them and needs to be eliminated, which they drive out by groaning,

καὶ πάλιν διὰ τῆς μεγάλης εἰσπνοῆς εἰσάγουσι καθαρὸν ἀέρα. καὶ ἔστιν ἡ ἀραιὰ ἀναπνοὴ ⟨. . .⟩ τῆς μεγάλης ἀναπνοῆς· προηγεῖται γὰρ ἡ ἀραιὰ καὶ ἕπεται ἡ μεγάλη.

Τετάρτη διαφορὰ τῆς δυσπνοίας ἐστὶν ἡ μικρὰ καὶ ἀραιὰ ἀναπνοή, ὅπερ κάκιστόν ἐστι σημεῖον· σημαίνει γὰρ αὐτὴ κατάπτωσιν ἐσχάτην καὶ ἀσθένειαν τῆς κινητικῆς δυνάμεως καὶ κατάσβεσιν καὶ κατάψυξιν καὶ νέκρωσιν τοῦ ἐμφύτου θερμοῦ.

Οὕτως σημειωσάμενος τὴν παρὰ φύσιν διάθεσιν τῆς ἀναπνοῆς σημειοῦται καὶ τὴν κατὰ φύσιν, ἐξαίρων καὶ ἐγκωμιάζων αὐτὴν λέγων οὕτως·

I 41 [5: 199,9 A.=II 122,14 L.] Εὔπνοιαν δὲ χρὴ νομίζειν κάρτα μεγάλην δύναμιν ἔχειν ἐς σωτηρίαν ἐν πᾶσι τοῖσιν ὀξέσι νοσήμασι

Τὸ λεγόμενον τοιοῦτόν ἐστιν, ὅτι θαυμαστὴ καὶ σωτήριός ἐστιν ἡ κατὰ φύσιν ἀναπνοή· δηλοῖ γὰρ ὅτι καλῶς καὶ ἰσχυρῶς διάκεινται αἵ τε κινητικαὶ δυνάμεις τῶν ἀναπνευστικῶν, ἀλλὰ καὶ τὸ ἔμφυτον θερμὸν δεόντως ῥιπιζόμενον καὶ οὐδεμία παρεκτροπὴ δυσκρασίας κακίστη σύνεστιν.

I 42 [5: 199,6 A.=II 122,11 L.] [Ἄλλως.] Πνεῦμα δὲ πυκνὸν μὲν ἐὸν καὶ τὰ ἑξῆς

Δεῖ εἰδέναι ὅτι ὁ Ἱπποκράτης ἀπὸ τοῦ ὑλικοῦ αἰτίου τὴν ἀναπνοὴν ἐδήλωσε· τὸ γὰρ πνεῦμα ὑλικὸν αἴτιόν ἐστι τῆς ἀναπνοῆς, ὡς ἴσμεν κατὰ τὴν ἐνέργειαν, καὶ διὰ τοῦτο καὶ τὴν προσηγορίαν οὕτως ἐποίησεν. καὶ
110 ἰδοὺ αὐτὸς μὲν | ὁ Ἱπποκράτης, ὡς καὶ ἐν τῇ θεωρίᾳ εἰρήκαμεν ὅτι οὐ περὶ πασῶν τῶν δυσπνοιῶν διαλέγεται οὐδὲ πάσαις ἐπεξέρχεται, ἀλλὰ μέμνηται τῆς πυκνῆς καὶ μεγάλης ἀναπνοῆς καὶ ἀραιᾶς· τὰς δὲ λοιπὰς παρῆκεν ἡμῖν ὑπογράψας μέθοδον ὥστε καὶ τῶν λοιπῶν δυσπνοιῶν τὴν ἐπεξεργασίαν ποιήσασθαι. καὶ ἤδη πεπράχαμεν, καθ' ὃν εἰρήκαμεν τρόπον.

I 43 [5: 199,8 A. = II 122,13 L.] Ψυχρὸν δὲ ἐκπνεόμενον ἐκ τῶν ῥινῶν καὶ ἐκ τοῦ στόματος ὀλέθριον πάνυ

Ψυχρὰ ἀναπνοὴ γίνεται ἐπὶ ἄκρᾳ καταβολῇ τῆς ζωτικῆς δυνάμεως καὶ ἐπὶ ὀλιγοσιτίᾳ καὶ καταψύξει καὶ οἱονεὶ νεκρώσει τοῦ ἐμφύτου θερμοῦ, ὅπερ ἐσχάτης ἀπωλείας ἐστὶ τεκμήριον· οἷον γὰρ εἰσπνεῖται, τοιοῦτον καὶ

4–7] *cf.* Gal. In Hipp. Progn. comm. I 24: CMG V 9,2 p. 238,24sq. De diff. respir. II 7: VII p. 849 K. In Hipp. Epid. III comm. III 78: CMG V 10,2,1 p. 170,19–21 13–16] *cf.* Gal. In Hipp. Progn. comm. I 25: CMG V 9,2 p. 239,12–20 19sq.] *cf.* Ioann. Comm. in Hipp. De morb. pop. VI: 124d7, 46sq. Pritchet 22 ἐν — εἰρήκαμεν] *supra,* p. 108,21–24

1 ἀναπνοῆς γ 2 *lacunam indicavi; exciderit* προτέρα *vel sim.* 5 ἐσχάτην] μεγάλην L 6 κινητικῆς] καθεκτικῆς L; *sed cf. infra, linn. 14 sq.* ἀπόσβεσιν γ 8 διάθεσιν τῆς ἀναπνοῆς] ἀναπνοὴν γ σημειοῦται *om.* L 10 Εὔπνοιαν — 16 σύνεστιν *post* τρόπον *(lin. 26) habent codd.*: *transposui* 11 εἰς L τοῖς γ 12 *post* νοσήμασι *add.* ὁπόσα σὺν πυ L 17 Ἄλλως *seclusi* 22 εἴρηκεν *codd.*: *correxi* 28 ὀλέθριον πάνυ *om.* γ πάνυ] κάρτα *Hipp.* 30 ἐμφύτου θερμοῦ] ἐμφυτευθέντος γ 31 οἷον — 114,2 τεκμήριον *om.* L

and again they introduce clean air by deep inhalation. The intermittent respiration is (prior to) the deep, because the intermittent comes first and the deep follows.

The fourth variety of dyspnoea is shallow and intermittent breathing, which is a very bad sign; for it means utter collapse and weakness of the kinetic faculty and extinction, cooling and mortification of the innate heat.

Having thus given the symptoms for the abnormal condition of respiration, he gives also those for the normal, which he regards very highly and commends in these words:

I 41 Good breathing must be considered to have a very great influence on recovery in all acute diseases

The meaning is this, that normal breathing is an excellent thing and contributes to recovery; for it shows that the kinetic faculties of the respiratory parts are healthy and strong, also that the innate heat is being properly fanned and that there is no serious abnormality in temperament.

I 42 When the breath is frequent, etc.

Note that Hippocrates expressed respiration here by means of the material cause; for breath is the material cause of breathing, as we know from the way it functions, and this explains his present use of the word. And note that Hippocrates himself, as we have said in the general discussion, does not describe or go through all the forms of dyspnoea, but mentions the frequent, deep and intermittent; he left the others out, having outlined a method for us to go through the remaining kinds of dyspnoea ourselves. This we have already done in the way we have given them.

I 43 But if the air exhaled from the nose and mouth is cold, it is a very deadly sign

Cold breath results from extreme failure of the vital faculty and from undernourishment, cooling and mortification, so to speak, of the innate heat, which is a sign of utter destruction, the air being exhaled

ἐκπνεῖται. πολλάκις δὲ τελευταῖον μετὰ τὴν ψυχρὰν ἀναπνοὴν δοκεῖ θερμὸν ἐκπνεῖσθαι, ὅπερ καὶ τοῦτο ἐσχάτης ἀπωλείας ἐστὶ τεκμήριον· δηλοῖ γὰρ καὶ αὐτὸ τὸ ἐγκαταλειφθὲν λείψανον τοῦ ἐμφύτου θερμοῦ διαφορηθῆναι. οὕτως γὰρ καὶ ἐπὶ τῆς κανδήλας ὁρῶμεν γινόμενον, ἣ τελευταῖον, ὅταν μέλλῃ ἀποσβέννυσθαι, μεγάλην φλόγα ἐξαίφνης ἐκλάμπει καὶ οὕτως σβέννυται.

I 44 [5: 199,10 A. = II 122,16 L.] Ὁκόσα σὺν πυρετοῖσίν ἐστι καὶ ἐν τεσσαράκοντα ἡμέρῃσι κρίνεται

Εἰπὼν ὅτι ἐν πᾶσι τοῖς ὀξέσι νοσήμασι τοῖς μετὰ πυρετοῦ ἀγαθὸν εἶναι τὴν εὔπνοιαν, οὐκ ἀντιδιέστειλε τοῖς χρονίοις νοσήμασιν, ὅτι τυχὸν
111 ἐπεὶ ἐν τοῖς ὀξέσι | νοσήμασιν ἡ εὔπνοια σωτήριός ἐστιν, ἤδη ἐν τοῖς χρονίοις οὐκ ἔστιν ἀγαθὸν ἡ εὔπνοια. καὶ γὰρ ἐπὶ τῶν χρονίων σωτήριός ἐστιν ἡ εὔπνοια πολλῷ μᾶλλον· ἀλλ' ἐπειδὴ εὑρίσκεται ἕτερα σημεῖα δηλωτικὰ ἐπὶ τῶν χρονίων νοσημάτων, αὐτὸ τοῦτο τὸ τεταλαιπωρηκέναι τὴν δύναμιν τῷ μήκει, διὰ τοῦτο ἐπὶ τῶν χρονίων νοσημάτων οὐκ εἶπεν ὅτι σωτήριός ἐστιν ἡ εὔπνοια, ἀλλὰ παρῆκεν. ἄλλως τε δὲ τὰ ὀξέα νοσήματα προέθετο σημειώσασθαι καὶ ἐπὶ τούτων ἔφη ὅτι σωτήριός ἐστιν ἡ εὔπνοια.

Εἶτα καὶ ἀποροῦσί τινες ὅτι «Τί δήποτε μνημονεύσας ὀξέων νοσημάτων τῆς τεσσαρακοστῆς ἐμνημόνευσε, τῶν ὀξέων νοσημάτων ἐντὸς τῆς τεσσαρεσκαιδεκάτης περιγραφομένων, ὡς αὐτὸς Ἱπποκράτης ἐν Ἀφορισμοῖς ἔφη ὅτι 'Τὰ ὀξέα τῶν νοσημάτων κρίνεται ἐν τεσσαρεσκαίδεκα ἡμέρῃσι';» καὶ λέγομεν ὅτι πλάτος ἐστὶν ἐν τοῖς ὀξέσι νοσήμασι· τῶν γὰρ ὀξέων νοσημάτων τὰ μέν ἐστι κατόξεα, τὰ μέχρι τῆς τετάρτης περιγραφόμενα, τὰ δὲ ἁπλῶς ὀξέα, τὰ μέχρι τῆς ἑβδόμης ἀφικνούμενα, τὰ δὲ ὀξέα ὁμωνύμως τῷ γένει, τὰ μέχρι τῆς τεσσαρεσκαιδεκάτης ἀφικνούμενα, τὰ δὲ μηκυνόμενα ὀξέα, τὰ μέχρι τῆς τεσσαρακοστῆς. καὶ τούτων τῶν μηκυνομένων ὀξέων πλείστη ἐστὶν ἡ διαφορά· τὰ μὲν γὰρ ἐκ μεταπτώσεως ὀξέα εἰσί, τὰ δὲ χρόνια, τὰ δὲ μηκυνόμενα, ἅτινα μέχρι τῆς τεσσαρακοστῆς ἀφικνοῦνται· τὰ δὲ ὑπερβαίνοντα τὴν τεσσαρακοστὴν ἡμέραν χρόνια κατατάσσονται. ὁ οὖν Ἱπποκράτης τῆς τεσσαρακοστῆς ἡμέρας ἐμνημόνευσεν, ἵνα ὑπογράψῃ πάντα τὰ ὀξέα χρόνια ἐντὸς περιγραφόμενα τῆς τεσσαρακοστῆς ἡμέρας.

XI

I 45 [6: 200,1 A. = II 122,18 L.] Οἱ δὲ ἱδρῶτες ἄριστοι μέν εἰσιν ἐν ἅπασι τοῖσιν ὀξέσι νοσήμασι

Νῦν τὴν σημείωσιν ποιεῖται ἀπὸ τῶν κενουμένων καὶ μεταχειρίζεται

19 ἐν Ἀφορισμοῖς] Hipp. Aph. II 23: IV p. 476,9sq. L.

1 ψυχρὰν] ψυχὴν γ: *corr. Dietz* 2 *post* γὰρ *add.* ὅτι γ 3 ἐδιεφορήθην γ 5 ἀποσβέννυται γ 6 πυρετοῖς γ 12 εὑρίσκει L 13sq. νοσημάτων – χρονίων *om.* γ 16 παρέθετο L 17 τινες *om.* γ Τί *om.* Pζ 18 τῆς[1] *om.* L σαρακοστῆς γ *(et ubique sine* τεσ*)* ἐμνημόνευσαι *(-σας?)* P: ἐμνημόνευσας ζ 20 ὅτι *om.* γ 21 ὀξέσι] ὀξέοις P *(e corr.)* ζ 25 τούτων] τὸ γ 27–29 σαρακοστ. *scr. et* τεσ *supra lin. ter inser.* L 33 πᾶσι τοῖς ὀξέοις γ

in the same condition as it is inhaled. And many times at the end, after cold breathing, the patient appears to exhale warm air; this, too, signifies complete destruction, showing that the very remnant of the innate heat is being dissipated. We see the same happen in the case of a candle; at the end, when it is just about to extinguish, it suddenly gives a great flame and then goes out.

I 44 Those that are accompanied by fever and come to a crisis in forty days

By stating that good breathing in all acute diseases accompanied by fever is a favorable symptom he does not make a contrast with the chronic; in other words, (he is not saying) that since good breathing in acute diseases indicates recovery, good breathing in the chronic is necessarily bad. In fact good breathing in the chronic is much more of a recovery symptom; however, since there are other indicative signs available in chronic diseases, (for example,) the very fact of the power's distress due to the long duration, for this reason he left out and did not mention that in the chronic good respiration is a salutary sign. Moreover, his original intention was to give the symptoms for acute diseases, and in them, he said, good breathing is an indication of recovery.

Then some raise the problem, "Why, in the context of acute diseases, did he mention the fortieth, seeing that the acute have a limit of fourteen days, as Hippocrates stated himself in the Aphorisms, 'Acute diseases come to a crisis within fourteen days'?" We reply that there are degrees in acute diseases: some acute diseases are very acute and are limited to four days, some generally acute and reach the seventh, others acute – with the same name as the class – extending to the fourteenth, others prolonged acute lasting until the fortieth. And there are very many different types of these prolonged acute, some being acute by change, some chronic, and others prolonged which extend to the fortieth day; but those that continue beyond the fortieth day are classed as chronic. Hippocrates, then, mentioned the fortieth day in order to indicate all the acute chronic diseases for which the fortieth day is the limit.

XI

I 45 The best sweats in all acute diseases are those

Now he makes the interpretation of symptoms derived from evacua-

τοὺς ἱδρῶτας. καὶ ἐπειδὴ ἱδρώτων μνήμην ἐποιησάμεθα, δεῖ ἡμᾶς εἰπεῖν τὰ τέσσαρα γενεσιουργὰ αἴτια τῶν ἱδρώτων, ποιητικόν, ὑλικόν, ὀργανικόν, |
112 τελικόν. καὶ ποιητικὸν μὲν αἴτιόν ἐστι τῶν ἱδρώτων οὐχ ἕν, ἀλλὰ πλείονα.

Ὧν πρῶτος τρόπος ποιητικοῦ αἰτίου ἐστὶ τῶν ἱδρώτων ὅτι δι' ἀσθένειαν καὶ ἀτονίαν καὶ καταβολὴν τῆς καθεκτικῆς δυνάμεως γίνονται οἱ ἱδρῶτες. τί γάρ; ὅτι τὸ λόγῳ τροφῆς φερόμενον ἐν ὅλῳ τῷ σώματι διὰ τὴν ἀσθένειαν οὐ κατέχεται, ὥστε ἀλλοιωθῆναι καὶ πεφθῆναι καὶ προστεθῆναι καὶ ἐξομοιωθῆναι, καὶ λοιπὸν μὴ κατεχόμενον τὸ λόγῳ τροφῆς φερόμενον κενοῦται ἱδρωτοειδῶς δίκην ἀψύχου.

Δεύτερος τρόπος ποιητικοῦ αἰτίου ἱδρώτων ⟨ὁ⟩ ἐπὶ πλημμελεῖ βλάβῃ τῆς ἀποκριτικῆς δυνάμεως γινόμενος. τί γάρ; ὅτι τῆς ἀποκριτικῆς δυνάμεως πλημμελῶς βεβλαμμένης, οὐκ ἀναμένει τὴν ἀλλοίωσιν καὶ τὴν πέψιν, ἀλλὰ πρὸ ὥρας ἐπεγειρομένη καὶ πλημμελῶς ἐνεργοῦσα ἐπεγείρεται καὶ ἀποκρίνει τὸ λόγῳ τροφῆς ⟨φερόμενον⟩ καὶ ποιεῖ τοὺς ἱδρῶτας.

Τρίτος τρόπος ποιητικοῦ αἰτίου τῶν ἱδρώτων ἐστὶν ὁ ἀπὸ τῶν ἔξωθεν βιαστικῶς προσομιλούντων καὶ προσπιπτόντων, ὥσπερ ἡλιοκαΐα· τῇ γὰρ προσομιλίᾳ τοῦ ἡλίου ἐπισπᾶται βίᾳ τινὶ τῇ οἰκείᾳ θερμότητι καὶ ποιεῖ τοὺς ἱδρῶτας. ἀλλὰ καὶ ἀλοιφαὶ θερμότεραι ποιοῦσιν ἱδρῶτας, καὶ τὰ θερμὰ καὶ δριμέα φάρμακα ἐπιτιθέμενα ποιοῦσιν ἱδρῶτας. τούτων δὲ ἓν εἶδός ἐστι καὶ τὸ λουτρόν· καὶ γὰρ τὸ λουτρὸν βίᾳ τινὶ ἐπισπᾶται τῇ θερμότητι τοῦ ἀέρος καὶ ποιεῖ τοὺς ἱδρῶτας.

Τέταρτος τρόπος ποιητικοῦ αἰτίου ἱδρώτων ὁ διὰ σύντηξιν τῆς πιμελῆς γινόμενος· καὶ γὰρ ἐπὶ δαπάνῃ καὶ συντήξει τῆς πιμελῆς γίνονται ἱδρῶτες, καθ' ἣν καὶ αἱ συγκοπαὶ ἐπακολουθοῦσι. γίνεται δὲ τοῦτο ἐπὶ ὀξεῖ καὶ διακαεῖ πυρετῷ καὶ ἐπὶ κακοηθείᾳ νοσήματος, λέγω δὴ ἡ σύντηξις τῆς πιμελῆς, καθ' ἣν καὶ αἱ συγκοπαὶ γίνονται καὶ οἱ ἱδρῶτες οἱ συγκοπτικοὶ λεγόμενοι.

Ὀργανικὸν δὲ αἴτιόν ἐστι τῶν ἱδρώτων οἱ πόροι, δι' ὧν παρεξέρχονται οἱ ἱδρῶτες. |
113 Ὑλικὸν δὲ αἴτιόν ἐστι πάντα τὰ ὑγρὰ ἤγουν πάντες οἱ χυμοὶ οἱ πλεονάζοντες, ὡς δηλοῦσιν ἐν τοῖς βαλανείοις ἀποξεόμενοι οἱ ἱδρῶτες κατά τε χρῶμα καὶ τὴν γεῦσιν καὶ τὴν ὄσφρησιν. ἀλλὰ καὶ τὰ ἱμάτια δηλοῦσι τὰ μετέχοντα τῶν ἱδρώτων, διάφορα χρώματα ἔχοντα, πῇ μὲν ξανθὸν χρῶμα, καὶ ἐνδείκνυται χολώδη τὴν ὕλην, πῇ δὲ πράσινα ἢ ὠχρά, τὰ δὲ ἰώδη ἔχοντα χρώματα, καὶ δὴ μελαγχολικὴν τὴν ὕλην ἐνδείκνυται, πῇ δὲ μέλανα, καὶ τοῦτο ⟨τὸ⟩ αὐτὸ ἐνδείκνυται. ἀλλὰ καὶ ἀπὸ τῆς γεύσεως, πῇ μὲν πικρά εἰσι, πῇ δὲ ὀξώδη, πῇ δὲ ἁλμυρά. ἀλλὰ καὶ ἀπὸ τῆς ὀσφρήσεως,

1 ἡμᾶς *om.* γ 2 γενεσιουργικὰ γ 3 τελικόν] ὑλικόν γ 4 ποιητικοῦ αἰτίου] ποιητικός L ἐστὶ *post* ἱδρώτων *trsp.* γ ὅτι *om.* γ 6 τὸ] τῶ LMP: *corr.* ζ 10 ὁ *addidi* 11 γινομένης L: γινομένων MP (ζ?): *correxi* 13 ἐπεγειρομένης MP: *ambig.* ζ καὶ[I] *om.* γ 14 τῶ *codd.*: *correxi* φερόμενον *addidi* 18 ἀλφαὶ L 22 *ante* ἱδρώτων *add.* τῶν γ σύνταξιν LP 23 συντήξει *(?)* M: συντάξει LP 25 σύνταξις L 28 παρέρχονται γ 30 δὲ *om.* L 31sq. ἐν – δηλοῦσι *om.* L 34 τὰ] *fort.* πῇ *scribendum est* 35 *post* ἔχοντα *add.* τὰ γ ἐνδείκνυνται γ 36 τὸ *addidi* ἐνδείκνυνται Pζ 37 ὀξώδη – ἁλμυρά] μέλανα καὶ ἁλμυρὰ ἀλλαχοῦ L

tions and he discusses sweats. And since we have mentioned sweats, we should give the four generating causes of sweats, the efficient, material, organic and final. As for the efficient cause of sweats, there is not one but several.

The first form of efficient cause is where the sweats develop because the retentive faculty is weak, toneless and in a state of collapse. Why? Because the matter conveyed in the form of nutriment throughout the body, due to weakness, is not retained so as to undergo conversion, coction, application and assimilation; then, not being held, the matter conveyed in the form of nutriment is evacuated as sweat like something inanimate.

The second form of efficient cause of sweats is that produced by a fault of irregularity in the excretory faculty. Why? Because when the excretory faculty is out of order on the excess side, it does not wait for conversion and coction (to finish) but, stimulated prematurely and working irregularly, it goes into action and excretes the matter conveyed in the form of nutriment, and produces the sweats.

The third form of efficient cause of sweats is forceful contact and impingement by external factors, e.g., the heat of the sun; for in contact with the sun, (the sun) by a certain force draws forth (the moisture) with its own heat and produces sweats. The hotter ointments also induce sweats, and so too do warm and pungent remedies when applied. The bath is an example of the latter; for the bath, too, has a certain power to attract (moisture) by the heat of the air and creates sweats.

The fourth form of efficient cause of sweats is that produced by melting of soft fat; for sweats do occur with the consumption and melting of soft fat, and syncope also results thereby. This occurs in acute and burning fever and in malignancy of a disease, I mean the melting of soft fat, which also is responsible for syncope and the so-called syncoptic sweats.

The organic cause of sweats are the pores through which the sweats pass out.

The material cause are all the fluids, i.e., all the humors which are in excess; this is obvious from the color, taste and smell of sweats wiped off in the baths. Clothes with sweat, too, prove it, having different colors; some are yellow, which points to bilious matter, some green or pale yellow, others verdigris, which means atrabilious matter, others are black and this indicates the same thing. In taste, too (there are differences), some being bitter, some acid and others salty. Also in smell, some being

πῆ μὲν δυσώδη, πῆ δὲ βρωμώδη, ἅτινα διαφόρων χυμῶν εἰσιν ἔκγονα.

Τελικὸν δὲ αἴτιόν ἐστι τῶν ἱδρώτων ἡ ἑπομένη εὐφορία καὶ δυσφορία.

Τούτων οὕτως εἰρημένων ἔλθωμεν εἰς τὴν σημείωσιν. καὶ σημειοῦται τοὺς ἱδρῶτας λέγων ὅτι σωτήριοι ἱδρῶτές εἰσιν, ἔνθα τὰ τέσσαρα ταῦτα συνέλθωσιν ἀλλήλοις καὶ συμπαρομαρτήσωσιν, ἡνίκα ἐν κρισίμῳ ἡμέρᾳ γένωνται ἱδρῶτες, ἡνίκα καὶ κατὰ παντὸς τοῦ σώματος, ἡνίκα καὶ θερμοὶ ὦσιν, ἡνίκα καὶ εὐφορία ἐπακολουθήσῃ· πάντως δὲ τούτοις καὶ ἡ εὐφορία ἐπακολουθεῖ. καὶ τὸ μὲν ἐν κρισίμῳ ἡμέρᾳ γίνεσθαι τοὺς ἱδρῶτας ἀγαθόν ἐστι· δηλοῖ γὰρ τὴν φύσιν τακτικῶς καὶ ἀβιάστως καὶ μετὰ πέψιν τὴν ὕλην ἐπιλαβομένην καὶ δι' ἱδρώτων ἐξωθῆσαι τὰ περιττώματα. τὸ δὲ κατὰ παντὸς τοῦ σώματος γίνεσθαι τοὺς ἱδρῶτας ἀγαθόν ἐστιν, ἐπειδὴ ὀξὺ νόσημα ὑπόκειται καὶ πυρετός· καὶ πάντως τὸ λόγῳ τροφῆς φερόμενον ἀπεπτεῖται καὶ γίνονται περιττώματα κατὰ παντὸς τοῦ σώματος, ἅτινα δι' ἱδρώτων δεῖ ἐκκριθῆναι, ὥστε ἀπαλλαγῆναι τὸν κάμνοντα τῆς νόσου. ἀλλὰ καὶ τὸ θερμοὺς εἶναι τοὺς ἱδρῶτας ἀγαθόν ἐστιν, ἐπειδὴ ὁμόστοιχοι εὑρίσκονται τῇ ὕλῃ, ἐν ᾗ τίκτονται· πυρετὸς γὰρ ὑπόκειται καὶ ζέσις, καὶ δηλονότι διὰ θερμῶν τόπων ποιοῦνται οἱ ἱδρῶτες τὴν πάροδον, καὶ διὰ τοῦτο δεῖ αὐτοὺς θερμοὺς εἶναι. ἐπὶ τούτοις δὲ πάντως
114 καὶ | εὐφορία ἕπεται.

Τὰ δ' ἐναντία τούτοις ἐπικίνδυνά εἰσιν· ἡνίκα μὴ ἐν κρισίμῳ ἡμέρᾳ οἱ ἱδρῶτες γένωνται μηδὲ κατὰ παντὸς τοῦ σώματος, ἀλλὰ μερικῶς καὶ ἐν τοῖς μορίοις γίνωνται καὶ ψυχροί εἰσιν οἱ ἱδρῶτες· ἐπὶ τούτοις ἐὰν καὶ δυσφορία ἐπακολουθήσῃ, κάκιστοί εἰσι καὶ ἐπικίνδυνοι. τὸ γὰρ μὴ ἐν κρισίμῳ ἡμέρᾳ γίνεσθαι τοὺς ἱδρῶτας δηλοῖ τὴν φύσιν πρὸ πέψεως τῶν ὑλῶν κινηθεῖσαν καὶ ἐρεθισθεῖσαν ἀπό τινων καὶ πρὸ ὥρας ἐπαναστᾶσαν καὶ ποιήσασαν τοὺς ἱδρῶτας, ὅπερ κάκιστόν ἐστι· δηλοῖ γὰρ ὅτι ἡ φύσις κατεκρατήθη ὑπὸ τῶν αἰτίων, καθ' ἃ οἱ ἱδρῶτες γεγόνασιν. ἀλλὰ καὶ οἱ ἐν μέρει τοῦ σώματος γινόμενοι ἱδρῶτες κάκιστοί εἰσι, τυχὸν οἱ περὶ τὴν κεφαλὴν καὶ τὸ πρόσωπον καὶ τὸν τράχηλον καὶ τὸν αὐχένα, ἐπειδὴ δηλοῖ ἀνάρροπον τὴν ὕλην· ὁ γὰρ πυρετὸς ἀναλύει μέρος τι τῆς ὕλης, καὶ ἀνάρροπον γίνεται ἐπὶ τὰ κυριώτερα μόρια καὶ ἐπὶ τὴν πρωτίστην ἀρχήν, λέγω δὴ τὸν ἐγκέφαλον, ὅπερ ὀλέθριόν ἐστιν. ἀλλὰ καὶ οἱ ψυχροὶ ἱδρῶτες κάκιστοί εἰσιν. ἀλλὰ δεῖ ἡμᾶς πρότερον εἰπεῖν, πῶς γίνονται. δεῖ εἰδέναι ὅτι οἱ ψυχροὶ ἱδρῶτες γίνονται ἐπὶ ἄκρᾳ καταβολῇ καὶ ἀσθενείᾳ καὶ ἐνδείᾳ τοῦ ἐμφύτου θερμοῦ· διὰ γὰρ οἰκείαν ἀσθένειαν καὶ διὰ τὴν ὀλιγότητα περὶ τὰ σπλάγχνα που καὶ περὶ τὸ βάθος ἐνειλίσσεται· τὰ δὲ ἐκτὸς μόρια τὰ περὶ τὴν ἐπιφάνειαν ψύχονται ἀμοιροῦντα τοῦ ἐμφύτου θερμοῦ· πυρετοῦ οὖν ὑποκειμένου χύσις γίνεται πάντως τῆς ὕλης· εἶτα τῇ χύσει φέρεται ἐπὶ τὴν ἐπιφάνειαν καὶ ψυχρὸν διϊδροῦται κεγχροειδῶς, ὡς ἀπὸ ἀψύχου ἐκκρινό-

1 βρομώδη *codd.*: *correxi* ἔγγονα γ 2 τῶν *om.* γ 3 εἰς] ἐπὶ γ 5 κρισίμη Pζ(M?) 6 γένηται ἱδρὼς L 7 ἡνίκα *om.* γ ἐπακολουθήσει γ 7 πάντως — 8 ἐπακολουθεῖ *om.* γ πάντως *scripsi (cf. infra, linn. 18 sq.)*: σπάνιος L 10 ἐπιλαβόμεν *(ambig.)* ζ: ἐπιλαβόμενοι M: ἐπιλαβόμενον P καὶ *om.* L 12 τῷ MP 13 ἀπαιτεῖται Pζ 16 ἐπειδὴ] ὥστε γ 22 τοῖσι L γένωνται γ 25 ἀπό] *fort.* ὑπό *scribendum est* καὶ^{II} *om.* γ 27 ἃ *scripsi*: ὧν *codd.* 28 οἱ] εἰ, *ut vid.*, L 34 sq. ἐμφύτου θερμοῦ] ἐμφυτευθέντος γ 36 καὶ *om.* L 37 ἀμοιροῦντα — θερμοῦ] ἀμοιροῦντος τοῦ ἐμφυτευθέντος γ 39 ἐκκρινομένου L

fetid and others stinking; all of these are produced by different humors.

The final cause of sweats is the resulting sense of well-being or discomfort.

This part of the discussion completed, let us turn to the symptoms. And he gives the symptoms for sweats, saying that those sweats indicate recovery in which the following four factors coincide and accompany each other: when sweats break out on a critical day, appear all over the body, are warm, and when a sense of well-being follows; and euphoria always results in such cases. It is a good sign when the sweats break out on a critical day; for it shows that nature has taken the matter in an orderly way, without force and after coction, and has expelled the residues through sweats. Sweating throughout the body also is a favorable symptom, because there is an underlying acute disease and fever; and so the matter conveyed in the form of nutriment of necessity remains undigested and residues develop all over the body; these, then, have to be shed by sweating, in order that the patient be rid of the disease. For sweats to be warm is also a good sign, since they come to be like the matter which produced them; for there is an underlying fever and seething heat, and since the sweats obviously make their way out through warm parts they must for this reason be warm themselves. And euphoria always follows these.

The opposite of these are dangerous: if sweats occur on a noncritical day and not throughout the body, but partially and in (certain) areas, and are cold; if on top of this a feeling of discomfort results, they are extremely bad and dangerous. For sweating on a noncritical day indicates that nature, moved and stimulated by something before the matter has been concocted, has gone to work prematurely and produced sweats, which is very bad; it means that nature has been overpowered by the causes which created the sweats. Very bad, too, are sweats that break out in a part of the body, e.g., around the head, face, throat or neck, for it means that the matter is tending upwards; for the fever releases part of the matter and it ascends to the more important parts and to the very first principle, namely the brain, and this is deadly. Cold sweats also are very serious. But first we should describe how they occur. It should be noted that cold sweats are caused by extreme failure, weakness and deficiency of the innate heat; because of its own weakness and deficiency (the heat) wraps itself around the viscera and the depths (of the body), while the outer parts at the surface, deprived of the innate heat, grow cold; and since there is an underlying fever, a flow of matter is bound to occur; then with the flow it comes to the surface and is exuded in beads of cold sweat, shed as from a lifeless body. This is how cold sweats develop.

μενον. καὶ οὕτως γίνονται οἱ ψυχροὶ ἱδρῶτες. κακὸν οὖν ἐν ὀξεῖ νοσήματι οἱ ψυχροὶ ἱδρῶτες· δηλοῖ γὰρ καταβεβλημένον τὸ ἔμφυτον θερμόν, ἐφ' ᾧ ὁ κίνδυνος πάρεστιν. ἐπὶ τούτοις δὲ πάντως ἕπεται δυσφορία. πλὴν καὶ τοῦτο δεῖ εἰδέναι, ὅτι οὐ πάντες οἱ ψυχροὶ ἱδρῶτες ἐπικίνδυνοί εἰσιν· ἐνδέχεται γὰρ διὰ ψυχροτέραν ὕλην βληχρὸν εἶναι τὸν πυρετὸν καὶ ψυχροὺς γενέ-
115 σθαι ἱδρῶτας, καὶ οὐκ ἔστιν ἐπι|κίνδυνον κατὰ τὸ εἰρημένον· «Οἱ ψυχροὶ ἱδρῶτες σὺν μὲν ὀξεῖ πυρετῷ θάνατον σημαίνουσι, σὺν δὲ πρηϋτέρῳ μῆκος νόσου.»

XII

I 46 [7: 200,8 A. = II 124,13 L.] Ὑποχόνδριον δὲ ἄριστον μὲν ἀνώδυνόν τε ἐὸν καὶ μαλθακὸν καὶ ὁμαλὸν καὶ ἐπὶ δεξιὰ καὶ ἐπ' ἀριστερά.

Νῦν σημειοῦται ὁ συγγραφεὺς τὸ ὀξὺ νόσημα ἀπὸ τῆς διαθέσεως τῆς ἐν τοῖς ὑποχονδρίοις συνισταμένης. καὶ εἰκότως μετὰ τοὺς ἱδρῶτας τὰ ὑποχόνδρια μετεχειρίσατο· οἱ γὰρ ἱδρῶτες τῆς τρίτης πέψεώς εἰσι περιττώματα, τὰ δὲ ὑποχόνδρια τὴν πέψιν τῶν χυμῶν ποιοῦνται. διαλέγεται οὖν περὶ ὑποχονδρίων καὶ λέγει ὅτι κάλλιστόν ἐστιν ὑποχόνδριον, ἐν ᾧ τὰ τέσσαρα ταῦτα συνέλθῃ, τὸ μαλθακόν, τὸ ἀνώδυνον, τὸ ὁμαλόν, τὸ ἀφλέγμαντον, τουτέστι τὸ μὴ ἔχον ζέσιν καὶ φλόγωσιν. τὰ δὲ ἐναντία τούτων ἐὰν συνέλθῃ, κάκιστόν ἐστι, τυχὸν ἐὰν συντεταμένον ἐστὶ τὸ ὑποχόνδριον καὶ ὀδύνη σύνεστι καὶ ζέσις καὶ φλόγωσις καὶ ἀνωμαλία. εἰ δὲ τὰ μὲν ὦσι, τὰ δὲ οὐκ ὦσιν, ἧττόν ἐστι κακόν. ἐν τῷ μεταξὺ δὲ τοῦ ἀρίστου καὶ τοῦ χειρίστου ἐστὶ τὸ τὰ ἀριστερὰ ὑποκεῖσθαι βεβλαμμένα, τυχὸν ὁ σπλήν, τὰ δὲ δεξιὰ ἀβλαβῆ, ἤγουν τὸ ἧπαρ· δηλοῖ γὰρ τὴν πρώτην ἀρχὴν τῆς πέψεως καλῶς διακεῖσθαι. εἶτα δεῖ ἡμᾶς εἰπεῖν καὶ τὴν αἰτίαν, καθ' ἣν κάλλιστόν ἐστιν ὑποχόνδριον, ἐὰν συνέλθῃ τὰ προειρημένα τέσσαρα σημεῖα. καὶ τὸ μὲν μαλθακὸν σημαίνει τὸ ἀπηλλαγμένον παντὸς ὄγκου παρὰ φύσιν, τυχὸν μήτε φλεγμονὴν ἔχον μήτε σκίρρον μήτε οἴδημα καὶ τὰ τοιαῦτα. ἀλλ' ἴσως ἐρεῖ τις ὅτι «Καὶ πόθεν δῆλον ὅτι οἴδημα οὐκ ἔστι; καὶ γὰρ τὸ οἴδημα ὄγκος μέν ἐστιν, εἴκει δὲ τῇ ἀφῇ, ὥσπερ καὶ τὸ μαλθακὸν εἴκει τῇ ἀφῇ· τὸ γὰρ μαλθακὸν τῷ συντεταμένῳ ἀντίκειται.» καὶ λέγομεν ὅτι οὐκ ἔστιν οἴδημα, ὡς δηλοῖ ἐκ τοῦ ὀξὺ εἶναι τὸ ἐξεταζόμενον νόσημα, ἐν δὲ ὀξεῖ νοσήματι
116 οὐδέποτε οἴδημα γίνεται ἐπὶ τὰ ὑποχόνδρια. ἀλλὰ καὶ τὸ | ἀνώδυνον ἀγαθόν ἐστι· δηλοῖ γὰρ ὅτι οὐδεμία δριμύτης πλεονάζει ἐν αὐτοῖς, ἀλλ' οὐδὲ πνεύματα ἐμφωλεύουσιν, ἀλλ' οὐδὲ πλῆθος χυμῶν πλεονάζει ἐν αὐτοῖς

6 τὸ εἰρημένον] Hipp. Aph. IV 37: IV p. 516,4sq. L. *cf.* Hipp. Progn. 6: p. 200,6sq. A. = II p. 124,6–8 L.

1 sq. οἱ ψυχροὶ ἱδρῶτες *post* οὖν *trsp.* γ 2 ᾧ] ὃ γ: ὧν L: *correxi* 4 sq. ἐνδέχεται γὰρ *om.* γ 5 ψυχροὺς] βληχρὰ L γενέσθαι] γεν *ante spat. circa 3 litt.* L 6 ἐπικίνδυνος γ 11 ὂν L καὶ ὁμαλὸν *om.* L, *sed cf. lin. 18* 11 sq. δεξιᾶ … ἀριστερᾶ γ 13 τῆς^{II}] τοῖς Pζ 14 συνισταμένοις Pζ: συνισταμένοις *in* -ης *corr.* M 17 ἐστιν *post* ὑποχόνδριον *trsp.* γ 22 τοῦ^{II} *om.* γ 23 βεβλαμμένος γ 24 ἀβλαβῶς *codd.*: *corr. Wk.* τῷ ἥπατι L 24 sq. καλῶς διακεῖσθαι *om.* L 29 Καὶ^{I} – γὰρ *om.* γ 30 εἴκει^{I}] ἥκει *codd.*: *corr. Dietz* εἴκει^{II}] ἥκει γ 32 *ante* ὀξεῖ *add.* τῷ γ

Cold sweats are an unfavorable sign, then, in acute disease, showing that the innate heat has failed, as a result of which the danger is created. In these circumstances a feeling of discomfort is sure to follow. However, it should also be realized that not all cold sweats are dangerous; for it is possible, on account of rather cold matter, that the fever be slight and cold sweats occur, and this is not dangerous, according to the words, "Cold sweats with acute fever mean death, with a milder (fever) prolonged illness."

XII

I 46 The hypochondrium is in the best condition when it is free from pain and soft and even on the right and left sides.

Our author now gives the symptoms for acute disease from the condition of the hypochondria. It is natural that after sweats he has taken up the subject of the hypochondria; for sweats are the residues of the third digestion and the hypochondria produce coction of the humors. He discusses the hypochondria, then, and tells us that the hypochondrium is in the best condition when the following four factors are present concurrently: softness, painlessness, evenness and freedom from inflammation, that is, absence of a seething and burning heat. But if the opposite of these occur together, it is very bad, that is, if the hypochondrium is taut, has pain, and a seething and burning heat, and is uneven. If some of these are present, but not the others, it is less serious. Between the best and the worst is the state in which the left side, i.e., the spleen, is affected while the right or liver is normal; for it means that the first principle of coction is working well. Next we should give also the reason why the hypochondrium is in the best condition if the four previously mentioned symptoms appear together. Being soft means that it is free of all abnormal swelling, which is to say that there is no inflammation, induration, tumor or the like. But someone may say, "How is it clear that there is no tumor? For while a tumor is a swelling, it does yield to pressure just as softness yields to pressure, softness being the opposite of tautness." We reply that there is no tumor, the proof being that the disease under consideration is acute and in acute disease a tumor never develops in the hypochondria. Painlessness also is a good sign, showing that the hypochondria have no excess of acrid matter, that there are no gases lurking inside and that there is no overflow of

παρατεῖνον, καὶ τῷ λόγῳ τούτῳ ἀνώδυνά εἰσιν. ἀλλὰ καὶ τὸ ἀφλέγμαντα εἶναι δηλοῖ ὅτι οὐδεμία ζέσις ἢ φλόγωσίς ἐστιν ἐν αὐτοῖς. καὶ δεῖ αὐτὰ καὶ ὁμαλὰ εἶναι, τουτέστιν ὅμοια καὶ ἴσα πάντῃ κατά τε ποσότητα καὶ κρᾶσιν· ἐνδέχεται γὰρ ὁμαλῶς διακεῖσθαι κατὰ τὸν ὄγκον καὶ μηδεὶς ὄγκος ὢν ἐν αὐτοῖς, ἀνωμάλως δὲ κεκρᾶσθαι. καὶ ταῦτα μὲν περὶ τῶν κατὰ φύσιν ὑποχονδρίων.

Εἴπωμεν δὲ καὶ τὴν αἰτίαν τῶν ποιούντων παρὰ φύσιν τὰ ὑποχόνδρια. τὸ δὲ παρὰ φύσιν καὶ νοσῶδες καὶ ἄχρηστον ἐκ τῶν ἐναντίων τεσσάρων συνίσταται, ἐκ τοῦ σκίρρου καὶ τῆς ὀδύνης καὶ τῆς ζέσεως καὶ τῆς ἀνωμαλίας. ταῦτα συνερχόμενα ἀλλήλοις καὶ ἐν τῷ ἅμα συνιστάμενα κάκιστον καὶ νοσῶδες τὸ ὑποχόνδριον ἀπεργάζονται. καὶ τὸ μὲν σκληρὸν ὑποχόνδριον ἢ μεγίστην φλεγμονὴν σημαίνει ἢ ἔμφραξιν, ἅπερ ἐπὶ δαψιλεῖ ὕλῃ γίνονται, καὶ κάκιστά εἰσι ταῦτα ἐν ὀξεῖ νοσήματι. ἀλλὰ καὶ ἡ ὀδύνη κακίστη ἐστὶ διά γε τὴν ὀδυνηρὰν διάθεσιν· οὐ πᾶσα γὰρ διάθεσις ὀδύνην ἐργάζεται, ἀλλὰ αἱ μέγισται διαθέσεις. ἄλλως τε δὲ κάκιστόν ἐστι τὸ ὀδυνᾶσθαι, ὅτι ἡ ὀδύνη ἐπιτείνει τὰ ῥεύματα· ἐπὶ δὲ τοῖς ῥευματισμοῖς αἱ δυνάμεις καταβάλλονται. ἀλλὰ καὶ ἡ φλόγωσις ἐν τοῖς ὑποχονδρίοις κακόν ἐστι· δηλοῖ γὰρ μεγάλην ζέσιν καὶ καῦσιν καὶ δραστήριον τὴν ποιήσασαν ὕλην καὶ ὑποκειμένην ἐν ᾧ ταῦτα γίνονται. ἀλλὰ καὶ τὸ ἀνώμαλον κακόν ἐστιν, ἐὰν ὄγκος ἐστὶν ἐν τῷ ὑποχονδρίῳ· μάλιστα δὲ κακόν ἐστιν, ἔνθα τὰ ἀμφότερα ὑποχόνδρια φλεγμαίνωσι. καὶ ἔστι τοῦτο ὁμαλὸν παρὰ φύσιν, ἐπειδὴ ἀμφότερα ὁμοίως ἐφλέγμαναν. μέσον δὲ τοῦ ἀρίστου καὶ τοῦ χειρίστου ἐστίν, ἐὰν τὰ μὲν μετέχωσι τοῦ πάθους, τὰ δὲ μὴ μετέχωσιν. εἶτα καὶ προσδιορίζεται ὅτι τὰ τέσσαρα σημεῖα κακά ἐστι μετὰ τῶν λοιπῶν, ἐπειδὴ ἐνδείκνυνται δαψίλειαν καὶ πλῆθος ὕλης, ἐφ' ᾗ οὐ μόνον τὸν πυρετὸν |
117 ἀνῆψεν, ἀλλ' ἀντήρκεσε καὶ τὰ πάθη ταῦτα ποιῆσαι, ὅπερ κάκιστόν ἐστιν ἐν ὀξεῖ νοσήματι. κακὰ δέ ἐστιν ἐν ἀρχῇ τῆς νόσου ταῦτα γινόμενα. ἀρχὴν δὲ ἀκουστέον ἐνταῦθα τὴν εἰκοστὴν ἡμέραν· ἡ γὰρ εἰκοστὴ ἡμέρα ἀκμή ἐστι τῆς φλεγμονῆς, ἀρχὴ δὲ τῆς ἀποστάσεως καὶ πυοποιήσεως. δεῖ γὰρ εἰδέναι ὅτι, ἐὰν ἔρρωται ἡ δύναμις καὶ ὡσαύτως μείνῃ ἡ ὀξύτης τοῦ πυρετοῦ μετὰ τὴν εἰκοστὴν ἡμέραν, εἰς πυοποίησιν τρέπεται τὸ ἀπόστημα. εἰ δέ γε ἀσθενής ἐστιν ἡ δύναμις καὶ ὑποχαλάσῃ ὁ πυρετὸς καὶ βληχρότερος γένηται μετὰ τὴν εἰκοστὴν ἡμέραν, ἢ θάνατον σημαίνει ἢ μῆκος νόσου, ὅπερ καὶ αὐτὸ κάκιστόν ἐστι. πολλάκις δὲ πρὸ τῆς κʹ ἡμέρας ἡ φύσις κριτικῶς κινουμένη, δι' αἱμορραγίας κενοῦσα τὴν ὕλην, ἀπαλλάσσει τοῦ πάθους τὸ ὑποχόνδριον. προγινώσκομεν δὲ τὴν μέλλουσαν κρίσιν δι' αἱμορραγίας γενέσθαι ἀπὸ ἕξ τινων· οἱ τοιοῦτοι κνῶνται τὴν ῥῖνα, τὰ μῆλα τοῦ προσώπου αὐτῶν ἐρυθραίνονται, πυραυγῆ καὶ ἐρυθρὰ φαντάσματα ὁρῶσιν, ἡλικία ἀκμαστική, κεφαλαλγία αὐτοῖς γίνεται ἄλογος καὶ ἀμβλυώττουσιν.

I 47 [7: 201,2 A. = II 126,3 L.] Εἰ δὲ καὶ σφυγμὸς ἐνείη ἐν τῷ

1 περιτείνοντα γ ἀφλέγμαντον γ 3 πάντῃ] κατὰ πάντα γ ποσότητα *scripsi*: ποιότητα *codd.* 4 κρίσιν γ 7 εἴπομεν γ 9 σκίρρους, *ut vid.*, L 14 γε] τε γ 15 αἱ *om.* L 18 κάκιστόν γ 19 γίνεται γ 21 τὰ *post* ἀμφότερα *trsp.* γ φλεγμήνωσι γ 22 ὁμοίως ἀμφότερα γ 30 μένει γ 31 τρέπει γ 32 ὑποχαλάσει γ 33 μῆκος] ὕπνος L 35 κενοῦσα] κινοῦσα L 37 κενῶνται L 39 ἀμβλυώττουσα γ 40 ἐνείη] εἴη L

humors causing them strain, and for this reason they are without pain. Being without inflammation means that there is no seething or burning heat in them. And they should be even as well, i.e., uniform and regular all over in both quantity and temperament, since it is possible for them to be even in bulk with no swelling, but to have an unbalanced te pera- ment. So much for the normal hypochondria.

Let us also explain the factors responsible for the abnormal hypochondria. The abnormal, diseased and useless hypochondrium is caused by the four opposite symptoms, namely induration, pain, seething heat and unevenness. When these appear together and develop at the same time they leave the hypochondrium in an extremely bad and morbid state. And the hard hypochondrium means either serious inflammation or a stoppage, which result from a superabundance of matter and are very dangerous symptoms in acute disease. Pain as well is an extremely bad sign because of the painful condition; for not every condition causes pain, but (only) the very serious. Besides, pain (in the hypochondrium) is highly dangerous because it increases the fluxes and these cause failure of the faculties. And burning heat in the hypochondria is bad, pointing to intense seething and burning heat and to the potency of the underlying and responsible matter in the place where this occurs. And unevenness is an unfavorable symptom, if there is a swelling in the hypochondrium; it is especially bad when both hypochondria are inflamed. This produces an abnormal evenness, since both are similarly inflamed. The condition midway between the best and the worst is where one (side of the hypochondrium) has the affection and the other not. Next he adds qualifying remarks to the effect that the four symptoms are bad in conjunction with the others, since they indicate an overflow and superabundance of matter which not only started the fever but was able as well to produce these affections; and this is highly dangerous in acute disease. And such conditions are bad when they arise at the beginning of the disease. The beginning here is to be understood as the twentieth day; for the twentieth day is the high point of the inflammation and the start of abscession and suppuration. For it should be noted that if the (body's) power is strong and the acuteness of the fever continues the same after the twentieth day, the abscess turns to suppuration. But if the power is weak and the fever abates and becomes slighter after the twentieth day, it signals either death or a prolonged illness, which also is a very bad sign. However, it often happens that before the twentieth day nature moves to crisis and evacuates the matter by haemorrhage, thus ridding the hypochondrium of its affection. An impending crisis by haemorrhage we predict from six indications: such people scratch the nose, their cheeks turn red, they see flaming fiery visions, they are in the prime age and suffer from unexplained headache and dim sight.

I 47 If there is pulsation as well in the hypochondrium, it

ὑποχονδρίῳ, θόρυβον σημαίνει ἢ παραφροσύνην.

Τινὰ τῶν ἀντιγράφων παλμὸν ἔχει. κακὸν δέ ἐστι σημεῖον· ὁ γὰρ παλμὸς ἐπὶ παχεῖ καὶ ψυχρώδει καὶ φυσώδει πνεύματι γίνεται. κακὸν οὖν ἐστι παλμὸν γίνεσθαι ἐν ὀξεῖ νοσήματι, ἐπειδὴ ξένον καὶ ἀλλότριόν ἐστι τὸ ἐπιγενόμενον σύμπτωμα. τινὰ δὲ εἰ δὲ καὶ σφυγμός ἐστι. κακὸν δέ ἐστι καὶ τοῦτο σημεῖον· δηλοῖ γὰρ ἢ θόρυβον, τουτέστι δυσφορίαν, τῷ κάμνοντι, ἀλλὰ καὶ τῷ τεχνίτῃ ἀγῶνα περὶ τὰ πρακτέα διὰ τὸ μέγεθος τοῦ πάθους. σφυγμὸν δὲ λέγει ἐνταῦθα τὴν σφυγματώδη ὀδύνην θλιβομένου καὶ στενοχωρουμένου τοῦ μεγάλου σφυγμοῦ, λέγω δὴ τῆς ἀρτηρίας. αὕτη γὰρ ἡ ἀρτηρία ἤγουν ἡ ἀορτὴ πλησιάζει τῷ στομάχῳ καὶ τῷ διαφράγματι καὶ τῷ ἥπατι.
118 τούτων οὖν φλεγμαινόντων τῶν ὑποχονδρίων ἐν | τῷ σφύζειν οὐ δύναται ἀβιάστως ἐν τῷ κατὰ φύσιν διασταλῆναι, ἀλλ' ἐν τῷ σφύζειν πλήττει τὸ φλεγμαῖνον μόριον καὶ ποιεῖ τὴν σφυγματώδη ὀδύνην, ὅπερ κάκιστόν ἐστιν ἐν ὀξεῖ νοσήματι· σημαίνει γὰρ παραφροσύνην, ἐπειδὴ ὁ ἐγκέφαλος συμπάσχει τοῖς νευρώδεσι μορίοις, ἔνθα ἢ πολλὰ νεῦρα καταφύονται ἢ μέγιστα. ἐπειδὴ οὖν ἐνταῦθα ὁ στόμαχος πολλὰ νεῦρα ὑποδέχεται, ἀλλὰ καὶ μέγιστα, ἐπὶ τῇ φλεγμονῇ τοῦ στομάχου ὁ ἐγκέφαλος ἄγεται εἰς συμπάθειαν διὰ τὴν συγγένειαν τῶν νεύρων, καὶ γίνεται ἡ παραφροσύνη. εἶτα ἐπειδὴ ἔφη ὅτι ἢ θόρυβον σημαίνει ἢ παραφροσύνην, καὶ προσδιορισμὸν τίθησι, πῶς ὀφείλομεν γνῶναι, εἴτε παραφροσύνη μέλλει γενέσθαι εἴτε θόρυβος. καὶ λέγει ὅτι δεῖ τοὺς ὀφθαλμοὺς θεωρῆσαι, καὶ εἰ μὲν ἀστήρικτοί εἰσι καὶ τρομωδῶς κινοῦνται, γίνωσκε ὅτι παραφροσύνην σημαίνει· ἡ γὰρ τοιαύτη κίνησις τῶν ὀφθαλμῶν ἐπὶ βλάβῃ τῶν κινούντων μυῶν γίνεται· ἡ δὲ βλάβη τῶν κινούντων μυῶν δηλοῖ τὸ πρῶτον γένος τοῦ νευρώδους γένους κακῶς διακείμενον· τὸ δὲ νευρῶδες γένος δηλοῖ τὸν ἐγκέφαλον βεβλαμμένον, ἐφ' ᾧ ἡ παραφροσύνη ἕπεται. εἰ δὲ κατὰ φύσιν κινοῦνται οἱ ὀφθαλμοί, θόρυβον σημαίνει καὶ δυσφορίαν τοῦ κάμνοντος καὶ ἀγῶνα τῷ τεχνίτῃ περὶ τὰ πρακτέα διὰ τὸ μέγεθος τῆς διαθέσεως. δεῖ δὲ καὶ τοῦτο εἰδέναι, ὅτι ἡ μανία ἐπιτεταμένη ἐστὶ παραφροσύνη.

I 48 [7: 201,4 A. = II 126,6 L.] Ἢν γὰρ αἱ ὄψιες πυκνὰ κινέωνται, μανῆναι τούτους ἐλπίς.

Ἐκ τούτου τοῦ ῥησειδίου κατασκευάζουσιν οἱ ἐξηγηταὶ ὅτι ἐν ἐγκεφάλῳ ἐστὶ τὸ ἡγεμονικόν· ἐὰν γὰρ ἡ βλάβη τῶν ὀφθαλμῶν δηλοῖ τὸν ἐγκέφαλον κακῶς διακείμενον, ἡ δὲ παραφροσύνη βλάβη ἐστὶ τοῦ ἡγεμο-

2sq.] *cf.* Gal. In Hipp. Progn. comm. I 28: CMG V 9,2 p. 245,11–13 19 καὶ – 26] *cf.* Gal. In Hipp. Progn. comm. I 28: CMG V 9,2 pp. 246,18–247,3 32–126,15] *cf.* Ioann. Comm. in Hipp. De morb. pop. VI: 143c8–15 Pritchet

4 ἐστι[I]] ἐπὶ L παλμὸν γίνεσθαι *om.* γ 5 τινὰ] ἀ *post spat. 3 litt.* L δὲ καὶ *sec. Hipp. scr. Dietz*: δὲ L: καὶ γ σφυγμὸν ἔχει γ 13 ἐστιν *post* νοσήματι *(lin. 14) trsp.* γ 15 *post* πολλὰ *add.* τὰ γ 16 *ante* πολλὰ *add.* καὶ γ 19 ὅτι *om.* γ 25 διακειμένου γ δηλοῖ] σημαίνει γ 29 ἐστὶ *post* μανία *(lin. 28) trsp.* γ 30 κινέονται γ 33 ἡ] ἢ MZ

means distress or delirium.

Some manuscripts have throbbing (instead of pulsation). This is a bad sign, since throbbing is caused by dense, cold and flatulent gas. Throbbing in acute disease, then, is dangerous because the symptom which develops is foreign and unusual. Some (copies) have If there is pulsation. And this, too, is a serious symptom, indicating both distress or discomfort for the patient and a struggle for the doctor in deciding what must be done, because of the magnitude of the condition. By pulsation here he means the throbbing pain produced by compression and constriction of the great pulse, in other words, of the (great) artery. For this artery, the aorta, runs close to the orifice of the stomach, the diaphragm and the liver. So when these parts of the hypochondrium are inflamed, (the artery,) unable to expand normally and without forcing during pulsation, strikes against the inflamed part when beating and produces the throbbing pain; this is a very bad sign in acute disease; for it means delirium, the brain being affected in sympathy with the nervous parts in which are implanted a large number of nerves or very important ones. Since the mouth of the stomach, then, has been given many and very important nerves, when the mouth of the stomach is affected by inflammation, the brain is made to sympathize due to the nerve relationship and delirium develops. Then, having said it means either distress or delirium he also specifies how we should recognize whether delirium is about to develop or distress. He says that it is necessary to observe the eyes; if they are unstable and trembling, you may conclude that it means delirium; for this type of eye movement is caused by damage in the kinetic muscles; and damage in the kinetic muscles indicates that the first class of nerves is in poor condition, which in turn means that the brain is damaged, and delirium follows as a result. On the other hand, if the eyes move normally it indicates distress and discomfort for the patient and a problem for the doctor in deciding the course of action to be adopted because of the seriousness of the condition. Note also that mania is a severe form of delirium.

I 48 For if the eyeballs move rapidly you may expect such patients to go mad.

The commentators use this text to argue that the brain is the seat of the governing principle; if a fault in the eyes, (they maintain,) indicates brain malfunction, and delirium is damage to the governing principle

νικοῦ, οὐκοῦν ἐν ἐγκεφάλῳ ἐστὶ τὸ ἡγεμονικόν. ὁ δὲ νέος ἐξηγητὴς λέγει ὅτι «Καὶ πόθεν δῆλον ὅτι ἐν καρδίᾳ οὐκ ἔστι ἡγεμονικόν; τί γάρ; ὅτι ἡ βλάβη τῶν ὀφθαλμῶν τὴν καρδίαν ἐνδείκνυται πεπονθέναι καὶ οὐ τὸν
119 ἐγκέφαλον, τρόπῳ | τοιούτῳ· πυρετὸς ὑπόκειται ὀξύς· ἐπὶ τῷ πυρετῷ βλάπτεται ἡ καρδία· ἐπὶ τῇ βλάβῃ τῆς καρδίας οὐ πέμπεται ζωτικὸς τόνος καὶ εὐκρασία ἐπὶ τὸν ἐγκέφαλον· ζωτικοῦ δὲ τόνου μὴ πεμπομένου οὐ τίκτεται ζωτικὸν πνεῦμα· τοῦ δὲ ζωτικοῦ πνεύματος μὴ τικτομένου, οὐ πέμπεται δῆλον ἐπὶ τοὺς ὀφθαλμούς, ἐν ᾧ ἔχουσι τὸ διογκοῦσθαι ἐν τῷ κατὰ φύσιν· καὶ ἰδοὺ ἡ βλάβη τῶν ὀφθαλμῶν δηλοῖ τὴν καρδίαν πεπονθυῖαν. βεβλαμμένης δὲ οὔσης τῆς καρδίας διὰ τῶν ἀρτηριῶν πέμπεται ἐπὶ τὸν ἐγκέφαλον, καὶ βλάπτεται ὁ ἐγκέφαλος καὶ ἐκ τοῦ σύνεγγυς μεταδίδωσι τῆς βλάβης καὶ τοῖς ὀφθαλμοῖς. καὶ κατὰ μὲν πρῶτον λόγον διὰ τὴν καρδίαν γέγονεν ἡ βλάβη καὶ τοῦ ἐγκεφάλου καὶ τῶν ὀφθαλμῶν. εἰ δὲ ταῦτα οὕτως, ἐν καρδίᾳ ἐστὶ τὸ ἡγεμονικόν.» καὶ μέχρι τοῦ νῦν ἐν δισταγμῷ ἐστιν ἡ τοιαύτη ζήτησις, εἴτε ἐν ἐγκεφάλῳ ἐστὶ τὸ ἡγεμονικὸν εἴτε ἐν καρδίᾳ.

I 49 [7: 201,9 A. = II 126,11 L.] Εἰ δὲ ὑπερβάλλοι εἴκοσιν ἡμέρας ὅ τε πυρετὸς ἔχων καὶ τὸ οἴδημα μὴ καθιστάμενον, εἰς διαπύησιν τρέπεται.

Ὁ Ἱπποκράτης πάντα ὄγκον οἴδημα καλεῖν εἴωθεν. καὶ δεῖ εἰδέναι ὅτι πάντες οἱ ὄγκοι ἢ διαφοροῦνται ἢ κατὰ ποιότητα μεταβάλλονται. καὶ οἱ μὲν διαφορούμενοι πέρας τὴν εἰκοστὴν ἡμέραν ἔχουσιν. οἱ δὲ κατὰ ποιότητα μεταβαλλόμενοι, εἰ μὲν ἔρρωται ἡ δύναμις καὶ ἡ σφοδρότης τοῦ πυρετοῦ ὡσαύτως μένει, μετὰ τὴν εἰκοστὴν ἡμέραν εἰς πυοποίησιν μεταβάλλει τοὺς ὄγκους· εἰ δὲ ἀσθενής ἐστιν ἡ δύναμις καὶ ὁ πυρετὸς βληχρότερος γένηται, μεταβάλλει μὲν τοὺς ὄγκους, ἀλλ' εἰς νοσώδη καὶ δυσώδη τινὰ ὑγρότητα.

XIII

I 50 [7: 202,1 A. = II 128,4 L.] Τὰ δὲ μαλθακὰ τῶν οἰδημάτων καὶ ἀνώδυνα καὶ τῷ δακτύλῳ ὑπείκοντα χρονιωτέρας

Νῦν ὁ συγγραφεὺς περὶ τοῦ οἰδήματος τοῦ ἐν τοῖς ὑποχονδρίοις σημειοῦται. καὶ τὴν ἑξηκοστὴν ἡμέραν ἀρχὴν τῆς πυοποιήσεως τίθησιν,

1 ὁ – ἐξηγητὴς] *v. supra*, p. 13 *cf. infra*, p. 256,32 Steph. Comm. in Hipp. Aph.: Escor. Σ. II. 10 fol. 69v 19] *v.* Gal. In Hipp. Progn. comm. I 29: CMG V 9,2 p. 247,8 *cf. infra*, pp. 184,21 sq.; 266,28 Steph. Comm. in Hipp. Aph.: Escor. Σ. II. 10 fol. 186v Pall. Comm. in Hipp. De morb. pop. VI: II p. 5,9sq. Dietz Ioann. Comm. in Hipp. De morb. pop. VI: 120c11sq. Pritchet 20 πάντες – μεταβάλλονται] *cf.* Gal. In Hipp. Progn. comm. I 31: CMG V 9,2 p. 248,10–22

2 ἡ *om.* L 3 ἐνδείκνυνται L πεπονθέναι] βεβλαμμένην γ 6 καὶ εὐκρασία *post* ἐγκέφαλον *trsp.* γ τίκτεται *post* πνεῦμα *(lin. 7) trsp.* γ 9 ἡ βλάβη *post* ὀφθαλμῶν *trsp.* γ δὲ *om.* γ 16 ὑπερβάλλει L 20 οἱ *om.* L 25 δυσώδη καὶ νοσώδη γ 29 χρονιωτέρας *om.* γ 31 εἰκοστὴν L

then the brain is the seat of the governing principle. The new commentator, however, says "What evidence is there that the governing principle is not situated in the heart? Why? Because eye damage means that the heart, not the brain, is affected, (and the proof is) as follows: there is acute fever; in the fever the heart is damaged; when the heart is damaged neither vital tone nor good temperament are transmitted to the brain; vital tone not being transmitted, no vital pneuma is produced; vital pneuma no longer produced, obviously none is sent to the eyes, which is their normal means of filling out; therefore eye damage means heart trouble. When the heart is out of order (the trouble) is transmitted through the arteries to the brain, then the brain is affected and, because of the proximity, passes on the fault also to the eyes. Therefore it is the heart which is primarily responsible for both brain and eye damage. This being the case, the heart is the seat of the governing principle." Thus the question remains unresolved up until now, whether the governing principle is situated in the brain or heart.

I 49 If the fever continues longer than twenty days and the tumor does not subside, it turns to suppuration.

Hippocrates usually calls every swelling a tumor. Note that all swellings either dissipate or undergo a change in quality. Those that dissipate have a limit of twenty days. Those that change in quality, when the (body's) power is strong and the fever's intensity remains constant, turn to suppuration after the twentieth day; however, if the power is weak and the fever becomes slighter, the swellings do change, but into a morbid and fetid fluid.

XIII

I 50 Tumors which are soft, painless and yield to the finger prolong

Here our author gives the symptoms from tumor in the hypochondria. He fixes the sixtieth day as the starting point of suppuration, since

120 ἐπειδὴ οὐ πέφυκε διαφορεῖσθαι | τὰ οἰδήματα διὰ τὴν ὕλην, ἀλλὰ πυοποιοῦνται. καὶ ἴσως ἀπορεῖ τις λέγων ὅτι «Καὶ πόθεν δῆλον ὅτι περὶ τοῦ κυρίως οἰδήματος διαλέγεται;» καὶ λέγομεν ὅτι ἐξ ὧν εἴρηκε δῆλον ὅτι περὶ τοῦ κυρίως οἰδήματος διαλεγόμενος· ἔφη γάρ· Τὰ δὲ μαλθακὰ τῶν οἰδημάτων καὶ ἀνώδυνα καὶ τῷ δακτύλῳ ὑπείκοντα καὶ τὰ λοιπά, ταῦτα δὲ πάντα οἰδήματός εἰσι χαρακτηριστικά. εἶτα καὶ ἀποροῦσι πάλιν ὅτι «Καὶ τί δήποτε περὶ ὀξέων νοσημάτων προθέμενος διαλεχθῆναι ὁ Ἱπποκράτης ἑξηκοστῆς ἡμέρας ἐμνημόνευσε, καίτοι τῶν ὀξέων νοσημάτων οὐδέποτε ἐν τῇ ἑξηκοστῇ ἡμέρᾳ περιγραφομένων, ἀλλὰ τῶν χρονίων ἐστὶν ἡ ἑξηκοστὴ ἡμέρα;» καὶ λέγομεν τούτου δύο αἰτίας, μίαν μὲν ὅτι πολλάκις οἱ συγγραφεῖς κατὰ παρέκβασιν ὑπερβαίνουσι τὴν τάξιν διὰ τὸ μηδὲν παραλιπεῖν. ἢ τοῦτο εἰπέ, ὅτι τῇ ἀκολουθίᾳ καὶ τῇ ὁμοιότητι παρακολουθοῦντες οἱ συγγραφεῖς παρεκβαίνουσι τοῦ οἰκείου σκοποῦ, ὅπερ νῦν πεποίηκεν ὁ Ἱπποκράτης. ἐπειδὴ γὰρ περὶ πυοποιήσεως φλεγμονῆς διελέγετο, ηὕρισκε καὶ τὸ οἴδημα πυοποιούμενον· διὰ τοῦτο τοῦ οἰκείου σκοποῦ μετῆλθε καὶ ἐπὶ τοῦτο μετήγαγε τὸν λόγον. δεῖ δὲ εἰδέναι ὅτι τὸ οἴδημα καὶ μακροχρόνιόν ἐστι διὰ τὴν ὕλην· ψυχρὸν γάρ ἐστιν. ἀλλὰ καὶ ἀκίνδυνον, ἐπειδὴ ἀνώδυνόν ἐστιν. οὐδὲν γὰρ οὕτως καταβάλλει τὰς δυνάμεις ὡς αἱ ὀδύναι.

Καὶ ἰστέον ὅτι πάντες οἱ ὄγκοι ἢ πρωϊαίτερον ἢ ὀψιαίτερον πυοποιοῦνται διά τε τὴν ὕλην καὶ διὰ τὸ μόριον. καὶ διὰ μὲν τὴν ὕλην τριχῶς, παρά τε τὸ ποσὸν καὶ ποιὸν καὶ τὴν σύστασιν τῆς ὕλης. καὶ παρὰ μὲν τὴν σύστασιν ἡ λεπτὴ ὕλη πρωϊαίτερον πυοποιΐσκεται, ἡ δὲ παχεῖα ὀψιαίτερον. παρὰ δὲ τὴν ποιότητα ἡ θερμὴ ὕλη πρωϊαίτερον, ἡ δὲ ψυχρὰ ὀψιαίτερον. παρὰ δὲ τὴν ποσότητα ἡ ὀλίγη ὕλη πρωϊαίτερον πυοποιΐσκεται, ἡ δὲ πολλὴ ὀψιαίτερον. τινὲς δὲ ἐκ τοῦ ἐναντίου λέγουσιν ὅτι ἡ πολλὴ ὕλη πρωϊαίτερον πυοποιΐσκεται, ἐπειδὴ τῷ πλήθει κατεπείγεται ἡ φύσις στενοχωρουμένη ὑπὸ
121 τοῦ πλήθους καὶ | κινουμένη συντόνως πρωϊαίτερον πυοποιεῖ αὐτήν. παρὰ δὲ τὸ πεπονθὸς διάφορον μόριον τριχῶς, παρά τε τὸ ἀξίωμα τοῦ μορίου καὶ παρὰ τὴν θέσιν καὶ παρὰ τὴν κρᾶσιν [καὶ παρὰ τὴν ἀξίαν]. καὶ παρὰ μὲν τὸ ἀξίωμα, τῶν κυριωτέρων μορίων μᾶλλον φροντίζουσα ἡ φύσις, ἐὰν ὑποστῇ ὄγκος τις ἐν κυρίῳ μορίῳ, κήδεται αὐτοῦ καὶ ἐπεγείρεται, ὥστε ἀπαλλάξαι αὐτὸ τῶν λυπούντων, καὶ πρωϊαίτερον πυοποιεῖ αὐτόν. εἰ δὲ ἀκυρότερόν ἐστι μόριον, οὐχ οὕτως φροντίζει αὐτοῦ καὶ ὀψιαίτερον πυοποιεῖ τὸν ὄγκον. διὸ μᾶλλον φροντίζει ἥπατος πάσχοντος ἤπερ γαστρὸς καὶ μᾶλλον κήδεται γαστρὸς ἤπερ σπληνὸς καὶ μᾶλλον σπληνὸς ἤπερ ἐντέρων. παρὰ δὲ τὴν θέσιν, ὅσα πλησιάζει κυρίοις μορίοις, πρωϊαίτερον πυοποιεῖ

1sq.] *cf.* Schol. R *in* Gal. In Hipp. Progn. comm. I 35: CMG V 9,2 p. 251 *ad* lin. 14

1 τὰ οἰδήματα *post* ἐπειδὴ *trsp.* γ 3 κυρίου *codd.*: *correxi* 4 δὲ *om.* L 5 *post* δακτύλῳ *add.* πιεζόμενα καὶ L *(ex Hipp.)*; *sed cf. supra, p. 126,29; infra, p. 130,31* 6 οἰδήματα L 12 κατακολουθοῦντες γ 15 διελέγετο *om.* L εὕρισκε γ 16 δὲ *om.* γ 17 ψυχρὰ L 18 ἀνώδυνόν] ἄνωθεν ὂν (ὂν *punctis del.?*) L 21 διὰ[II] *om.* γ 25 τὴν *om.* L 29 τριχῶς *scripsi*: τετραχῶς *codd.* 30 καὶ[II] – ἀξίαν *seclusi* *post* ἀξίαν *add.* γοῦν L 30sq. καὶ[III] – ἀξίωμα *om.* L 33 αὐτὸ] αὐτῷ *codd.*: *corr. Dietz* αὐτόν] αὐτὸ γ 35 *post* ἥπατος *add.* ἢ L 37 πυοποιεῖται L

these tumors are not able to dissipate due to the matter, but turn to suppuration. Here someone may object, "How can you be sure that he is talking about tumor in the strict sense?" Our answer is that it is clear from his own words that he is discussing tumor in the strict sense; for he said, Tumors which are soft, painless and yield to the finger, etc., and all these are tumor characteristics. Then a further problem is raised, "If his original proposal was to discuss acute diseases, why did Hippocrates mention the sixtieth day, despite the fact that the sixtieth day is never a limit for acute diseases, but applies to the chronic?" We offer two reasons for this; first, many times writers by a digression, to avoid omitting anything, go beyond the limit (of their topic). Alternatively, you may say that authors stray outside the subject proper when they follow through and continue on the same line of thought, which is what Hippocrates has just done. Since he has been describing inflammation turned to suppuration, he came also upon suppurating tumor; for this reason he went beyond his subject proper and diverted the discussion to this point. And note that the tumor lasts a long time, too, because of the matter, since it is a cold thing. However, being painless it is without danger. For there is nothing that weakens the faculties as pains do.

Note that all swellings suppurate sooner or later depending on the matter and the part. The matter determines this in three ways, by its quantity, quality and consistency. By consistency: thin matter suppurates sooner, dense later. By quality: warm matter sooner, cold later. By quantity: little matter suppurates sooner, much later. But on this point some maintain the opposite, that a large quantity of matter suppurates sooner, since nature is pressured by the abundance, being constricted by it, and moving under strain it brings about suppuration earlier. The different part affected in three ways, by its importance, position and temperament. By importance: seeing that nature has greater concern for the more important parts, if an important part is affected by a swelling it is concerned about it and, going into action to rid it of the offending matter, it suppurates the swelling sooner. But if it is a less important part, (nature) is not so concerned for it and suppurates the swelling later. For this reason, when they are affected, (nature) is more concerned about the liver than about the stomach, and cares more about the stomach than the spleen and more about the spleen than the intestines. By position: the nearer they are to important parts the quicker (nature) suppurates

τοὺς ὄγκους, τυχὸν τὰ παρακείμενα μόρια τῷ διαφράγματι καὶ ἥπατι καὶ καρδίᾳ καὶ τοῖς τοιούτοις. φροντίζει γὰρ ἡ φύσις, ἵνα μὴ ἐκ τοῦ σύνεγγυς μετασχῇ τῆς κακίας τὰ κύρια μόρια, καὶ πρωϊαίτερον πυοποιεῖ αὐτά. εἰ δὲ ἀφεστήκασιν, ὀψιαίτερον πυοποιοῦνται. διὰ δὲ τὴν κρᾶσιν, τὰ μὲν θερμότερα πρωϊαίτερον πυοποιοῦνται, τὰ δὲ ψυχρότερα ὀψιαίτερον. καὶ τὰ μὲν μαλθακὰ καὶ μανὰ πρωϊαίτερον διὰ τὴν θερμότητα, τὰ δὲ σκληρὰ καὶ πυκνὰ ὀψιαίτερον διὰ τὴν ψυχρότητα, ὥσπερ νεῦρα καὶ μύες καὶ τὰ τοιαῦτα. τινὲς καὶ ἐνταῦθα ἐκ τοῦ ἐναντίου λέγουσιν ὅτι τὰ πυκνὰ καὶ στεγανά, ἐπειδὴ ἐναποκέκλεισται τὸ ἐν αὐτοῖς θερμόν, πρωϊαίτερον πυοποιοῦνται, κατὰ τὸ εἰρημένον ἐν ἄλλοις ὑπὸ τοῦ Ἱπποκράτους· «Ὁκόσα πεπαίνεσθαι χρή, ἐγκατακεκλεῖσθαι χρή». οὕτως δὲ καὶ ἐν τῇ συνηθείᾳ ποιοῦμεν· τὰ δεόμενα πυοποιήσεως οὐ τοῖς διαφοροῦσι κεχρήμεθα, ἀλλὰ τοῖς πυκνοῦσιν.

Εἶτα καὶ προσδιορισμὸν τίθησιν. ἐπειδὴ γὰρ περὶ οἰδήματος αὐτῷ ὁ λόγος, λέγει καί, ποία ἀρίστη ἐστὶ ῥῆξις ἐπὶ τῶν ἀποστημάτων· φησὶ γὰρ ὅτι Ὁκόσα ἔσω ῥήγνυται, ἄριστά ἐστι. καὶ ἵνα σαφῶς τοῖς λεγομένοις παρακολουθήσωμεν, δεῖ εἰδέναι ὅτι αἱ ῥήξεις τῶν ἀποστημάτων ἢ
122 ἐντὸς γί|νονται ἢ ἐκτὸς ἢ κατὰ τὸ συναμφότερον, καὶ ἐντὸς καὶ ἐκτός. καὶ ἡ μὲν ἐπὶ τὰ ἐκτὸς γινομένη ῥῆξις πασῶν ἀγαθωτέρα καὶ ἀκίνδυνός ἐστιν. ἡ δὲ κατὰ τὸ συναμφότερον χειρίστη πασῶν ἐστιν. ἡ δὲ ἐπὶ τὰ ἐντὸς μέσως πώς ἐστι τούτων· πρὸς μὲν τὴν ἐπὶ τὰ ἐκτὸς ῥῆξιν χείρων ἐστί, πρὸς δὲ τὴν κατὰ τὸ συναμφότερον εὐιατοτέρα ἐστὶ καὶ ἀκίνδυνος, ἐπειδὴ ἡ κατὰ τὸ συναμφότερον γινομένη ῥῆξις οὐ μόνον ἐπὶ τὰ ἐντὸς μολύνει τὸ ἔμφυτον θερμόν, ἀλλὰ καὶ ἐπὶ τὰ ἐκτὸς συριγγοῖ τοὺς τόπους ἐκείνους καὶ κατανέμεται. ὅταν οὖν ὁ Ἱπποκράτης ἐπαινῇ τὴν ἐπὶ τὰ ἐντὸς ῥῆξιν, ἀρίστην αὐτὴν ὑποτιθέμενος, οὐ πρὸς τὴν ἔξωθεν γινομένην ῥῆξιν παραβάλλων ταῦτα λέγει, ἀλλὰ τὴν πρὸς τὸ συναμφότερον γινομένην.

I 51 [7: 202,1 A. = II 128,4 L.] Τὰ δὲ μαλθακὰ τῶν οἰδημάτων καὶ ἀνώδυνα καὶ τῷ δακτύλῳ ὑπείκοντα χρονιωτέρας τὰς κρίσιας ποιέεται

Οὐ ταὐτολογεῖ ἐνταῦθα ὁ Ἱπποκράτης εἰπὼν μαλθακὰ καὶ πάλιν τῷ δακτύλῳ ὑπείκοντα· ἀλλ' ἵνα ἐπίτασιν τῆς ὁμαλότητος δηλώσῃ, ἔφη καὶ τῷ δακτύλῳ ὑπείκοντα, ἐπειδὴ οὐ πᾶν μαλθακὸν ὑπείκει τῷ δακτύλῳ. τῷ δὲ εἰπεῖν τὰς κρίσιας ποιέεται τὴν πυοποίησιν ἐδήλωσε, τουτέστιν ὅτι χρονιωτέρας τὰς πυοποιήσιας ποιέεται ἐπὶ τῶν οἰδημάτων.

9sq. τὸ εἰρημένον] Hipp. Epid. VI 2,16: V p. 284,13 L. 15 Ὁκόσα–ῥήγνυται] Hipp. Progn. 7: p. 203,3sq. A. = II p. 130,7 L. 18sq.] *cf.* Gal. In Hipp. Progn. comm. I 41: CMG V 9,2 p. 255,15sq.

5 προιαίτερα ... ὀψιαίτερα γ 6 καὶ πυκνὰ *om.* L 7 πρωιαίτερον L; *cf. supra, p. 14* 10 ἐν ἄλλοις *om.* L ὁπόσα γ 11 χρή] δεῖ γ 14 ἐστὶ *om.* γ 15 ῥήγνυνται γ 16 ἀποστήσεων γ 17 ἐντὸς ... ἐκτός^{I}] ἐκτὸς ... ἐντὸς γ 18 γενομένη γ ἐστιν *ante* καὶ *trsp.* γ 20 χεῖρον *codd.*: *corr. Nickel* 22 γενομένη Mζ 24 ἐπαινεῖ γ ὑποθέμενος γ 25 λέγη L 28 *post* ἀνώδυνα *add.* ἐόντα γ *post* δακτύλῳ *add.* πιεζόμενα καὶ L *(ex Hipp.); cf. lin. 31sq.; supra, p. 128,5* 31 ὁμαλότητος] *fort.* μαλ(θ)ακότητος *scribendum est* 32 μαλακὸν γ 33 τῷ] τὸ *codd.*: *correxi* 34 ποιεῖται γ

their swellings, in other words, the parts bordering on the diaphragm, liver, heart and the like. For nature is concerned that the important parts, due to their proximity, might contract the malady, and so it suppurates them sooner. If they are distant, on the other hand, they are suppurated later. By temperament: the warmer suppurate sooner, the colder later. (Thus) those that are soft and loose (in texture) suppurate sooner because of the heat, while the hard and solid because of the cold suppurate later, for example, nerves and muscles and the like. Here again some take the opposite view that the solid and impervious suppurate sooner, seeing that the heat in them is closed up, just as Hippocrates says in another place, "Anything which must be brought to maturation should be kept enclosed". And this is what we do in everyday practice; on the parts requiring suppuration we use solidifying, not dissipating, remedies.

Then he adds a specific point. Since he is on the topic of tumors he also tells us which kind of breaking is best in abscesses; he says, Those which break inwards are the best. And in order to follow his meaning fully, we should note that abscesses erupt inwards or outwards or in both directions, inwards and outwards. Breaking to the outside is best of all and is without danger. Breaking both ways is worst of all. And breaking to the inside is somewhere between these: compared to breaking outwards it is more serious, while compared to both directions it is more easily cured and less dangerous; this is so because an abscess which erupts both ways not only pollutes the innate heat on the inside, but it also on the outside forms fistulas in these places and spreads itself about. When Hippocrates, then, lauds inward breaking, classing it as best, he says this comparing it, not to breaking outwards, but to breaking in both directions.

I 51 Tumors which are soft, painless and yield to the finger prolong the crises

By saying soft and then yield to the finger Hippocrates is not repeating himself here; rather, he said and yield to the finger in order to indicate a high degree of evenness, since not every soft body gives way to the finger. And by mentioning crises he referred to suppuration, in other words, tumors make the suppurations more prolonged.

καὶ σκόπησον ὅτι τὸ τῆς κρίσεως ὄνομα οἱ παλαιοὶ οὐ μόνον ἐπὶ τῶν ὀξέων νοσημάτων τιθέασιν, ἀλλὰ καὶ ἐπὶ τῶν χρονίων, ὥσπερ ἐνταῦθα.

I 52 [7: 202,4 A.=II 128,8 L.] Καὶ τοῦτο καὶ τὸ ἐν τῇ ἄλλῃ κοιλίῃ κατὰ τὸ αὐτό.

Ἰστέον ὅτι ὁ Ἱπποκράτης κοιλίαν οὐ μόνον τὴν γαστέρα καὶ τὰ ἔντερα καὶ τὸν θώρακα καλεῖ, ἀλλὰ καὶ τὸν σπλῆνα καὶ τὸ ἧπαρ κοιλίας καλεῖ ἐνταῦθα· περὶ γὰρ τῶν ὑποχονδρίων αὐτῷ ὁ λόγος.

XIV

I 53 [7: 203,6 A.=II 130,9 L.] Τὸ δὲ πύον ἄριστόν ἐστι λευκόν τε καὶ λεῖον καὶ ὁμαλὸν καὶ ἥκιστα δυσῶδες.

Διαλεχθεὶς ὁ Ἱπποκράτης περὶ τῶν πυοποιουμένων εἰς τὰ ὑποχόν-
123 δρια ἀποστημάτων νῦν σημειοῦται αὐτὰ | καὶ ἀπὸ τοῦ κενουμένου, τουτέστι τοῦ πύου. καὶ λέγει, ποῖον ἄριστόν ἐστι, καί φησιν ὅτι τὸ ἄριστον πύον λευκόν τε εἶναι καὶ λεῖον καὶ ὁμαλὸν καὶ ἥκιστα δυσῶδες, ὅπερ γίνεται καὶ ἐπὶ ἰσχύϊ δυνάμεως καὶ συμμετρίᾳ τοῦ ἐμφύτου θερμοῦ.

Λοιπὸν δεῖ ἡμᾶς καὶ τὰς αἰτίας εἰπεῖν. ἀλλ' ἵνα τοῦτο σαφῶς διαγνῶμεν, δεῖ ἡμᾶς ἐπιμνησθῆναι, τίνων μεμαθήκαμεν ἐν Φυσικοῖς, ὅτι τέσσαρές εἰσιν αἱ φυσικαὶ δυνάμεις καὶ ὅτι ἡ ἀλλοιωτικὴ δύναμίς ἐστιν ἡ ἀλλοιοῦσα καὶ πέττουσα καὶ ἐξομοιοῦσα τὴν τροφὴν ὁμοίαν τῷ τρεφομένῳ μορίῳ. ἀλλὰ καὶ τοῦτο ἴσμεν, ὅτι τὰ μόρια πρὸς ἑαυτὰ ἐξομοιοῦσι τὴν τροφὴν καὶ οὕτως τρέφονται· οὐδὲν γὰρ ἄλλο ἐστὶ θρέψις ἢ ὁμοίωσις τοῦ τρέφοντος πρὸς τὸ τρεφόμενον. ἀλλὰ καὶ τοῦτο ἴσμεν, ὅτι τὰ στερεὰ μόρια λευκά ἐστιν, ὥσπερ χόνδροι καὶ νεῦρα καὶ ὑμένες καὶ φλέβες καὶ ἀρτηρίαι καὶ τὰ τοιαῦτα, καὶ ὅτι ἐκ σπέρματος ἔχοντα τὴν γένεσιν ἐκ σπέρματος καὶ τρέφονται· τὸ γὰρ λόγῳ τροφῆς φερόμενον ἐν αὐτοῖς αἷμα, ἐξομοιοῦσιν αὐτὸ πρὸς τὴν οἰκείαν φύσιν καὶ ἐκσπερματοῦσι καὶ οὕτως τρέφονται.

Τούτων οὕτως εἰρημένων σαφὴς καὶ δήλη γέγονεν ἡμῖν ἡ αἰτία, καθ' ἣν λευκὸν γίνεται τὸ πύον. τοῦτο δὲ τὸ συρρεῦσαν αἷμα ἐν τοῖς ὑποχονδρίοις καὶ ποιῆσαν τὴν φλεγμονὴν ἢ σήπεται ἢ πέττεται. καὶ εἰ μὲν ἀσθενὴς ἐστιν ἡ δύναμις καὶ τὸ ἔμφυτον θερμὸν ἐξέστη τῶν οἰκείων ὅρων, τουτέστι τῆς εὐκρασίας, καὶ δύσκρατον γέγονε, τότε οἷον ὡς ἐπὶ ἀψύχου τινὸς ἀπρονόητον μένον σήπεται. εἰ μέντοι ἔρρωται ἡ δύναμις καὶ τὸ ἔμφυτον

17 ἐν Φυσικοῖς] *v. supra*, p. 13 n. 3 ὅτι – 22] *cf.* Gal. In Hipp. Progn. comm. I 42: CMG V 9,2 p. 256,4–15 De fac. nat. I 11: Scr. min. III p. 119 Helmr. = II pp. 25sq. K. 27–134,15] *cf.* Gal. In Hipp. Progn. comm. I 42: CMG V 9,2 pp. 256,1–257,25

1 τῶ . . . ὀνόματι *codd.*: *correxi* 3 καὶ[II] *om.* γ 4 κοιλία L 5 *post* γαστέρα *add.* ἀλλὰ γ 7 ἐνταῦθα καλεῖ γ *post* καλεῖ *add.* ὁ ἱπποκράτης L 10 τε *om.* γ *ante* ἥκιστα *add.* ὡς L *(ex Hipp.); sed cf. lin. 14; infra, pp. 134,7; 136,25* 23 καὶ[VI] *om.* L; *cf. supra, pp. 14 sq.* 24 ἔχουσα Μζ 25 αὐτὸ] αὐτῶ γ 30 ἔμφυτον θερμὸν] ἐμφυτευθὲν γ ἔξεστι γ 31 ἐπὶ *scripsi*: ἀπὸ *codd.* 32–134,1 ἔμφυτον θερμὸν] ἐμφυτευθὲν γ

Observe, too, that the ancients use "crisis" not only of acute, but of chronic diseases as well, as in the present instance.

I 52 And a tumor in any other part of the cavity will fare likewise.

Note that by cavity Hippocrates means not just the stomach, intestines and thorax, but also calls here the spleen and the liver cavities, seeing that he is on the subject of the hypochondria.

XIV

I 53 The pus is best when white, uniform, even and least foul-smelling.

Having discussed suppurated abscesses in the hypochondria Hippocrates now gives the symptoms for them from the evacuated matter as well, that is, from the pus. He tells us which kind is the most favorable saying, The pus is best when white, uniform, even and least foul-smelling, which is the case when the power is strong and the innate heat temperate.

Next we should give the causes. But in order to understand the subject fully, it is necessary to recall some things we learned in the Physics: that there are four natural faculties and that the converting faculty is the one which converts, concocts and assimilates the nutriment to the part nourished. We know, too, that the parts are nourished by assimilating the nutriment to themselves; for nourishing is nothing other than the assimilation of nutrient to the nourished. This we have learned as well, that the solid parts, such as cartilage, nerves, membranes, veins, arteries, etc., are white and being generated from sperm they are also nourished by sperm; for they are nourished by assimilating to their own nature and converting to semen the blood conveyed to them in the form of nutriment.

In light of these remarks it becomes clear and obvious what causes the pus to be white. Now the flow of blood in the hypochondria responsible for the inflammation either decomposes or is concocted. If the power is weak and the innate heat exceeds its proper bounds, that is to say, (the limits of) good temperament, becoming distempered, then (the blood) is left neglected as in a lifeless body and decomposes. However, if the power

θερμὸν εὐκράτως διάκειται, ὡς προνοούμενον τότε τὸ αἷμα πέττεται, καὶ τὸ ἄριστον πύον γίνεται. χαρακτηρίζεται δὲ ἀπὸ τῆς εὐκρασίας. ἐὰν γὰρ ἀσθενῶς διάκειται ἡ δύναμις καὶ τὸ ἔμφυτον θερμὸν τῆς οἰκείας κράσεως ἐξέστηκε, τότε πέττεται μέν, ἀλλὰ τὸ χείριστον καὶ δυσῶδες γίνεται πύον. εἰ μέντοι ἔρρωται ἡ δύναμις καὶ εὐκράτως διάκειται τὸ ἔμφυτον θερμόν, ὡς ἂν ἐπίμικτον ἔχον τὴν ποιητικὴν αἰτίαν καὶ ἐπαμφοτερίζουσαν, τότε τὸ
124 ἄριστον πύον γίνεται, ὅπερ | αὐτὸς ἔφη ἥκιστα δυσῶδες. ἐπειδὴ δὲ τὸ συρρεῦσαν αἷμα ἔξω τῶν ἀγγείων γενόμενον παρὰ φύσιν λοιπόν ἐστι καὶ οὐχ αἷμά ἐστι κυρίως, διὰ τοῦτο ἧττον μετέχει δυσωδίας. λευκὸν οὖν τὸ πύον γίνεται, ἐπειδὴ εἰς τὸ χρῶμα τῶν στερεῶν ἄγεται. ἡ γὰρ μεταβολὴ τοῦ συρρεύσαντος αἵματος ἐν τοῖς ὑποχονδρίοις τοῦ τὴν φλεγμονὴν ἐργασαμένου, ἡνίκα εἰς πυοποίησιν τρέπεται, ἐν τοῖς στερεοῖς γίνεται, ὥσπερ καὶ τὸ σπέρμα ἐν αὐτοῖς τοῖς στερεοῖς μεταβάλλεται. ἀλλὰ τὸ μὲν σπέρμα ὑπὸ τοῦ κατὰ φύσιν αἵματος γίνεται τοῦ λόγῳ τροφῆς φερομένου ἐν τοῖς στερεοῖς μορίοις, καὶ οὕτως μεταβαλλόμενον εἰς σπέρματος φύσιν ἀποσπερματοῦται· τὸ δὲ πύον ἀπὸ ἀχρήστου ὕλης καὶ ἀπρονοήτου γίνεται. ἄριστον δὲ πύον λέγομεν αὐτὸ παραβάλλοντες πρὸς τὸ κάκιστον πάντῃ πύον. λοιπὸν δὲ ὅτι ἄριστον καὶ κατὰ φύσιν λέγομεν πύον διὰ τὴν ἐπικράτειαν τῆς [τε] δυνάμεως καὶ τὴν εὐκρασίαν τοῦ ἐμφύτου θερμοῦ. ἐπειδὴ δὲ ἐξ ἀχρήστου ὕλης γίνεται, διὰ τοῦτο δυσῶδές ἐστιν ὀλίγον. διὰ τοῦτο καὶ δεύτερον πλοῦν λέγομεν τὴν φύσιν ὁδεύειν ἐπὶ τῆς πυοποιήσεως, διὰ τὸ ἀνεπιτηδείως ἔχειν τὴν ὕλην πρὸς τὸ τὴν ἀκριβῆ πέψιν καὶ ἀλλοίωσιν ἐπιδέξασθαι.

Καὶ ἴσως ἀπορεῖ τις λέγων ὅτι «Ἐπειδὴ ἡ φλεγμονὴ μάλιστα ἐν ταῖς σαρξὶ συνίσταται, ἔδει ποτὲ καὶ ἐρυθρὸν γενέσθαι τὸ πύον ὀφειλουσῶν τῶν σαρκῶν πρὸς τὴν ἑαυτῶν φύσιν ἐξομοιῶσαι τὸ συρρεῦσαν αἷμα.» καὶ λέγομεν ὅτι τὸ αἷμα, ἡνίκα πλεονάζῃ κατὰ ποσότητα, διηθεῖται ἐκ τῶν ἀγγείων κατὰ ἀπολακτισμόν τινα καὶ φέρεται εἰς τὰς κενὰς χώρας· εἶτα ἐνεχθὲν εἰς τὰς κενὰς χώρας καὶ ἀπρονόητον μένει καὶ σήπεται καὶ σηπόμενον δαπανᾷ τὰς παρακειμένας σάρκας. ἐπειδὴ δέ εἰσιν ἶνες ἐν αὐταῖς καὶ ὑμένες, ταῦτα δὲ ὡς δυσπαθῆ οὐ πάσχουσί τι, ἀλλὰ μένουσι καὶ πρὸς τὴν οἰκείαν φύσιν ἐξομοιοῦσι καὶ λευκὸν ἀπεργάζονται ἐκεῖνο τὸ αἷμα, τὸ τηνικαῦτα πύον.

Ἀλλ' ἴσως ἀπορήσει τις λέγων ὅτι «Ὅλη οὖν ἡ σὰρξ δαπανᾶται. καὶ
125 μὴν ὁρῶμεν ἐπὶ τῶν ἑλκῶν | ὅτι πολλάκις αἱ σάρκες οὐδὲ φθείρονται οὐδ' ἶνες πάντῃ διαφθείρονται· ἐπεί τοί γε πῶς τὰ ἕλκη σαρκοῦνται ἀπὸ τοῦ πάντῃ μὴ ὄντος; ἐὰν γὰρ μηδόλως ἐστὶ σὰρξ περιλειφθεῖσα, οὐκοῦν οὐδὲ σαρκοῦνται· ἀλλὰ μὴν σαρκοῦνται, καὶ ἐμμένει σάρξ, καθ' ἣν ἀναπληροῦται ἡ δαπανηθεῖσα σὰρξ ἐπὶ τῶν ἑλκῶν.» καὶ λέγομεν ὅτι, εἰ καὶ μένουσι σάρκες

1 τὸ^{I} *om.* γ πέττεται] σήπεται L 3 ἔμφυτον θερμὸν] ἐμφυτευθὲν γ 6 ἀνεπίμικτον LPζ: *corr.* M; *cf. infra, p. 136,30* ἔχειν *codd.*: *corr. Dietz* ἐπαμφοτερίζον *codd.*: *corr. Wk.; cf. infra, p. 136,30* τὸ *om.* γ 7 δὲ] καὶ MP 14 τοῦ^{II}] τῷ M *(ex* τοῦ *mut.)* P 15 καὶ *om.* γ 16 ὕλης ἀχρήστου γ 17 πάντῃ κάκιστον γ 18 τε *secl. Kollesch* 19 τῆς εὐκρασίας L: τῆς εὐκράτου γ: *corr. Wk.; cf. infra, p. 136,30* 20 ἐλέγομεν γ 22 τὸ *om.* L 24 ὀφειλόντων γ 26 ἡνίκα τὸ αἷμα γ πλεονάζει γ ποιότητα γ 27 sq. εἶτα – χώρας *om.* L 28 καὶ^{I} *om.* γ σηπομένου γ 29 παρει μένας *spat. circa 3 litt. rel.* L δέ *om., ut vid.,* L ἶναι γ 31 ἐκεῖνο τὸ αἷμα *post* ἐξομοιοῦσι *trsp.* γ *ante* πύον *add.* τὸ γ 32 ἀπορήσει *ex* -ήσοι, *ut vid., corr.* P: ἀπορήσοι ζ: ἀπορήσ *(ambig.)* M 34 ἶναι γ πάντῃ *om.* γ 36 ἀλλὰ μὴν σαρκοῦνται *om.* γ

is strong and the innate heat temperate, the blood in that case receives attention, is concocted and the best pus forms. (Pus of this kind) is characterized by the balanced blend. For if the power is weak and the innate heat exceeds its proper temperament, then (the blood) does undergo concoction, but the resulting pus is extremely bad and fetid. If, however, the power is strong and the innate heat temperate, the efficient cause being mixed and ambivalent, then the best pus develops, which he himself described as least foul-smelling. And since the blood which overflows the vessels is abnormal really and not blood in the strict sense, this explains the slight fetidness. Pus, then, turns white because the color of the solid parts is imposed on it. For when the flood of blood in the hypochondria responsible for the inflammation turns to suppuration, the transformation takes place in the solid parts, just as the semen also is converted in the solid parts themselves. But whereas semen is produced from the normal blood conveyed in the form of nutriment to the solid parts, undergoing its change and conversion to sperm there, pus comes from useless and neglected matter. And when we speak of the best pus we are comparing it to the very worst kind. Secondly, we call the pus best and normal because it has been produced under the influence of strong (body) power and temperate innate heat. However, since it issues from useless matter, it is slightly fetid for this reason. This also explains why we say that nature is using its second option in suppurating, the matter being unfit to undergo concoction and conversion in the strict sense.

Someone may raise the problem that "Since inflammation occurs mostly in the flesh, the pus should sometimes be red also, seeing that the flesh ought to assimilate the flood of blood to its own nature." Our answer is that when there is an excessive quantity of blood it percolates from the vessels in a kind of haemorrhage and is conveyed to the vacant areas; once brought to the vacant areas it lies unattended and decomposes, and decomposed it consumes the surrounding flesh. But since the flesh contains sinews and membranes, these, being durable, are in no way affected but remain intact and assimilate to their own nature and whiten that blood, which by then is pus.

However, someone may object and say, "The whole flesh, then, is consumed. But in fact we see in ulcers that frequently neither is the flesh destroyed nor are the sinews in any way affected; but how do ulcers receive flesh from what does not at all exist? For if absolutely no flesh is left, surely they will not be healed over; the fact is, however, that they are healed and flesh does remain, with which the consumed flesh is restored in ulcers." We say that, even if some flesh survives, it is, neverthe-

τινές, ἀλλ' οὖν αἱ σάρκες εὐπαθεῖς εἰσι, καὶ ὡς εὐπαθεῖς οὐκ ἐξομοιοῦσιν ὡς πρὸς τὴν οἰκείαν φύσιν καὶ ἐρυθρὸν ποιοῦσι τὸ πύον· ἀλλ' αἱ ἶνες ἰσχυραὶ οὖσαι καὶ δυσπαθεῖς πρὸς τὴν οἰκείαν φύσιν ἐξομοιοῦσι τὸ αἷμα ἐκεῖνο, καὶ λευκὸν τὸ πύον γίνεται. ὅθεν ἐὰν ἐν ἥπατι ὑποσταίη φλεγμονή, ἡ πυοποίησις οὐ γίνεται ἀκριβὴς λευκὴ διὰ τὸ πλεῖστον τοῦ παρεγχύματος τοῦ ἥπατος σαρκῶδες εἶναι· ὀλίγας δὲ ἶνας ἡ φύσις ἐν αὐτῷ ἐνέθηκε, καὶ διὰ τοῦτο οὐκ ἀκριβῶς λευκὸν γίνεται τὸ πύον διὰ τὴν ὀλιγότητα τῶν ἰνῶν. αὕτη οὖν ἐστιν ἡ αἰτία, καθ' ἣν λευκὸν γίνεται τὸ πύον καὶ ἧττον δυσῶδες.

I 54 [7: 203,6 A. = II 130,10 L.] Καὶ λεῖον

Τὸ λεῖον κατὰ τὸν χρόνον δεῖ νοῆσαι, ὅτι δεῖ λευκὸν εἶναι τὸ πύον ἀείσε καὶ μὴ ποτὲ μὲν λευκόν, ποτὲ δὲ φαιὸν ἢ τρυγῶδες καὶ τὰ τοιαῦτα.

I 55 [7: 203,6 A. = II 130,10 L.] Καὶ ὁμαλόν

Τὸ ὁμαλόν, δεῖ αὐτὸ κατὰ τὸ ὁμοιομερὲς ὑπολαβεῖν· τοῦτο δὲ διττόν ἐστι κατὰ τὴν σύστασιν καὶ κατὰ τὸν χρόνον. καὶ κατὰ μὲν τὴν σύστασιν, ἵνα μὴ τὸ μὲν αὐτοῦ μέρος ἐστὶ παχύ, τὸ δὲ λεπτόν, ἀλλ' ὅμοιον κατὰ πᾶν ἑαυτό. κατὰ δὲ τὸν χρόνον, ἵνα μὴ ποτὲ μὲν φαιόν ἐστι, ποτὲ δὲ ἀμόργη καὶ τὰ τοιαῦτα, ἀλλὰ κατὰ πᾶν ἑαυτὸ λευκότατον δεῖ εἶναι. τοῦτο ἔστι τὸ ἄριστον πύον καὶ κατὰ φύσιν. τὸ δὲ παρὰ φύσιν ἐστὶ τὸ μὴ ὂν λευκὸν μηδὲ λεῖον, ἀλλὰ σήμερον μὲν τρυγῶδες, αὔριον δὲ κυανοῦν, ποτὲ δὲ μελάντερον καὶ τὰ τοιαῦτα. ἀλλὰ καὶ ἀνώμαλον αὐτὸ δεῖ εἶναι κατά τε τὴν σύστασιν καὶ τὸν χρόνον· ποτὲ μὲν γὰρ παχύ, ποτὲ δὲ λεπτόν, ποτὲ δὲ ἐκτετηκὸς καὶ
126 τὰ τοιαῦτα. | ἔστι δὲ καὶ μέσον πύον· τούτου δὲ πολλή ἐστιν ἡ διαφορὰ πρὸς τὴν κρᾶσιν τούτων ἢ ἐκείνων καὶ παρὰ τὸ μᾶλλον καὶ ἧττον γινόμενον πρὸς τὸ πλησιάζον.

I 56 [7: 203,6 A. = II 130,10 L.] Καὶ ἥκιστα δυσῶδες

Δεῖ εἰδέναι ὅτι τριττή ἐστιν ἡ πέψις· πρώτη μὲν ἡ κατὰ φύσιν, ὥσπερ ἡ χυλοποίησις καὶ ἡ ἐξαιμάτωσις, δευτέρα δὲ ἡ παρὰ φύσιν, ὥσπερ ἡ σῆψις, καὶ τρίτη πέψις ἐστὶν ἡ μέση τούτων, καθ' ἣν τὸ πύον γίνεται. τοῦτο δὲ τὸ πύον ἥκιστά ἐστι δυσῶδες διὰ τὴν ἐπικράτειαν τῆς [τε] δυνάμεως καὶ τὴν εὐκρασίαν τοῦ ἐμφύτου θερμοῦ. ἀλλ' ἐπειδὴ ἐπίμικτός ἐστιν καὶ ἐπαμφοτερίζει ἡ ποιητικὴ αἰτία, ἄχρηστός ἐστιν ἡ ὕλη· διὰ τοῦτο ἧττον μετέχει δυσωδίας. ἐπεὶ οὖν ταῦτα εἴρηται, ἐν οἷς σὺν θεῷ καὶ τὸ πρῶτον τμῆμα πληροῦται.

26–28] *cf.* Steph. Comm. in Hipp. Aph.: Ambros. S 19 sup. fol. 54v

1 εὐπαθεῖς[I]] εὐπειθεῖς MV: -ει- *in* -α- *corr.* PY 2 ποιῆσαι γ ἶναι γ 4 ἐν *om.* L ἡ πυοποίησις] ἡ πυοποιηθῇ γ 5 ἀκριβῶς *Dietz* 7 αὐτὴ γ 11 ἀείσε *ante* εἶναι *(lin. 10) trsp.* γ 13 αὐτὸ] αὐτῷ *post* ὁμοιομερὲς *trsp.* γ 13 sq. τοῦτο – τὸν *om.* γ 16 ἑαυτῷ L ἀμοργῇ γ 17 ἑαυτῷ *codd.*: *correxi ante* δεῖ *fort. excidit* ἀεὶ 20 κατά τε] καὶ τὰ τοιαῦτα L 23 sq. καὶ[I] – πλησιάζον *om.* γ 29 τε *secl. Kollesch* 29 sq. τῆς εὐκρασίας L: *om.* γ: *corr. Wk.*; *cf. supra, p. 134,19* 30 καὶ *om.* L

less, delicate and as such does not assimilate the pus to its own nature and make it red; sinews, on the other hand, being tough and resistant assimilate that blood to their own nature and the pus becomes white. For this reason if there is inflammation in the liver, the pus does not become exactly white, since the greater part of the liver's substance consists of flesh; and nature placed few sinews in it, and hence the pus does not become exactly white because of the fewness of the sinews. This, then, is the reason why the pus becomes white and slightly fetid.

I 54 And uniform

Uniform must be understood in a temporal sense to mean that the pus should be white all the time, not sometimes white, sometimes grey or having the color of wine dregs and so on.

I 55 And even

Even should be taken to refer to homogeneity; and this can be observed in two ways, in consistency and time. (To be even) in consistency one part of the pus should not be thick and another thin, but the whole should be similar throughout. In a temporal sense (even means) that the pus should not be at one time grey and at another purple and so on, but be completely white throughout. This is the best and normal kind of pus. Pus is abnormal, on the other hand, when it is neither white nor uniform but has the color of wine dregs today, is dark blue tomorrow, at another time blackish, etc. And it will necessarily be uneven both in consistency and in a temporal sense: sometimes thick, sometimes thin, at other times soft and so forth. There is also an intermediate pus of which there are many varieties depending on the blend of these or those (elements) and on the degree of assimilation to its surroundings.

I 56 And least foul-smelling

Note that there are three types of coction; the first is normal, namely conversion to chyle and blood making; the second is abnormal, viz. decomposition; the third coction is intermediate between those two and is the one which creates pus. This pus is least foul-smelling because the power has been strong and the innate heat temperate. But since the efficient cause is mixed and ambiguous, the matter is worthless and hence slightly fetid. This said, then, the first section is completed with the help of God.

ΑΡΧΗ ΣΥΝ ΘΕΩΙ ΤΟΥ ΔΕΥΤΕΡΟΥ ΤΜΗΜΑΤΟΣ

I

II 1 [8: 203,8 A. = II 130,12 L.] Οἱ δὲ ὕδρωπες οἱ ἐκ τῶν ὀξέων νοσημάτων πάντες κακοί.

Ἀρχόμενος τοῦ δευτέρου τμήματος ὁ Ἱπποκράτης τὴν τῶν ὑδέρων μεταχειρίζεται διδασκαλίαν, ἵνα συνάφειαν χαρίσηται τὰ μέλλοντα πρὸς τὰ φθάσαντα, ἐπειδὴ καὶ ὁ ὕδερος πάθος ἐστὶν ἐν τοῖς ὑποχονδρίοις συνιστάμενον. καὶ μηδεὶς ὑπολάβῃ ὅτι περὶ χρονίων νοσημάτων διαλέγεται ὁ Ἱπποκράτης, καίτοι προθέμενος περὶ ὀξέων διαλαβεῖν· ἀλλὰ περὶ τῶν
127 ὀξέων νοσημάτων διαλεγόμενος | διαλαμβάνει καὶ περὶ τῶν ἐκ μεταπτώσεως ὀξέων, καθάπερ καὶ τοῦτο νῦν δείκνυσιν αὐτοῦ ἡ ῥῆσις· ἔφη γὰρ Οἱ δὲ ὕδρωπες οἱ ἐκ τῶν ὀξέων νοσημάτων. ἰδοὺ περὶ τῶν ἐκ μεταπτώσεως ὀξέων διαλέγεται καὶ οὐ περὶ τῶν χρονίων.

Οὔτε γὰρ τοῦ πυρὸς ἀπαλλάττουσιν ἐπώδυνοί τέ εἰσι καὶ κάρτα θανατώδεις. καὶ καλῶς ἐπώδυνοί εἰσι· τοῦ γὰρ ὑγροῦ ἀθροισθέντος ἀθρόως περὶ τὰ ὑποχόνδρια τείνονται καὶ τῇ τάσει κινδυνεύοντα διαρραγῆναι τῇ ὀδυνηρᾷ συναισθήσει ὀδυνῶνται.

Οὔτε τοῦ πυρὸς ἀπαλλάττουσιν. τοῦτο δοκεῖ μὴ κυρίως ἀληθὲς εἶναι· ἐρεῖ γάρ τις ὅτι «Πῶς οὐκ ἀπαλλάσσονται τοῦ πυρετοῦ, εἴ γε τοσούτου ὑγροῦ ἐστιν ἄθροισις; τὸ γὰρ ὑγρὸν σβέννυσι τὴν δυσκρασίαν καὶ παύει τὸν πυρετόν.» πρὸς ὅ τινες ἀπολογοῦνται ὅτι «Διὰ τοῦτο οὐκ ἀπαλλάσσονται τοῦ πυρετοῦ οἱ ὑδεριῶντες, ἐπειδὴ ὁ πυρετὸς δι' ὅλου τοῦ σώματός ἐστιν ἐκτεταμένος, τὸ δὲ ὑγρὸν ἐν ἑνὶ μορίῳ ἐστὶ συναθροιζόμενον· καὶ οὐ δύναται ἡ μερικὴ συναγωγὴ τοῦ ὑγροῦ ἀπαλλάξαι τὴν δυσκρασίαν ὅλου τοῦ σώματος καὶ παῦσαι τὸν πυρετόν.» ἐπιπόλαιος δέ ἐστιν ἡ ἀπολογία αὕτη· ἐρεῖ γάρ τις πρὸς αὐτοὺς ὅτι «Κἂν ἐν ἑνὶ μορίῳ ἐστὶν ἡ συναγωγὴ τοῦ ὑγροῦ, ἀλλ' οὖν ἐν αὐτῇ τῇ ἑστίᾳ, λέγω δὴ περὶ τὰ ὑποχόνδρια καὶ τὴν καρδίαν ἐστί· καὶ ἐὰν τὴν καρδίαν καθυγράνῃ καὶ ἀποσβέσῃ, κατὰ συμβεβηκὸς καὶ ἡ ἐν ὅλῳ τῷ σώματι δυσκρασία ἀποπαύσεται.» διὸ δεῖ τὴν ἀληθεστέραν εἰπεῖν αἰτίαν, ὅτι κἂν πολλοῦ ὑγροῦ ἐστι συνάθροισις ἐπὶ τῶν ὑδεριώντων, ἀλλὰ λοιπὸν οὐ παύει τὸν πυρετόν, ἐπειδὴ τῇ φαντασίᾳ καὶ μόνῃ

8 μηδεὶς ὑπολάβῃ] *cf.* Gal. In Hipp. Progn. comm. II 1: CMG V 9,2 pp. 259,8–260,7

8 ὑπολάβοι Pζ 10 νοσημάτων διαλεγόμενος] τῶν ἐκ μεταπτώσεως διαλέγεται L καὶ – 11 ὀξέων *om.* L μεταπτώσεων γ 11 νῦν καὶ τοῦτο γ 12 *post* νοσημάτων *add.* πάντες κακοί γ μεταπτώσεων γ 13 χρόνων Pζ 16 γείνονται M: γίνονται P 18 *post* τοῦτο *add.* μοι L ἀληθῶς γ 19 *post* τις *add.* καὶ γ 23 δὲ] γὰρ γ 26 ἐστιν *om.* γ 27 ἑστίᾳ] αἰτία γ 28 *post* κατὰ *add.* τὸ γ 29 ἀποπαύεται γ 31 λοιπὸν *om.* γ

THE BEGINNING, WITH GOD'S HELP, OF THE SECOND SECTION

I

II 1 All dropsies which result from acute diseases are bad.

Hippocrates begins the second section by giving instruction on dropsies, in order to establish a continuity between what is to come and what has gone before, since dropsy also is a condition that develops in the hypochondria. But no one should suppose that, despite his original proposal to deal with acute, Hippocrates is discussing chronic diseases; the fact is that in discussing the acute he also deals with those conditions which result from a change in the character of acute diseases, and his present words bear this out; for he said, Dropsies which result from acute diseases. So he is talking not about chronic diseases, but about those which develop from a change in acute diseases.

For not only do they fail to get rid of the fever, but they are also painful and very deadly. He has a good reason for saying they are painful; for when the fluid accumulates all at once around the hypochondria, they are subjected to strain, and running the risk of being ruptured from the strain they are pained by the accompanying painful sensation.

Not only do they fail to get rid of the fever. This might appear to be not strictly true; for someone will say, "How can they fail to get rid of the fever, if there is so much fluid accumulated? For the fluid will quench the distemper and stop the fever." Some answer this by saying, "The reason why people with this complaint are not cured of the fever is that the fever is spread over the whole body, while the fluid is gathered in one part; and the localized accumulation of fluid cannot cure the distemper of the whole body and stop the fever." But this is a superficial reply; for someone will say to them, "Even though the accumulation of fluid is in one part, nevertheless it is in the very hearth (of the body), I mean around the hypochondria and the heart; and if it wets the heart well and quenches it, the distemper of the whole body also will be cured as a result." Wherefore it is necessary to give the reason that is closer to the truth; even though a large quantity of fluid gathers in dropsy cases, it does not stop the fever, being moist in

φαίνεται ὑγρόν· ἐπεί τοί γε τῇ δυνάμει κακόχυμον ὂν καὶ ἁλμυρόν, θερμόν ἐστι καὶ ξηρὸν καθάπερ καὶ ἐπὶ τοῦ θαλασσίου ὕδατος ἔχει. καὶ διὰ τοῦτο δὴ καὶ τὸ ὑγρὸν τὸ ἀθροιζόμενον ἐπὶ τῶν ὑδεριώντων τῇ μὲν φαντασίᾳ
128 ὑγρὸν φαίνεται, τῇ δὲ δυνάμει θερμαίνει καὶ ξηραίνει διὰ τὸ | μετέχειν κακοχυμίας τινὸς καὶ ἁλμυρότητος καὶ σηπεδόνος· καὶ διὰ τοῦτο οὐ παύει τὸν πυρετόν. ἀλλὰ καὶ διψώδεις εἰσὶν οἱ ὑδεριῶντες· καὶ ἐπὶ τῇ δίψῃ πάλιν τὸ αὐτὸ ἄπορον δοκεῖ εἶναι καὶ ἡ αὐτὴ λύσις.

Εἶτα λοιπὸν λέγει, πῶς γίνονται οἱ ὕδρωπες. καί φησιν ὅτι Ἄρχονται δὲ οἱ πλεῖστοι ἐκ τῶν κενεώνων τε καὶ τῆς ὀσφύος, οἱ δὲ καὶ ἀπὸ τοῦ ἥπατος. κενεῶνας δὲ καλεῖ ἐκεῖνα τὰ μόρια τὰ ἀπὸ τοῦ τελευταίου πλευροῦ μέχρι τοῦ ὀστοῦ τῆς λαγόνος· δοκεῖ γὰρ ταῦτα παρὰ πάντα τὰ μόρια τά τε ὑπερκείμενα ἢ ὑποκείμενα, τυχὸν θώρακα καὶ ὑποχόνδρια καὶ γαστέρα καὶ κύστιν, κενότερα εἶναι. ἐπεί τοί γε καὶ ταῦτα οὐκ εἰσι κενά, ἀλλὰ περιέχουσι τὰ λεπτὰ ἔντερα καὶ τὰ μεσεντέρια. ἁπλῶς οὖν αὐτὸς λέγει ὅτι ἄρχονται ἢ ἀπὸ τοῦ ἥπατος ἢ ἀπὸ τῶν κενεώνων. σὺ δὲ εἰπὲ ὅτι «Καὶ πᾶς ὕδερος ἐπὶ ἀσθενείᾳ τοῦ ἥπατος γίνεται καὶ ἐπὶ ἀποτυχίᾳ τῆς αἱματοποιητικῆς δυνάμεως.» ἀλλὰ καὶ τοῦτο ἢ κατὰ πρωτοπάθειαν ἢ κατὰ συμπάθειαν γίνεται. καὶ κατὰ συμπάθειαν διαφόρως· ἢ γὰρ διὰ γειτνίασιν συμπάσχουσι τὰ μόρια ἢ διὰ συγγένειαν μεγίστων ἀγγείων, λέγω δὴ ἀξιολόγων φλεβῶν ἢ ἀρτηριῶν ἢ νεύρων καὶ τῶν τοιούτων.

Εἶτα λοιπὸν συνελόντες οἱ ἐξηγηταὶ τὸν περὶ τῶν ὑδέρων λόγον εἰς τέσσαρα κεφάλαια τὴν πᾶσαν θεωρίαν συνάγουσι. καὶ ἀρκτέον ἀπὸ τοῦ πρώτου κεφαλαίου καὶ λεκτέον· «Τί ἐστιν ὕδερος;» ὕδερός ἐστι συναγωγὴ ὑγροῦ παρὰ φύσιν μεταξὺ περιτοναίου καὶ ἐντέρων, πρὸς ἀντιδιαστολὴν τῆς ὑγροκήλης· καὶ γὰρ κἀκείνη συναγωγή ἐστιν ὑγροῦ, ἀλλ' οὐχὶ μεταξὺ περιτοναίου καὶ ἐντέρων, ἀλλ' ἐν ἄλλοις μορίοις. ἀλλὰ δοκεῖ ἀτελῶς ἔχειν τὸν ὁρισμόν, ἐπειδὴ τὸν ἀνὰ σάρκα ὕδερον οὐ περιλαμβάνει· ὁ γὰρ ἀνὰ σάρκα ἐν τῷ παντὶ σώματι οὔσης τῆς βλάβης γίνεται, οὐ μὴν μεταξὺ περι-
129 τοναίου καὶ ἐντέρων. | διὸ δεῖ εἰπεῖν ὅτι ὕδερός ἐστι συναγωγὴ ὑγροῦ παρὰ φύσιν μεταξὺ περιτοναίου καὶ ἐντέρων ἢ ἐν τῷ σαρκώδει μέρει τῶν μυῶν.

Δεύτερον κεφάλαιόν ἐστιν, ἐν ᾧ δεῖ ἡμᾶς τὰ μόρια εἰπεῖν, ἐν οἷς συνίσταται ὁ ὕδερος· ἢ γὰρ μεταξὺ περιτοναίου καὶ ἐντέρων ἢ ἐν τοῖς κενεῶσι καὶ ἐν τῇ ὀσφύϊ. λοιπὸν δεῖ εἰπεῖν τὸν τρόπον τῆς γενέσεως τῶν ὑδέρων. ἀλλὰ πρὸ τούτου δεῖ ἡμᾶς λῆμμά τι προσλαβεῖν ἔχον οὕτως· δεῖ εἰδέναι ὅτι μετὰ τὸ παρασχεθῆναι τὴν τροφὴν ἐν τῇ γαστρὶ ἀλλοιοῦται καὶ πέττεται· εἶτα μετὰ τὸ πεφθῆναι καὶ ἀλλοιωθῆναι καὶ χυλοποιηθῆναι τὸ μὲν λευκότερον καὶ λιπαρώτερον εἰς τροφὴν κέχρηται ἡ γαστὴρ τῆς ἑαυτῆς

10–14] *cf.* Gal. In Hipp. Progn. comm. II 1: CMG V 9,2 p. 260,11–17 *infra*, p. 156,14–16 15–20] *cf.* Gal. In Hipp. Progn. comm. II 1: CMG V 9,2 pp. 260,20–261,1 27–29] *cf.* [Gal.] Def. med. 279: XIX p. 424 K.

8 οἱ *om.* Pζ ὅτι *om.* γ 15 Καὶ *om.* γ 16 ἐξαιματοποιητικῆς L 18 γίνεται *om.* γ 19 συμπάσχοντα *codd.*: *corr. Dietz* συγγένειαν *om.* L 20 καὶ] ἢ L 22 εἰσάγουσι L 23 λεκτέον] εἰπεῖν γ 25 οὐχὶ] οὐ Pζ: *om.* M 32 τὰ μόρια *om.* L 33 *post* ἐντέρων *add.* συνίσταται γ 35 *post* ἡμᾶς *add.* εἰπεῖν L λήμματι *codd.*: *corr. Dietz* προλαβεῖν γ 37 καὶ ἀλλοιωθῆναι *om.* γ

appearance only; the fact is that, being in effect unwholesome and salty, it is hot and dry, just like sea-water. For this reason, then, the fluid that accumulates in dropsy cases is moist in appearance, but in effect it warms and dries, since it partakes of a certain unwholesomeness and saltiness and decay; and because of this it does not stop the fever. Dropsy subjects are also prone to thirst, which seems to raise the same problem, but the solution also is the same.

Next he explains how dropsies develop. He says, The majority originate in the flanks and loins, but some also in the liver. By flanks (*keneōnes*) he means those areas between the last rib and the iliac bone, these parts appearing emptier (*kenotera*) than any others either above or below, namely the thorax, hypochondria, belly and bladder. However, even these are not vacant, but contain the small intestines and the mesenteries. He states, then, in a general way that (dropsies) begin either in the liver or in the flanks. But you may say, "All dropsy is caused by weakness of the liver and failure of the faculty which produces blood." And this results from either a primary or a sympathetic affection. If by a sympathetic affection, it happens in different ways; the parts sympathize either because of their proximity to, or because of their connection with, major vessels, I mean important veins or arteries or nerves and the like.

Then the commentators giving a succinct account of dropsies, draw together the entire subject in four chapters. We must begin with the first chapter and ask, "What is dropsy?" Dropsy is an abnormal accumulation of fluid between the peritoneum and the intestines; this distinguishes it from hydrocele which, while it also is an accumulation of fluid, collects somewhere other than between the peritoneum and intestines. However, the definition appears to be incomplete, as it does not include (the type known as) anasarca; anasarca develops when the fault is in the whole body and not in the area between the peritoneum and intestines. So we must define dropsy as an abnormal accumulation of fluid between the peritoneum and intestines or in the fleshy part of the muscles.

The second chapter is where we must name the parts in which dropsy is found; (it develops) either between the peritoneum and intestines or in the flanks and loin. Next we should describe the way in which dropsies are produced. However, we must first admit an assumption which is as follows: after nutriment is supplied to the stomach, we must know that it undergoes conversion and digestion; then when it has been digested, converted and made into chyle, the stomach uses the whiter and richer

οὐσίας — τὸ γὰρ ἔνδον τῆς γαστρὸς μέρος ἀπὸ τοῦ χυλοῦ τρέφεται —, τὸ δὲ λοιπὸν μέρος τοῦ χυλοῦ ὡς περίττωμα ἀποβάλλεται καὶ φέρεται διὰ τῶν μεσαραίων, καὶ ἕλκει τὸ ἧπαρ πρὸς ἑαυτὸ καὶ ἀναφέρεται. εἶτα δευτέραν πέψιν ἀναδέχεται, καὶ πρὸς τὴν οἰκείαν φύσιν καὶ οὐσίαν ἐξομοιοῖ αὐτό. εἶτα πάλιν τὸ ἧπαρ κρατεῖ τὸ ἀρκοῦν πρὸς τροφὴν αὐτοῦ καὶ τὸ λοιπὸν ὡς περίττωμα ἀπωθεῖ διὰ τῶν φλεβῶν ἐπὶ τὸ πᾶν σῶμα, καὶ οὕτως τρέφονται πάντα τὰ μόρια. ἐὰν οὖν συμβῇ τὴν ἀλλοιωτικὴν δύναμιν τοῦ ἥπατος κακῶς διατεθῆναι — κακῶς δὲ διατίθεται κατὰ δύο τρόπους ὡς πρὸς τὰ νῦν λεγόμενα· ἢ γὰρ ὁμοιομερῶς βλάπτεται ἢ ὀργανικῶς· καὶ ὁμοιομερῶς μὲν κατὰ δυσκρασίαν τινά, ὀργανικῶς δὲ ἢ δι' ἔμφραξιν ἢ δι' ὄγκον τινά —, κακῶς οὖν διατιθεμένης τῆς ἀλλοιωτικῆς δυνάμεως τοῦ ἥπατος ἀποτυγχάνει ἡ ἐξαιμάτωσις, καὶ ἀπεπτεῖται. καὶ τὸ μὲν λεπτομερὲς αὐτοῦ διεξέρχεται τὸν ὑμένα τοῦ ἥπατος, ἐπειδὴ λεπτός ἐστι, καὶ φέρεται ἀτμοειδῶς ἐν μέσῳ περιτοναίου καὶ ἐντέρων. εἶτα λοιπὸν οὗτος ὁ
130 ἀτμὸς λαμβάνων ἀείσε προσθήκην στέγεται ὡς ἐπὶ τὸν | περιτόναιον, ἐπειδὴ οὐ διεξέρχεται τὸν περιτόναιον, στεγανοῦ αὐτοῦ ὄντος, καὶ τῇ προσθήκῃ παχύνεται καὶ δίκην ὑετοῦ ἀντικαταρρεῖ, καὶ οὕτως ἀθροίζεται καὶ ποιεῖ τὸν ὕδερον. οὕτω γὰρ καὶ ἐπὶ τῶν βαλανείων ἔστιν ἰδεῖν· οἱ γὰρ ἀτμοὶ γινόμενοι περὶ τὴν ὀροφὴν παχύνονται καὶ σταλαγμοὶ γινόμενοι ἀντικαταρρέουσι δίκην ὑετοῦ, ὡς εἴρηται. εἷς οὖν τρόπος ὑδέρου οὗτος ὁ ἐπὶ ἀσθενείᾳ τῆς ἀλλοιωτικῆς δυνάμεως γινόμενος τοῦ ἥπατος.

Γίνεται ὕδερος καὶ κατὰ ἕτερον τρόπον, ἐπὶ ἀσθενείᾳ τῆς καθεκτικῆς δυνάμεως. τί γάρ; ὅτι ἐὰν ἀσθενὴς ᾖ ἡ καθεκτικὴ δύναμις, μετὰ τὸ ἄρξασθαι τὴν ἀλλοιωτικὴν ἀλλοιοῦν καὶ μεταβάλλειν τὸν χυλὸν καὶ ἐξαιματοῦν αὐτόν, πρὸ ὥρας ἐπεγειρομένη ἡ καθεκτικὴ ἐξαφεῖ αὐτό, καὶ φέρεται δι' ὧνπερ ἀνῆλθεν ὁδῶν, ἐπὶ γαστέρα λέγω καὶ ἔντερα, καὶ ποιεῖ ἡπατηρὰν δυσεντερίαν ἐοικυῖαν πλύματι κρεῶν νεοσφαγῶν, ἐπειδὴ ἀρχὴν λαμβάνει πέψεως ἤγουν ἐξαιματώσεως ὑπὸ τῆς ἀλλοιωτικῆς, οὐ τελείως δέ, διὰ τὸ τὴν καθεκτικὴν δύναμιν ἐξεῶσαι πρὸ ὥρας. ὅθεν τῷ χρόνῳ ἀτροφοῦντα ἐπὶ τῇ ἡπατηρᾷ δυσεντερίᾳ πάντως ὕδερος ἐπιγίνεται, καὶ οὕτως ἀπόλλυνται. καὶ ἀναλογεῖ ἡ μὲν διάρροια τῆς γαστρὸς τῇ ἡπατηρᾷ δυσεντερίᾳ, ἡ δὲ ἐκχόλωσις τῷ ὑδέρῳ· εἴ τι γάρ ἐστι διάρροια γαστρὸς ἐπὶ τῇ ἀποτυχίᾳ τοῦ χυλοῦ, τοῦτο ἐπὶ τοῦ ἥπατος ἡ δυσεντερία, καὶ εἴ τί ἐστιν ἐκχόλωσις ἐπὶ τῆς γαστρός, τοῦτο ἐπὶ τοῦ ἥπατος ὕδερός ἐστιν. εἶτα καὶ ἀποροῦσιν ὅτι «Διὰ τί ἐπὶ τῇ ἀποτυχίᾳ τῆς γαστρὸς οὐ γίνεται ὕδερος καίτοι δαψιλοῦς οὔσης τῆς ὕλης ἐπὶ τῆς γαστρός;» καὶ λέγομεν ὅτι, ἐπειδὴ στεγανός ἐστιν ὁ ὑμὴν ἤγουν ἡ οὐσία τῆς γαστρός, οὐκ ἰσχύει ἀτμοειδῶς διεξελθεῖν, ἀλλ' ἐκεῖσε στέγεται καὶ τῷ βάρει κενοῦται κάτωθεν καὶ ποιεῖ διάρροιαν, οὐ μὴν ὕδερον.

Τρίτον ἐστὶ κεφάλαιον, ἐν ᾧ δεῖ ἡμᾶς τὰς διαφορὰς τῶν ὑδέρων ζητῆσαι.

4 καὶ[I] *om.* γ καὶ οὐσίαν *post* αὐτό *trsp.* L 5 κρατεῖ τὸ ἧπαρ γ 8 κατὰ] διὰ γ ὡς] ὅσον γ 11sq. τοῦ ἥπατος *om.* γ 13 ἐπειδὴ λεπτός ἐστι *om.* L 15 sq. ἐπειδὴ — περιτόναιον *om.* γ 16 ὄντος αὐτοῦ γ 20 δίκην ὑετοῦ *post* εἴρηται *trsp.* γ 25 ἐξαφῆ *codd.*: *correxi* αὐτῶ γ: *fort.* αὐτόν *scribendum est* 26 γαστρὶ ... ἐντέροις γ 27 πλύμα γ 29 ἐξῶσαι L ἀτροφοῦντα] *sc.* τὰ μόρια *(cf. infra, p. 144,21)*: ἀτροφοῦνται MPV 34 τῇ γαστρὶ *codd.*: *correxi* 37 ἡ *om.* γ 39 οὐ μὴν ὕδερον *om.* γ

part as nutriment for its own substance — chyle being the nutrient of the inside of the stomach —, while the remainder of the chyle is rejected as a residue; this is conveyed through the mesaraics and is attracted by and received into the liver. Next it undergoes a second digestion and the liver assimilates it to its own nature and substance. Then again the liver takes from it an amount sufficient for nourishment and expels the rest as a residue through the veins all over the body, and thus all the parts are nourished. If, then, it should happen that the liver's converting faculty is defective — and as far as the present discussion is concerned, it is put out of order in two ways: for it is impaired either homogeneously or organically; and homogeneously by a distemper, organically by a stoppage or a swelling — if, then, the liver's faculty of conversion is damaged, blood formation fails and (the chyle) is not concocted. Then the thin part seeps through the liver's membrane, due to its fineness, and is conveyed in vapor form to the area between the peritoneum and the intestines. Next this vapor, which is constantly being added to, is held in by the peritoneum, being unable to penetrate it, since it is impervious; then it condenses by addition, falls like rain, and thus accumulates and produces dropsy. The same process can be observed in the baths also: the vapors that gather around the ceiling condense, form drops and fall like rain, as we have described. This, then, is one way that dropsy is produced, namely from weakness of the liver's converting faculty.

Dropsy is produced in another way also, by weakness of the retentive faculty. Why? Because, if the retentive faculty is weak, after the converting has begun to change and convert the chyle and make it into blood, the retentive is stimulated prematurely and expels it; it is conveyed back, by the way it came, i.e., to the stomach and the intestines, causing dysentery of the liver like water in which freshly slaughtered meat has been washed; (this happens) because (the chyle) begins to be digested, i.e., formed into blood, by the converting faculty, but it is not completed, since the retentive faculty expels prematurely. The result is that through time the dysentery of the liver causes the parts to be without nutriment, dropsy inevitably follows and thus the patients die. And there is a correspondence between diarrhoea of the stomach and dysentery of the liver on the one hand, and between eccholosis and dropsy on the other; for diarrhoea of the stomach from failure of the chyle is analogous to dysentery in the liver, while eccholosis of the stomach corresponds to dropsy in the liver. Here the question is raised, "Why is dropsy not occasioned by failure (of chyle) in the stomach, even though the stomach contains a large quantity of matter?" Our reply is that, since the membrane or substance of the stomach is impervious, (the matter) cannot penetrate in vapor form, but is held in there and is evacuated downwards because of its weight; this produces diarrhoea, not dropsy.

In the third chapter we must examine the different kinds of dropsy.

131 καὶ δεῖ εἰδέναι ὅτι ὕδερος ἢ με|ταξὺ περιτοναίου καὶ ἐντέρων συνίσταται ἢ ἐν ὅλῳ τῷ σώματι. καὶ εἰ μὲν μεταξὺ περιτοναίου καὶ ἐντέρων συσταίη, ἢ ὑγρὸν μόνον ἐστὶ τὸ ἀθροιζόμενον καὶ ποιεῖ τὸν ἁπλῶς ὕδερον, ἢ μετὰ τοῦ ὑγροῦ καὶ πνεῦμά τι· καὶ ἢ τὸ ὑγρὸν ἐπικρατεῖ καὶ ποιεῖ τὸν ἀσκίτην, ἢ τὸ πνεῦμα ἐπικρατεῖ καὶ ποιεῖ τὸν τυμπανίαν. εἰ δὲ ἐν ὅλῳ τῷ σώματί ἐστιν ἡ βλάβη, ἢ ὑγροῦ μόνον ἐστὶ συνάθροισις καὶ ποιεῖ τὸν λεγόμενον λευκοφλεγματίαν ἤγουν τὸν ἀνὰ σάρκα· εἰ δὲ μετὰ τοῦ ὑγροῦ καὶ πνεύματά εἰσι συναναπεπλεγμένα, ποιεῖ τότε τὴν ὑδαλέαν λεγομένην ἕξιν.

Καὶ ἀποροῦσιν ὅτι «Ἐπὶ μὲν τῶν ἄλλων ὑδέρων, οἳ μεταξὺ περιτοναίου καὶ ἐντέρων ⟨συνίστανται, ἐπὶ ἀσθενείᾳ τῆς ἀλλοιωτικῆς δυνάμεως τοῦ ἥπατος γίνονται· οἱ δὲ ἐν ὅλῳ τῷ σώματι⟩ συνιστάμενοι οὐκ ἐπὶ ἀσθενείᾳ τῆς ἀλλοιωτικῆς δυνάμεως τοῦ ἥπατος γίνονται, ἀλλ' ἐπὶ βλάβῃ τῆς ἐν ἑκάστῳ μορίῳ ἀλλοιωτικῆς δυνάμεως· πῶς οὖν ὁ Ἱπποκράτης λέγει πάντα ὕδερον ἐπὶ ἀσθενείᾳ τῆς ἀλλοιωτικῆς δυνάμεως τοῦ ἥπατος γίνεσθαι;» καὶ λέγομεν ὅτι, ἐὰν καλῶς ἔχῃ ἡ ἀλλοιωτικὴ δύναμις τοῦ ἥπατος καὶ δεόντως γίνεται ἡ πέψις καὶ ἡ ἐξαιμάτωσις, ἔδει μὴ γενέσθαι ὕδερον, ἀλλ' ἄλλο τι πάθος· ἐὰν γὰρ ἐν ὅλῳ τῷ σώματί ἐστιν ἡ βλάβη καὶ οὐχὶ ἐν ἥπατι, ἔδει τυχὸν σαπῆναι καὶ ἀνάψαι πυρετὸν ἢ ἕτερον ποιῆσαι νόσημα. ἀλλὰ καὶ ὁ ἀνὰ σάρκα ὕδερος ἐπὶ ἀσθενείᾳ τῆς ἀλλοιωτικῆς δυνάμεως τοῦ ἥπατος γίνεται· ἐπὶ γὰρ τῇ ἀσθενείᾳ λεπτὸν καὶ ὑδαρὲς τὸ αἷμα γίνεται καὶ ὀλίγον, καὶ ἐντεῦθεν διὰ τὴν ὀλιγότητα ἀτροφοῦσι τὰ μόρια, καὶ ἐπὶ τῇ ἀτροφίᾳ γίνεται ὁ ἀνὰ σάρκα ὕδερος ἀτόνως καὶ αὐτῶν διατιθεμένων. οὐκοῦν πᾶς ὕδερος ἐπὶ ἀσθενείᾳ τῆς ἀλλοιωτικῆς δυνάμεως γίνεται.

Τέταρτόν ἐστι κεφάλαιον, ἐν ᾧ δεῖ ἡμᾶς τὰ αἴτια εἰπεῖν τοῦ ὑδέρου. δεῖ εἰδέναι ὅτι δύο εἰσὶν αἴτια τὰ ποιητικὰ τοῦ ὑδέρου, ψῦξις καὶ ἡ παρὰ φύσιν θερμότης. καὶ πῶς γίνεται ὕδερος ἐπὶ καταψύξει; εἴρηται ἡμῖν ὅτι ἐπὶ ἀσθενείᾳ τῆς ἀλλοιωτικῆς δυνάμεως τοῦ ἥπατος γίνεται. ἡ δὲ θερμότης ποιεῖ ὕδερον τρόπῳ τοιούτῳ· ἡ θερμότης ἢ κατὰ φύσιν ἐστὶν ἢ παρὰ φύσιν·
132 καὶ ἡ μὲν κατὰ φύ|σιν θερμότης ζωοποιητική ἐστι τοῦ ἡμετέρου σώματος, ἡ δὲ παρὰ φύσιν φθαρτική ἐστι καὶ ἀναστοιχειωτική. αὕτη οὖν ἡ παρὰ φύσιν θερμότης διαφορητική ἐστι τοῦ κατὰ φύσιν θερμοῦ, καθ' ἣν καὶ ἀπεψίαι τὸ τηνικαῦτα γίνονται. οὕτως γοῦν συμβαίνει ἡμᾶς ἐν τῷ θέρει ἐκλύτους καὶ χαύνους εἶναι ⟨διὰ τὸ⟩ ὑπὸ τῆς παρὰ φύσιν, λέγω δὴ τῆς ἐκτὸς θερμότητος, δραστηρίου τυγχανούσης, διαφορεῖσθαι τὸ κατὰ φύσιν ἡμῖν θερμόν. ἀλλὰ καὶ οἱ πυρέσσοντες διὰ τοῦτο ἁδροτέρας τροφὰς πέψαι οὐ δύνανται, ἐπειδὴ διαφορεῖται ἡ κατὰ φύσιν θερμότης, καθ' ἣν αἱ πέψεις γίνονται· καὶ τῷ λόγῳ τούτῳ λεπτῇ τροφῇ τρέφομεν αὐτούς. ἐὰν οὖν συμβῇ δυσκρασίαν γενέσθαι ἐν τῷ ἥπατι, διαφορεῖ τὸ κατὰ φύσιν θερμὸν τὸ ἐν τῷ ἥπατι· τούτου διαφορουμένου ψύχεται, καὶ ἀποτυχία γίνεται τῆς ἐξαι-

1–7] *cf.* Steph. Comm. in Hipp. Aph.: Escor. Σ. II. 10 fol. 72r; 258r

1 *ante* ὕδερος *add.* ὁ γ 5 ἐπικρατεῖ *om.* γ 6 *fort.* μόνου *scribendum est* 7 ἤγουν – σάρκα *om.* L 9 οἱ *codd.*: *corr. Wk.* 10 sq. συνίστανται – σώματι *add. Wk.* 15 ἔχει MPY 19 ὕδερος *om.* γ 22 αὐτὸν διατιθέμενον (-μένου γ) *codd.*: *correxi* 25 αἴτια *post* ποιητικὰ *trsp.* γ 26 *post* ἐπὶ^{I} *add.* τῇ γ 27 τοῦ ἥπατος] ὁ ὕδερος γ 33 διὰ τὸ *add. Wk.* 34 ἡμῶν γ: *fort.* ἐν ἡμῖν *scribendum est; sed cf. infra, p. 220,24* 37 τρεφόμενα L ἑαυτοὺς Pζ

And note that dropsy forms either between the peritoneum and intestines or throughout the body. If it forms between the peritoneum and intestines, the accumulation either consists of fluid alone and produces simple dropsy or it contains some gas along with the fluid; and either there is a preponderance of fluid, which causes ascites, or the gas predominates to produce tympanias. On the other hand, if the fault is all over the body, either there is an accumulation of fluid alone creating the so-called leucophlegmatias, i.e., anasarca, or a mixture of fluid and gases which in that case produces the so-called hydalean condition.

Here the problem is posed, "In the case of the other dropsies which form between the peritoneum and intestines the cause is weakness of the liver's converting faculty, while those that develop all over the body are not produced by a weakness of the liver's converting faculty, but by damage to the converting faculty of each part. How can Hippocrates, then, state that all dropsy is caused by weakness of the liver's converting faculty?" Our response is that, if the liver's converting faculty is working well and digestion and blood formation are normal, the result should not be dropsy, but some other affection; for if the fault is in the whole body and not in the liver, the matter should, for example, decompose and touch off fever or bring about some other disease. Anasarca dropsy, too, results from weakness of the liver's converting faculty; for because of the weakness the blood becomes thin, watery and scarce and then due to the scarcity the parts are deprived of nutriment and lack of nourishment brings on anasarca, the parts having been left in a toneless state. The conclusion, then, is that every form of dropsy is caused by weakness of the (liver's) converting faculty.

The fourth chapter is where we must discuss the causes of dropsy. Observe that there are two efficient causes of dropsy, cold and abnormal heat. How is dropsy caused by cold? We have already explained that it is brought about by weakness of the liver's converting faculty. Heat, on the other hand, produces dropsy in the following way: heat is either normal or abnormal, and while the normal heat vitalizes our bodies, the abnormal destroys and dissolves them. This abnormal heat, then, dissipates the normal heat and a further result is indigestion. In the same way during the summer we are left weak and sluggish because the abnormal, i.e., external, heat being potent dissipates the natural heat in us. This is also the reason why those with fever are unable to digest the more solid foods, since the normal heat which promotes digestions is dissipated; and because of this we feed them light nourishment. If a distemper, then, arises in the liver, it dissipates the natural heat which is in the liver; when this is dissipated (the liver) turns cold, blood

ματώσεως, καὶ γίνεται ὁ ὕδερος· ὡς ἐντεῦθεν πάλιν τὸν ὕδερον ἐπὶ ψύξει κατὰ πρῶτον λόγον γίνεσθαι.

II 2 [8: 203,8 A. = II 130,12 L.] Οἱ δὲ ὕδρωπες οἱ ἐκ τῶν ὀξέων νοσημάτων γινόμενοι πάντες κακοί. οὔτε γὰρ τοῦ πυρὸς ἀπαλλάττουσιν ἐπώδυνοί τέ εἰσι κάρτα καὶ θανατώδεις.

Ἐντεῦθεν ἀπορία ἀναφαίνεται τοιαύτη, ὅτι «Πῶς τὰ ἐναντία ἐν τῷ αὐτῷ συνίστανται; ὁ γὰρ πυρετὸς θερμόν τι χρῆμά ἐστι καὶ ξηρόν, ὁ δὲ ὕδερος ψυχρόν ἐστι πάθος καὶ ὑγρόν.» πρὸς ὅ τινες λέγουσιν ὅτι «Ἡ χολὴ θερμή ἐστι καὶ ξηρὰ καὶ δριμεῖα· ἀλλὰ καὶ ὁ πυρετὸς ὑπὸ τοιαύτης ὕλης ἀνάπτεται· καὶ κατὰ πρωτοπάθειαν ἡ χολὴ τὸν πυρετὸν ἐξάπτει, τὸν δὲ ὕδερον ποιεῖ ἡ χολὴ κατὰ συμπάθειαν. θερμὴ γὰρ οὖσα διαφορεῖ τὸ κατὰ φύσιν θερμὸν τοῦ ἥπατος, καὶ ἐντεῦθεν καταψύχεται καὶ ἀποτυγχάνει ἡ ἐξαιμάτωσις, καὶ λεπτὸν καὶ δίυγρον γίνεται τὸ αἷμα καὶ ἀτμοειδῶς φέρεται μεταξὺ περιτοναίου καὶ ἐντέρων καὶ ποιεῖ τὸν ὕδερον.» ἀνατρέπουσι δὲ αὐτούς τινες λέγοντες ὅτι «Ἐὰν δραστήριος τοσοῦτόν ἐστιν ἡ θερμότης τῆς χολῆς, ὥστε τὸ κατὰ φύσιν θερμὸν διαφορῆσαι καὶ κατα-
133 ψῦξαι τὸ ἧπαρ, ἔδει τῇ | δραστηρίῳ δυνάμει καὶ αὐτὸ τὸ ὑγρὸν ἐκδαπανῆσαι καὶ ξηρὸν ποιῆσαι νόσημα, οὐ μὴν ὑγρόν, λέγω δὴ ὕδερον.» διὸ δεῖ εἰπεῖν αἰτίαν τοιαύτην, ὅτι κατὰ διαφέροντα μόρια τἀναντία συνίστανται· ἡ μὲν δυσκρασία ἤγουν ὁ πυρετὸς ἐν τῇ καρδίᾳ καὶ ἐν τῷ ἀρτηριώδει γένει — καὶ κατὰ σχέσιν τινὰ καὶ τὸ πᾶν σῶμα μετέχει τῆς θερμασίας —, τὸν δὲ ὕδερον μεταξὺ περιτοναίου καὶ ἐντέρων συστῆναι. πῶς δὲ ὅλως γίνονται τὰ ἐναντία δεῖ εἰπεῖν. ἡ χολὴ κατὰ μὲν τὴν ποιότητα τὸν πυρετὸν ἀνάπτει, τῇ δὲ ποσότητι βαρύνει τὰς ἐν ἥπατι δυνάμεις καὶ καταπνίγει καὶ καταβάλλει, καὶ ἐπὶ τῇ καταβολῇ ἀποτυγχάνει ἡ ἐξαιμάτωσις καὶ γίνεται ὕδερος.

II 3 [8: 203,9 A. = II 130,14 L.] Ἄρχονται δὲ οἱ πλεῖστοι ἐκ τῶν κενεώνων τε καὶ τῆς ὀσφύος, οἱ δὲ καὶ ἀπὸ τοῦ ἥπατος.

Εἰρηκὼς ὁ Ἱπποκράτης ὅτι Ἄρχονται οἱ πλεῖστοι ἐκ τῶν κενεώνων τε καὶ τῆς ὀσφύος, τὸ κατὰ συμπάθειαν ἐδήλωσεν· εἰρηκὼς δὲ οἱ δὲ καὶ ἀπὸ τοῦ ἥπατος, τὸ κατὰ πρωτοπάθειαν. πᾶς γὰρ ὕδερος ἢ κατὰ συμπάθειάν ἐστιν ἢ κατὰ πρωτοπάθειαν τοῦ ἥπατος.

II

II 4 [8: 203,10 A. = II 130,15 L.] Ὁκόσοισι μὲν οὖν αἱ ἀρχαὶ ἐκ τῶν κενεώνων τε καὶ τῆς ὀσφύος γίνονται

2 *ad* γίνεσθαι *des.* YW 3 ἄλλο *in mg.* L 4 γινόμενοι *om.* γ 5 ἐπώδυνοί — θανατώδεις *om.* γ 7 χρῆμά *om.* γ 9 *post* ὑπὸ *add.* τῆς γ 11 ἐξάπτει] ἀνάπτει γ 12 τοῦ ἥπατος θερμόν γ 15 τινες αὐτοὺς γ λέγοντες *om.* γ ἐστι τοσοῦτον γ 17 δραστηρία L; *sed cf. lin. 15; supra, p. 122,18; 144,34* 32 *post* πρωτοπάθειαν *add.* γίνεται γ 35 γίνονται] οἱ δὲ καὶ ἀπὸ τοῦ ἥπατος γ; *cf. supra, lin. 28*

formation fails and dropsy develops; so again we see that dropsy is caused in a primary way by cold.

II 2 All dropsies resulting from acute diseases are bad. For not only do they fail to get rid of the fever, but they are also extremely painful and deadly.

Here the following problem arises, "How can opposites coexist in the same (person)? For fever is a hot and dry thing, and dropsy is a cold and wet affection." To which some say, "Bile is hot, dry and pungent; but fever is touched off by such matter; and bile ignites the fever as a primary affection, while it produces dropsy as a sympathetic affection. For (bile) being hot dissipates the liver's normal heat; then (the liver) turns cold and blood formation fails; this makes the blood thin and watery and it is conveyed in vapor form between the peritoneum and intestines and creates dropsy." Some, however, refute them saying, "If the heat from bile is so effective that it can dissipate the normal heat and cool the liver, it ought with its potent power to completely consume the fluid itself and produce a dry disease, not a wet one, I mean dropsy." For this reason we must give the following explanation: the opposites are in different parts of the body; the distemper or fever is in the heart and in the arterial class – and by some sort of relationship even the whole body has a share of the heat –, while the dropsy is located between the peritoneum and intestines. But we should describe how the opposites arise in the first place. Fever is touched off by the bile's quality, while the quantity oppresses, smothers and disables the faculties of the liver; collapse (of the faculties) causes failure of blood formation and the result is dropsy.

II 3 The majority start in the flanks and loin, but some also in the liver.

When Hippocrates said, The majority start in the flanks and loin, he was indicating sympathetic affection, while but some also in the liver (refers to) primary affection. You see, every dropsy is either a sympathetic or primary affection of the liver.

II

II 4 In cases where they begin in the flanks and loin

Μεμαθήκαμεν ἀνωτέρω ὅτι ὁ κατὰ πρωτοπάθειαν ὕδερος τοῦ ἥπατος γίνεται, ἡνίκα ἐν αὐτῷ συσταίη τῷ ἥπατι τὸ πάθος, φλεγμονὴ τυχὸν ἢ σκίρρος ἢ οἴδημα ἢ ἔμφραξις ἢ ἕτερος ὄγκος ἢ δυσκρασία θερμὴ ἢ ψυχρά· τότε γὰρ καταβάλλονται αἱ φυσικαὶ δυνάμεις τοῦ ἥπατος, μάλιστα δὲ ἡ ἀλλοιωτικὴ αὐτοῦ δύναμις, καὶ ἀποτυγχάνει ἡ ἐξαιμάτωσις καὶ ἀπεπτεῖ⟨ται⟩, καὶ γίνεται τὸ αἷμα λεπτὸν καὶ ὑδαρές, καὶ ἀτμοειδῶς διηθεῖται καὶ φέρεται μεταξὺ περιτοναίου καὶ ἐντέρων, καὶ γίνεται ὕδερος ὁ κατὰ πρωτοπάθειαν τοῦ ἥπατος.

Ὁ δὲ ὕδερος ὁ κατὰ πρωτοπάθειαν τῶν κενεώνων γινόμενος, ἤγουν ὁ κατὰ συμπάθειαν τοῦ ἥπατος, γίνεται, ἡνίκα ἐν τοῖς μορίοις ἐκείνοις ἐστὶ
134 τὸ πάθος, τουτέστιν ἐν τοῖς κενεῶσι καὶ ἐν | τῇ ὀσφύϊ. καὶ ποῖά εἰσι τὰ μόρια; ἐγὼ λέγω· ἡνίκα ἐστὶν ἐν τοῖς μεσαραϊκοῖς ὄγκος ἢ φλεγμονὴ ἢ ἔμφραξις, ἢ δυσκρασία ἐν τοῖς νεφροῖς ἢ ἐν τῷ σπληνὶ ἢ ἐν τῇ γαστρὶ ἢ ἐν τοῖς ἐντέροις· τότε γὰρ πάντως συμπάσχει τὸ ἧπαρ, ἢ διὰ τὴν γειτνίασιν, ὥσπερ γαστὴρ καὶ τὰ μεσάραια, ἢ διὰ τὸ τῶν ἀγγείων μέγεθος· ἀξιολόγους γὰρ φλέβας πέμπει ἐπὶ τὰ προειρημένα μόρια διὰ τὴν θρέψιν, καὶ ἐντεῦθεν ἄγεται εἰς συμπάθειαν τούτοις τὸ ἧπαρ. τί γάρ; ὅτι μεταλαμβάνει τῆς δυσκρασίας τὸ ἧπαρ καὶ καταβάλλονται αὐτοῦ αἱ φυσικαὶ δυνάμεις, καὶ μάλιστα ἡ ἀλλοιωτική, καὶ ἀπεπτεῖται τὸ αἷμα καὶ λεπτὸν καὶ ὑδαρὲς γίνεται καὶ ἀτμοειδῶς φέρεται μεταξὺ περιτοναίου καὶ ἐντέρων, καὶ γίνεται ὁ ὕδερος ὁ κατὰ συμπάθειαν τοῦ ἥπατος.

Λοιπὸν σημείωσιν ἡμῖν παραδίδωσι, πόθεν ἔχομεν γνῶναι, εἴτε κατὰ πρωτοπάθειαν εἴτε κατὰ συμπάθειαν τοῦ ἥπατος ἐγένετο ὁ ὕδερος. καί φησιν ὅτι Ὁκόσοισι μὲν τῶν ὑδέρων ἐκ τῶν κενεώνων τε καὶ τῆς ὀσφύος ἄρχονται, οἵ τε πόδες οἰδαίνουσι. καὶ οἱ πόδες οἰδαίνουσι τρόπῳ τοιούτῳ· οἱ πόδες πολὺ ἀφεστήκασι τῆς καρδίας καὶ ἄσαρκοι σχεδόν εἰσιν· ὀστώδεις γάρ εἰσι καὶ δῆλον καὶ ψυχροί. ἀλλὰ καὶ αὐτοῦ τοῦ ἐμφύτου θερμοῦ στερίσκονται· περὶ γὰρ τὰ πεπονθότα μόρια ἐναπασχολεῖται πρὸς ἄμυναν τοῦ λυποῦντος. κἀντεῦθεν στερισκόμενοι τῆς ἀκτινοειδοῦς ἐλλάμψεως τοῦ ἐμφύτου θερμοῦ, καταβάλλονται αἱ ἐν αὐτοῖς φυσικαὶ δυνάμεις, καὶ τὸ τηνικαῦτα τὸ λόγῳ τροφῆς φερόμενον ἐν αὐτοῖς ἀπεπτεῖται καὶ εἰς ἀτμοὺς καὶ εἰς παχέα πνεύματα ἀναλύεται, καὶ οὕτως οἰδαίνουσιν οἱ πόδες. ἢ καὶ ἄλλως· πολλάκις ἰχῶρές τινες ἀπορρέουσιν ἐκ τῆς φλεγμονῆς καὶ παχέα πνεύματα καὶ ὡς κατωφερῆ φέρονται ἐπὶ τοὺς πόδας, καὶ τῷ λόγῳ τούτῳ οἰδαίνουσιν οἱ πόδες. αἱ δὲ χεῖρες οὐκ οἰδαίνουσι, καίτοι καὶ αὐτῶν πόρρω ἀφεστηκυιῶν, καὶ ὀστώδεις εἰσίν, ἀλλὰ καὶ τοῦ ἐμφύτου θερμοῦ ὡσαύτως ἐστέρηνται, διά τε τὴν ὕλην καὶ διὰ τὴν θέσιν· καὶ διὰ μὲν τὴν ὕλην,
135 ἐπειδὴ παχέα εἰσὶ τὰ πνεύματα· λοιπὸν δὲ καὶ | οἱ ἰχῶρες ἐπὶ τὰ κάτω

1 ἀνωτέρω] *cf. supra*, p. 142,7–18

1 ὕδερος *om.* L 2 γίνεται *ante* τοῦ *(lin. 1) trsp.* γ συσταίη *post* ἥπατι *trsp.* γ 3 σκίρος γ ψυχρὴ γ 5 ἀπεπτεῖ *codd.*: *correxi* 6 τὸ αἷμα *om.* L 10 γίνεται *om.* γ 11 ἐν^{II} *om.* γ 12 ἐστὶν *scripsi; cf. infra, p. 150,13*: ὁ L: *om.* γ 16 εἰρημένα γ διὰ τὴν θρέψιν *om.* L; *sed cf. infra, p. 186,12* 17 sq. τί — ἧπαρ *om.* L 21 ὁ^{I} *om.* L 24 ὅτι *om.* γ μὲν *om.* L 25 οἱ — οἰδαίνουσι] οἰδαίνουσι οἱ πόδες γ 27 ἐμφύτου] ἐμφυτευθέντος MV 29 στερισκόμενα L 30 αἱ *om.* L αὐταῖς γ 33 πολλάκις *om.* γ 36 ἀφεστηκότων γ 37 διὰ^{II} *om.* γ 38 οἱ *om.* L

We learned earlier that dropsy as a primary affection of the liver occurs when the affection is in the liver itself, for example, inflammation or induration or tumor or stoppage or any other swelling or a hot or cold distemper; in such cases the natural faculties of the liver are disabled, especially its faculty of conversion; then blood formation fails and the blood is not concocted, but becomes thin and watery; this seeps through in vapor form, is conveyed (to the area) between the peritoneum and the intestines, and dropsy as a primary affection of the liver develops.

Dropsy as a primary affection of the flanks, or, in other words, as a sympathetic affection of the liver, occurs when the affection is in those parts, namely in the flanks and loin. And which are the parts? I will name them: (the condition arises) when there is swelling or inflammation or stoppage in the mesenteries or distemper in the kidneys or spleen or stomach or intestines; in those cases the liver is sure to be affected sympathetically either because of the proximity (of the parts), for example, of the stomach and mesenteries, or because of the magnitude of the vessels; for the liver sends important veins to the parts we have mentioned for the purpose of nourishing, and so it is affected in sympathy with them. Why? Because the liver receives some of the distemper and its natural faculties collapse, particularly that of conversion; coction of the blood does not take place and it becomes thin and watery; it is conveyed in vapor form between the peritoneum and intestines and dropsy as a sympathetic affection of the liver develops.

Next (Hippocrates) gives us symptoms for distinguishing whether the dropsy has arisen as a primary or a sympathetic affection of the liver. He says, In cases where they begin in the flanks and loin, the feet swell. And the feet swell in the following way: the feet are located a long way from the heart and are practically fleshless; for they are bony and obviously cold too. But as well they are deprived of the innate heat itself, since it is fully occupied around the affected parts warding off the offending matter. So, deprived of the innate heat's radiation, their natural faculties are overcome; then the matter conveyed in them in the form of nutriment is not digested, but is dissolved into vapors and dense gases, and in this way the feet swell. Or (it can also be explained) in another way: oftentimes the inflammation gives off certain serous fluids and dense gases; these being heavy travel down to the feet and for this reason the feet swell. The hands, however, are not subject to swelling, despite the fact that they, too, are distant (from the heart), are bony and are likewise deprived of innate heat due to their matter and position; to the matter, because the gases are

βρίθουσιν· ἀλλὰ καὶ διὰ τὴν θέσιν, ὅτι ὑψηλοτέραν θέσιν ἔχουσιν αἱ χεῖρες.

Ἀλλ' ἴσως ἀπορήσει τις λέγων ὅτι «Καὶ ἐπὶ τῇ πρωτοπαθείᾳ τοῦ ἥπατος οἰδαίνουσιν οἱ πόδες καὶ οὐ μόνον ἐπὶ τῶν κενεώνων πασχόντων.» καὶ λέγομεν ὅτι κἂν ἐν τῇ πρωτοπαθείᾳ τοῦ ἥπατος οἰδαίνουσιν οἱ πόδες, τελευταῖον καὶ μετὰ πολὺν χρόνον ἐπὶ τῇ πρωτοπαθείᾳ· ἐπὶ δὲ τῶν κενεώνων εὐθὺς ἐξ ἀρχῆς οἰδαίνουσιν οἱ πόδες ἐπὶ τῇ πρωτοπαθείᾳ τῶν κενεώνων, ἐπειδὴ ἔγγιστά εἰσιν οἱ πεπονθότες τόποι. καὶ διὰ τοῦτο ἑτοίμως μεταλαμβάνουσιν οἱ πόδες καὶ εὐθέως οἰδαίνουσιν. ἐπὶ δὲ τῇ πρωτοπαθείᾳ τοῦ ἥπατος μετὰ χρόνον τινὰ οἰδαίνουσι, διὰ τὸ πόρρω ἀφεστάναι τὸ ἧπαρ ἀπὸ τῶν ποδῶν.

Λέγει καὶ δεύτερον σημεῖον, καί φησιν ὅτι καὶ διάρροιαι πολυχρόνιοι γίνονται αὐτοῖς. καὶ ἡ διάρροια γίνεται αὐτοῖς, ἡνίκα ἢ φλεγμονὴ ἢ ὄγκος τις ἢ ἔμφραξίς ἐστιν ἐν τοῖς μεσαραίοις ἢ ἐν τῇ νήστει [ἢ ἐν τοῖς μεσεντερίοις]· τὸ τηνικαῦτα γὰρ οὐκ ἀνάγεται ὁ χυλὸς εἰς ἧπαρ, καὶ βλάπτεται ἡ ἑλκτικὴ δύναμις, ἀλλὰ καὶ δι' ὧν διοδεύει τόπων ἐμπεφραγμένων ὄντων, ἀνοίγεται ὁ πυλωρός, καὶ ἄγεται ὁ χυλὸς ἐπὶ τὰ ἔντερα καὶ καθυγραίνει τὴν κόπρον, καὶ γίνεται διάρροια. ἢ καὶ ἄλλως διάρροια ἐπιγίνεται αὐτοῖς· ἐξ αὐτῆς πολλάκις τῆς δυσκρασίας φέρονται ἰχῶρές τινες ἐπὶ τὰ ἔντερα καὶ δάκνουσι καὶ ἀνιῶσι, καὶ πρὸ ὥρας ἐπεγειρομένη ἡ ἀποκριτικὴ δύναμις ποιεῖ τὴν διάρροιαν. ἢ καὶ ἄλλως γίνεται αὐτοῖς διάρροια· ἐξ αὐτῆς τῆς δυσκρασίας πολλάκις μεταλαμβάνουσι τὰ ἔντερα, καὶ τὸ τηνικαῦτα κακῶς διατίθενται αἱ ἐν αὐτοῖς φυσικαὶ δυνάμεις, καὶ ἀπεπτεῖται τὸ λόγῳ τροφῆς φερόμενον ἐν αὐτοῖς καὶ φέρεται ἄπεπτον καὶ ποιεῖ τὴν διάρροιαν. αὕτη δὲ ἡ διάρροια εἰς οὐδὲν λυσιτελεῖ τοῖς ὑδεριῶσιν, ὅθεν ἐπιφέρει λέγων ὅτι οὔτε τὰς ὀδύνας λύουσιν οὔτε τὴν γαστέρα λαπάσσουσι, τυχὸν συμπέττουσι. ποίῳ δὲ λόγῳ αἱ ὀδύναι γίνονται; φανερόν ἐστι τῇ δήξει τῆς κακοχυμίας καὶ τῇ τάσει· τὸ γὰρ ὑγρὸν τὸ παρὰ
136 φύσιν | περίτασιν ποιεῖ. ἡ οὖν διάρροια οὐ παύει τὰς ὀδύνας, ἀλλ' οὐδὲ τὴν γαστέρα λαπάττει, ἐπειδὴ οὐ κενοῦται ἐκεῖνο τὸ ὑγρὸν τὸ παρὰ φύσιν τὸ ὂν μεταξὺ περιτοναίου καὶ ἐντέρων καὶ γαστρός, ἀλλ' ἐκεῖνο κενοῦται τὸ χρηστόν, λέγω δὴ ὁ χυλός. ὅθεν σὺν τούτῳ καὶ ὁ ζωτικὸς τόνος συνεκκρίνεται, τὸ δὲ παρὰ φύσιν μένει ἐν οἷς τόποις ἠθροίσθη.

Εἶτα λέγει καὶ τρίτον σημεῖον, ὅτι βὴξ αὐτοῖς πρόσεστιν. ἀλλὰ τοῦτο τὸ σημεῖον κοινόν ἐστιν, ἐπειδὴ καὶ ἐν τῇ πρωτοπαθείᾳ τοῦ ἥπατος βὴξ προσγίνεται. ἀλλὰ διαφέρουσιν ὅτι ἐπὶ τῶν κατὰ πρωτοπάθειαν τοῦ ἥπατος εὐθέως ἐξ ἀρχῆς ἡ βὴξ προσγίνεται αὐτοῖς. τί γάρ; ὅτι ἐπὶ τῆς φλεγμονῆς καὶ τοῦ ὄγκου τοῦ ἐν ἥπατι ὠθεῖται τὸ διάφραγμα καὶ ἀποστενοῦται ὁ θώραξ, ὡς νομίζειν τοὺς οὕτω πάσχοντας ὅτι περιουσία ὕλης

36–152,2] *cf.* Gal. In Hipp. Progn. comm. II 3: CMG V 9,2 pp. 262,21–263,12

2 ἀπορεῖ γ 3 οἱ πόδες *om.* γ 4 *post* κἂν *add.* καὶ L; *cf. supra, pp. 14 sq.* ἐν] ἐπὶ γ 6 *post* εὐθὺς *add.* οἱ PV 6 sq. ἐπὶ – κενεώνων *om.* γ 8 sq. ἐπὶ – οἰδαίνουσι *om.* γ 11 καί[I]] δὲ PV: *om.* M πολυχρόνιαι L 12 ἢ] ἡ L 13 τις *om.* γ 13 sq. ἢ[IV] – μεσεντερίοις *secl. Kollesch* 14 μεσεντέροις L 15 καὶ *om.* L 23 ἐν αὐτοῖς φερόμενον γ 28 sq. ἀλλ' – λαπάττει *om.* γ 34 τὸ *om.* γ ἐν] ἐπὶ γ 35 τῶν] τῷ L 36 sq. τοῦ ὄγκου καὶ τῆς φλεγμονῆς *codd.*: *transposui; cf. infra, p. 152,13*

dense and the serous fluids sink downwards; and to position, because the hands have a higher place.

But someone may object, "The feet swell with a primary affection of the liver as well, and not just when the flanks are affected." We reply that, even though a primary affection of the liver does produce swollen feet, it happens at the end and after a considerable time in the case of primary affection; but in a primary affection of the flanks the feet swell straightaway, since the affected parts are very near. So this is why the condition is readily passed on to the feet and they swell immediately. With a primary affection of the liver, on the other hand, (the feet) swell after some time, because the liver is far distant from the feet.

He gives also a second sign and says, and they have prolonged bouts of diarrhoea. Now diarrhoea develops in them when there is inflammation or a swelling or a stoppage in the mesaraics or in the jejunum; in these circumstances the chyle fails to reach the liver and the attractive faculty is put out of order, and since the parts through which (the chyle) passes are blocked, the pylorus opens, the chyle enters the intestines soaking the feces, and diarrhoea results. Or they can get diarrhoea in another way also: frequently certain serous fluids from the distemper itself are conveyed to the intestines and cause stinging and irritation, and the excretory faculty, prematurely activated, produces diarrhoea. Or diarrhoea develops in them for another reason: oftentimes the intestines receive part of the distemper itself; the natural faculties there are then poorly disposed and the matter conveyed to them in the form of nutriment is not digested and is carried along unconcocted and produces diarrhoea. Such diarrhoea, however, in no way benefits dropsy subjects, which is why he goes on to say, they neither get rid of the pains nor soften the bowels; (by soften) he means promote concoction. For what reason do the pains occur? Obviously because of the stinging and strain of the unwholesome humors; for the abnormal fluid causes distension. The diarrhoea, then, does not stop the pains, nor does it soften the bowels, since that abnormal fluid between the peritoneum, intestines and stomach is not evacuated; however, that useful fluid, namely the chyle, is passed off. And hence the vital tone is evacuated along with it, but the abnormal stays in the places where it has accumulated.

Then he gives a third symptom, that coughing occurs in these cases. But this sign is common (to both types), since coughing is present as well when the liver is primarily affected. However, there is a difference in that, when there is a primary affection of the liver, coughing develops in them right at the outset. Why? Because the inflammation and swelling of the liver push the diaphragm and the thorax is contracted, so that those affected in this way think that there is a superabundance of

ἐστί, καὶ ὑπ' αὐτῆς ἐνδελεχοῦνται καὶ βήττουσι, προσδοκῶντες ἀπαλλαγῆναι τῆς τοιαύτης ἐνδελεχείας. καὶ οὐδὲν ὠφελοῦσι, μηδὲν ἀναπτύοντες ἀξιόλογον, ὡς αὐτὸς παρακατιών φησιν. ἐπὶ δὲ τῇ πρωτοπαθείᾳ τῶν κενεώνων τελευταῖον ἐπιγίνεται αὐτοῖς ἡ βήξ, ὅπερ κάκιστόν ἐστι σημεῖον ἐσχάτης ἀπογνώσεως· δηλοῖ γὰρ ὅτι τοσοῦτον ἐπλημμύρησεν ἡ παρὰ φύσιν ὑγρότης κατὰ ποσότητα, ὅτι οὐκ ἀρκεῖται στεχθῆναι μεταξὺ περιτοναίου καὶ ἐντέρων καὶ γαστρός, ἀλλὰ λοιπὸν καὶ ἐπὶ τὰ ἀναπνευστικὰ ἐχώρησε κἀκείνων λοιπὸν ἐπιλαμβάνεται, ὅπερ ἐσχάτης ἐστὶν ἀπογνώσεως τὸ σημεῖον τοῦτο.

Οὕτως σημειωσάμενος τὸν κατὰ πρωτοπάθειαν τῶν κενεώνων γινόμενον ὕδερον, νῦν σημειοῦται καὶ τὸν ἐπὶ πρωτοπαθείᾳ τοῦ ἥπατος γινόμενον ὕδερον. καί φησιν ὅτι βὴξ ἐξ ἀρχῆς αὐτοῖς προσγίνεται τῷ λόγῳ τῆς φλεγμονῆς τοῦ ἥπατος· ὑπὸ γὰρ τῆς φλεγμονῆς καὶ τοῦ ὄγκου τοῦ ὄντος ἐν ἥπατι ὠθεῖται τὸ διάφραγμα καὶ κατασπᾶται, καὶ ἀποστενοῦται ὁ θώραξ καὶ ὁ πνεύμων καὶ ἡ τραχεῖα ἀρτηρία, καὶ ὡς ἐν στενοχωρίᾳ 137 τυγχάνοντα, προσκρούει | τὸ πνεῦμα καὶ ποιεῖ ἦχον, καὶ οὕτως βήττουσι. διὰ τοῦτο οὖν βήττουσιν εὐθέως κατ' ἀρχὰς μὴ ἀναφέροντες ἀξιόλογόν τι, εἰ μή τι τῶν εὑρισκομένων σιέλων. καὶ διὰ τοῦτο οὐκ ἀναφέρουσιν, ἐπειδὴ οὐκ ἔστιν ἐν τοῖς ἀναπνευστικοῖς ἡ ὕλη, ἀλλ' ἐν τοῖς θρεπτικοῖς.

Δεύτερον σημεῖον, ἡ κοιλία αὐτῶν ξηραίνεται διὰ τὴν ζέσιν τῆς φλεγμονῆς τῆς ἐν ἥπατι ἐξαναλισκούσης τὴν ἰκμάδα τὴν ἐν γαστρί, καὶ ἐξ ἀνάγκης ξηραίνεται ἡ κόπρος, καὶ οὐκ ἀποπατοῦσι. κἂν γὰρ περιουσία ὑγροῦ ἐστιν, οὐκ ἐν τῷ κύτει τῆς γαστρὸς περιέχεται, ἀλλ' ἐν τοῖς μεταξὺ χωρίοις περιτοναίου καὶ ἐντέρων.

Τρίτον σημεῖον, ὅτι καὶ ἐπὶ τούτων οἱ πόδες οἰδίσκουσι. καὶ κατὰ τὸν αὐτὸν τρόπον καὶ ἐνταῦθα οἰδαίνουσι, καθ' ὃν τρόπον καὶ ἐπὶ τῇ πρωτοπαθείᾳ τῶν κενεώνων, ὡς ἤδη εἴρηται. πλὴν ἐπὶ τούτων καὶ αἱ χεῖρες καὶ τὸ δέρμα τοῦ παντὸς σώματος οἰδαίνουσι. καὶ τίνι λόγῳ ταῦτα οἰδαίνουσιν; ἐπεὶ ἀποτυχία ἐστὶ τῆς ἐξαιματώσεως, λεπτὸν καὶ ὑδαρές ἐστι τὸ αἷμα, ἐξ οὗ τρέφονται, καὶ ἐντεῦθεν οἰδαίνουσιν.

Τέταρτον σημεῖόν ἐστιν, ὅτι ἐπάρματά τινα γίνονται αὐτοῖς ἐν τοῖς δεξιοῖς καὶ ἐν τοῖς ἀριστεροῖς, γινόμενα καὶ πάλιν παυόμενα· τελευταῖον μέντοι γίνονται μέν, οὐ παύονται δέ, ἀλλὰ μένουσι. γίνονται δὲ τὰ ἐπάρματα ὑπὸ ὑγρότητός τινος καὶ ὑπὸ πνευμάτων πολλῶν. καὶ τίνι λόγῳ κατ' ἀρχὰς μὲν γίνονται καὶ παύονται, τελευταῖον δὲ γίνονται μέν, οὐ παύονται δέ; τοῦτο πρὸς τὸ ἔμφυτον θερμόν· κατ' ἀρχὰς ἐρρωμενέστερόν ἐστι, κἂν ἔπαθέ τι, καὶ ἡνίκα γένωνται τὰ ἐπάρματα ταῦτα, τὸ ἔμφυτον θερμὸν διαφορεῖ αὐτά. τελευταῖον μέντοι, ἐπειδὴ ἀδρανέστερόν ἐστι τὸ ἔμφυτον

3 αὐτὸς – φησιν] Hipp. Progn. 8: p. 204,5 A. = II p. 132,2 L. (*infra*, p. 156,22 sq.) 27 εἴρηται] *cf. supra*, p. 148,24–32

1 προσδοκοῦντες L 3 φησιν] ἐρεῖ γ 4 τελευταία γ γίνεται γ 6 τεχθῆναι L: στερχθῆναι γ: *corr. Dietz* 8 ἐστὶν *post* ἀπογνώσεως *trsp.* γ 12 ὕδερον *om.* γ 15 καὶ^{III} *om.* L 16 ἀναβήττουσι γ 18 σιάλων γ 21 *post* ἐν^{II} *add.* τῇ L; *cf. supra, pp. 14 sq.* 22 ἀποπατοῦται γ 23 *post* ἐν^{II} *add.* τῷ L 25 οἰδίσκουσι *om.* L 26 ἐπὶ] ἐν γ 27 ὡς *om.* L 30 οὗ] ὧν *codd.*: *correxi* 34 τινος] πολλῆς γ 38 ἐστι *om.* L 38–154,1 ἔμφυτον θερμόν] ἐμφυτευθὲν γ

matter, and, being bothered by it, they cough in the hope of getting rid of this nuisance. But they are of no help to themselves, for, as he goes on to tell us, they fail to get up anything appreciable. In a primary affection of the flanks, on the other hand, coughing develops in them at the end; this is a very bad sign meaning complete hopelessness; for it shows that the abnormal fluid has been so excessive in quantity that it could not be contained between the peritoneum, the intestines and the stomach, but eventually reached even the respiratory system and took over those parts; and this is a sign of complete hopelessness.

Having thus given us the symptoms for dropsy which has resulted from a primary affection of the flanks, he now does the same also for dropsy from a primary affection of the liver. He says that coughing develops at the start in these cases because of the inflammation of the liver; for the diaphragm is forced and compressed by the inflammation and the swelling in the liver, and the thorax, lungs and trachea are compressed; and being in a confined space they collide with the air and produce a noise, and thus the patients cough. This is why they cough right from the start without bringing up anything worth talking about, apart from some saliva which is encountered. And the reason why they fail to expectorate is that the matter is not in the respiratory, but in the digestive, parts.

The second symptom is that their bowels are dried up on account of the seething heat of the inflammation in the liver which consumes the stomach's moisture; the feces necessarily become dry and are not passed off. For, even if there is a surplus of fluid, it is not contained in the hollow of the stomach, but in the areas between the peritoneum and intestines.

The third symptom is that in these cases also the feet swell. And they swell here for the very same reason as in a primary affection of the flanks, which we have already described. However, here the hands as well and the skin of the entire body swell. For what reason do these swell? Since blood formation fails, these areas are nourished by thin and watery blood, and hence they swell.

The fourth symptom is that they develop swellings both on the right and left hand sides (of the belly) which come and go away again; eventually, however, they come to stay and do not disappear. The swellings are caused by a certain fluid and many vapors. Now, why do they appear and disappear in the beginning, but eventually come and do not disappear? This is determined by the innate heat; at the outset the innate heat is more powerful, even if it is somewhat affected, and it is able to dissipate these swellings when they appear. In the end, however, since it has become weaker, there is almost a danger that the innate

θερμόν, σχεδὸν κίνδυνός ἐστιν καὶ τοῦ ἀποσβεσθῆναι αὐτό· καὶ γίνονται μὲν τὰ ἐπάρματα, οὐ παύονται δέ, ἐπειδὴ οὐκ ἰσχύει τὸ ἔμφυτον θερμὸν αὐτὰ διαφορῆσαι. πλὴν καὶ ἐπὶ τῶν κατὰ πρωτοπάθειαν τῶν κενεώνων γίνονται
138 τὰ ἐπάρματα ταῦτα, ἀλλ' οὐ παύονται. ἀλλὰ | καὶ ἄλλως διαφέρουσιν, ὅτι ἐπὶ τῶν κατὰ πρωτοπάθειαν τοῦ ἥπατος εἴκουσι τῇ ἁφῇ καὶ κοιλαίνονται, ἐπὶ δὲ τῶν κατὰ πρωτοπάθειαν τῶν κενεώνων τὰ ἐπάρματα οὐκ εἴκουσι τῇ ἁφῇ, ἀλλ' ἀντίτυπα μένουσιν ὡς ἐπὶ λίθου. καὶ τίνι λόγῳ ταῦτα γίνονται; λέγομεν ὅτι ἐν μὲν τῇ πρωτοπαθείᾳ τοῦ ἥπατος τὰ ἐπάρματα ὑπὸ φλεγματικωτέρας ὕλης γίνονται· ἡ δὲ τοιαύτη ὕλη μαλακή ἐστι, καὶ διὰ τοῦτο εἴκουσι τῇ ἁφῇ καὶ κοιλαίνονται· ἐπὶ δὲ τῇ πρωτοπαθείᾳ τῶν κενεώνων οὐκ εἴκουσι τὰ ἐπάρματα τῇ ἁφῇ, ἐπειδὴ ὑπὸ παχέων πνευμάτων γίνονται· τὰ δὲ παχέα πνεύματα τὰ ἐνισχόμενα οὐκ εἴκουσι τῇ ἁφῇ, δίκην ἀσκοῦ ἀκριβῶς πεφυσημένου.

Δεύτερόν ἐστι κεφάλαιον, ἐν ᾧ καὶ ἕτερα σημεῖα ἡμῖν παραδίδωσι, μὴ μόνον ἐπὶ τῶν ὑδεριώντων θεωρούμενα, ἀλλὰ καὶ ἐπὶ ἑτέρων ὀξέων νοσημάτων. ὧν πρῶτόν γε σημεῖον λέγει τοιοῦτον, ὅτι κάκιστόν ἐστιν ἐπὶ τῶν ὀξέων νοσημάτων τὸ κατεψυγμένα ἔχειν τὰ ἄκρα, κεφαλὴν λέγω καὶ χεῖρας καὶ πόδας, τὴν δὲ κοιλίαν καὶ τὰς πλευρὰς καὶ τὰ σπλάγχνα καὶ τὸν θώρακα θερμὰ ἔχειν καὶ διακαίεσθαι· δηλοῖ γὰρ ἢ μεγάλην φλεγμονὴν ἢ ἐπιτεταμένην ὀδύνην ἢ καὶ ἀμφότερα. ἐπὶ γὰρ τῇ φλεγμονῇ καὶ τῇ ὀδύνῃ τῶν σπλάγχνων ὀλίγον αἷμα φέρεται ἐπὶ τὸ πᾶν σῶμα πρὸς ἀποτροφὴν τῶν μορίων· τὸ δὲ πλεῖστον τοῦ αἵματος φέρεται, ἔνθα ἡ φλεγμονὴ καὶ ἡ ὀδύνη, καὶ ἐκεῖσε συρρεῖ. καὶ διὰ τοῦτο τὰ μὲν ἄκρα ψύχονται· ἔνθα δέ ἐστιν ἡ φλεγμονή, τυχὸν ἐν τοῖς σπλάγχνοις, διὰ τοῦτο διακαίονται. ἀγαθὸν δέ ἐστι σημεῖον καὶ ἄριστον τὸ ὁμαλῶς καὶ ὁμοτίμως θερμὸν εἶναι τὸ πᾶν σῶμα καὶ μαλθακόν· δηλοῖ γὰρ ὅτι οὐκ ἔστι φλεγμονὴ ἢ ὀδύνη, ἀλλ' οὐδὲ ὀξὺς πυρετός· ἐπὶ γὰρ τοῦ ὀξέος πυρετοῦ, κἂν ὁμοτίμως θερμὸν γίνηται τὸ πᾶν σῶμα, ἀλλ' ὅμως ἐκείνη ἡ θερμότης οὐκ ἔστι μαλθακή, ἀλλὰ κατάξηρος καὶ ἐπιτεταμένη.

Δεύτερον σημεῖον, κακόν ἐστιν ἐπὶ τῶν ὀξέων νοσημάτων τὸ δυσκι-
139 νήτως ἔχειν ἐν τῷ στρέφεσθαι καὶ συστέλ|λειν τὰ μόρια, πόδας λέγω καὶ χεῖρας, καὶ ἐν τῷ μετεωρίζεσθαι, τυχὸν ἐν τῷ ἀνακαθέζεσθαι· δηλοῖ γὰρ ἐσχάτην ἀσθένειαν τῆς συνεκτικῆς δυνάμεως τῆς ἐν ἑκάστῳ μορίῳ συνεχούσης καὶ στηριζούσης τὸ σῶμα· ταύτης γὰρ ἀσθενούσης οὐκ ἀντέχεται τὸ σῶμα, ἀλλὰ τῷ βάρει δυσκινητεῖ. ἢ τοῦτο, ὅτι ἡ δυσκινησία γίνεται ἀσθενούσης τῆς ψυχικῆς δυνάμεως, ἐν ᾗ κατὰ προαίρεσιν κινοῦνται τὰ μόρια· ταύτης γὰρ ἀσθενούσης οὐ κινοῦνται κατὰ προαίρεσιν, ὅπερ κά-

16 λέγει] Hipp. Progn. 9: p. 204,9sq. A. = II p. 132,6sq. L. 20–24] *cf.* Gal. In Hipp. Progn. comm. II 4: CMG V 9,2 pp. 264,23–265,11 24–29] *cf.* Gal. In Hipp. Progn. comm. II 5: CMG V 9,2 p. 265,16–21

1 *post* σχεδὸν *add.* καὶ MP, δὲ V καὶ τοῦ *om.* L καὶ[II] *om.* γ 2 αὐτὸ γ 4 ἀλλ'] καὶ γ 5 *post* ὅτι *add.* καὶ L ἥκουσι γ 6 τὰ ἐπάρματα *om.* γ 7 ἀντίτυποι γ 8 ὅτι *om.* L ἐν] ἐπὶ γ 12 τὰ[II] *om.* γ 15sq. ἕτερα ὀξέα νοσήματα L 16 γε *om.* γ κακόν γ 18 καὶ τὰς πλευρὰς *om.* γ 27 ὀξέος] ὀξέου γ γίνεται γ 32 ἀνακαθίζεσθαι γ 34 οὐ κατέχεται MP *(deest* V*)* 35 *post* τοῦτο *add.* ἡ γ 36 τῆς *om.* γ ᾗ] ᾧ *codd.*: *correxi*

heat will be extinguished altogether; and the swellings appear but do not go away, since the innate heat is not powerful enough to dissipate them. In cases of primary affection of the flanks, on the other hand, while these swellings develop, they do not go away. And there is also the other difference that, in primary affections of the liver, the swellings yield to pressure and become dented, while, in primary affections of the flanks they do not give way to pressure, but remain rigid like a stone. Why does this happen? We say that in a primary affection of the liver the swellings are produced by rather phlegmatic matter; this matter is soft, hence (the swellings) yield to pressure and dent; but in a primary affection of the flanks the swellings do not give way to pressure, since they are produced by dense vapors; and dense vapors which are held in (tight) do not yield to pressure, just as in the case of a bag that has been blown up hard.

In the second chapter (of this section) he presents to us other symptoms which can be observed not only in dropsies, but in other acute diseases as well. The first he gives is that it is a very bad sign in acute diseases when the extremities, namely the head, hands and feet, are cold, while the belly, sides, viscera and thorax are hot and burning; for it indicates either severe inflammation or intense pain or even both. For when there is inflammation and pain in the viscera, little blood gets around the rest of the body to nourish the parts; but most of the blood goes to the site of the inflammation and pain and circulates there. Hence the extremities, on the one hand, turn cold; but the parts with inflammation, e.g. the viscera, become hot for this reason. And it is a good and excellent symptom when the entire body is evenly and equally hot and soft; for it indicates the absence of inflammation or pain and also of acute fever; for in acute fever, even though the whole body becomes equally warm, nevertheless that heat is not softening but very dry and intense.

The second symptom is that in acute diseases it is bad if the patient has difficulty in turning and gathering together the parts, I mean the legs and arms, and in raising himself, that is, in sitting up; for it means extreme weakness of the sustaining faculty which holds together and supports the body in each of its parts; for when this is weak, the body cannot support itself, but is hampered in movement by its own weight. Alternatively (you could say) this, that the difficulty in movement is caused by weakness of the psychic faculty which controls the voluntary motion of the parts; for when this (faculty) loses power, they do not move in response to the will, which is a very bad sign, since it means

κιστόν ἐστιν, ἐπειδὴ μεγάλην βλάβην ἐνδείκνυται τῆς ἀρχῆς τῶν νεύρων, λέγω δὴ τοῦ ἐγκεφάλου, καὶ αὐτῶν τῶν νεύρων.

Τρίτον σημεῖον, κακόν ἐστι τὸ πελιδνοῦσθαι ἢ μελαίνεσθαι τὰ ἄκρα ἐπὶ τῶν ὀξέων νοσημάτων· δηλοῖ γὰρ ἢ μεγίστην ὀδύνην ἢ θάνατον· ἐπὶ γὰρ τοῦ θανάτου ἐλάχιστος πυρετὸς περὶ τὰ σπλάγχνα τὸ τέως ἐμφωλεύει ἐκ τοῦ ἐμφύτου θερμοῦ, καὶ ὡς ἐπὶ τὰ ἐκεῖ λοιπὸν καὶ τὰ μόρια συντρέχουσι καὶ δοκοῦσιν ἀνασπᾶσθαι, προσδοκῶντα τυχεῖν τῆς ἑαυτῶν σωτηρίας. ἀλλὰ καὶ ἐπὶ τῶν ὀδυνῶν τῶν ἐπιτεταμένων, ὡς ἐπὶ κωλικῆς διαθέσεως καὶ τῶν νεφριτικῶν καὶ τῶν τοιούτων, τὰ μόρια συντρέχουσιν ὡς ἐπὶ τὸ ὀδυνώμενον μόριον, διὰ τὸ καὶ τὴν φύσιν ἐκεῖσε συννεύειν καὶ συντρέχειν.

II 5 [8: 203,10 A. = II 130,15 L.] Ὁκόσοισι μὲν οὖν τῶν ὑδέρων ἐκ τῶν κενεώνων τε καὶ τῆς ὀσφύος

Κενεῶνας εἴωθε καλεῖν ὁ Ἱπποκράτης ἐκεῖνο τὸ χωρίον τὸ ἀπὸ τῆς ἐσχάτης πλευρᾶς μέχρι τοῦ ὀστοῦ τῆς λαγόνος, ἐπειδὴ κενότερον δοκεῖ εἶναι ὡς πρὸς τὰ ὑπερκείμενά τε καὶ ὑποκείμενα. ὡς δὲ τῷ Γαληνῷ δοκεῖ, ἐν τούτοις τοῖς κενεῶσι περιέχεται ἡ νῆστις, αἱ μεσαραϊκαὶ φλέβες καὶ οἱ νεφροί. τούτων οὖν φλεγμαινόντων ἢ καὶ ἑνὸς ἢ καὶ δύο, ἔστιν ὅτε δὲ καὶ ὅλων, μεταλαμβάνει τῆς κακίας τὸ ἧπαρ καὶ βλάπτεται ἡ ἀλλοιωτικὴ δύναμις αὐτοῦ· καὶ ἐντεῦθεν ἀποτυγχάνει ἡ ἐξαιμάτωσις, καὶ γίνεται ὕδερος ὁ κατὰ πρωτοπάθειαν μὲν τῶν κενεώνων, κατὰ συμπάθειαν δὲ τοῦ ἥπατος. |

140 **II 6** [8: 204,4 A.=II 132,1 L.] Βῆξαί τε θυμὸς γίνεται αὐτέοισι καὶ ἀποπτύουσιν οὐδὲν ἄξιον λόγου

Θυμὸν ἐνταῦθα ἀκουστέον τὴν ἐπιθυμίαν. τί γάρ; ὅτι οἱ κατὰ πρωτοπάθειαν τοῦ ἥπατος ὑδεριῶντες, ὠθούμενον τὸ διάφραγμα ὑπὸ τῆς φλεγμονῆς τοῦ ἥπατος, στενοχωρεῖται ὁ πνεύμων καὶ ἐπιθυμοῦσι βήττειν· οὐδὲν δὲ ἀναφέρουσι βήττοντες, ἐπειδὴ οὐκ ἔστιν ἡ ὕλη ἐν τοῖς ἀναπνευστικοῖς, ἀλλ' ἐν ἄλλοις μορίοις, λέγω δὴ καὶ ἐν τοῖς θρεπτικοῖς καὶ ἐν τῷ ὑμένι τῷ περικειμένῳ τῷ ἥπατι· καὶ ἐκεῖσε σφηνοῦται, καὶ βήττοντες οὐδὲν ἀναπτύουσιν ἄξιον λόγου. ὀλίγιστον δὲ ὑγρὸν ἀναφέρουσιν· οὐδὲ γὰρ πάντῃ ἀμοιροῦσιν ὑγρότητος τὰ ἀναπνευστικὰ μόρια, ἀλλὰ περιγράφεται λεπτὸν πάντως ὑγρὸν καὶ ἐν τῷ θώρακι καὶ ἐν τῷ πνεύμονι καὶ ἐν τῇ τραχείᾳ ἀρτηρίᾳ. βήττοντες οὖν, ἐκ τούτων τῶν μορίων ὑγρὸν λεπτὸν μεθίεται ὀλίγιστον, καὶ τοῦτο ἀποπτύουσιν, οὐ μὴν ἐκ τῆς ὕλης, ἐπειδὴ ἐν ἄλλοις μορίοις ἐστὶν ἐσφηνωμένη.

14–18] Gal. In Hipp. Progn. comm. II 1: CMG V 9,2 p. 260,11–17 *cf. supra*, p. 140,10–14 24–26] *cf.* Gal. In Hipp. Progn. comm. II 3: CMG V 9,2 p. 262,19–22 30–32] *cf.* Gal. In Hipp. Progn. comm. II 3: CMG V 9,2 p. 263,11–13

3 πελιοῦσθαι γ 5 ἐλάχιστον PV τὸ] τῶ γ 7 προσδοκοῦντα *codd.*: *correxi (cf. supra, p. 152,1)* 8 ἀλλὰ – 11 συντρέχειν *om.* L 12 οὖν *om.* γ ὑδέρων] ὑδρώπων *Hipp.* 13 ὀσφύος *om.* L 16 τε *om.* γ 17 φλέβαι γ 18 νεφροί *om.* γ ¦(*spat. vac. in* PV) καὶ^{I} *om.* γ ὅτε *om.* γ 20 ὕδερος *post* μὲν (*lin.* 21) *trsp.* γ 22 ἐγγίνεται γ 27 δὲ] γὰρ γ 28 καὶ^{I} *om.* γ θρεπτικοῖς] ἀναπνευστικοῖς L 34 ἐστὶ μορίοις γ

serious damage in the nerve source, that is the brain, and in the nerves themselves.

The third symptom is that in acute diseases it is bad if the extremities turn livid or black; for it means either very severe pain or death; you see, in the case of death, at the beginning there is a tiny amount of fever from the innate heat lurking around the viscera; so the parts too shrink and seem to pull themselves towards that area in the hope of finding their salvation. And in the case of intense pains too, such as the colic, nephritis and so on, the parts contract towards the pained part, because nature also converges on and musters at that spot.

II 5 In those dropsies, then, which (begin) in the flanks and loin

Flanks (*keneōnes*) is the usual term in Hippocrates for the area between the last rib and the iliac bone, since it appears to be emptier (*kenoteron*) than the parts above and below. But as Galen sees it, these flanks contain the jejunum, the mesaraic veins and the kidneys. When one of these, then, becomes inflamed, or two or, as sometimes happens, even all (three), the liver contracts the malady and its converting faculty is damaged; whereupon blood formation fails, and dropsy as a primary affection of the flanks and a sympathetic affection of the liver develops.

II 6 They have a mind to cough, but get up nothing worth speaking of

By mind here we should understand desire. Why (does this happen)? Because in those who have dropsy from a primary affection of the liver the diaphragm is pushed up by the inflammation of the liver and the lungs are compressed, so they desire to cough; but in coughing they do not bring up anything, since the matter is not in the respiratory parts, but elsewhere, namely in the digestive parts and in the membrane surrounding the liver; it is wedged in there and by coughing they spit up nothing worth mention. However, they do bring up a very small quantity of fluid; for the respiratory parts are not entirely devoid of moisture, but the thorax, lungs and trachea contain a very thin fluid. In coughing, then, a trace of thin fluid is discharged from these parts and this they bring up, but not indeed from the (morbid) matter, seeing that it is lodged in other parts.

II 7 [9: 204,9 A.=II 132,6 L.] Κεφαλὴ δὲ καὶ χεῖρες καὶ πόδες ψυχρὰ ἐόντα κακὸν τῆς τε κοιλίας καὶ τῶν πλευρῶν

Ἀποροῦσιν ὅτι «Οὐκ ἔστι τοῦτο ἀληθές, οὐδὲ πάντως κακόν ἐστι τὸ τὰ ἄκρα ψύχεσθαι· ἐνδέχεται γὰρ ψύχεσθαι τὰ ἄκρα καὶ ἐν χειμῶνι καὶ ἐν γεροντικῇ ἡλικίᾳ, ἀλλὰ καὶ ἐν ταῖς εἰσβολαῖς τῶν παροξυσμῶν. εἰ δὲ χρόνιον νόσημα, λειφαιμοῦντα τὰ ἄκρα καταψύχονται, καὶ οὐκ ἔστι κακὸν ἢ ἐπικίνδυνον. πῶς οὖν ἔφη ὁ Ἱπποκράτης ὅτι κακόν ἐστι τὸ ψύχεσθαι τὰ ἄκρα;» πρὸς ὃ ἀπολογούμεθα ὅτι ὁ Ἱπποκράτης ἐνταῦθα περὶ ὀξέος νοσήματος ἐξετάζων ἐκάκισε τὸ τὰ ἄκρα ψύχεσθαι. τί γάρ; ὅτι ὀξὺ νόσημα ὑπέθετο καὶ διακαῆ πυρετὸν καὶ φλογώδη ζέσιν· καὶ ἐὰν τούτων ὑποκειμένων ψυχρὰ ἔσονται τὰ ἄκρα, πῶς οὐκ ἔσται κακόν; δηλοῖ γὰρ ἀσθένειαν καὶ καταβολὴν τοῦ ἐμφύτου θερμοῦ καὶ ἧτταν τῆς φύσεως· καὶ πῶς οὐκ ἔστι κακὸν τὸ τοιοῦτον; |

141 **II 8** [9: 204,12 A.=II 132,8 L.] Στρέφεσθαι δὲ χρὴ ῥηϊδίως τὸν νοσέοντα καὶ ἐν τοῖσι μετεωρισμοῖσιν ἐλαφρὸν εἶναι.

Μετεωρισμὸν καλεῖ ὁ Ἱπποκράτης τὴν ἀβίαστον κίνησιν, ἵνα ἀβιάστως ἀνακαθέζηται ὁ νοσέων καὶ στρέφηται. τί γάρ; δηλοῖ ῥώμην καὶ ἰσχὺν τῆς κινητικῆς δυνάμεως καὶ αὐτῆς τῆς ἀρχῆς, λέγω δὴ τοῦ ἐγκεφάλου. οἱ γὰρ περὶ Διοκλέα, ἡ κίνησις διττή ἐστιν, ἐκ φέροντος καὶ φερομένου. καὶ φέρον μὲν ἐκάλουν τὴν δύναμιν τὴν κινητικήν, φερόμενον δὲ τὸ σῶμα· ὑπὸ γὰρ τῆς δυνάμεως φέρεται τὸ σῶμα, ἐπεί τοί γε ὅσον πρὸς ἑαυτὸ τὸ σῶμα βαρύ ἐστι καὶ βριθον.

II 9 [9: 204,13 A.=II 132,10 L.] Καὶ τὸ ὅλον σῶμα καὶ τὰς χεῖρας καὶ τοὺς πόδας, ἐπικινδυνότερον

Ἀποροῦσιν ὅτι «Εἰπὼν καὶ τὸ ὅλον σῶμα, τί δήποτε ἐπήγαγε καὶ τὰς χεῖρας καὶ τοὺς πόδας καὶ ἰδίᾳ καὶ χωρὶς εἶπεν; τί γὰρ οὐκ ἠδύνατο εἰπεῖν καὶ τὸ ὅλον σῶμα, ἀλλ' ἰδίᾳ καὶ χωρὶς ἔφη αὐτά;» πρὸς οὓς λέγομεν ὅτι κατ' ἐξοχὴν τοῦτο πεποίηκεν· ἐπειδὴ γὰρ μάλιστα ἐν τούτοις τοῖς μορίοις, χεῖρας λέγω καὶ πόδας, διαφαίνεται τὸ ἐπικινδυνότερον σημεῖον καὶ ἡ κακία τοῦ πάθους ἐν αὐτοῖς θεωρεῖται, καὶ διὰ τοῦτο κατ' ἐξοχὴν ἐμνημόνευσεν αὐτῶν.

II 10 [9: 205,2 A.=II 132,13 L.] Μελαινόμενοι δὲ παντελῶς οἱ δάκτυλοι ἢ οἱ πόδες ἧσσον ὀλέθριοι τῶν πελιδνῶν.

4–6 ἐπικίνδυνον] *cf.* Gal. In Hipp. Progn. comm. II 4: CMG V 9,2 p. 264,14–18 19 οἱ – Διοκλέα] Gal. In Hipp. Progn. comm. II 6: CMG V 9,2 p. 267,1–8 ἡ – 20] *cf.* Steph. Comm. in Hipp. Aph.: Ambros. S 19 sup. fol. 8ᵛ

2 τῆς – πλευρῶν *om.* γ 4 ψύχεσθαι[I] – ἄκρα *om.* γ 5 παροξυνόντων γ 6 λειφαιμοῦνται γ 8 ἀπολογούμεθα] λέγομεν L ὀξέων νοσημάτων γ 14 δὲ *om.* γ ῥηϊδίως *om.* L 15 νοσοῦντα L τοῖς L ἐλαφρὸν εἶναι *om.* γ 17 στρέφεται PV: στρέφεσθαι M 17 sq. ἰσχὺν καὶ ῥώμην γ 19 οἱ] *cf. infra, pp. 188,34 sq.; 210,10* 20 sq. ὑπὸ – σῶμα[I] *om.* γ 23 ὅλον] ἄλλο *codd. Hipp. praeter* X (σῶμα πᾶν) 26 εἶπεν *scripsi*: εἰπεῖν *codd.* 33 ἢ οἱ πόδες *om.* γ

II 7 It is a bad sign if the head, hands and feet are cold, while the belly and sides

The objection is raised that "This is not true, nor is it necessarily a bad symptom if the extremities are cold; for the extremities can become cold in the winter and in old age and also with the onset of paroxysms. And if the disease is a chronic one, the extremities grow cold from lack of blood, which is not bad or dangerous. Why did Hippocrates, then, say that it is bad if the extremities are cold?" To this we answer that Hippocrates here disapproves of cold extremities in the context of acute disease. Why? Because he has proposed to discuss acute disease attended by burning fever and fiery-hot seething; and if, in these circumstances, the extremities turn cold, how can it fail to be a dangerous symptom? For it means that the innate heat has become weak and has collapsed and that nature has been defeated; how could this not be bad?

II 8 The patient ought to turn easily and be light when raising himself up.

By raising up Hippocrates means unforced movement, by which the patient can sit up and turn without straining. Why? Because it shows that the kinetic faculty is strong and vigorous and also the principal part itself, namely the brain. For according to the school of Diocles movement consists of two elements, a carrier and a carried. The kinetic faculty they designated as the carrier and the body as the carried; for it is the faculty which conveys the body, seeing that by itself the body is heavy and pulls downward.

II 9 The whole body and the hands and feet, it is fairly dangerous

The question is raised, "After saying the whole body why did he go on to mention and the hands and feet apart and separately? Why could he not say the whole body, but mentions these on their own?" Our answer is that he does it to highlight them, since it is particularly in these parts, the hands and feet, that the rather dangerous symptom manifests itself and the malignancy of the affection is observed; this is why he gives them prominent mention.

II 10 But if the fingers or the feet turn completely black, they are less deadly than the livid.

Ἡ μέλανσις ἐπίτασίς ἐστι τῆς πελιδνώσεως· πρότερον πελιδνοῦνται καὶ οὕτως μελαίνονται. καὶ ἀποροῦσί τινες ὅτι «Ἐὰν ἡ μέλανσις ἐπίτασίς ἐστι τῆς πελιδνώσεως, πῶς ἔφη ὁ Ἱπποκράτης καὶ οἱ δάκτυλοι πελιδνούμενοι, προσδόκιμος ὁ θάνατος, μελαινόμενοι δὲ παντελῶς οἱ δάκτυλοι καὶ οἱ πόδες, ἧσσον ὀλέθριοι τῶν πελιδνῶν;» καὶ λέγομεν ὅτι ἡ μέλανσις διττή ἐστιν, ἡ μὲν κατὰ ἐπίτασιν τῆς πελιδνώσεως γίνεται, ἡ δὲ οὐχί. καὶ εἰ μὲν κατ' ἐπίτασιν, ἐνδείκνυται μεγίστην σηπεδόνα, ἥτις κα-
142 κίστη ἐστί. γίνεται μέλανσις καὶ κριτικῶς, ἡνίκα ὀξέος ὑποκειμένου νοσή|ματος ἐπεγερθῇ ἡ φύσις κριτικῶς καὶ ἀπορρίψῃ τὴν ὕλην ἐπὶ τὰ ἄκρα· καὶ ἐκεῖνα μὲν μελαίνονται, ἔστι δ' ὅτε καὶ ἀποπίπτουσιν ὑπὸ τῆς ἐκριφείσης κακοχυμίας, ὁ δὲ ἄνθρωπος περισῴζεται τοῦ κινδύνου καὶ ἐλευθεροῦται. ὁ οὖν Ἱπποκράτης ταύτην τὴν μέλανσιν ἐνταῦθα ἐκάλεσεν ἧσσον ὀλέθριον τῶν πελιδνῶν. ἐπεί τοί γε ἐνδέχεται αὐτὴν τὴν ἐκριφεῖσαν ὕλην κριτικῶς ἧττον μετέχειν κακίας καὶ πελιδνοῦσθαι τὰς χεῖρας καὶ τοὺς πόδας, οὐ μὴν μελανθῆναι.

III

II 11 [10: 205,9 A.= II 134,5 L.] Περὶ δὲ ὕπνου ὥσπερ καὶ κατὰ φύσιν ἡμῖν ξύνηθές ἐστι, τὴν μὲν ἡμέρην

Ἐντεῦθεν ἐπὶ τὴν ἀρχὴν τῶν νεύρων ἐπάνεισιν ὁ Ἱπποκράτης, φημὶ δὴ τὸν ἐγκέφαλον, καὶ τοῦτον σημειοῦται ἀπὸ τῆς βλάβης τῆς ἐνεργείας· περὶ γὰρ ὕπνου διαλέγεται, ὁ δὲ παρὰ φύσιν ὕπνος ἐν βλάβαις τῶν ψυχικῶν ἐνεργειῶν θεωρεῖται, φημὶ δὴ τῆς κοινῆς αἰσθήσεως, ἤγουν τῶν κατὰ μέρος αἰσθήσεων, εἴ γε ἐδείχθη ἐν ἑτέροις πάσαις ταῖς κατὰ μέρος αἰσθήσεσι συνεργοῦσα καὶ ἡ κοινὴ αἴσθησις, ὧν ἡ ἠρεμία τὸν ὕπνον ἐργάζεται. τριττὸς δὲ ὁ ὕπνος, ἢ κατὰ φύσιν ἢ παρὰ φύσιν ἢ μεταξὺ ἀμφοτέρων. ἀλλ' ἐπειδὴ περὶ ὕπνου ὁ λόγος, φέρε τὰ τέσσαρα γενεσιουργὰ αἴτια τῶν ὕπνων προδιασκεψώμεθα.

Καὶ ποιητικὸν μὲν αἴτιόν ἐστιν ἡ ἠρεμία τῶν κατὰ μέρος αἰσθήσεων καὶ τῆς κοινῆς αἰσθήσεως. καὶ ὅτι ποιητικὸν μὲν αἴτιόν ἐστι τοῦ ὕπνου ἡ ἠρεμία τῶν κατὰ μέρος αἰσθήσεων καὶ τῆς κοινῆς αἰσθήσεως πάντες ὡμοφώνησαν. περὶ δὲ ἕτερόν τι ἀμφιβάλλουσιν οἱ ἰατροὶ καὶ οἱ φιλόσοφοι, περὶ τῆς ἐνεργείας καὶ τῆς ἠρεμίας, εἴ γε ἀμφότερα ὑπὸ φύσεως καὶ κατὰ πρῶτον λόγον ἐπιτελοῦνται. καὶ οἱ μὲν ἰατροὶ ἀμφότερα ὑπὸ φύσεως λέγουσιν ἐπιτελεῖσθαι καὶ κατὰ πρῶτον λόγον, δεικνύντες τὸν τρόπον τοῦτον· ἡ φύσις πολλὴν πρόνοιαν καὶ φροντίδα περὶ τῶν ὑπ' αὐτῆς γινομένων ποιεῖται, καὶ ποιήσα-
143 σα | τὴν ἐνέργειαν ἐπετήδευσε καὶ τὴν ἠρεμίαν, ἵνα μὴ τῇ ἀενναῷ κινήσει καὶ ἐνεργείᾳ φθείρωνται τὰ μόρια καὶ ἐν αὐτοῖς καταβληθῶσιν αἱ δυνάμεις. διό,

1 πρότερον — 3 πελιδνώσεως *om.* γ 4 παντελῶς *om.* γ 5 πελιῶν γ 8 ἐστί *om.* γ ὀξέου γ 9 ἀπορρίψει γ 11 καὶ ἐλευθεροῦται *om.* γ 18 σύνηθές L τὴν μὲν ἡμέρην *om.* γ 19 ἐνταῦθα P: ἐν τῷ θέ *(sic)* V 21 *ante* τῶν *add.* ταῖς L; *cf. supra, pp. 14 sq.* 23 συναισθήσεων L γε] δὲ γ συνεργοῦσι γ 24 ἡ[II] *om.* L 26 γενεσιουργικὰ γ διασκεψώμεθα L 29 μὲν *om.* γ ἐστι *post* ἠρεμία *trsp.* γ τοῦ ὕπνου *om.* L 32 γε] ἔστιν L 37 φθείρονται MP

Blackening is an intense form of lividness; first they become livid and then black. Here some raise the problem that "If blackness is a higher degree of lividness, how could Hippocrates say, If the fingers become livid, you may expect death, but if the fingers and the feet turn completely black, they are less deadly than the livid?" We say that there are two kinds of blackening — the one results from an intensity of lividness, the other does not. If it is the former, it means very extensive putrefaction, which is highly dangerous. But blackening is also produced by crisis when, in an acute disease, nature is aroused to crisis and expels the matter to the extremities; these parts turn black and sometimes even fall off because of the morbid humors discarded in them, but the patient is saved from the danger and is freed. This is the blackening, then, that Hippocrates here characterized as less dangerous than the livid. However, it can also happen that the matter itself which is expelled during crisis has a lesser share of the morbidity and the hands and feet turn, not black, but livid.

III

II 11 In the matter of sleep, the patient should follow the normal habit; during the day

At this point Hippocrates passes on to the nerve principle, namely the brain, and he gives for it symptoms from impaired function; for he is discussing sleep, and abnormal sleep is observed in impairments of the psychic functions, I mean of the common sense or the particular senses, it having been shown elsewhere that the common sense works in conjunction with all the particular senses, whose resting produces sleep. There are three kinds of sleep, normal, abnormal and intermediate. And since we are on the subject, let us first examine the four generative causes of sleeps.

The efficient cause is the resting of the particular senses and of the common sense. And everyone agrees that the efficient cause of sleep is the resting of the particular senses and of the common sense. It is about another matter, that of function and rest, that doctors and philosophers dispute, whether both are produced by nature and in a primary way. On the one side doctors claim that both are primary products of nature; and their proof is as follows: nature shows great thought and concern for the things she makes, so having created function she also provided for rest, in order to prevent the destruction of the parts and the collapse of the faculties in them from endless movement and activity.

ὡς εἴρηται, καὶ τὴν ἐνέργειαν καὶ τὴν ἠρεμίαν κατὰ πρῶτον λόγον ἐποίησεν ἡ πάνσοφος φύσις, ἵνα μετὰ τὴν ἐνέργειαν ἠρεμοῦντα, ἀνάπαυλαν καὶ ἀνακωχὴν λαμβάνοντα, ἐν αὐτοῖς αἱ δυνάμεις πάλιν πρὸς ὁρμὴν τῆς ἐνεργείας ἀκόπως ἐπιβαίνωσιν. ἢ οὐχ ὁρῶμεν τὰ ἀγαθὰ τὰ γινόμενα ἐν τοῖς ὕπνοις, τὴν διάφορον πέψιν καὶ τὴν διάκρισιν τῶν χυμῶν καὶ τὰ τοιαῦτα; ὅθεν τινὲς τὸν ὕπνον οὐκ ἠθέλησαν ἠρεμίαν καλέσαι, ἀλλ' ἐπιτεταμένην κίνησιν τῶν φυσικῶν δυνάμεων.

Οἱ δὲ φιλόσοφοι λέγουσι κατὰ πρῶτον λόγον τὴν ἐνέργειαν ἀποτελεῖσθαι ὑπὸ τῆς φύσεως, τὴν δὲ ἠρεμίαν παρακολούθημά τι εἶναι, κατασκευάζοντες οὕτως, ὅτι ἡ φύσις διὰ τοῦτο ἐποίησε καὶ τὴν διάφορον ποικιλίαν τῶν μορίων κατεσκεύασε, διὰ τὴν ἐνέργειαν, ἵνα ἀμέμπτως καὶ κατὰ πρῶτον λόγον ἐπιτελῆται ἡ ἐνέργεια, ἡ δὲ ἠρεμία παρακολουθεῖ, ἵνα μετὰ τὴν ἐνέργειαν καὶ ἠρεμῶσι τά τε μόρια καὶ αἱ δυνάμεις.

Καὶ ἐπειδὴ φύσεως ἐμνημονεύσαμεν, τριττὴ δέ ἐστιν αὕτη, εἴπωμεν, ὑπὸ ποίας φύσεως προνοίᾳ ἐπιτελεῖται ἡ ἠρεμία, ἤγουν ὁ ὕπνος. ἔστι γὰρ ἡ φυτικὴ ψυχή, ἔστιν ἡ λογικὴ ψυχή, ἔστι καὶ ἡ ἄλογος ψυχή. ὑπὸ ποίας ἄρα τούτων ἐπιτελεῖται ὁ ὕπνος; καὶ ὑπὸ μὲν τῆς φυτικῆς οὐδαμῶς, ἐπεὶ ὤφειλον καὶ τὰ φυτὰ ὑπνοῦν· ἀλλ' ὑπὸ τῆς λογικῆς οὐδαμῶς, ἐπεὶ ὤφειλε μόνος ὁ ἄνθρωπος ὑπνοῦν· οὐκοῦν προνοίᾳ τῆς ἀλόγου ψυχῆς. διάφοροί εἰσιν ἐν αὐτῇ δυνάμεις κινητικαί· ἔστι γὰρ ζωτική, ἔστι καὶ κινητική. ὑπὸ ποίας ἄρα τούτων ἐπιτελεῖται ὁ ὕπνος; ὑπὸ μὲν τῆς ζωτικῆς οὐδαμῶς· αὐτὴ γὰρ ἀεὶ ἐνεργεῖ κατά τε τὴν σφυγμικὴν καὶ τὴν ἀναπνευστικήν. ἀλλ' ἴσως ἀπορεῖ τις λέγων ὅτι «Καὶ πῶς οὐ φθείρονται τῇ ἀενάῳ κινήσει καὶ ἐνεργείᾳ;» καὶ
144 λέγομεν ὅτι οὐκ ἔστι μία καὶ ἡ αὐτὴ κίνησις, ἀλλὰ | δύο ἐναντίαι· μεταξὺ δὲ δύο ἐναντίων κινήσεων πάντως μεταξυλαβεῖται ἠρεμία. ἐπὶ μὲν τῆς σφυγμικῆς ἔστι συστολὴ καὶ διαστολή, καὶ ἐν τῷ μέσῳ, ἐν ᾧ ἀλλήλας διαδέχονται, ἔστιν ἠρεμία. ἀλλὰ καὶ ἐπὶ τῆς ἀναπνοῆς ἔστιν εἰσπνοὴ καὶ ἐκπνοή, καὶ μεταξυλαβεῖται ἠρεμία. ἐν ταύταις οὖν ταῖς εἰρημέναις ἀνακωχὴν λαμβάνουσαι αἱ ζωτικαὶ δυνάμεις ἀποτελοῦσι τὴν οἰκείαν ἐνέργειαν. ἀλλ' οὐδὲ ὑπὸ τῆς κινητικῆς δυνάμεως ἀποτελεῖται ὁ ὕπνος, ἐπειδὴ αἱ καθ' ὁρμὴν κινήσεις προαιρέσει δουλεύουσιν, ὁ δὲ ὕπνος προαιρέσει οὐ δουλεύει. λείπεται οὖν προνοίᾳ ὑπὸ τῆς ἀλόγου ψυχῆς καὶ τῆς κατὰ μέρος αἰσθήσεως καὶ τῆς κοινῆς αἰσθήσεως ἐπιτελεῖσθαι τὸν ὕπνον. κατὰ συμβεβηκὸς δὲ καὶ ὑπὸ τῆς ἠρεμίας τῆς φαντασίας καὶ τῆς μνήμης ἐπιτελεῖται ὁ ὕπνος. τί γάρ; ἠρεμουσῶν τῶν αἰσθήσεων οὐκ ἀναπέμπονται τύποι ἐπὶ τὴν φαντασίαν, ἐν ᾗ ὤφειλον φαντασθῆναι, καὶ ἐντεῦθεν ἠρεμεῖ· καὶ ἰδοὺ κατὰ μὲν πρῶτον λόγον ὑπὸ τῶν αἰσθήσεων ἐπιτελεῖται ὁ ὕπνος· κατὰ συμβεβηκὸς δὲ καὶ ὑπὸ τῆς ἠρεμίας τῆς φαντασίας καὶ τῆς μνήμης.

2 ἠρεμοῦνται γ 3 λαμβάνωνται γ 12 ἐπιτελεῖται MP παρακολουθῆ *codd.*: *corr. Wk.* 13 ἠρεμοῦσι *codd.*: *correxi* 14 *post* ἐπειδὴ *add.* δὲ L 14 *et* 15 φύσεως] *fort.* ψυχῆς *scribendum est* 14 εἴπομεν γ 16 sq. ἄρα τούτων] ὅτι τοῦτο γ 17 καὶ *om.* γ φυσικῆς γ 17 sq. ἐπεὶ – οὐδαμῶς *om.* γ 18 ὑπὸ *scripsi*: ἐπὶ L 20 αὐτῷ *codd.*: *correxi* *post* ζωτική *fort. exciderunt* ἔστι καὶ γνωστική *vel sim. (cf. infra, lin. 31–p. 164,7)* 20 sq. ἄρα τούτων] ὅτι τοῦτο γ 21 ἀεὶ γὰρ αὐτὴ γ 23 ὅτι *om.* L κινήσει καὶ *om.* γ συνεργεία γ 24 ἐναντία γ 28 λαμβάνουσιν γ 29 ἀποτελοῦσαι γ 30 κινητικῆς *scripsi*: ζωτικῆς *codd.* 31 λείπεται] λοιπὸν γ 33 τελεῖσθαι γ 35 τῇ φαντασία *codd.*: *correxi* 35 sq. ἐν ῷ ὤφειλε *codd.*: *correxi*

On this account, as we said, the very wise nature produced both function and rest in a primary way, so that after their activity (the parts) might rest, get a break and relief, and their faculties proceed unwearied to start their work again. Do we not see the useful things which take place during sleep, the various digestions, the separation of humors and so forth? For this reason some have wanted to characterize sleep, not as rest, but as an intense activity of the natural faculties.

Philosophers, for their part, maintain that function is a primary effect of nature, while rest is a by-product; they argue like this: when nature provided the great variety of parts, she did so for the sake of function, in order that function be produced perfectly and primarily; rest, on the other hand, follows as a secondary product, so that, after their work, the parts and faculties might get a respite.

And since we have spoken of nature, and it is threefold, let us discuss which nature takes care of the production of rest or sleep. There is the vegetative soul, the rational soul and the irrational soul. Which of these, then, is responsible for sleep? Certainly not the vegetative, for, (if that were so,) vegetation also ought to sleep; and surely not the rational, since, (in that case,) man should be the only one to sleep; so (it is produced), then, by the care of the irrational soul. The irrational has different kinetic faculties; for there is the vital and the kinetic. Which of these, then, produces sleep? It could never be the vital, since it is always working in the pulse and in respiration. But someone may raise a problem and ask, "How is it that these (systems) are not destroyed by the endless movement and function?" We say that there is not just the one and the same movement, but two opposites; and between the two contrary motions a rest is always taken. In pulsation there is systole and diastole together with a pause in the middle, when the one takes over from the other. In respiration, too, there is inhalation and exhalation and in between a rest is taken. So in these two cases we have cited the vital faculties carry out their proper function by taking a pause. But sleep is not produced by the kinetic faculty either, since appetitive movements work subject to choice, while sleep does not. It is left, then, that sleep is brought about as a provision of the irrational soul, the particular senses and the common sense. But it is also produced accidentally by the resting of the imagination and memory. Why? Because when the senses are resting, impressions are not transmitted to the imagination, where they would be developed, and so it remains quiet; we see, then, that sleep is produced primarily by the senses and accidentally by the resting of imagination and memory.

Ἀλλ' ἴσως ἀπορεῖ τις λέγων ὅτι «Εἰ οὖν ἡ φαντασία ἐν τοῖς ὕπνοις ἠρεμεῖ, πῶς ὀνειρώττομεν ἐν τοῖς ὕπνοις, εἰ μὴ ὅτι τῆς φαντασίας ἐνεργούσης;» καὶ λέγομεν ὅτι ἐν τῷ κατὰ φύσιν ὕπνῳ ἡ φαντασία πάντως ἠρεμεῖ, ὅθεν οὐδὲ ὀνειρώττομεν ἐν τῷ κατὰ φύσιν ὕπνῳ· εἰ μὴ γὰρ αἱ αἰσθήσεις πέμπουσι τοὺς τύπους τῇ φαντασίᾳ, οὐκ ἐνεργεῖ. τούτων δὲ ἠρεμουσῶν ἐν τῷ ὕπνῳ καὶ ἡ φαντασία ἠρεμεῖ καὶ ἡ μνήμη ἐν τῷ κατὰ φύσιν ὕπνῳ. οὐδὲν γάρ ἐστι φαντασία ἢ μονὴ καὶ στάσις τῶν φαντασθέντων.

Ὑλικὸν δὲ αἴτιόν ἐστι τοῦ ὕπνου ἡ ἀναπεμπομένη χρηστὴ ὑγρότης, ἥτις φερομένη ἐπὶ τοὺς πόρους τῶν νεύρων καὶ περὶ τὰς ῥίζας αὐτῶν παρεμποδίζει καὶ παρακωλύει διεξελθεῖν τὸ ψυχικὸν πνεῦμα· τούτου γὰρ κωλυομένου, οὐ διοδεύει καὶ διαλάμπεται ἀκτινοειδῶς ταῖς αἰσθήσεσιν, ἀλλ' ἠρεμίαν ἔχουσιν, ὅπερ ὁ κατὰ φύσιν ἐστὶν ὕπνος. καλῶς δὲ εἴπομεν ὅτι πα-
145 ρακωλύει διεξελ|θεῖν τὸ ψυχικὸν πνεῦμα· οὐδὲ γὰρ πάντῃ ἐμφράττει τὰς ῥίζας τῶν νεύρων καὶ τοὺς πόρους ἡ χρηστὴ ὑγρότης, ἀλλ' ἐπιπολαίως, ὥστε μοῖρά τις τοῦ ψυχικοῦ πνεύματος διεξέρχεται. οὕτως γὰρ καὶ ἐπὶ τῶν ἐκτὸς ὁρῶμεν ἐπὶ τοῦ ἡλίου, ἡνίκα καθαρὸν νέφος ὑποδράμῃ τῷ ἡλίῳ, τὴν μὲν ἀκτῖνα αὐτοῦ κωλύει διεξελθεῖν, τὸ δὲ φῶς διεξέρχεται καὶ ποιεῖ τὴν ἡμέραν. οὕτως οὖν καὶ ἐνταῦθα διεξέρχεται μοῖρά τις τοῦ ψυχικοῦ πνεύματος, ὡς δηλοῖ τὸ ἐν τῷ ὑπνώττειν ἡμᾶς συγγινώσκειν πολλάκις τὰ γινόμενα καὶ τὰ λεγόμενα ἀκούομεν, ἐν οἱῳδήποτε ὑπνοῦντες οἴκῳ. εἰ δὲ ἀχλυωδέστερον καὶ παχύτερόν ἐστι τὸ ὑγρὸν καὶ μείζων ἡ ἔμφραξις γένηται, τότε οὐχ ὕπνος ἐστὶ σχεδόν, ἀλλ' ἀποπληξία ἢ κῶμα καὶ τὰ τοιαῦτα. ὥσπερ πάλιν ἐπὶ τοῦ ἡλίου, ἐὰν νέφος ζοφῶδες καὶ παχὺ ὑποδράμῃ αὐτόν, τότε οὐ μόνον τὴν ἀκτῖνα κωλύει, ἀλλὰ καὶ τὸ φῶς, ὡς δοκεῖν ἡμᾶς ὁρῶντας πολλάκις τοῦτο γινόμενον ἐν ἡμέρᾳ ὡς ἑσπέραν εἶναι. εἰ δὲ γεωδέστερόν ἐστι τὸ ὑγρόν, παντελῆ ποιεῖται τὴν ἔμφραξιν καὶ θάνατον ἐπιφέρει, οὐ μὴν ὕπνον. οὕτως γὰρ καὶ ὁ ἥλιος ὑπόγειος γινόμενος καὶ σκεπόμενος ὑπὸ τοῦ πάχους τῆς γῆς, στερεῖται ὁ ἀὴρ οὗτος τοῦ φωτίζοντος, καὶ γίνεται ἡ νύξ. τοῦτο οὖν καὶ τὸ ὑλικόν ἐστιν αἴτιον, ἡ χρηστὴ ὑγρότης.

Ὀργανικὸν δὲ αἴτιόν ἐστιν αὐτὸς ὁ ἐγκέφαλος, ἐν ᾧ χορηγεῖται ἡ ὑγρότης.

Τελικὸν δὲ αἴτιόν ἐστι, δι' ὃ ἐγένετο αὐτὸς ὁ ὕπνος, λέγω δὴ διὰ τὴν ἀνάπαυλαν τῶν δυνάμεων.

Δεύτερόν ἐστιν κεφάλαιον, ἐν ᾧ δεῖ ἡμᾶς τέσσαρά τινα περὶ τοῦ ὕπνου εἰπεῖν καὶ ζητῆσαι, τὸ ποσὸν τοῦ ὕπνου, τὸ ποιόν, τὸν καιρόν, τὸν τρόπον τῆς χρήσεως.

8–12] *cf.* Steph. Comm. in Hipp. Aph.: Ambros. S 19 sup. fol. 29r

1 Εἰ *om.* γ 2 *ante* πῶς *add.* καὶ γ 4 αἱ *om.* L 5 τύπους] ὕπνους L δὲ *om.* MP 9 περὶ *om.* L 11 διοδεύει καὶ *om.* γ 12 ὕπνος ἐστίν γ 14 τῶν νεύρων *post* πόρους *trsp.* γ ἐπιπόλαιος γ: ἐπιπόλως L: *corr. Dietz* 16 τῷ ἡλίῳ] *fort.* τὸν ἥλιον *scribendum est (cf. infra, lin. 23)* 18 *post* τις *add.* ψυχικὴ L 19 συγγινώσκειν ἡμᾶς γ 19 sq. τὰ λεγόμενα καὶ τὰ γινόμενα L 20 οἴκῳ ὑπνοῦντες γ 23 τότε] ποτὲ L; *cf. supra, pp. 14 sq.* 24 ὁρᾶν *codd.*: *correxi* 26 ποιεῖ γ 27 καὶ γὰρ L ὑπόγειος] ὑπόϋλος γ γενόμενος γ τάχους γ 28 ἐστέρηται γ 29 ἐστιν *om.* γ 32 ὃ] οὗ *codd.*: *correxi* 35 εἰπεῖν καὶ *om.* γ

But someone may object that "If, then, the imagination is at rest during sleep, how are dreams possible in sleep without the imagination being active?" We reply that during normal sleep the imagination is always quiet, with the result that we do not have dreams either in normal sleep; for, unless the senses transmit the impressions to the imagination, it does not work. And since the senses are inactive during sleep, both imagination and memory rest in normal sleep. You see, imagination is simply the continuance and holding of the imagined objects.

The material cause of sleep is the useful moisture transmitted upwards which, when conveyed to the ducts of the nerves and around their roots, partially hinders and prevents the psychic pneuma from passing out; for when this (pneuma) is obstructed, it is unable to make its way through to irradiate the senses; instead they experience the rest that constitutes normal sleep. And we had good reason to say that the useful moisture partially prevents the passage of the psychic pneuma; for the blockage of the nerve roots and ducts is not complete but superficial, with the result that a certain amount of the psychic pneuma makes its way through. We see a similar phenomenon also in the world around us in the case of the sun; when a bright cloud floats below the sun, the rays are prevented from getting through, but the light penetrates to give us daylight. In the same way here, too, a part of the psychic pneuma penetrates, and this is proved by the fact that while sleeping we are often conscious of what is going on (around us) and hear what is being said, no matter in what house we are sleeping. However, if the moisture is on the dense and thick side and the obstruction becomes greater, then (what results) is scarcely sleep, but apoplexy or coma or the like. Again the same happens in the case of the sun; if a thick dark cloud passes underneath, then it blocks not only the rays but the light as well, so that frequently, when we see this happen during the day, we think that it is evening. But if the moisture is on the earthy side, it causes total stoppage and brings on death, not sleep. It is the same with the sun as well; once it sinks below the horizon and is covered by the dense earth, our sky is left without its source of light and night falls. This useful moisture, then, is the material cause.

The organic cause is the brain itself to which the moisture is supplied.

The final cause is that for which sleep itself is produced, namely the resting of the faculties.

The second chapter is where we have to discuss and examine four things concerning sleep: quantity of sleep, quality, time and mode of use.

Καὶ ἀρκτέον ἀπὸ τοῦ ποσοῦ. τὸ ποσὸν τοῦ ὕπνου μήτε πολὺ δεῖ εἶναι
146 μήτε βραχύ· ὁ γὰρ πολὺς ὕπνος περιττωματικὸν τὸ σῶμα δη|λοῖ καὶ αὐτὴν τὴν ἀναπεμπομένην ὑγρότητα. ὁ δὲ βραχὺς ὕπνος δηλοῖ ἔνδειαν ὑγρότητος καὶ λεπτὴν καὶ ἀερώδη φύσιν τοῦ ὑγροῦ· τὸ τηνικαῦτα γὰρ ἑτοίμως διαφορεῖται, καὶ διὰ τοῦτο βραχὺς γίνεται ὁ ὕπνος. ἀλλὰ δεῖ μέσον αὐτὸν εἶναι, μήτε πολὺν μήτε βραχύν.

Κατὰ δὲ ποιότητα, οὐ δεῖ τὸν ὕπνον βαθὺν εἶναι καὶ καταφορικόν· κακὸν γάρ ἐστι· δηλοῖ γὰρ παχεῖαν τὴν ὑγρότητα. ἀλλ' οὔτε ἐπιπόλαιον δεῖ εἶναι τὸν ὕπνον καὶ ἑτοιμοεγρήγορον· δηλοῖ γὰρ λεπτὴν τὴν ὑγρότητα καὶ εὐδιαφόρητον. ἀλλὰ δεῖ αὐτὸν μέσως πως εἶναι.

Κατὰ δὲ τὸν καιρόν, δεῖ ἐν τῇ νυκτερινῇ ὥρᾳ ἐπιτελεῖσθαι τοὺς ὕπνους· τότε γὰρ ἐπιτηδειότης ἐστὶ τῆς ἠρεμίας ἐπὶ παντὸς ζῴου.

Ἀλλ' ἴσως ἐρεῖ τις ὅτι «Καὶ πῶς τινας ὁρῶμεν τῶν τεχνιτῶν ἐν μὲν τῇ νυκτὶ κάμνοντας, ἐν δὲ τῇ ἡμέρᾳ ὑπνοῦντας, καὶ ὑγιεινῶς διάγοντας, ὥσπερ μάγκιπες καὶ χαλκεῖς;» πρὸς ὅ φαμεν ὅτι ἐν τοῖς χρόνοις τοῦ Ἱπποκράτους πάντες εὐτάκτως ἐβίουν καὶ οὐκ ἦν τοιαύτη κατάστασις, ἀλλὰ κοσμίως ἔζων. οὕτως γὰρ καὶ ἐπὶ τῶν ἐκτὸς ὁρῶμεν ὅτι ἀνίσχοντος τοῦ ἡλίου καὶ ἡμέρας γινομένης πάντα τὰ ζῷα ἐπὶ τὰ πλεῖστα ὁρμῶσι πρὸς τὴν ἐνέργειαν· ὑπὸ γῆν δὲ γινομένου τοῦ ἡλίου πάλιν ἐν ἡσυχίᾳ διάγουσι τὰ ζῷα. οὕτως καὶ οἱ τότε ἄνθρωποι κοσμικὴν τάξιν ἐφρόντιζον καὶ ἐν μὲν τῇ νυκτὶ ὕπνουν, ἐν δὲ τῇ ἡμέρᾳ ἐνήργουν. δεῖ γὰρ εἰδέναι ὅτι ἐν τῇ νυκτί ἐστιν ὁ κατὰ φύσιν ὕπνος, ἐπειδὴ τοῦ ἡλίου ὑπὸ γῆν γινομένου στερεῖται ὁ ἀὴρ τοῦ φωτίζοντος καὶ πρὸς ἐνέργειαν ποιοῦντος τὰς αἰσθήσεις κινεῖσθαι. τί γάρ; ὅτι ἀπόντος τοῦ φωτίζοντος οὐκ ἀντιλαμβάνονται αἱ αἰσθήσεις περὶ τὰ αἰσθητὰ καὶ λοιπὸν ἠρεμοῦσι, καὶ διὰ τοῦτο ἐν νυκτὶ μάλιστα ἐπιτελεῖται ὁ κατὰ φύσιν ὕπνος. ἢ καὶ ἄλλως· ἑκάστη νὺξ πρὸς τὴν οἰκείαν ἡμέραν ψυχροτέρα ἐστίν· ἐν γοῦν τῇ νυκτὶ ὑπὸ τῆς ψύξεως στεγνοῦται ἡ ἐπιφάνεια τοῦ δέρματος, καὶ
147 τῇ στεγνώσει περιστέλλεται τὸ ἔμφυτον θερμὸν καὶ συννεύει | ἐπὶ τὸ βάθος· δηλονότι καὶ ἡ φύσις συννεύει ἐπὶ τὸ βάθος· καὶ λοιπὸν οὐκ ἐλλάμπεται ταῖς αἰσθήσεσι, καὶ τὸ τηνικαῦτα ὁ κατὰ φύσιν ὕπνος ἕπεται τῇ νυκτί. ἵνα δὲ ἐπὶ τὸ τελειότερον ἀγάγωμεν τὸν λόγον, δεῖ ἡμᾶς ἐκ διαιρέσεως προελθεῖν καὶ εἰπεῖν οὕτως, ὅτι ὁ ὕπνος ἢ καὶ ἐν ⟨τῇ⟩ νυκτὶ καὶ ἐν τῇ ἡμέρᾳ ἐπιτελεῖται, καὶ ἔστι κακός· δηλοῖ γὰρ ἢ ἀποπληξίαν ἢ κάρον ἢ κῶμα ἢ ἕτερόν τι τοιοῦτον· ἔστι δ' ὅτε καὶ θάνατον ἐπιφέρει. ἢ οὐδὲ ἐν τῇ νυκτὶ οὐδὲ ἐν τῇ ἡμέρᾳ. οὗτος δὲ οὐκ ἔστιν ὕπνος, ἀλλ' ἀγρυπνία, ὅπερ καὶ τοῦτο κακόν ἐστι· δηλοῖ γὰρ ἐπιτεταμένην ξηρότητα καὶ ἐλαχίστην ὑγρότητα, ἥτις καὶ αὐτὴ λεπτὴ οὖσα διαφορεῖται, καὶ διὰ τοῦτο οὐχ ὑπνοῦσιν. ἢ ἐν τῇ νυκτὶ ἐπιτελεῖται, καὶ ἔστιν οὗτος ἀγαθὸς ὕπνος καὶ κατὰ φύσιν, ὡς ἤδη ἡ αἰτία εἴρηται

15 ἐν – 17] *cf.* Gal. In Hipp. Progn. comm. II 11: CMG V 9,2 p. 270,5sq. Steph. Comm. in Hipp. Aph.: Escor. Σ. II.10 fol. 252r

1 πολὺν γ εἶναι] εἰδέναι L 2 βραχύν PV 4 λεπτοῦ καὶ ἀερώδους *codd.*: *correxi* 8 γὰρ^{II}] δὲ γ 9 ἑτοιμοεγρήγορτον PV *(deest* M*)* 11 τὸν ὕπνον γ 15 μάγκυπες MP: μάγγιπες L: *corr.* V 16 πάντως L ἐβίων PV 18 ἐπὶ *scr.* *Dietz*: ἐπείτοι *codd.* 22 φωτίζοντος *scripsi*: φωτίζειν *codd.* 23 ποιοῦντος] οὐ ποιεῖ L 28 ἔμφυτον θερμόν] ἐμφυτευθὲν γ 30 ὁ] καὶ L 31 προαιρέσεως γ 32 καὶ^{II} – νυκτὶ *om.* L τῇ^{I} *add.* M 33 ἢ κῶμα *om.* γ 38 ὕπνος *om.* γ

We should start with quantity. The quantity of sleep should be neither great nor small; for much sleep indicates that the body and the transmitted moisture itself contain a lot of residues. Short sleep, on the other hand, means that the moisture is deficient and that the composition of the moisture is thin and rarefied; for in that state it dissipates easily, thus causing the sleep to be short. But sleep should be moderate, neither long nor short.

In quality sleep should not be deep or heavy; (sleep of this kind) is bad; for it means that the moisture is dense. But neither should sleep be light and easily disturbed; for it shows that the moisture is thin and dissipates readily. But it should be somewhere in between.

As for the time, sleep should be taken during the night hours, since all living creatures find this a suitable period for resting.

But someone may say, "How is that we see some craftsmen, such as bakers and smiths, who work at night, sleep during the day, and lead healthy lives?" Our answer is that in Hippocrates' day, all lived well-ordered and regular lives and such a state of affairs did not exist. Thus, in the world about us, too, we see that, when the sun comes up and day breaks, all animals generally speaking start their activities; but once the sun goes below the horizon the animals are at rest again. In the same way also the men of those times cared about an ordered system, so they slept at night and were active during the daytime. For it should be noted that night is the time for normal sleep, since, once the sun goes below the earth, the sky loses the source of light which also stimulates the senses into activity. Why? Because, in the absence of the light source, the senses cannot grasp sensible objects and so they rest; this explains, then, why normal sleep is achieved above all during the nighttime. Or (it may be explained) in another way: every night is colder than its corresponding day; during the night, then, the skin's surface is closed up by the cold, and because of the closing the innate heat gathers itself together and converges on the interior; – and nature also obviously converges on the interior; – and so it does not irradiate the senses; hence normal sleep comes at night. But in order to make the discussion more complete, we must proceed from the following division and say that sleep is either achieved both during the night and day, which is bad; for it indicates apoplexy or torpor or coma or another similar condition; sometimes it even brings on death. Or (it is obtained) neither at night nor during the day. But this is not sleep, it is insomnia, which again is a bad symptom; for it means extreme dryness and a very small supply of moisture and even this dissipates because of its thinness, and for this reason they do not sleep. Or it is achieved at night, and this is good and normal sleep for the reason we gave earlier. Or it is achieved

πρόσθεν. ἢ ἐν τῇ ἡμέρᾳ ἐπιτελεῖται μόνον. οὗτος δὲ ἧττόν ἐστιν ἀγαθὸς ὡς πρὸς τὸν ἐν νυκτὶ ἐπιτελούμενον· τῶν δὲ ἄλλων καλλίων ἐστὶν οὗτος. τί γάρ; ὅτι πολλάκις διά τινα ἐπιτεταμένην ὀδύνην ἢ φροντίδα τινὰ οὐκ ἐκοιμήθησαν ἐν τῇ νυκτί, καὶ ὅπερ ἐν τῇ νυκτὶ σφάλμα γέγονε, δέον ἐν τῇ ἡμέρᾳ ἀναπληρωθῆναι τὸ σφαλὲν καὶ ἀνάπαυλαν καὶ ἄνεσιν γενέσθαι τῶν δυνάμεων. πλὴν καὶ τοῦτο δεῖ σε εἰδέναι, ὅτι καὶ τῆς ἡμέρας κάλλιόν ἐστιν ἐν τῷ ἑωθινῷ ὑπνῶσαι, ἐπειδὴ τὸ ψυχρότερόν ἐστι τὸ ἑωθινὸν τῆς ἡμέρας.

Ὁ δὲ τρόπος τῆς χρήσεως τοῦ ὕπνου ἐστίν, ἵνα εἱρμῷ τινι καὶ ἀκολουθίᾳ καὶ συνέχεια φυλάττηται ἐν τῷ ὕπνῳ καὶ μὴ διακόπτεσθαι τὸν ὕπνον· ὁ γὰρ εἱρμῷ τινι καὶ ἀκολουθίᾳ γινόμενος ὕπνος χρηστὴν ὑγρότητα ἐνδείκνυται. ὁ δὲ διακοπτόμενος ὕπνος δηλοῖ λεπτὴν τὴν ὑγρότητα καὶ εὐδιαφόρητον· καὶ καθ' ἣν διεφορήθη, διακόπτεται ὁ ὕπνος, καὶ διϋπνίζονται. ἢ πολλάκις διακόπτεται ὁ ὕπνος ὑπὸ φροντίδος πολλῆς. τί γάρ; κοιμᾶται, καὶ αὐτὴ ἡ φροντὶς διϋπνίζει αὐτόν, καὶ πάλιν κοιμᾶται, καὶ πάλιν ἡ φροντὶς διϋπνίζει αὐτόν, καὶ οὕτως διακόπτεται ὁ ὕπνος. |

IV

148 **II 12** [11: 206,3 A.=II 134,13 L.] Διαχώρημα δὲ ἄριστόν ἐστι μαλθακόν τε καὶ συνεστηκὸς καὶ τὴν ὥρην ἥνπερ καὶ ὑγιαίνοντι διεχώρει, πλῆθος δὲ πρὸς λόγον τῶν εἰσιόντων.

Μεμαθήκαμεν ὅτι τριττή ἐστιν ἡ πέψις· ἔστι γὰρ πρώτη ἡ χυλοποίησις, ἧς περίττωμά ἐστιν ἡ κόπρος· δευτέρα δὲ πέψις ἡ ἐν ἥπατι γινομένη, ἡ ἐξαιμάτωσις, ἧς περίττωμά ἐστι τὸ οὖρον· τρίτη πέψις ἐστὶν ἡ ἐν ἑκάστῳ μορίῳ, ἤγουν ἡ ἐν τῷ παντὶ σώματι, πέψις καὶ ἐξομοίωσις, ἧς περίττωμά ἐστιν ἡ ἄδηλος διαπνοή. νῦν οὖν περὶ τοῦ περιττώματος τῆς πρώτης πέψεως διαλέγεται, λέγω δὴ τῆς κόπρου. καὶ τοῦτο σημειοῦται ἀπὸ ἕξ τινων, ἀπὸ τῆς ποσότητος, ἀπὸ τῆς συστάσεως, ἀπὸ τοῦ καιροῦ, ἀπὸ τῆς χροιᾶς, ἀπὸ τῆς ὀσμῆς, ἀπὸ τοῦ τρόπου τῆς ἐκκρίσεως.

Ἀπὸ τῆς ποσότητος, πῶς τὸ κατὰ φύσιν διαχώρημα οὐ πρὸς τὴν ποσότητα τῆς παρεχομένης τροφῆς δέον προσέχειν, ἀλλὰ πρὸς τὴν φύσιν αὐτῆς τῆς παρεχομένης τροφῆς. τινὰ μὲν γὰρ τῶν τροφῶν πολὺ μὲν τρέφουσι καὶ πολὺ ἔχουσι τὸ χρηστόν, ὀλίγον δὲ τὸ περίττωμα, ὥσπερ κρέα καὶ ὄρνεα καὶ τὰ τοιαῦτα· τινὰ δὲ τοὐναντίον ὀλίγον τρέφουσιν, ἐπειδὴ ἐλάχιστον ἔχουσι τὸ χρηστόν, ὥσπερ καὶ λάχανα καὶ φακῆ καὶ τὰ ὄσπρια. καὶ τοῦτο ἔστιν, ὅπερ λέγει ὁ Ἱπποκράτης, πλῆθος δὲ πρὸς λόγον τῶν εἰσιόντων.

Ἀπὸ δὲ τῆς συστάσεως, τὸ κατὰ φύσιν διαχώρημα οὔτε ἔξυγρον καὶ ὑδαρὲς θέλει εἶναι οὔτε μὴν σκληρὸν καὶ συνεστραμμένον, ἀλλὰ μέσως πως.

20–24] *cf.* Steph. Comm. in Hipp. Aph.: Ambros. S 19 sup. fol. 37^{v}

3 ὅτι *om.* γ ἐκοιμήθη γ 4 ἐν τῇ ἡμέρᾳ *om.* L 5 σφάλμα L 7 τὸ^{I} *om.* γ 8 ἀκολουθία *codd.*: *correxi* (*cf. lin. 10*) 15 *post* ὕπνος *add.* αὐτῶν γ 18 ὧραν L 19 πλῆθος – εἰσιόντων *om.* γ 20 πέψις] περίττωσις γ 21 περίττωμά] περίττωσις γ ἡ^{III} *om.* γ 23 περίττωμά] περίττωσις γ 30 περιεχομένης *codd.*: *correxi* 33 καὶ^{I} *om.* γ

only during the day. Compared to night sleep this is less good, but better than the others. Why? Because it often happens that an intense pain or some worry has prevented them from sleeping during the night, and it is then necessary that what was lost in the night be restored during the day and that the faculties have rest and relaxation. But you should be aware of this also, that during the day it is better to sleep in the morning, this being the cooler part of the day.

As to mode of use, in sleep, by means of a certain sequence and coherence, continuity should be preserved and sleep should not be broken; for sleep which has a certain sequence and coherence points to a useful moisture. But interrupted sleep means that the moisture is thin and easily dissipated; and according as it is dissipated, the sleep is broken and waking follows. Or oftentimes sleep is broken by serious worry. Why? Because (the person) is sleeping, then the worry itself wakes him; he goes back to sleep, but again is awakened by the worry, and in this way the sleep is interrupted.

IV

II 12 The excrement is best when it is soft, has consistency and is passed at the time usual for the patient before his illness; the quantity (should be) in proportion to the amount of nourishment taken.

We have learned that there are three digestions; the first is conversion to chyle, and excrement is the residue; second, the digestion that occurs in the liver, i.e. blood formation, with urine as residue; third, that which takes place in each part, in other words, digestion and conversion throughout the body, whose residue is the invisible transpiration. In the present instance, then, he is discussing the residue of the first digestion, namely excrement. And he gives the symptoms for it from six factors: from quantity, consistency, time, color, smell and the mode of excretion.

From quantity: (he tells us) that for normal excrement one should consider not the amount, but the nature, of the food administered. For some foods are highly nutritious and have much that is useful, but little residue, such as meat and fowl and the like; but some on the contrary, such as vegetables, lentil soup and pulse, are poor nutrients, since they have very little that is useful. This is what Hippocrates means by the quantity in proportion to the amount of nourishment taken.

From consistency: normal excrement should be neither very moist and watery nor hard and condensed, but somewhere in between.

Ἀπὸ δὲ τοῦ καιροῦ, τὸ κατὰ φύσιν διαχώρημα δεῖ ἐν τῷ ἑωθινῷ καιρῷ τῆς ἡμέρας ἀποπατεῖσθαι· μετὰ γὰρ τὴν πέψιν καὶ τὴν διάκρισιν, τότε εἰς ἀποπάτησιν τρέπονται οἱ ἄνθρωποι.

Ἀπὸ δὲ τῆς χροιᾶς, δεῖ τὸ κατὰ φύσιν διαχώρημα ὅσον πρὸς ἑαυτὸ
149 λευκὸν εἶναι, ἐπειδὴ καὶ ὁ χυλὸς τοι|οῦτός ἐστιν. ἀλλ' ἐπειδὴ ἀπὸ χολῆς χρώννυται, δεῖ αὐτὸ ὑπόξανθον εἶναι καὶ ὑπέρυθρον.

Ἀπὸ δὲ τῆς ὀσμῆς, τὸ κατὰ φύσιν διαχώρημα οὐ θέλει εἶναι οὔτε δυσωδέστατον οὔτε εὔοσμον· τὸ γὰρ δυσωδέστατον δηλοῖ μεγάλην σηπεδόνα ἐν τῇ γαστρὶ καὶ ἐν τοῖς ἐντέροις· τὸ δὲ εὐῶδες διαχώρημα δηλοῖ ὅτι καὶ τὰ χρηστὰ μετὰ τῶν ἀχρήστων συνεκκρίνεται· ἀλλὰ δεῖ αὐτὸ ὀλίγης μετέχειν δυσωδίας, ὡς αὐτός φησι καὶ ἥκιστα δυσῶδες.

Ἀπὸ δὲ τοῦ τρόπου τῆς ἐκκρίσεως, δεῖ τὸ κατὰ φύσιν διαχώρημα μήτε μετὰ τρυσμοῦ τινος ἢ πνεύματος ἢ μετά τινος ὀδύνης ἐκκρίνεσθαι, μήτε μετὰ τεινεσμοῦ τινος καὶ συντάσεως, ἀλλὰ δεῖ αὐτὸ ὁμαλῶς καὶ ἀδιακόπως ἐκκρίνεσθαι.

Λοιπὸν δὲ δεῖ ἡμᾶς καὶ τὴν αἰτίαν ⟨τῆς ἀμετρίας⟩ ἑκάστου ἀποδοῦναι. καὶ τέως τῆς κατὰ ποσότητα εἴπωμεν τὰ αἴτια. γίνεται πολὺ τὸ διαχώρημα ἢ δι' ἀσθένειαν τῆς καθεκτικῆς δυνάμεως, μὴ ἰσχυσάσης κατασχεῖν, ἀλλ' ἐξεῶσαι· καὶ τὸ τηνικαῦτα καὶ τὰ χρηστὰ μετὰ τῶν ἀχρήστων συνεκκρίνονται. ἢ διὰ βλάβην τινὰ τῆς ἀναδόσεως· βλάπτεται δὲ ἡ ἀνάδοσις ἢ δι' ἀσθένειαν τῆς ἐν ἥπατι ἑλκτικῆς, μὴ ἰσχυούσης ἕλξαι, ἢ δι' ἔμφραξιν ἢ φλεγμονὴν τῶν μεσαραϊκῶν φλεβῶν· τὸ τηνικαῦτα γὰρ ἐνδεὴς γίνεται ἡ ἀνάδοσις, καὶ ἐξ ἀνάγκης καὶ ὁ χυλὸς φέρεται μετὰ τῆς κόπρου καὶ συνεκκρίνεται, καὶ πολὺ γίνεται τὸ διαχώρημα. ἢ δι' ἐπιρροὴν χυμῶν τινων ἐπὶ τὴν γαστέρα, ἀπὸ τοῦ παντὸς σώματος συρρυέντων. τί γάρ; ὅτι συνεκκρίνονται καὶ οἱ χυμοὶ οὗτοι μετὰ τῆς κόπρου καὶ γίνεται πολὺ τὸ διαχώρημα. ὀλίγον δὲ γίνεται ἢ διὰ πλημμελῆ βλάβην τῆς καθεκτικῆς δυνάμεως, πλέον κατέχουσα τοῦ δέοντος· ἀναδίδοται γὰρ τὸ πλεῖστον μέρος τοῦ χυλοῦ, καὶ ὀλίγον γίνεται τὸ διαχώρημα. ἢ διὰ πλημμελῆ βλάβην τῆς ἑλκτικῆς δυνάμεως τοῦ ἥπατος, ἐπὶ πλέον τοῦ δέοντος ἕλκοντος, καὶ ἐντεῦθεν
150 γίνεται ὀλίγον τὸ διαχώ|ρημα. ἢ διὰ θερμὴν δυσκρασίαν τῶν μεσαραϊκῶν φλεβῶν· σχεδὸν δὲ ἡ αὐτή ἐστιν αἰτία· καὶ ἐνταῦθα γὰρ ἕλκει ἡ θερμὴ δυσκρασία τὸ ὑγρόν, ἤγουν τὸν χυλόν, καὶ ἐξαναλίσκει καὶ δαπανᾷ πλέον τοῦ δέοντος, καὶ ὀλίγον γίνεται τὸ διαχώρημα.

Τῆς δὲ κατὰ σύστασιν ἀμετρίας, τίς ἡ αἰτία τοῦ δίυγρον καὶ ὑδαρὲς γίνεσθαι τὸ διαχώρημα ἢ σκληρὸν καὶ ξηρόν; καὶ ὑγρὸν καὶ ὑδαρὲς γίνεται τὸ διαχώρημα δι' ἀσθένειαν τῆς ἀλλοιωτικῆς δυνάμεως, μὴ ἰσχυούσης ἀλλοιῶσαι καὶ χυμῶσαι καὶ πέψαι, ἀλλ' ἐξεῶσαι· τὸ τηνικαῦτα γὰρ ἔξυγρον γίνεται τὸ διαχώρημα, ὥσπερ ἐν ταῖς κοιλιακαῖς διαθέσεσιν. ἢ διὰ πλημμελῆ

11 καὶ – δυσῶδες] *cf.* Hipp. Progn. 7; 11: pp. 203,6sq.; 206,12sq. A. = II pp. 130,10sq.; 136,7 L.

5 καὶ *om.* γ   τοιοῦτόν PV   10 ἐκκρίνεται L   14 τενισμοῦ γ   16 δὲ *om.* γ   τῆς ἀμετρίας *add. Wk.*   17 εἴπομεν γ   18 καθεκτικῆς] ἀποκριτικῆς γ   19 ἐξεᾶσαι γ; *sed cf. infra, lin. 38*   συνεκκρίνεται γ   20 τινὰ *del.* L   τῆς *om.* γ   28 κατέχουσιν *scr. et post* δέοντος *trsp.* γ; *sed cf. e. g. infra, pp. 172,8sq.; 194,32sq.*   35 τοῦ] τὸ L   38 ἐξεώσης L; *sed cf. supra, lin. 19*

From time: normal excrement should be passed in the morning part of the day; for it is after digestion and separation that people go to stool.

From color: normal excrement as such ought to be white, since this is also the color of the chyle. But seeing that it is tinted by bile, it should show traces of yellow and red.

From smell: normal excrement should be neither very fetid nor sweet-smelling; for the very fetid means serious putrefaction in the stomach and intestines, while sweet-smelling excrement shows that the useful matter is being evacuated along with the useless; but it should be slightly fetid, as he himself says, in the least degree foul-smelling.

From the mode of excretion: normal excrement should be passed without any (rumbling) noise or wind or any kind of pain; nor should there be any straining or exertion, but it should be eliminated evenly and without breaking.

Next we must give the cause of irregularity in each case. And first let us name the causes of (irregular) quantity. The excrement becomes large either because of a weakness of the retentive faculty, when it is not able to retain but releases, in which event the useful is passed out along with the useless matter. Or by a fault in the distribution; and the distribution is impaired either by a weakness in the liver's attractive (faculty), when it is incapable of attracting, or by a stoppage or inflammation in the mesaraic veins; for in that case the distribution becomes deficient, so that the chyle also is inevitably carried along with the excrement and is passed out with it, and the excrement becomes large. Or by an influx of humors to the stomach flowing together from all over the body. Why? Because these humors are passed out along with the excrement and it becomes large. It becomes small, on the other hand, either due to a fault of irregularity in the retentive faculty, when it holds longer than it should; for most of the chyle is distributed and the excrement becomes small. Or due to a fault of irregularity in the liver's attractive faculty; it attracts more than it should and so the excrement becomes small. Or due to a hot distemper in the mesaraic veins, for practically the same reason (as in the previous case); for here also the fluid, i.e. the chyle, is attracted by the hot distemper which uses up and consumes more than it should, and the excrement becomes small.

In the matter of irregular consistency, what causes the excrement to become very moist and watery or hard and dry? Moist and watery excrement results from a weakness in the converting faculty, when it is not strong enough to convert, form humor or digest, but expels (the matter); in these circumstances the excrement becomes very moist, as in cases of gastric disturbance. Or due to a fault of irregularity in the

βλάβην τῆς καθεκτικῆς δυνάμεως, μὴ τὸν δέοντα καιρὸν κατέχουσα, ἐν ᾧ ὤφειλεν ἡ ἀλλοιωτικὴ δύναμις ἐνεργῆσαι, ἀλλὰ πρὸ ὥρας ἐξεῶσα φέρεται δίυγρον. ἢ δι' ἐνδεῆ ἀνάδοσιν. τί γάρ; ὅτι ἐνδεοῦς τῆς ἀναδόσεως γινομένης φέρεται καὶ ὁ χυλὸς καὶ ἐξυγραίνει τὸ διαχώρημα. ἢ διὰ κακοχυμίαν, ἀπὸ τοῦ παντὸς σώματος ἐπὶ τὴν γαστέρα συρρέουσαν· τὸ τηνικαῦτα γὰρ συνεκκρίνονται τῷ περιττώματι καὶ ἐξυγραίνουσιν αὐτό. ξηρὸν δὲ γίνεται τὸ διαχώρημα ἢ διὰ θερμὴν δυσκρασίαν τοῦ ἥπατος καὶ τῶν περὶ τὴν γαστέρα χωρίων, [καὶ] ἐκδαπανώσης τὸ ὑγρόν. ἢ διὰ πλημμελῆ βλάβην τῆς καθεκτικῆς δυνάμεως, πλέον τοῦ δέοντος κατέχουσα· τὸ τηνικαῦτα γὰρ ἀναδίδοται τὸ ὑγρόν, καὶ κερδαίνει τι ἐξ αὐτοῦ, καὶ ξηρὸν γίνεται τὸ διαχώρημα.

Τῆς δὲ κατὰ τὸν καιρόν, τοῦ πρὸ ὥρας ἐκκρίνεσθαι τὸ διαχώρημα αἰτία καθέστηκεν ἡ καθεκτικὴ δύναμις, διὰ πλημμελῆ βλάβην, πρὸ πέψεως ἐπεγειρομένη καὶ ἐξεῶσα πρὸ τοῦ δέοντος καιροῦ. ἢ διὰ πλημμελῆ βλάβην τῆς ἀποκριτικῆς, πρὸ ὥρας ἐπεγειρομένης καὶ ἀποκρινούσης τὸ διαχώρημα. ἢ δι' ἐπιρροὴν κακοχυμίας φερομένης ἐπὶ τὴν ἀποκριτικὴν δύναμιν καὶ μαστιζούσης αὐτήν, πρὸ ὥρας ἐπεγειρομένη πρωϊαίτερον ἐκκρίνει τὸ διαχώρημα.
151 ὀψιαίτερον δὲ ἀπωθεῖται ἡ κόπρος ἢ διὰ πλημμελῆ βλάβην τῆς καθε|κτικῆς δυνάμεως, πλέον τοῦ δέοντος κατέχουσα, τυχὸν μετὰ τὴν πέψιν. ἢ διὰ πλημμελῆ βλάβην τῆς ἀποκριτικῆς, μὴ ἐπεγειρομένης εἰς τὸν δέοντα καιρὸν καὶ ἀποκρινούσης τὸ διαχώρημα, ἀλλ' ἐμβραδυνούσης.

Ἀπὸ δὲ τοῦ χρώματος, ὅσον πρὸς ἑαυτὸ ἔδει λευκὸν εἶναι, ἐπειδὴ καὶ ἡ γαστὴρ καὶ τὰ ἔντερα λευκά εἰσιν, ἀλλὰ καὶ ὁ χυλὸς λευκός. ἀλλ' ἐπειδὴ δύο ἀγγεῖα ἀπὸ τῆς χοληδόχου κύστεως ἐκφύονται, καὶ τὸ μὲν μεῖζον φέρεται ἐπὶ τὰ ἔντερα, τὸ δὲ μικρότερον ἐπὶ τὴν γαστέρα χάριν τοῦ χρωννύειν τὴν κόπρον, διὰ τοῦτο δεῖ τὴν κόπρον ὑπόξανθον καὶ ὑπέρυθρον εἶναι.

Ἀπὸ δὲ τοῦ τρόπου τῆς ἐκκρίσεως, ὅτι δεῖ εὐφόρως ἐκκρίνεσθαι καὶ ὁμαλῶς. τὸ δὲ μετὰ τρυσμοῦ καὶ πνευμάτων καὶ τεινεσμῶν γίνεται τρόπῳ τοιούτῳ· τὸ μὲν μετὰ τρυσμοῦ δηλοῖ περιουσίαν φλέγματος ἐν τοῖς ἐντέροις καὶ ἐν τῷ ἀπευθυσμένῳ ἐγκειμένην· τηνικαῦτα γὰρ ἀποστενοῖ τὴν διέξοδον τοῦ διαχωρήματος· λοιπὸν καὶ προσαναλύει τι μέρος τοῦ φλέγματος, καὶ τῇ τοιαύτῃ κινήσει τίκτονται πνεύματά τινα καὶ ποιοῦσι τὸν τρυσμόν. τὸ δὲ μετὰ φυσῶν ἐκκρίνεσθαι δηλοῖ περιουσίαν πνευμάτων ἢ ὑπὸ ψυχρᾶς δυσκρασίας τῆς γαστρὸς γεννηθέντων ἢ διὰ τροφὰς τοιαύτας παρασχεθείσας. τὸ δὲ μετὰ τεινεσμοῦ ἐκκρίνεσθαι δηλοῖ ἢ φλεγμονὴν ἢ ἕλκος γινόμενον ἐν τοῖς τόποις ἐκείνοις. τί γάρ; ὅτι ἀπὸ τῆς φλεγμονῆς ἰχῶρές

2 δύναμις *om.* L διενεργῆσαι γ 3 *post* ἐνδεοῦς *add.* οὔσης L 5 συρρέουσι γ 8 καὶ *seclusi* ἐκδαπανώσης] *cf. e. g. supra, p. 170,28; infra, p. 194,32 sq.* 9 κατέχουσι γ 10 *post* αὐτοῦ *fort. excidit* τὸ σῶμα *vel sim.* 13 sq. πρὸ – βλάβην *om.* LM 14 ἐπεγειρομένη *scripsi*: ἐπεγειρομέν *(ambig.)* V: ἐπεγειρομένης P 16 *post* ἐπιρροὴν *add.* καὶ L μαστιζούσης] μὴ βασταζούσης L 17 ἐπεγειρομέν *(ambig.)* V: ἐπεγειρομένης P 19 τυχὸν] λοιπὸν γ 20 τῆς – ἐπεγειρομένης] τῆς ἐπεγειρομένης τῆς ἀποκριτικῆς δυνάμεως γ 23 ἐστιν γ 28 τῆς *post* δὲ *habent codd.*: *trsp. Dietz* 31 ἐν *om.* L ἐγκείμενα M: ἐγκείμενοι P: ἐγκείμεν *(ambig.)* V 32 προαναλύει γ 33 τινα] πολλὰ γ; *sed cf. infra, p. 174,15* 34 φυσῶν] φύσιν γ 35 ψυχρᾶς] χρᾶς L γεννηθέντα L

retentive faculty, when it fails to hold long enough for the converting faculty to go into action, but expels prematurely and (the excrement) passes soaking wet. Or due to defective distribution. Why? Because, the distribution being defective, the chyle also is carried along and it soaks the excrement. Or due to a flood of unwholesome humors to the stomach from all over the body; for these are then shed along with the residue and wet it thoroughly. The excrement becomes dry, on the other hand, either because of a hot distemper in the liver and in the areas around the stomach, which consumes the moisture. Or from a fault of irregularity in the retentive faculty, when it overretains; for in that event the moisture is distributed, (the body) obtains some of it (?) and the excrement becomes dry.

As for (irregularity) in time, premature passing of excrement is caused by a fault of irregularity in the retentive faculty, when it is roused before digestion and expels before the proper time. Or by a fault of irregularity in the excretory, when it is stimulated prematurely and passes the excrement. Or by an influx of bad humors which reaches the excretory faculty and stimulates it; then aroused before its time, it eliminates the excrement early. Delayed passing of the excrement, on the other hand, results either from a fault of irregularity in the retentive faculty, when it holds longer than it should, i.e. after digestion. Or from a fault of irregularity in the excretory, when it is not stimulated to pass the excrement at the proper time, but lags behind.

On the point of color, (excrement) considered on its own ought to be white, since the stomach and the intestines are white and the chyle too is white. But since two vessels grow out of the gallbladder, and the larger travels to the intestines and the smaller to the stomach, for the purpose of tinting the excrement, for this reason the excrement should be yellowish and reddish.

With regard to mode of excretion, (the matter) should be excreted easily and evenly. But passing accompanied by noise, wind and straining happens as follows: noisy elimination indicates an overabundance of phlegm lying in the intestines and rectum; for in that case it narrows the passageway of the excrement; then also a part of the phlegm dissolves and in this activity are produced certain gases which produce the noise. Passing with wind means an excess of gases produced either by a cold distemper of the stomach or by the provision of gassy foods. Elimination with straining indicates either inflammation or ulceration in those parts (mentioned above). Why? Because serous discharges from the inflamma-

τινες ἀποστάζουσιν ἐπὶ τὸ ἀπευθυσμένον καὶ δάκνουσι καὶ ποιοῦσι τεινεσμόν.

II 13 [11: 206,5 A. = II 134,15 L.] Τοιαύτης γὰρ ἐούσης τῆς διεξόδου ἡ κάτω κοιλίη ὑγιαίνοι ἄν.

Ἰστέον ὅτι κάτω κοιλίαν τὴν γαστέρα καὶ τὰ ἔντερα ἐκάλεσε νῦν πρὸς ἀντιδιαστολὴν τοῦ θώρακος. τί οὖν φησιν; ὅτι ἐὰν κατὰ φύσιν ὄντος τοῦ διαχωρήματος ἐν τῇ διεξόδῳ, ἡ γαστὴρ καὶ τὰ ἔντερα ὑγιῶς διάκεινται. πλὴν οὐκ ἀντιστρέφει· οὐδὲ γὰρ εἰ ὑγιῶς διάκεινται γαστὴρ καὶ τὰ ἔντερα,
152 ἤδη καὶ τὰ διαχωρήματα κατὰ φύσιν εἰσίν· | ἐνδέχεται γὰρ καὶ κακοχυμίαν τινὰ ἀπὸ τοῦ παντὸς σώματος συρρεῖν ἐπὶ τὴν γαστέρα ⟨καὶ τὰ ἔντερα⟩ καὶ ῥευματίζειν αὐτὰ καὶ ἐκκρίνεσθαι κακόχυμον.

II 14 [11: 206,6 A. = II 134,16 L.] Συμφέρει μήτε τρύζειν μήτε πυκνόν τε ἐὸν καὶ κατ' ὀλίγον διαχωρέειν.

Τὸ μετὰ τρυσμοῦ διαχώρημα κάκιστόν ἐστι· γίνεται γὰρ πνευμάτων τινῶν προσαναλυομένων καὶ συνεκκρινομένων τῷ διαχωρήματι. ἢ πολλάκις φλεγμονώδης τις ὄγκος ἐστὶ περὶ τὸ ἀπευθυσμένον, καὶ στενοχωρούμενον τὸ διαχώρημα μετὰ τρυσμοῦ διεξέρχεται.

Τοῦτο δὲ δεῖ εἰδέναι, ὅτι κατὰ τὸν νόμον τῶν συμπλοκῶν ἓξ γίνονται ἀντιθέσεις. καὶ αἱ μὲν δύο οὐ συνίστανται, αἱ δὲ λοιπαὶ τέσσαρες συνίστανται. καί εἰσιν αἱ συνιστάμεναι αὗται, πολλὰ πολλάκις, ὅπερ καὶ χειρίστη ἐστὶ πασῶν τῶν συζυγιῶν. τί γάρ; ὅτι καὶ τὸ πολλὰ κενοῦσθαι καταβάλλει τὴν δύναμιν, ἀλλὰ καὶ τὸ πολλάκις, τῇ συνεχεῖ ἐξαναστάσει καταβάλλεται ἡ δύναμις. πολλὰ ὀλιγάκις· αὕτη ἧττόν ἐστι κακόν· κατὰ γὰρ τὸ πολλὰ κενοῦσθαι καὶ μόνον λυπεῖ τὴν δύναμιν. εἶτα ὀλίγα πολλάκις· αὕτη πλεῖόν ἐστι χειρίστη, πλὴν καὶ αὕτη κατὰ μίαν ἀντίθεσιν λυπεῖ τὴν δύναμιν· τῇ γὰρ συνεχείᾳ τῆς ἐξαναστάσεως καταλύεται ἡ δύναμις. εἶτα ὀλίγα ὀλιγάκις· αὕτη πασῶν καλλίστη ἐστίν, ἐπειδὴ κατ' ἄμφω οὐ λυπεῖ τὴν δύναμιν. τὸ δὲ πολλὰ ὀλίγα καὶ τὸ πολλάκις ὀλιγάκις οὐ συνίστανται.

II 15 [11: 206,11 A. = II 136,6 L.] Παχύνεσθαι χρὴ τὸ διαχώρημα πρὸς τὴν κρίσιν ἰούσης τῆς νόσου.

Καλῶς ἔφη παχύνεσθαι καὶ οὐχὶ σκληρύνεσθαι· τὸ γὰρ παχὺ τῇ φύσει ἐστί, τὸ δὲ σκληρὸν ἐν δυσκρασίᾳ θεωρεῖται. τί οὖν ἔφη αὐτός; ὅτι ἐὰν λεπτόν ἐστι τὸ διαχώρημα, δεῖ παχύνεσθαι αὐτὸ ἐν τῇ κρίσει ἰούσης τῆς

5sq.] *cf.* Gal. In Hipp. Progn. comm. II 13: CMG V 9,2 p. 271,17–19 6 ὅτι – 11] *cf.* Gal. In Hipp. Progn. comm. II 13: CMG V 9,2 p. 271,19–24

4 κοιλία L ὑγιαίνη L 5 νῦν *om.* γ 8 εἰ *om.* γ διάκειται γ 9 καὶ[II] *om.* γ 10 καὶ τὰ ἔντερα *addidi* 11 αὐτὴν γ 12 *post* Συμφέρει *add.* δὲ L 13 ὂν L 14 κακόν γ 16 φλεγμαινώδης γ 21 καὶ] *fort.* κατὰ *scribendum est; cf. lin. 23sq. et 25* 24 εἶτα – 26 δύναμιν *om.* γ πολλάκις *scripsi*: ὀλιγάκις L 26 συνεχεῖ ἐξαναστάσει γ 27 αὕτη – 202,39 πνεύμονα *om.* L

tion drip into the rectum, sting it and produce straining.

II 13 For when the passage is like this, the lower cavity is in a healthy state.

Note that here he used lower cavity to indicate the stomach and intestines as distinct from the thorax. What, then, is he saying? If the excrement is normal in passage, the stomach and intestines are in a healthy state. The converse, however, does not hold; for even if the stomach and intestines are in good health, the excrements are not necessarily normal; you see, it is possible also for bad humors to flow together from all over the body into the stomach and intestines, subject them to a flux and cause an unwholesome discharge.

II 14 It is good to pass without noise, not frequently, and in small quantities.

Passing with noise is very bad; for it happens when certain gases are released and are passed out along with the excrement. Or many times there is an inflamed swelling around the rectum, and since the excrement is compressed, it passes out with a noise.

Now it should be noted that, going by the law of combinations, there are six (pairs of) opposites. And while two of these do not exist, the remaining four do exist. The (four) real ones are these: a large quantity frequently, and this is the worst of all the combinations. Why? Because not only does evacuation in large quantity destroy the power (of the body), but frequent evacuation too destroys the power because of the constant rising. A large quantity infrequently, which is less serious; for only evacuation in large quantity harasses the power. Next a small quantity frequently; and this is far worse, except that in this combination too (only) one of the opposites harasses the power; for the power is destroyed by the constant rising. Then a small quantity infrequently, which is the best combination of all, since it harasses the power with neither (of the opposites). A large quantity in small amounts and often infrequently do not exist.

II 15 The excrement should thicken as the disease advances to crisis.

He is right to say thicken and not harden, since thickness is normal, while hardness is observed in distemper. What was (Hippocrates) saying then? That if the excrement is thin, it should thicken as the disease

νόσου. σὺ δὲ εἰπὲ ὅτι «Ὥσπερ τὸ λεπτὸν παχύνεσθαι χρή, οὕτω καὶ τὸ
153 παχὺ δεῖ λεπτύνεσθαι, ἐν τῇ κρίσει | ἰούσης τῆς νόσου.» ἡ γὰρ φύσις ἐκ τῶν ἀντικειμένων σπουδάζει ἐπὶ τὸ σύμμετρον ἄγειν τοῦ λεπτοῦ καὶ παχέος.

II 16 [11: 206,13 A. = II 136,7 L.] Ἐπιτήδειον δὲ καὶ ἕλμινθας στρογγύλας διεξιέναι μετὰ τοῦ διαχωρήματος πρὸς τὴν κρίσιν ἰούσης τῆς νόσου.

Ἰστέον ὅτι μετὰ τῶν ἄλλων περιττωμάτων εἰ καὶ ἕλμινθες συνεκκρίνονται ἐν τῇ ἀκμῇ τοῦ νοσήματος, ἡνίκα πρὸς τὴν κρίσιν ἰούσης τῆς νόσου, ἀγαθόν ἐστι καὶ ὡς σημεῖον καὶ ὡς αἴτιον. καὶ ὡς μὲν σημεῖον, ὅτι δηλοῖ τὴν ὕλην ἐκκρινομένην, ὡς δὲ αἴτιον, ὅτι δηλοῖ ἀποκαθαίρεσθαι τὸ σῶμα ἀπὸ τῆς νοσοποιοῦ αἰτίας. εἰ δέ γε ἀπέπτου οὔσης τῆς ὕλης ἐκκρίνονται ἕλμινθες, κακόν ἐστι, τουτέστιν ἐν τῇ ἀρχῇ καὶ ἀναβάσει τοῦ νοσήματος· δηλοῖ γὰρ μεγίστην σηπεδόνα, καθ' ἣν αἱ ἕλμινθες γίνονται.

Καὶ ποιητικὸν μὲν αἴτιον τῶν ἑλμίνθων ἐστὶν αὐτὴ ἡ ἐπιφοιτῶσα διαπλαστικὴ δύναμις, καθ' ἣν γίνονται αἱ ἕλμινθες. ὑλικὸν δὲ οἱ ὠμοὶ καὶ παχεῖς χυμοί. ὀργανικὸν δέ, τοῦτο αἴτιον διάφορόν ἐστιν, ἐπειδὴ καὶ τὸ εἶδος τοῦ σχήματος τῶν ἑλμίνθων διάφορόν ἐστιν· αἱ μὲν γὰρ ἀσκαρίδες ἐν τῷ ἀπευθυσμένῳ γεννῶνται, αἱ δὲ πλατεῖαι ἐν τοῖς παχυτέροις ἐντέροις, αἱ δὲ στρογγύλαι ἐν τοῖς λεπτοῖς ἐντέροις. τελικὸν δὲ αἴτιον ἐν τοῖς παρὰ φύσιν οὐκ ἔστι ζητῆσαι, ἐπειδὴ οὐ συνίσταται.

Περὶ δὲ τοῦ σχήματος τῶν ἑλμίνθων πολλὴ διαφωνία γέγονεν. τινὲς γὰρ λέγουσιν ὅτι πρὸς τὴν θέσιν τῶν ἐντέρων σχηματίζονται, καὶ τοσοῦτον ὅτι καὶ ἀνεμοῦνται αἱ στρογγύλαι, ὡς ἂν ἐν τοῖς λεπτοῖς ἐντέροις γενομένων αὐτῶν. ἕτεροι δὲ λέγουσιν ὅτι καὶ αἱ πλατεῖαι ἀνεμοῦνται, εἰ καὶ σπανίως. διὸ ἕτεροί φασιν ὅτι, ἐὰν πρὸς τὴν θέσιν τῶν ἐντέρων σχηματίζωνται, οὐκοῦν ἔμφραξις γενήσεται ἤπερ ἕλμινθες. ἀλλὰ δεῖ εἰπεῖν ὅτι πρὸς τὴν θέσιν τῆς ὕλης σχηματίζονται αἱ ἕλμινθες καὶ τὰ ἔντερα συμβάλλονται
154 πρὸς τὸ σχῆμα· — ὡς ὀρ|γανικὸν συνεισάγουσί τι μέρος· — ὅθεν καὶ ὡς ἀκατίδες ἐκκρίνονται καὶ ἐκτὸς ἀπειλοῦνται.

Ἀλλ' ἴσως ἐρεῖ τις· «Διὰ τί μόνων τῶν στρογγύλων ἑλμίνθων ἐμνημόνευσεν ὁ Ἱπποκράτης, τὰς δὲ ἄλλας παρῆκε;» καὶ λέγομεν ὅτι ἀμφότεραι ὑπὸ παχείας ὕλης γίνονται. ἐνταῦθα μέντοι περὶ ὀξέος νοσήματος αὐτῷ ὁ λόγος· ἐν δὲ ὀξεῖ νοσήματι οὐκ ἔστιν εὑρεῖν τοσαύτην παχεῖαν ὕλην ὥστε ποιῆσαι πλατεῖαν ἕλμινθα ἢ ἀσκαρίδας, ἀλλ' ἐπ' ὀλίγον ἔστιν εὑρεῖν παχεῖαν τὴν ὕλην, καθ' ἣν αἱ στρογγύλαι γίνονται ἕλμινθες, καὶ διὰ τοῦτο

17–19] *cf.* Steph. Comm. in Hipp. Aph.: Escor. Σ. II. 10 fol. 49^r 19sq.] *cf.* Steph. Comm. in Hipp. Aph.: Escor. Σ. II. 10 fol. 48^r

4 ἑλμίνθ *(ambig., sic)* γ: *corr. Dietz* 7 ἕλμινθαι PV: *ambig.* M: *corr. Dietz* 8 ἡνίκα — ἰούσης] *cf. supra, p. 174,6* 11 τὸ *om.* M 12 ἕλμινθαι MP: ἕλμινθες *in* -οι *mut.* V: *correxi* 13 αἱ *om.* M 13 *et* 15 ἕλμινθοι γ: *correxi* 20 οὐ *om.* P 24 *post* εἰ *add.* δὲ M 25 σχηματίζονται P 26 *et* 27 ἕλμινθοι γ: *correxi* 28 *post* ὡς^{I} *add.* γὰρ P συνάγουσι P 29 εὐκατίδες V: ἀκτίδες P: *corr.* M 30 μόνον M 31 ἀμφότεροι γ: *correxi* 34 ἀσκαρίδες γ: *corr. Dietz* ἐπ'] μετ' V 35 ἕλμινθαι γ: *correxi* *post* ἕλμινθες *iter. linn. 34 sq.* ἢ — ἕλμινθες PV

goes to the crisis. But you may say that "Just as the thin should thicken, so should the thick also become thinner as the disease goes to crisis." For nature is concerned to go from the opposites to the right proportion of the thin and thick.

II 16 It is a favorable sign when round worms are passed in the excrement, as the disease advances to crisis.

Note that, if, along with the other residues, worms also are passed at the climax of the disease, as the disease advances to crisis, this is good both as a symptom and as a cause. As a symptom, because it means that the matter is being eliminated, and as a cause, since it indicates that the body is getting rid of the disease-producing cause. But if worms are passed when the matter is still unconcocted, it is a bad symptom, i.e. at the beginning and during the heightening of the disease; for it means serious putrefaction which is responsible for the worms.

The efficient cause of worms, by which they come to be, is the formative faculty itself frequenting (the body). The material (cause), the crude and dense humors. Organically there are various causes, since the kind of worms' shapes too is varied; for ascarides are produced in the rectum, flat (worms) in the large intestines and the round in the small intestines. As for the final cause, we do not look for one in abnormal conditions, since none exists.

On the question of shape of worms there is a lot of disagreement. For some claim that they are shaped according to the layout of the intestines; and (they have a point) in so far as the round are vomited, implying that they are formed in the small intestines. But others say that the flat too are vomited, even if rarely. Hence others say that, if their shape is determined by the layout of the intestines, surely there will be a blockage rather than worms. But it must be stated that the worms are shaped according to the structure of the matter and the intestines contribute to the shape; – as the organic cause they contribute a part; – hence too they are passed like millepedes and unroll outside.

But someone may remark, "Why did Hippocrates mention only the round worms, leaving out the others?" We reply that both (the round and the others) are produced by thick matter. Here, however, he is discussing acute disease; and in acute disease it is not possible to find matter of the thickness sufficient for producing the flat worm or ascarides, but it is possible to find matter of the slight thickness by which the round

αὐτῶν ἐμνημόνευσεν ὁ Ἱπποκράτης, ὡς ἂν ὑπὸ ἥττονος παχείας ὕλης γινόμεναι.

II 17 [11: 207,1 A. = II 136,9 L.] Λαπαρήν τε εἶναι τὴν κοιλίην καὶ εὔογκον

Καλῶς τὸ λαπαρὴν εἶναι τὴν κοιλίην καὶ εὔογκον ἐπαινεῖ· τὸ γὰρ λαπαρόν ἐστι τὸ ὁμαλὸν καὶ τὸ μαλακόν, ὅπερ ἀντίκειται τῷ συντεταμένῳ· τὸ δὲ εὔογκον δηλοῖ τὸ εὔσαρκον, ᾧπερ ἀντίκειται τὸ συντετηκός. ταῦτα οὖν βέλτιόν ἐστιν ἐν ταῖς νόσοις θεωρεῖσθαι, ὥς φησι καὶ ἐν Ἀφορισμοῖς, ὅτι «Ὁκόσοισι περὶ τὸν ὀμφαλὸν καὶ τὸ ἦτρον πάχος ἔχειν, βέλτιόν ἐστι, τὸ δὲ σφόδρα λεπτὸν καὶ ἐκτετηκός, μοχθηρόν.»

V

II 18 [11: 207,1 A. = II 136,10 L.] Ὑδαρὲς δὲ κάρτα ἢ λευκὸν ἢ χλωρὸν ἰσχυρῶς ἢ ἀφρῶδες διαχωρέειν, πονηρὰ ταῦτα.

Νῦν περὶ τοῦ παρὰ φύσιν διαχωρήματος διαλέγεται, καὶ παραδίδωσιν ἡμῖν τρεῖς διαφοράς. καὶ τέως λέγει διαφορὰν τοιαύτην, ὅτι, ἐὰν τὸ διαχώρημα ὑδαρές ἐστιν ἢ λευκὸν ἢ ὠχρὸν ἢ ἀφρῶδες, πονηρά ἐστι ταῦτα πάντα. καὶ ἡ αἰτία ἑκάστου δήλη· τὸ μὲν ὑδαρὲς ⟨δηλοῖ⟩ ἀποτυχίαν τῆς χυλοποιήσεως καὶ χυμώσεως καὶ τῆς πέψεως, καὶ τὸν πρέποντα κόσμον οὐκ ἐδέξατο· τὸ δὲ λευκὸν δηλοῖ ἔμφραξιν τῶν ἀπὸ τῆς χοληδόχου κύστεως
155 φερομένων ἀγγείων ἐπὶ γαστέρα, καὶ διὰ τοῦτο οὐ φέρεται χολὴ ἐπὶ | τὴν γαστέρα καὶ λευκὸν ἐκκρίνεται τὸ διαχώρημα. τὸ δὲ χλωρὸν δύο σημαίνει, ἢ τὸ ὠχρὸν ἢ τὸ ἰῶδες, ἅπερ καὶ ταῦτα κάκιστά ἐστι· δηλοῦσι γὰρ ἢ ἐπιρροὴν χολώδους ὕλης ἐπὶ τὴν γαστέρα ἢ ἐν αὐτῇ τῇ γαστρὶ γινομένην κατὰ περιουσίαν καὶ οὕτως ἐκκρινόμενα. τὸ δὲ ἀφρῶδες, καὶ τοῦτο διττόν ἐστι· γίνεται γὰρ ἀφρῶδες ἢ ὑπὸ πνευμάτων τινῶν συναναπλεκομένων ὑγρῷ καὶ ὑμενούντων αὐτό· γίνεται ἀφρῶδες καὶ ὑπὸ θερμότητος, καθάπερ καὶ ἐπὶ τῶν ἐκτὸς ἔστιν ἰδεῖν, ὅτι ἀφρὸς γεννᾶται ὑπὸ πνευμάτων, ἡνίκα δραστήριος ἄνεμος πνεύσῃ ἐπὶ τὴν θάλασσαν, συναναπλέκεται τῷ ὕδατι καὶ ὑμενοῦται αὐτὸ καὶ γίνεται ἀφρὸς ἐν τοῖς κύμασιν. ὑπὸ δὲ τῆς θερμότητος γίνεται ἀφρός, καθάπερ ἐπὶ τῶν ζωμευομένων κρεῶν ἐν τοῖς χαλκίοις ἢ ἐν ταῖς χύτραις τῇ περιουσίᾳ τῆς θερμότητος ἀφρὸς γίνεται.

Λέγει δὲ καὶ δευτέραν διαφορὰν τῶν παρὰ φύσιν διαχωρημάτων, ἥτις καὶ μᾶλλόν ἐστι χειρίστη. καί φησιν ὅτι κάκιστά ἐστι διαχωρήματα, ἡνίκα

5 τὸ[II]–7] *cf.* Gal. In Hipp. Progn. comm. II 19: CMG V 9,2 p. 275,16sq. 8 ἐν Ἀφορισμοῖς] Hipp. Aph. II 35: IV p. 480,10–12 L. 17 τὸ – 31] *cf.* Gal. In Hipp. Progn. comm. II 20: CMG V 9,2 p. 276,1–10 26–31] *cf.* Steph. Comm. in Hipp. Aph.: Ambros. S 19 sup. fol. 52[r]

1 αὐτῶν *om.* M 5 κοιλίαν V 7 ὅπερ γ: *corr. Dietz* 8 βελτίονα V 9 καὶ] ἢ P 17 δηλοῖ *coni. Dietz* 24 καὶ[I]] κἂν M ἐκκρινόμενα P: *ambig.* MV 27 *ante* ὑπὸ *add.* καὶ M 28 πλεύσει γ: *corr. Dietz* συναναπλέκονται PV: *corr.* M: συναναπλέκοντος *coni. Dietz* 29 ὑμενοῦται *scripsi*: ὑμενοῦντος M: ὑμενοῦσιν V: ὑμένου *(sic)* P δὲ *om.* V 30 ζωμένων P 32 περὶ P

worms are produced; this is why Hippocrates mentioned them, as being produced from matter of a lesser thickness.

II 17 The belly should be slack and well-rounded

He does well to praise the slack and well-rounded belly; for slack means even and soft, which is the opposite of taut, while well-rounded stands for fullness of flesh, the opposite of emaciated. It is better, then, when these are observed in diseases, as he says in the Aphorisms also, that "It is better to have the umbilical area and lower abdomen filled out; when they are very thin and emaciated, it is a bad sign."

V

II 18 If the excrements are very watery or white or very green or frothy, they are bad.

At this point he discusses abnormal excrement, and he teaches us three varieties. And first he mentions this variety, that if the excrement is watery or white or pale yellow or frothy, these are all bad. And the cause of each is evident; the watery indicates failure of conversion to chyle and humor and of digestion, and it has not received its proper composition; the white points to a stoppage in the vessels leading from the gallbladder to the stomach; as a result, no bile is conveyed to the stomach and the excrement is passed white. Green stands for two colors, either pale yellow or verdigris, both of which also are very bad; for they mean either a flow of bilious humor to the stomach or an overflow arising in the stomach itself, and so (the excrement) is passed (with these colors). As for the frothy, it also comes about in two ways; for the frothy is produced either by gases, when they combine with moisture and coat it with a film; or it becomes frothy under the influence of heat, just as also in the case of external phenomena it can be seen that froth is produced by winds: when a strong gust blows on the sea it mixes with the water, covers it with a film and froth appears on the waves. And froth is created by heat, just as when meat is being boiled for soup in cauldrons or pots the superabundance of heat produces a froth.

He mentions also a second variety of abnormal excrements, which is much worse. He says that the excrements are worst when the excrement

ὀλίγον ἕπεται τὸ διαχώρημα καὶ λευκὸν καὶ γλίσχρον καὶ ὑπόχλωρον καὶ λεῖον. αὕτη δὲ ἡ διαφορὰ διττὴν ἔχει τὴν ἰδέαν· ἑκάστη δὲ ἰδέα ἐπὶ ἐκτήξει τῆς πιμελῆς γίνεται. ἡ δὲ αἰτία ἡ ἑτέρα ἐστὶν ἡ κατ' ἐπίτασιν ἔκτηξις τῆς πιμελῆς, ἥτις ἐστὶ τὸ ὑπόχλωρον καὶ λεῖον. κατ' ἐπίτασιν τῆς πιμελῆς γίνεται ἡ ἔκτηξις, καὶ οἷον ἐπὶ παλαιοπαθείᾳ ⟨καὶ προγεγενημένῃ⟩ ἐκτήξει τῆς πιμελῆς γίνεται. οὕτως γὰρ ἐὰν ἀποτεθῇ στέαρ ἢ πιμελή, χλωρὸν γίνεται ἤγουν ὠχρόν· οὕτως οὖν καὶ ἐνταῦθα, ἐὰν ὑπόχλωρον εἴη τὸ διαχώρημα, ἐπὶ προγεγενημένῃ ἐκτήξει καὶ παλαιοπαθείᾳ τῆς πιμελῆς γίνεται. εἰ δὲ μὴ τὸ χλωρὸν τὸ ὠχρὸν νοήσωμεν. ἀλλὰ καὶ τὸ ἰῶδες τῷ αὐτῷ γίνεται τρόπῳ. τὸ δὲ λεῖον γίνεται, ἡνίκα κατὰ πᾶν ἑαυτὸ ἀλλοιωθῇ καὶ ὁμαλὸν γένηται. ἀλλὰ τὸ λεῖον ἢ κατὰ φύσιν γίνεται ἢ παρὰ φύσιν. καὶ τὸ μὲν κατὰ φύσιν ⟨. . .⟩, ὥσπερ ἡ χυλοποίησις καὶ ἡ ἐξαιμάτωσις·
156 ταῦτα γὰρ κατὰ πάντα λεῖα καὶ ὁμαλὰ γίνονται τῆς ἀλλοιωτι|κῆς ἰσχυσάσης. τὸ δὲ παρὰ φύσιν λεῖον κάκιστόν ἐστι· δηλοῖ γὰρ δραστήριον τὴν νοσοποιὸν αἰτίαν, καθὸ ἴσχυσε πᾶσαν τὴν ὕλην πρὸς τὴν ἑαυτῆς κακίαν ἐκλειῶσαι. διὸ οὐ δεῖ ἐν τοῖς παρὰ φύσιν κατὰ πᾶν ἑαυτὸ λεῖον εἶναι τὸ διαχώρημα, ἀλλὰ κατά τι καὶ ἀδρομερὲς ἔχειν· δηλοῖ γὰρ ὅτι κατά τι μὲν ἐκρατήθη ἡ δύναμις, λέγω δὴ κατὰ τὸ λεῖον, κατά τι δὲ κρατεῖ, λέγω δὴ κατὰ τὸ ἀδρομερές.

Τὸ δὲ γλίσχρον διαχώρημα γίνεται ἐπὶ τῇ ἐκτήξει τῆς πιμελῆς, ἀλλ' ἔστιν ὅτε διαχώρημα γλίσχρον γίνεται, ἡνίκα καὶ τὰ ἐδηδεσμένα, τυχὸν αἱ παρεχόμεναι τροφαὶ φύσει γλίσχραι ὦσι· τὸ τηνικαῦτα γὰρ γίνεται γλίσχρον τὸ διαχώρημα. διακρίνομεν δὲ τοῦτο τῇ ποσότητι· εἰ μὲν γὰρ διὰ τὴν ἔκτηξιν τῆς πιμελῆς γένηται γλίσχρον τὸ διαχώρημα, κατ' ὀλίγον γίνεται ἡ ἔκκρισις· εἰ δὲ διὰ τὴν φύσιν τῶν τροφῶν, ἀθρόως γίνεται ἡ διέξοδος τῶν γλίσχρων διαχωρημάτων.

'Αλλ' ἴσως ἀπορεῖ τις λέγων ὅτι «'Ενδέχεταί ποτε καὶ ⟨διὰ⟩ δραστήριον καὶ ἐπιτεταμένην ἔκτηξιν τῆς πιμελῆς γενέσθαι ἀθρόαν ἔκκρισιν τῶν γλίσχρων διαχωρημάτων.» ἀλλὰ λέγομεν ὅτι τοῦτο διαστέλλομεν τῇ δυσωδίᾳ· εἰ μὲν γὰρ διὰ τὴν ἔκτηξιν τῆς πιμελῆς γίνεται ἀθρόα ἡ ἔκκρισις τῶν γλίσχρων διαχωρημάτων, δυσωδέστατά εἰσιν· εἰ δὲ διὰ τὴν φύσιν τῶν παρεχομένων τροφῶν, οὐκ εἰσὶ δυσώδη οὕτως· εἰ δὲ διὰ παχεῖς καὶ ὠμοὺς χυμούς – ἐνδέχεται γὰρ καὶ τοιούτους ἐκκρίνεσθαι καὶ γλίσχρα τὰ διαχωρήματα –, ἀλλὰ καὶ ἐπὶ τούτων ἧττον μετέχουσι δυσωδίας.

Λέγει δὲ καὶ τρίτην ἰδέαν διαχωρημάτων, καί φησιν ὅτι τὰ μέλανα διαχωρήματα καὶ τὰ πελιδνὰ καὶ τὰ ἰώδη καὶ τὰ κάκοσμα δηλοῦσι μεγίστην σηπεδόνα. τὸ μὲν γὰρ μέλαν διαχώρημα δηλοῖ περιουσίαν τῆς μελαίνης χολῆς, ἀλλ' ὑφειμένως καὶ ἐπ' ἔλαττον· τὸ δὲ ἰῶδες πάλιν περιουσίαν

2–9] *cf.* Gal. In Hipp. Progn. comm. II 21: CMG V 9,2 p. 276,13–23 10sq.] *cf.* Gal. In Hipp. Progn. comm. II 21: CMG V 9,2 p. 277,1sq. 20–34] *cf.* Gal. In Hipp. Progn. comm. II 21: CMG V 9,2 p. 277,9–16 *et* Schol. R *ad* p. 276,23

1 ἕπεται ὀλίγον M 5 καὶ προγεγενημένῃ *add. Wk.* (*cf. infra, lin. 8*) 10 ἑαυτῷ γ: *correxi* 11 γένηται] γίνεται P 12 *lacunam indicavi; exciderunt* λεῖον ἀγαθόν ἐστι· δηλοῖ γὰρ τὰς πέψεις γινομένας κατὰ φύσιν *vel sim.* 14 λεῖον *om.* M 15 καθ' ὃν γ: *corr. Dietz* 16 οὐ *om.* V πάντα ἑαυτῷ γ: *corr. Wk.* 23 ποιότητι γ: *correxi* 27 διὰ *add. Dietz*

is small, white, viscous, greenish and smooth. And this variety has two forms; and each form is caused by melting of soft fat. In the one, that of greenish and smooth, the cause is an intense melting of soft fat. The melting of the soft fat is intense and (this type of excrement) results, so to speak, from an old affection and a pre-existing melting of soft fat. For just as suet or lard when kept turn green or pale yellow, so here also, if the excrement is greenish, the cause is a pre-existing melting and an old affection of soft fat. And if not green, we will find it pale yellow. The verdigris, too, is produced in the same way. The smooth, on the other hand, is found when (the excrement) has been converted throughout itself and has become even. Now, smoothness is either normal or abnormal. The normal . . ., namely conversion to chyle and blood formation; for these become completely smooth and even when the converting (faculty) is strong. The abnormal smooth, for its part, is very bad, since it means that the disease-producing cause is potent to the extent that it was able to reduce all the matter to its own unnatural condition. Because of this the excrement in abnormal conditions should not be smooth throughout itself, but should have some coarseness too; for it indicates that while the faculty has been overcome in one respect, namely smoothness, it has prevailed in another, I mean with regard to coarseness.

Viscous excrement is caused by melting of soft fat, but sometimes an excrement is made viscous when the victuals, i.e. the foods given, also are of a viscous nature; for in that case the excrement becomes viscous. And we distinguish this type by the quantity; for if the cause of viscosity of the excrement is melting of fat, the evacuation is slight; but if the nature of the foods is responsible, there is copious passing of the viscous excrements.

But perhaps someone will raise a problem and say, "It is sometimes also possible for a strong and intense melting of soft fat to produce a copious discharge of viscous excrements." We reply that we tell the difference from the malodor; for if the discharge of viscous excrements is copious because of the melting of soft fat, they are most fetid; but if because of the nature of the food given, they are not so fetid; and if the cause is thick and crude humors – since these, too, can be passed and make the excrements viscous –, the odor is less foul here also.

He distinguishes a third variety of excrements saying that excrements which are black or livid or verdigris or fetid point to very great putrefaction. For the black excrement means that there is an overabundance of black bile, but one which is moderate and slight; again, the

τῆς ἰώδους χολῆς δηλοῖ· τὰ δὲ κάκοσμα καὶ ἰώδη διαχωρήματα, ὡς προείρηται, δηλοῦσι μεγίστην σηπεδόνα. ταῦτα δὲ ἔστιν ὅτε ἕκαστον ἰδίᾳ καὶ
157 χωρὶς ἐκκρίνονται· ἔστι δὲ ὅτε καὶ συμπλέκονται ἀλλήλοις, ἡνίκα | λέγονται καὶ πολυποίκιλα, ἡνίκα καὶ αἷμα σύνεστι καὶ ξύσματα λευκὰ καὶ μέλανα καὶ ἀφρώδη. παγκάκιστόν ἐστι τὸ τοιοῦτον διαχώρημα· δηλοῖ γὰρ εὐθέως ὅτι χρονίσαι ἔχει τὸ νόσημα. δηλοῖ γὰρ καὶ διάφορα πάθη, ἐπειδὴ καὶ διάφοροι κακοχυμίαι, καθ' ἣν πολυποίκιλα τὰ διαχωρήματα ἐκκρίνονται, ἀλλὰ καὶ περισπασμὸν τῆς φύσεως· [ἐκκρίνονται καὶ] περιδονεῖται γὰρ πρὸς ἑκάστην κακοχυμίαν, ὅπερ παγκάκιστόν ἐστι. χρόνιον δέ, ὅτι καὶ θερμὰ ἐκκρίνονται καὶ ψυχρά, καὶ τῇ ψύξει χρονίαν ἐνδείκνυται τὴν νόσον.

Λέγει καὶ τετάρτην [τὴν] διαφοράν, ὅτι τὰ διαχωρήματα πάντως μετὰ πνευμάτων ἐκκρίνονται ἢ ἐπέχονται. καὶ ἐκκρινόμενα ἢ μετὰ ψόφου ἐκκρίνονται ἢ ἀψοφητί. καὶ εἰ μὲν μετὰ ψόφου, δηλοῦσιν ἢ παραφροσύνην ἢ μεγίστην ὀδύνην οὖσαν ἐν τοῖς ὑποχονδρίοις, εἰ μή τι ὁ ἄρρωστος ἑκὼν μετὰ ψόφου ἐκκρίνει· τότε γὰρ οὐδὲν δηλοῦσιν. πλὴν δεῖ εἰδέναι ὅτι τινὲς τῶν ἀνθρώπων ἀναισχυντοῦντες καὶ μὴ ποιούμενοι λόγον, ἐπὶ οἱουδήποτε προσώπου τύχῃ, μετὰ ψόφου ἀπολύουσι τὰ πνεύματα, ὡς εἴρηται, μηδένα λόγον προσποιούμενοι, ἀλλ' ἀναιδῶς ἀπολύουσι τὰ πνεύματα μετὰ ψόφου τινός. τινὲς δὲ αἰδέσιμοι καὶ λόγον ποιούμενοι τῶν θεωρούντων αἰσχυνόμενοι μᾶλλον ἐπέχουσι τὰ πνεύματα καὶ αἱροῦνται κινδύνοις περιπεσεῖν ἤπερ μετὰ ψόφου ἐᾶσαι ἢ ἀπολῦσαι τὰ πνεύματα. ἐὰν οὖν τις τῶν αἰδεσίμων ἀνθρώπων ἐν τῷ νοσεῖν μετὰ ψόφου ἀπολύει τὰ πνεύματα, ἔσο γινώσκων ἢ παραφροσύνην ὁ τοιοῦτος ἢ ὀδύνην μεγίστην ἐνδείκνυται, καθ' ἣν ἐπικήδεται ἀπολύειν ψοφώδη πνεύματα, ὥστε παρηγορηθῆναι αὐτὸν ἐκ τῆς ὀδύνης. εἰ δέ γέ ἐστιν ἐκ τῶν ἀναισχύντων [καὶ ἀδεσίμων] καὶ μὴ ποιούντων λόγον, ἀλλ' ἐν συνηθείᾳ ἐστὶ τοῦ μετὰ ψόφου ἀπολύειν τὰ πνεύματα, οὐδὲν κερδαίνεις ἐκ τῆς σημειώσεως ταύτης· οὐδὲ γὰρ συμβάλλεταί σοι πρὸς εὔκλειαν. δεῖ δὲ εἰδέναι ὅτι ἐν τῷ καθόλου τὰ μετὰ ψόφου πνεύματα ἐκκρινόμενα ἐν-
158 δείκνυνται ἢ παχέα πνεύματα ἐκκρι|νόμενα ἢ στενοχωρίαν τῶν ὀργάνων, δι' ὧνπερ διεξέρχονται τὰ πνεύματα. τί γάρ; ὅτι παχέων ὄντων τῶν διεξερχομένων πνευμάτων, ἐν τῇ διεξόδῳ στενοχωρούμενα καὶ ὡς ἀπὸ στενοῦ διεξερχόμενα διὰ τοῦ ἀπευθυσμένου ψόφον ἀπεργάζονται. κάλλιον οὖν ἐστι τὰ πνεύματα διεξέρχεσθαι καὶ ἐκκρίνεσθαι ἤπερ ἐπέχεσθαι· ἐπεχόμενα γὰρ τὰ πνεύματα μεγάλας ὀδύνας ἐμποιοῦσι καὶ ἐπάρματα ἀπεργάζονται. ὀδύνας μέν, ἐπεχόμενα τῇ τάσει· τῇ γὰρ τάσει κίνδυνός ἐστι τοῦ ἀπορραγῆναι καὶ λυθῆναι τὴν συνέχειαν τῶν μορίων· τὰ δὲ κυρτώματα ἤγουν τὰ ἐπάρματα τῇ ἐποχῇ τῶν πνευμάτων γίνονται, ἡνίκα ἐμφραγῶσι

5 δηλοῖ — 7 ἐκκρίνονται] *cf.* Gal. In Hipp. Progn. comm. II 23: CMG V 9,2 p. 278,3–6 13–21] *cf.* Gal. In Hipp. Progn. comm. II 24: CMG V 9,2 p. 278,12–22 28 sq.] *cf.* Gal. In Hipp. Progn. comm. II 24: CMG V 9,2 p. 278,19sq.

2 ὅτι PV: *corr.* M 7 sq. ἀλλὰ — ἐκκρίνονται *om.* M 8 ἐκκρίνονται καὶ *seclusi* 11 τὴν *om.* M, *seclusi* 13 *post* ἐκκρίνονται *add.* ἢ ἐπέχονται P 14 ὁ ἑκὼν ἄρρωστος PV: *trsp.* M 18 ἀποδύουσι V 18 sq. μετὰ ψόφου τινός *post* ἀναιδῶς *trsp.* M 21 ψήφου P 24 ἀπολύον M 25 καὶ ἀδεσίμων *(sic)* PV: *om.* M, *seclusi* 26 εἰσὶν γ: *correxi* τοῦ] τὸ γ: *corr. Dietz* 28 ἐνδείκνυται M 29 στενόχωρα γ: *corr. Dietz* 30 τῶν *om.* M

verdigris means an overabundance of verdigris-colored bile; the fetid and verdigris excrements, as already mentioned, are signs of serious putrefaction. Now these excrements are passed sometimes separately and individually; at other times in combination with one another, in which case they are also designated much-variegated, when there is a mixture of blood with white, black and frothy scrapings. Such an excrement is extremely bad, being an immediate indication that the disease will be chronic. It also points to the presence of various affections, since the unwholesome humors, which cause the passing of much-variegated excrements, are also of different kinds; further, it shows that nature is distracted; for she goes around from one unwholesome humor to another, which is an extremely dangerous sign. (Now such excrement means) a chronic (illness) because both hot and cold matter is eliminated and coldness shows that the disease is chronic.

He gives a fourth variety (and says) that excrements in every case are either passed with wind or retained with it. And if passed, they are passed either with noise or silently. If with noise, it means either delirium or severe pain in the hypochondria, unless the patient passes with noise intentionally, in which case it shows nothing. However, one should be aware that some people have no shame and show no regard, but no matter in whose presence they may be, they let off wind with a noise; they have no consideration, as we have said, but shamelessly release the wind with a noise. Others, however, have decency and, showing regard for those around them, they hold the wind out of a sense of shame and choose to fall into dangers rather than let off or release the wind with noise. If, then, one of those with decency releases wind with noise during illness, this will tell you that he is delirious or that he has an intense pain, which makes him want to release wind with noise, in order to get relief from the pain. But if he is one of those who have no shame or regard for others and is in the habit of letting off wind with noise, the observation will not help you in any way, not even to enhance your reputation. It should be noted that, in general, wind passed with noise means either that the gases being passed are dense or that the organs through which the gases emerge are constricted. Why? Because, when the emerging gases are dense, they are compressed on the way out, and since they pass out from a narrow space through the rectum, they make a noise. It is better, then, for wind to pass out and be eliminated than to be retained. For gases held inside cause intense pains and produce swellings. Pains, because they are retained under pressure; for the strain threatens to rupture and destroy the integrity of the parts; bulges or swellings, on the other hand, are created by retained gases when they become blocked up and closed inside the

τὰ πνεύματα καὶ στεχθῶσιν ἐν τοῖς ὑποχονδρίοις. τὰς οὖν ὀδύνας καὶ τὰ ἐπάρματα οἱ ψόφοι τῶν πνευμάτων καὶ οἱ βορβορυγμοὶ λύουσι. κάλλιόν ἐστι τὰ πνεύματα μετὰ ψόφου ἐκκρινόμενα, μετὰ κόπρου καὶ οὔρου ἐκκρίνεσθαι μᾶλλον· δηλοῖ γὰρ ὅτι πάντα τὰ περιττώματα ἐκκρίνονται καὶ οὐδὲν ὑπολέλειπται αἴτιον τὸ ὀφεῖλον ἐνδελεχῆσαι.

II 19 [11: 207,5 A. = II 138,2 L.] Τὰ δὲ ποικίλα χρονιώτερα μὲν τουτέων, ὀλέθρια δὲ οὐδὲν ἧττον.

Φησὶν ὁ ἐξηγητὴς ὅτι «Οὐ προσδέχομαι τὸ λέγειν τὸν Ἱπποκράτην ὅτι τὰ ποικίλα διαχωρήματα χρονιώτερά ἐστιν ὅλως· ἐπὰν ποικίλα, αὐτόθι ἐπίκειται ὁ θάνατος. ἀλλ' οὐδὲ τοῦτο δέχομαι, τὸ λέγειν αὐτὸν ὅτι τὰ ποικίλα διαχωρήματα διαφόρους ἐνδείκνυνται διαθέσεις, ἐπειδὴ διάφορός ἐστιν ἡ κακοχυμία· ἐνδέχεται γὰρ μίαν διάθεσιν ὑποκεῖσθαι καὶ ποικίλα ἐκκρίνεσθαι διαχωρήματα. οὕτως γὰρ ὑπόκειται εἷς πυρετὸς καὶ τῷ χρόνῳ κατὰ μέρος διάφορον ἐγέννησε κακοχυμίαν. οὕτως οὖν καὶ ἐπὶ τῶν ἐκτὸς ἔστιν ἰδεῖν, ὅτι ἑνὸς ὄντος τοῦ πυρὸς ἐν τῷ ἕψειν τὰ φάρμακα τῷ χρόνῳ διάφορον χρῶμα ἀναδέχεται πρὸς τὴν ἕψησιν.»

II 20 [11: 207,10 A. = II 138,10 L.] Τοὺς δὲ ἐκ τῶν ὑποχονδρίων πόνους τε καὶ τὰ κυρτώματα, ἢν νεαρά τε εἴη καὶ μὴ σὺν φλεγμονῇ, λύει βορβορυγμὸς ἐπιγενόμενος

Δεῖ εἰδέναι ὅτι κυρτώματα καλεῖ ὁ Ἱπποκράτης τὰ ἐπάρματα
159 ἤγουν τὰ οἰδήματα· οὕτω γὰρ εἴωθεν ὁ Ἱπ|ποκράτης πάντα ὄγκον οἴδημα ὀνομάζειν. ἐὰν οὖν ἔστιν ἔπαρμα ἤγουν οἴδημα νεαρόν, τουτέστι πρόσφατον, βορβορυγμὸς γενόμενος λύει τὸ οἴδημα καὶ τὸ ἔπαρμα τῇ ὑποχαλάσει διαφορουμένων τῶν πνευμάτων τῶν ἄνευ φλεγμονῆς· ἡ γὰρ φλεγμονὴ ἐπὶ παχείᾳ ὕλῃ γίνεται, καὶ ὁ βορβορυγμὸς οὐ λύει ἐπιγενόμενος. ἀλλὰ καὶ τὸ οἴδημα τὸ χρονιώτερον οὐ λύει, ἐπειδὴ τῷ χρόνῳ προσλαμβάνει ὑγρότητά τινα. ἀλλὰ δεῖ αὐτό, ὡς εἴρηται, πρόσφατον εἶναι, ἤγουν τὸ ἔπαρμα, καὶ νεαρόν· τότε γὰρ οἱ βορβορυγμοὶ ἐπιγενόμενοι λύουσιν αὐτό.

VI

II 21 [12: 208,4 A. = II 138,15 L.] Οὖρον γὰρ ἄριστόν ἐστιν, ὅταν λευκή τε ἡ ὑπόστασις εἴη καὶ λείη καὶ ὁμαλὴ παρὰ πάντα τὸν χρόνον

2–5] *cf.* Gal. In Hipp. Progn. comm. II 25: CMG V 9,2 p. 279,16–18 8–12] *cf. supra*, p. 182,3–7 20–24] *cf.* Gal. In Hipp. Progn. comm. II 25: CMG V 9,2 p. 279,7–10 21 sq.] *cf. supra*, p. 126,19

1 στεχθῶσιν *ex* τεχθῶσιν *corr.* P: τεχθῶσιν M: στερχθῶσιν V οὖν *om.* M 3 κόπρου *scripsi (cf. Hipp., p. 208,1 A.)*: ψόφου γ 14 καὶ *om.* M 22 ὀνομάζειν] καλέειν M ἐπάρματα γ: *correxi* 27 δεῖ] δὴ γ: *corr. Dietz* 31 γὰρ] δὲ *Hipp.* ἐστιν ἄριστον V

hypochondria. Both pains and swellings, then, are relieved if the wind is passed with noise and rumbling. It is better to eliminate wind with noise, but more so to pass it along with feces and urine; for this shows that all the residues are being evacuated and no cause has been left behind which would continue (to create trouble).

II 19 Variegated (excrements) indicate an illness longer than these, but are no less dangerous.

The commentator says, "I do not agree with Hippocrates' assertion that the variegated excrements always mean prolonged illness; for, if they are variegated, there is an immediate threat of death. Nor do I accept his claim that variegated excrements indicate different conditions caused by the variety of unwholesome humors; for it is possible for variegated excrements to be passed when there is a single underlying condition. Thus there is one fever, but through time it has created in turn a variety of unwholesome humors. We see this also in external phenomena, that in boiling drugs there is one fire, but through time, they assume a different color relative to the boiling."

II 20 Pains and bulges in the hypochondria, if recent and free from inflammation, are relieved when rumbling supervenes

Note that by bulges Hippocrates means swellings or tumors; for Hippocrates has the habit of calling any swelling a tumor. If, then, there is a swelling or tumor which is recent, i.e. fresh, a supervening rumbling will cure the tumor or swelling; it releases pressure by dispersing the gases (of swellings) free from inflammation; for inflammation is produced by dense matter and a supervening rumbling will not remove it. Neither will it end a tumor of some standing, since it accumulates a certain moisture with the passage of time. Rather it, i.e. the swelling, as we have said, should be fresh and recent, in which case it will be relieved by supervening rumblings.

VI

II 21 Urine is best when the sediment is white, smooth and even all along

Νῦν περὶ τῶν οὔρων διαλαμβάνει. τὸ δὲ οὖρον, ὡς ἴσμεν, περίττωμά ἐστι τῆς δευτέρας πέψεως. καὶ ἵνα σαφῶς τοῖς λεγομένοις παρακολουθήσωμεν, ἐκ διαιρέσεως προαγάγωμεν τὸν λόγον οὕτως· τὸ οὖρον εἰς δύο διαιρεῖται, ⟨εἰς χύμα καὶ παρέγχυμα. καὶ τὸ μὲν παρέγχυμα εἰς τρία διαιρεῖται⟩· εἰ μὲν γὰρ ἐπιπολάζει καὶ ἄνω περιφέρεται, λέγεται νεφέλη, δίκην τοῦ ἐπιπροσθοῦντος νέφους ἐπιπολάζοντος τῷ ἀέρι· ἢ βρίθει ἐν τῷ κλοκίῳ καὶ ὑφιζάνει καὶ λέγεται ὑπόστασις· ἢ ἐν τῷ μέσῳ ἐστὶ καὶ λέγεται ἐναιώρημα. τὸ δὲ χύμα ἐστὶν αὐτὴ ἡ ὑγρότης τοῦ οὔρου. δεῖ γὰρ εἰδέναι ὅτι αὐτοὶ οἱ τέσσαρες χυμοὶ ἐν τῷ ἥπατι γεννῶνται. καὶ οἱ μὲν δύο χυμοὶ ἔχουσι δοχεῖα καὶ καθαρτήρια, δι' ὧνπερ ἀποκαθαίρονται, ὁ μὲν μελαγχολικὸς ὑπὸ τοῦ σπληνός, ἡ δὲ ξανθὴ χολὴ ὑπὸ τῆς χοληδόχου κύστεως. τὸ δὲ αἷμα ἀναδίδοται διὰ τῶν φλεβῶν ἐπὶ τὸ πᾶν σῶμα διὰ τὴν θρέψιν· σὺν δὲ τῷ αἵματι ἀναδίδοται καὶ ὀρῶδές τι ὑγρόν· ἀλλὰ καὶ φλέγμα συναναδίδοται, οὐχ ἁπλῶς καὶ ὡς ἔτυχεν, ἀλλ' ἑκάτερον δι' ἀναγκαίαν χρείαν. τὸ μὲν ὀρῶδες ὑγρόν, ἐπειδὴ τὸ αἷμα φύσει ἀργόν ἐστι καὶ δυσπόρευτον, συναναδίδοται τὸ ὑγρόν, ἵνα ποδηγήσῃ καὶ εὔρουν ποιήσῃ τὸ αἷμα, ὡς αὐτὸς Ἱπποκράτης ἀλλαχοῦ λέγει, ὅτι «Ὑγρασίη τροφῆς ὄχημα.» ταύτην οὖν 160 τὴν χρείαν ποιεῖ τὸ | ὀρῶδες ὑγρόν. ἀλλὰ καὶ τὸ φλέγμα μεγίστην χρείαν ποιεῖται ἀναδιδόμενον σὺν τῷ αἵματι, ἵν' ὅταν λεῖψις τοῦ αἵματος γένηται ἐν ταῖς λιμαγχονίαις καὶ ἐν ταῖς περιστάσεσιν, αὐτὸ τὸ φλέγμα ἡμίπεπτον αἷμα φύσει τυγχάνον τὴν χρείαν ποιῆται τῆς τροφῆς. ἔγνωμεν οὖν, ποίαν ἀποτελεῖ ἑκάτερον χρείαν. τὸ οὖν ὀρῶδες ὑγρὸν μετὰ τὸ ποιῆσαι τὴν χρείαν καὶ ὁδηγῆσαι τὸ αἷμα λοιπὸν ὡς περίττωμα φέρεται διὰ τῶν φλεβῶν ἐκείνων ἐπὶ νεφρούς, δι' ὧνπερ ἡ τροφὴ φέρεται ἐν αὐτοῖς, ἐπειδὴ χαίρουσιν οἱ νεφροὶ τῇ ποιότητι τοῦ οὔρου, καὶ μετὰ τὸ ἐνεχθῆναι εἰς τοὺς νεφροὺς φέρεται ἐπὶ τὴν κύστιν καὶ οὕτως ἀπουρεῖται. καὶ τοῦτο τὸ ὀρῶδες ὑγρὸν ἤγουν τὸ οὖρον λέγεται χύμα.

Σημειοῦται οὖν τὸ κατὰ φύσιν οὖρον. καὶ λέγει ὅτι δεῖ τὸ ἄριστον οὖρον λευκὴν ἔχειν τὴν ὑπόστασιν καὶ λείην καὶ ὁμαλὴν παρὰ πάντα τὸν χρόνον· τὸ δὲ χύμα ἤγουν τὸ ὑγρὸν ὑπόπυρρον καὶ ὑπόξανθον δεῖ εἶναι.

Καὶ ἐπεξέλθωμεν ἑκάστου τὴν αἰτίαν. διὰ τί λευκὴ ἡ ὑπόστασις θέλει εἶναι; τοῦτο κατὰ δύο αἰτίας. πρῶτον μὲν ὅτι ἢ διαδιδράσκει μέρος τι τοῦ συναναδιδομένου φλέγματος καὶ φέρεται μετὰ τοῦ οὔρου καὶ γίνεται λευκὴ ἡ ὑπόστασις, ἐπειδὴ λευκόν ἐστι τὸ φλέγμα. ἢ δι' ἕτερον τρόπον λευκὴ γίνεται ἡ ὑπόστασις, ἐπειδὴ περίττωμά ἐστι τῶν στερεῶν τῆς τρίτης πέψεως· ἐπειδὴ γὰρ τὰ στερεὰ ἀπὸ σπέρματος τρέφονται, τὸ δὲ σπέρμα λευκόν ἐστι φύσει, τοῦτο οὖν τὸ περίττωμα ἀλᾶται καὶ πλανᾶται τῇδε

5–8 οὔρου] *v. e.g.* [Gal.] De urinis compend.: XIX p. 606 K. 17 Ἱπποκράτης] Hipp. De alim. 55: CMG I 1 p. 84,22

2 παρακολουθήσομεν M 4 εἰς[I] – διαιρεῖται *addidi* 6 κλωβίῳ (-οβ- M) γ: *corr. Dietz* 13 *post* συναναδίδοται *fort. exciderunt fere* τῷ αἵματι· ταῦτα δὲ συναναδίδοται 14 sq. οὐχ – συναναδίδοται *om.* M 16 *post* αὐτὸς *add.* ὁ P 21 ποιεῖται γ: *correxi* 23 ὁδηγῆσαι *coni. Dietz*: ὁδηγήσῃ M: ὁδηγήσει P: ὁδηγήσ *(ambig.)* V 25 νεφροὶ] νέοι γ: *corr. Dietz* νεφροὺς] νέους γ: *corr. Dietz* 29 ἔχει V: ἔχον P: *corr.* M περὶ P 38 ἀλᾶται *coni. Wk.*: ἄλεται P: ἄλεται V: ἄγεται M

Here he takes up the subject of urines. And urine, as we know, is the residue of the second digestion. And in order to follow clearly the text, we will lead off the discussion with the following division: urine is divided into two: the fluid and the deposit. The deposit is divided into three varieties; for if it is at the surface and floats on top, it is called a cloud, like an opaque cloud floating on the air; or it sinks down in the urinal and settles and is called a sediment; or it is in the middle and is termed a suspension. The fluid, on the other hand, is the urine's liquid itself. For it should be noted that the four humors themselves are produced in the liver. And two of the humors have receptacles and purifiers through which they are cleaned out, black bile by the spleen, yellow bile by the gallbladder. Blood, on the other hand, is distributed for nourishing through the veins to every part of the body; and a certain serous liquid as well is transmitted along with the blood; phlegm, too, is distributed; (and they are distributed) not haphazardly and without purpose, but each for a necessary function. For blood being by nature slow and hard to move, the serous liquid is distributed with it to lead the way and make the blood easy-flowing, just as Hippocrates says elsewhere, "Moisture is the vehicle of nourishment." So this is the function of the serous fluid. And phlegm also is distributed with the blood to perform a very important task, so that, when blood fails in cases of weakening from hunger or in difficult circumstances, the phlegm itself, being by nature semi-concocted blood, might perform the function of nourishing. We have learned, then, the job that each performs. When the serous liquid, then, has finished its work of conducting the blood, it is eventually conveyed as a residue to the kidneys through those same veins which bring them nutriment, the kidneys having an affinity for the quality of urine, and after it is conveyed to the kidneys it goes to the bladder and is thus eliminated as urine. This serous liquid or urine is what is called the fluid.

He gives, then, the symptoms for normal urine. He says that the best urine should have a sediment which is white, smooth and even all along, while the fluid or liquid should be reddish and yellowish.

We will discuss the cause of each. Why should the sediment be white? There are two reasons for this. First, either because a part of the phlegm distributed (with the blood) breaks loose, is carried along with the urine and the sediment turns white, since the phlegm is white. Or the sediment becomes white in another way, because it is the residue of the third digestion in the solid parts; for since the solid parts are nourished by sperm, and the sperm is white by nature, this residue, then, strays and

κἀκεῖσε, καὶ ἡ φύσις λοιπὸν σὺν τῷ οὔρῳ ἐκκρίνει αὐτὸ καὶ ὑφίσταται καὶ λευκὴ γίνεται ἡ ὑπόστασις.

Καὶ λεῖον· λεῖον λέγει τὸ ὁμοιομερές, τὸ κατὰ πᾶν ἑαυτὸ ὅμοιον, καὶ μὴ τὸ μὲν αὐτοῦ πεπεμμένον ἐστί, τὸ δὲ ἄπεπτον, καὶ τὸ μὲν αὐτοῦ λεπτόν, τὸ δὲ παχύ, καὶ τὸ μὲν αὐτοῦ λευκόν, τὸ δὲ οὐ λευκόν.

Ἀλλὰ καὶ ὁμαλὸν αὐτὸ δεῖ εἶναι. ὁμαλὸν λέγει εἶναι τὸ κατὰ τὸν
161 χρόνον, | ὅτι δεῖ τὴν ὑπόστασιν ἀείσε τοιαύτην εἶναι, τυχὸν κατὰ φύσιν· τοῦτο γὰρ ἐνδείκνυται ἰσχὺν καὶ ἐπικράτειαν τῶν δυνάμεων.

Τὸ δὲ χρῶμα ὑπέρυθρον καὶ ὑπόξανθον θέλει εἶναι τοῦ χύματος· καὶ ὑπέρυθρον μέν, ἐπειδὴ ὀρὸς μετὰ τοῦ αἵματος ἐκκρίνεται καὶ ἐξυδαροῦται τὸ αἷμα καὶ οὐκέτι ἐρυθρὸν ἐκκρίνεται, ἀλλ' ὑπέρυθρον· τὸ δὲ ὑπόξανθον, ἐπειδὴ καὶ μέρος τι τῆς χολῆς συνεκκρίνεται καὶ ἐξυδαροῦται καὶ ὑπόξανθον ἐκκρίνεται τὸ οὖρον.

Εἶτα καὶ ἀποροῦσιν ὅτι «Ἐπὰν χολὴ συνεκκρίνεται καὶ γίνεται ὑπόξανθον τὸ οὖρον, διὰ τί καὶ ὁ μελαγχολικός ποτε οὐ συναναδίδοται καὶ οὕτως χρώννυσι τὸ οὖρον;» καὶ λέγομεν ὅτι ὁ μελαγχολικὸς βαρύς ἐστι καὶ βρίθει ὥσπερ κόνις ἤγουν στακτή· ἄλλως τε δὲ ἀποκαθαίρεται καὶ φθάζει ἀποκαθαρθῆναι ὡς γεώδης καὶ βαρὺς καὶ οὐ συναναδίδοται, ⟨ὥστε⟩ χρῶσαι τὸ οὖρον ἐν τῷ κατὰ φύσιν.

Καὶ ἀποροῦσι πάλιν ὅτι «Τὸ κατὰ φύσιν οὖρον, πῶς ἐπὶ πάσης ἡλικίας καὶ ὥρας καὶ χώρας τὸ αὐτὸ ἔχομεν λέγειν κατὰ φύσιν, εἴ γε διάφορός ἐστιν ἡ ἡλικία καὶ ἑκάστης ἡλικίας διάφορός ἐστι καὶ ἡ κρᾶσις, ἀλλὰ καὶ τοῦ θέρους ἄλλη ἐστὶ κρᾶσις καὶ ἐν χειμῶνι ἄλλη καὶ ἐπὶ τῶν ἄλλων καιρῶν ὡσαύτως, ἀλλὰ καὶ ἑκάστη χώρα ἰδίαν κρᾶσιν ἔχει;» καὶ ἀπολογούμεθα οὕτως, ὅτι ἐπὶ τῶν τελείων αἱ τέλειαι σημειώσεις ἀποτελοῦνται· ἐπὶ οὖν τῶν ἀκμαστικῶν τὸ κατὰ φύσιν ἁρμόζει μᾶλλον οὖρον· τοῦ οὖν εἴδους φυλαττομένου τοῦ κατὰ φύσιν οὔρου διαφορὰς ἐπιδέχεται κατά τε τὸ χρῶμα καὶ τὴν σύστασιν παρὰ τὸ μᾶλλον καὶ ἧττον, καὶ ἐπὶ πάσης ἡλικίας καὶ ὥρας καὶ χώρας φυλάττεται τὸ κατὰ φύσιν οὖρον. οὕτως γοῦν ἐπὶ παίδων ἐπ' ἔλαττον λευκότερα εὑρίσκονται τὰ οὖρα, καὶ οὐχ ὥσπερ ἐπὶ τῆς ἀκμαστικῆς ἡλικίας, οὕτως ὑπέρυθρον καὶ ὑπόξανθον. ἀλλὰ καὶ ἐπὶ τῶν γερόντων ἔτι μικρὸν λευκότερον ἐκκρίνεται. οὕτως γὰρ καὶ κατὰ τὴν ὑπόστασιν εὑρίσκομεν γινόμενον· τῶν ἁβροδιαίτων ἢ πολλὰ ἐσθιόντων πολλὴ γέγονεν ἡ ὑπόστα-
162 σις ἐν τῷ | οὔρῳ, καὶ οὐ λέγομεν αὐτὸ παρὰ φύσιν. ἀλλὰ καὶ οἱ ὀλίγην τροφὴν λαμβάνοντες, ὀλίγη γίνεται αὐτῶν καὶ ἡ ὑπόστασις, καὶ οὐ λέγομεν ὅτι οὐκ ἔστι κατὰ φύσιν, ἐπειδὴ ἀποθεωροῦμεν εἰς τὴν ὀλιγότητα τῶν τροφῶν. ἀλλὰ καὶ οἱ μέσως πως διαιτώμενοι, μέσως πως καὶ ἡ ὑπόστασις ἐκκρίνεται.

Δεύτερόν ἐστι κεφάλαιον, ἐν ᾧ ⟨περὶ⟩ τοῦ παρὰ φύσιν διαλέγεται οὔρου ὁ Ἱπποκράτης. ἀλλὰ πρὸ τούτου τέσσαρά τινα δεῖ ἡμᾶς ζητῆσαι. πρῶτον, διὰ τί τὸ οὖρον σημειούμεθα· δεύτερον, εἰ ἐπὶ πάντων τῶν νοσημάτων ἁρμόζει ἡ τῶν οὔρων σημείωσις καὶ πάντα σημειούμεθα δι' αὐτῶν· τρίτον, τὸν πρέποντα καιρόν, ἐν ᾧ ἡ ἀπόθεσις τοῦ οὔρου γίνεται· καὶ τέταρ-

3 πάντα ἑαυτῶ γ: *correxi* 17 στάκτη γ: *corr. Dietz* *ante* ἄλλως *add.* καὶ M 18 ὥστε *addidi* 32 ἐκκρίνονται M 33 γινόμενα M: γινόμεν *(ambig.)* V 34 αὐτὴν M 39 περὶ *add. Dietz* 41 εἰ *om.* V

wanders all over until nature finally eliminates it in the urine, and it settles and the sediment becomes white.

And smooth: by smooth he means homogeneous; (the urine) should be uniform throughout, and not with some parts digested and others not, some thin and others dense, some white and others not white.

And it should also be even. Even he means in a temporal sense; the sediment should be of that kind, i.e. normal, all the time; for this indicates that the faculties are strong and in control.

The color of the fluid should be reddish and yellowish; reddish, since serum is passed with the blood and waters it down, so that it is not passed red but reddish; and yellowish, because some (yellow) bile also is passed with it and waters it, and the urine is passed yellowish.

Here the problem is raised that "If (yellow) bile is passed along with it and the urine becomes yellowish, why does black bile, too, not sometimes get distributed with it and color the urine accordingly?" We reply that black bile is heavy and sinks like dust or lye of ashes; moreover, it is cleared out, and it succeeds in being cleansed because of its earthiness and weight; and it is not distributed so as to color the urine under normal circumstances.

Again the problem is posed, "With regard to normal urine, how can we speak of the same thing as normal for every age, season and region, if it is true that there are different age groups and each age also has a distinct temperament, and summer has one temperament and winter another and the other seasons likewise, and each region too has its peculiar temperament?" Our answer is as follows, that the most wholesome symptoms are produced in the fully-grown, so that normal urine is more appropriate to those in their prime; but normal urine can admit of differences of more or less in color and composition without losing its normal character, so that for every age group, season and region normal urine is preserved. Accordingly, you will find the urines of children slightly whiter and not so much reddish and yellowish like those of the prime age. And in the old it is passed slightly whiter still. And the same thing we find happening in the sediment also: those who eat rich foods or in great quantities have a large sediment in their urine, but we do not regard it as abnormal. And those who eat little have a small sediment, and we do not say that it is not normal, since we consider the small quantity of food. And for the group whose diet is moderate, the sediment, too, is average.

In a second chapter Hippocrates discusses abnormal urine. But before this it is necessary to ask four questions. First, why do we observe urine symptoms? Second, are the symptoms from urines appropriate for all diseases and do we obtain from them symptoms for all (diseases)? Third, when is the proper time for passing urine? And fourth, what does

τον, τί βούλεται λέγειν ὁ Ἱπποκράτης διὰ ῥησειδίου, ἐν ᾧ φησιν ὅτι παρὰ πάντα τὸν χρόνον, ἔστ' ἂν κριθῇ ἡ νοῦσος.

Καὶ ἀρκτέον ἀπὸ τοῦ πρώτου· τὴν ἀπὸ τῶν οὔρων σημείωσιν ποιούμεθα, ἵνα γνῶμεν τὰς φυσικὰς δυνάμεις τὰς ἐν ἥπατι καὶ ἐν ταῖς φλεψί.

Δεύτερον δέ, εἰ πάντα τὰ νοσήματα ἐκ τῶν οὔρων δυνάμεθα σημειώσασθαι. καὶ λέγομεν ὅτι οὐ πάντα, ἀλλὰ μόνα τὰ θρεπτικά· καὶ τὸ θρεπτικὸν ἧπαρ καὶ φλέβες. κατὰ οὖν πρῶτον λόγον ἡ ἀπὸ τῶν οὔρων σημείωσις τὴν δευτέραν πέψιν ἤγουν τὴν ἐξαιμάτωσιν, τὸ πῶς διάκεινται αἱ ἐν αὐτοῖς δυνάμεις, δηλοῖ, εἰ μὴ ὅτε συμπαθήσωσι τό τε ἧπαρ καὶ αἱ φλέβες τοῖς ἀναπνευστικοῖς ἢ τῷ ἐγκεφάλῳ, καὶ ὡς ὁμοιοπαθοῦντα, συμβάλλεται ἡ τῶν οὔρων σημείωσις.

Τρίτον, δεῖ ἡμᾶς ζητῆσαι τὸν πρέποντα καιρὸν τῆς ἀποθέσεως τῶν οὔρων. πρέπων καιρός ἐστι μετὰ τὸ κατὰ λόγον γενέσθαι τὴν δευτέραν πέψιν, λέγω δὴ τὴν ἐν ἥπατι, τυχὸν μετὰ τὴν κατὰ λόγον ἐξαιμάτωσιν, τότε ἐστὶν ὁ πρέπων καιρὸς τῆς ἀποθέσεως τοῦ οὔρου. παρὰ φύσιν δὲ
163 καιρός ἐστιν ἡ πρὸ πέψεως τῆς δευτέρας | ἀπόθεσις τοῦ οὔρου· οὐδὲν γὰρ ἐνδείκνυται πρὸς σημείωσιν· λεπτὸν γὰρ καὶ ἄπεπτον καὶ ἀχόλωτον εὑρίσκεται, δίκην τῶν πολλὰ ἐσθιόντων. ἀλλὰ καὶ κατὰ χρόνον τῆς πέψεως ἐὰν ἀπωθεῖται τὸ οὖρον, παρὰ φύσιν ἐστὶ καὶ οὐδὲν ἐνδείκνυται, ἐπειδὴ οὐ χολοῦται καὶ οὕτως ἐκκρίνεται. ἀλλὰ καὶ ἡ ἐν τῷ κλοκίῳ ἀπόθεσις, οὐ δεῖ ἐγχρονίζειν καὶ μετὰ μίαν ἡμέραν ἐνδείκνυσθαι· οὐδὲ τότε γὰρ συμβάλλεται εἰς σημείωσιν· τῷ γὰρ χρόνῳ ἀποψύχεται καὶ νεκροῦται καὶ χύσιν ὑφίσταται. ἀλλ' οὐδὲ ἡ πρόσφατος ἀπόθεσις συμβάλλεταί σοι εἰς σημείωσιν, ἐπειδὴ ἔτι ἀδιάκριτόν ἐστι καὶ συγκεχυμένον.

Τέταρτόν ἐστιν, ἐν ᾧ δεῖ ἡμᾶς ζητῆσαι, τί βούλεται λέγειν ὁ Ἱπποκράτης τὸ τοιοῦτον δεῖ εἶναι παρὰ πάντα τὸν χρόνον, ἔστ' ἂν κριθῇ ἡ νοῦσος. καί τινές φασιν ὅτι παρὰ πάντα τὸν χρόνον λέγει, ὡς ἂν δεῖ αὐτὸ παρὰ πάντα τὸν χρόνον τοῦ νοσήματος εἶναι κατὰ φύσιν, ὅπερ παρὰ τὰ πράγματά ἐστιν· οὔτε γὰρ ἀρχὴ διαφανήσεται πρὸς σημείωσιν οὔτε ἀνάβασις οὔτε ἀκμή, ἐὰν κατὰ φύσιν ἐστὶ τὸ οὖρον· λοιπὸν δὲ ὅτι κατὰ φύσιν ὄντος τοῦ οὔρου οὐδὲ νόσημα ὑποστήσεται. καὶ λέγομεν ὅτι ταῦτα νόει λέγειν δυνατὸν Ἱπποκράτην, ὅτι ἐὰν μέλλῃ σωτήριον εἶναι τὸ νόσημα, ἐν τῇ ἀρχῇ δεῖ εἶναι ἴχνη τινὰ πέψεως ἐν τῷ οὔρῳ, ἵνα τυχὸν λευκότερον μέν ἐστι τὸ οὖρον, ἔχῃ δὲ καὶ τὴν ὑπόστασιν ἢ νεφέλιον· εἶτα ἐν τῇ ἀναβάσει δεῖ αὐτὸ πλεῖον χρώννυσθαι, καὶ τὴν ὑπόστασιν δεῖ ἐναιώρημα γενέσθαι· ἐν δὲ τῇ ἀκμῇ καὶ ἐν αὐτῇ τῇ κρίσει δεῖ αὐτὸ κατὰ φύσιν εἶναι, τυχὸν λευκὸν καὶ λεῖον καὶ ὁμαλὸν καὶ ὑπέρυθρον καὶ ὑπόξανθον.

Τούτων οὕτως εἰρημένων σημειοῦται τὰ παρὰ φύσιν οὖρα. ταῦτα δὲ πολλὴν ἔχουσι τὴν διαφορὰν κατά τε τὸ χύμα καὶ τὸ παρέγχυμα, λέγω δὴ τὸ νεφέλιον καὶ τὸ ἐναιώρημα. ἀλλὰ πρότερον περὶ τοῦ χύματος διαλέγεται,

27–29] *cf.* Gal. In Hipp. Progn. comm. II 26: CMG V 9,2 p. 281,6–8

2 περὶ MP: *corr.* V πάντων M 4 φλεψί *scripsi (cf. infra, p. 200,21)*: φλέβαις γ 9 δηλοῦσιν γ: *correxi* 10 ὁμοιοπαθοῦντας V 15 sq. παρὰ — οὔρου *om.* V 16 ἡ] ὁ M τῆς δευτέρας] δευτέρα P 18 κατὰ χρόνον *scripsi*: μετὰ χρόνου γ 26 περὶ MP: *corr.* V τὸν *om.* V 27 περὶ MP: *corr.* V 28 παρὰ[II]] περὶ MP: *corr.* V 31 οὐδὲ *ex* οὐδὲν *corr.* P: οὐδὲν M 32 ἱπποκράτης γ: *corr.* *Dietz*

Hippocrates mean by the phrase in which he says all along, until the disease reaches a crisis?

Starting with the first, we take symptoms from urines in order to discover (the condition of) the natural faculties in the liver and veins.

Secondly, can we give the symptoms for all diseases from urines? The answer is not all, but only for those of the digestive parts, which means the liver and the veins. Urine symptoms, then, give us primary information on the second digestion, that is, blood-formation; (they tell us) how the faculties in the liver and veins are working, unless sometimes the liver and veins be affected in sympathy with the respiratory parts or the brain; then the urine symptoms are helpful for these parts which are affected in the same way (as the liver and veins).

Thirdly, we must consider the proper time for passing urines. The proper time is after normal second digestion, I mean coction in the liver, has taken place, in other words, after normal conversion to blood – then is the proper time for passing the urine. But if the urine is passed prior to second digestion, the time is abnormal; for it gives nothing in the way of symptoms, since it is thin, unconcocted and not converted to bile, as happens in the case of those who eat great quantities. Urine is also abnormal if it is eliminated during the time of digestion, and it shows nothing, since it is not converted to bile but is passed in that state. And the deposit in the urinal: it should not continue long there and (be examined to) show signs after one day; for then it does not help with symptoms; for through time it grows cold, mortifies and turns to sediment (?). On the other hand, neither will a fresh deposit (of urine) help you with symptoms, since it is still unseparated and confused.

The fourth is where we must ask what Hippocrates means when he says that it should be of such a kind all along, until the disease reaches a crisis. According to some he uses all along in the sense that it should be normal for the duration of the disease; but this misses the point; for, if the urine is normal, no beginning will show through to be observed nor heightening nor acme; moreover, there won't even be a disease, since the urine is normal. We say that you may consider the possible meaning of Hippocrates to be as follows, that if the disease is going to prove curable, in the beginning the urine should show some traces of concoction; the urine should, for example, be on the white side and have a sediment or cloud; then during the heightening it should get more color and the sediment should become a suspension; and during the acme and the crisis itself it should be normal, that is, white, smooth, even, reddish and yellowish.

After this he gives the symptoms of abnormal urines. And these show many varieties in respect to both fluid and deposit, i.e. cloud and suspension. But first he deals with the fluid which is subject to many abnorma-

164 πολλὰς ἔχον παρεκτροπάς. καί φησιν ὅτι τὸ ξανθὸν | οὖρον καὶ πυρρὸν παρὰ φύσιν εἰσί· τὸ μὲν γὰρ ξανθὸν ἐνδείκνυται περιουσίαν χολώδους ὕλης, ὅπερ κάκιστόν ἐστι· τὸ δὲ πυρρὸν ἧττόν ἐστι κακόν, ἐπειδὴ ἐνδείκνυται περιουσίαν αἵματος, τὸ δὲ αἷμα φίλιον ἡμῖν ἐστιν· ἀλλ' ὅμως κακόν ἐστιν, ἐπειδὴ ἐνδείκνυται τὸ αἷμα λεπτὸν ὂν καὶ ἄπεπτον καὶ ἀκατέργαστον καὶ τὸν πρέποντα κόσμον μὴ δεξάμενον. καὶ τὸ τηνικαῦτα ὡς λεπτὸν καὶ ὑδαρὲς συνεκκρίνεται τῷ ὀρώδει ὑγρῷ καὶ ποιεῖ πυρρὸν τὸ οὖρον. ἀλλὰ καὶ τὸ πολὺ καὶ τὸ ὀλίγον οὖρον κάκιστόν ἐστι· τὸ μὲν γὰρ πολὺ ἐνδείκνυται ἀπεψίαν, καὶ τῇ ἀπεψίᾳ ἐξ ἀνάγκης πολλὰ γεννῶνται τὰ περιττώματα· τὸ δὲ ὀλίγον ἐνδείκνυται ὅτι οὐ πάντα τὰ περιττώματα κενοῦνται, ἀλλ' ἐνδομυχοῦσι διαλανθάνοντα καί πού ποτε ἀθροίζονται. κακὰ οὖν εἰσι καὶ τὸ μέλαν καὶ τὸ πελιόν· ταῦτα γὰρ ἐνδείκνυνται ἢ μεγίστην ζέσιν καὶ φλόγωσιν θερμότητος οὖσαν ἐν τῷ βάθει ἢ ἐπιτεταμένην σηπεδόνα ἢ ἀπόψυξιν καὶ νέκρωσιν. ἀλλὰ καὶ τὸ λευκὸν οὖρον καὶ παχὺ δίκην τρυγίας κακόν ἐστιν, ἐπειδὴ ἐνδείκνυται μεγίστην ἀπεψίαν τῶν ὑλῶν, καθ' ἣν ταῦτα ἐκκρίνεται. ἀλλὰ καὶ τὸ λεπτὸν καὶ ὑδατῶδες καὶ διαυγὲς καὶ στίλβον οὖρον κακόν ἐστι· καὶ τοῦτο γὰρ ἀπεψίαν ἐνδείκνυται. ἀλλὰ καὶ πνευμάτων τινῶν συναναπεπλεγμένων τῷ οὔρῳ, καὶ τῇ τάσει ποιοῦσιν αὐτὸ στίλβον δίκην ἀκόνης.

Ἀλλὰ καὶ τὸ παρέγχυμα ἔχει διαφοράς· τὸ γὰρ νεφέλιον ἐνδείκνυται περιουσίαν πνευμάτων. ἀλλὰ καὶ τὸ ἐναιώρημα παρὰ φύσιν ἐστίν· ἐνδείκνυται γὰρ καὶ αὐτὸ περιουσίαν πνευμάτων, ἀλλ' ἐπ' ἔλαττον, ὅθεν καὶ ἧττον κακόν ἐστιν. ἐνδέχεται δέ ποτε καὶ τὸ νεφέλιον καὶ τὸ ἐναιώρημα κατὰ κρᾶσιν μὴ εἶναι παρὰ φύσιν, ἀλλὰ κατὰ φύσιν. εἰ μὲν αὐχμηρά ἐστιν ἡ ἕξις τοῦ σώματος καὶ τὰ σύστοιχα θερμότερα ἐπιτεταμένως, τότε νεφέλιον γίνεται·
165 εἰ δὲ ὑφειμένη ἐστὶν ἡ ξηρότης τῆς | ἕξεως καὶ τὰ σύστοιχα ἧττόν ἐστι θερμά, ἐναιώρημα γίνεται ἡ ὑπόστασις.

Ταῦτα εἰρηκὼς λέγει καὶ ἕτερα παρὰ φύσιν οὖρα ἐν τῇ ὑποστάσει συνιστάμενα. καί φησιν ὅτι κακαί εἰσιν αἱ κριμνώδεις ὑποστάσεις· ἐπὶ γὰρ ἀνωμάλῳ ἐκτήξει ἐκκρίνονται, ἐπὶ πυρώδει καὶ φλογώδει θερμότητι γινομένης τῆς ἐκτήξεως. ἡ δὲ ἔκτηξις γίνεται τῆς νεοπαγοῦς σαρκὸς καὶ αὐτῆς τῆς σαρκός, καὶ λοιπὸν ἐν τοῖς τοιούτοις κριμνώδη ἐκκρίνονται ἐν τοῖς οὔροις. ἀλλὰ καὶ ἐπὶ παχεῖ αἵματι κριμνώδη ἐκκρίνονται ἐν τοῖς οὔροις· ἀνώμαλός ἐστιν ἡ ἔκτηξις, ὅτι τὰ μὲν λεπτὰ ἐμφέρονται, τὰ δὲ παχέα· ἐρυθρὰ δέ ἐστι τὰ οὖρα καὶ τὰ κριμνώδη τὰ ἐμφερόμενα κατὰ τὴν ὑπόστασιν. κριμνώδεις δὲ λέγονται αἱ τοιαῦται ὑποστάσεις δίκην τῶν κρίμνων τῶν ἀπὸ τῶν πεφρυγμένων κριθῶν καὶ ἀλεσθέντων καὶ διαλαθόντων τινῶν ἁδρομερῶν.

Λέγει καὶ ἑτέραν διαφοράν, ὅτι καὶ ἡ πεταλώδης ὑπόστασις κακίστη ἐστί· καὶ αὕτη γὰρ ἐπὶ ἐκτήξει ἐκκρίνεται τῶν στερεῶν κατ' ἐπίτασιν τῆς πυρώδους καὶ φλογώδους θερμότητος.

Ἀλλὰ καὶ τὰ πιτυρώδη κακά ἐστιν, ἐπειδὴ καὶ ταῦτα ἐπὶ ἐκτήξει τῶν στερεῶν μορίων ἐκκρίνονται κατ' ἐπίτασιν μεγίστην τῆς φλογώδους καὶ

28–36] *cf.* Gal. In Hipp. Progn. comm. II 28: CMG V 9,2 p. 283,5–21 40–194,1 θερμότητος] *cf.* Gal. In Hipp. Progn. comm. II 28: CMG V 9,2 p. 284,10–12

2 γὰρ *om.* M 4 ὅλως γ: *corr. Dietz* 5 ὄντα γ: *corr. Dietz* 7 τὸ ὀρῶδες ὑγρὸν γ: *correxi* 9 τὰ *om.* V 12 ἢ *om.* M 20 περὶ P παραφύσιον M 29 ἐκτήξει *scripsi*: ἐκταράξει γ 41–194,1 πυρώδους καὶ φλογώδους M

lities. He says that yellow and red urine are abnormal; for the yellow indicates a superabundance of bilious matter, which is a very bad sign; the red is not as serious, since it means a superabundance of blood, and blood is congenial to us; but it is a bad sign all the same, being an indication that the blood is thin, unconcocted, undigested and has not reached its proper state. Then, because it is thin and watery, it is passed out along with the serous fluid and makes the urine red. Copious and small urines also are very unfavorable symptoms; for the copious points to indigestion and indigestion of necessity gives rise to many residues; the small, on the other hand, means that not all the residues are emptied out, but have been missed and are lurking inside and are gathering at some spot. Dangerous, too, are the black and livid; for these point to a severe seething and inflamed heat deep in the interior or intense putrefaction or cooling and mortification. And urine which is white and dense as dregs is bad, since it means serious indigestion of the substances, which causes these (urines) to be passed. And thin, watery, translucent and glistening urine is bad, this also being a sign of indigestion. When certain gases are mixed with the urine, they make it glisten like a whetstone, because of the strain.

There are differences in the deposit too; for the cloud indicates a superabundance of gases. The suspension as well is abnormal, since it also means a surplus of gases, but a smaller one; hence it is not as serious. On the other hand, it is sometimes possible for both cloud and suspension to be, not abnormal, but normal in temperament. If the condition of the body is dry and the concomitant factors very much on the warm side, then a cloud develops; while if the dryness of the condition is less intense and the concomitant factors less hot, the deposit becomes a suspension.

Having said this he mentions also other urines that are abnormal in sediment. He says that meal-like sediments are bad, since they are passed due to an irregular melting which is produced by a fiery and inflamed heat. The melting is of newly formed tissue and of the flesh itself, and so in such cases meal-like particles are passed in the urines. Thick blood, too, causes meal-like particles to be passed in the urines; the melting is uneven, since it involves both fine and thick particles; and the urines and meal-like particles contained in the sediment have a red color. Deposits of this kind are called meal-like from the resemblance to the coarse grains of meal which escape when barley is being roasted and ground.

He distinguishes another variety and says that the flaky sediment is very bad; for it is passed due to a melting of the solid parts which is caused by an intensification of the fiery and inflamed heat.

And urines with bran-like sediments are unfavorable, since they, too, are passed due to a melting of the solid parts produced by an in-

πυρώδους θερμότητος. πιτυρώδη δὲ ὀνομάζονται, ἐπειδὴ ἐοίκασι πιτύροις.

Καὶ ἀποροῦσί τινες· «Εἴ γε τὸ ὑπέρυθρον καὶ ὑπόξανθον ὑπό τε τοῦ αἵματος καὶ τῆς χολῆς χρωννύντων αὐτὸ τοιοῦτον γίνεται, ὑπέρυθρον μὲν ὑπὸ τοῦ αἵματος χρωννυμένου, ὑπόξανθον δὲ ὑπὸ τῆς χολῆς, τί δήποτε μὴ ὥσπερ τὸ χύμα χρώννυται καὶ ἡ ὑπόστασις χρώννυται καὶ γίνεται ὑπόπυρρον ἢ ὑπόξανθον, ἀλλὰ μένει λευκή;» καὶ λέγομεν ὅτι οἱ τοιοῦτοι χυμοὶ λεπτομερεῖς εἰσι καὶ λοιπὸν ἑτοίμως διεισκρίνονται καὶ διεισέρχονται εἰς τὸ
166 ὀρῶδες ὑγρὸν καὶ ἀναχύνονται ἐν αὐτῷ καὶ | διὰ τοῦτο χρώννυσιν αὐτό. ἡ δὲ ὑπόστασις κάτω ὑφίσταται· λοιπὸν δὲ καὶ παχεῖά ἐστι, καὶ οὐ φθάνουσιν εἰσκριθῆναι ἐν τῇ ὑποστάσει ὥστε χρῶσαι αὐτήν, καὶ διὰ τοῦτο λευκὴ εὑρίσκεται.

Καὶ πάλιν ἀποροῦσιν ὅτι «Ἐπὶ τῆς νεφελώδους ὑποστάσεως καὶ τοῦ ἐναιωρήματος τί ἔχετε εἰπεῖν, ἐπειδὴ ταῦτα ἐμφέρονται καὶ ἐπιπολάζουσι, καὶ μὴν ὁρῶμεν λευκὰ καὶ αὐτὰ ὄντα;» πρὸς ὃ ἀπολογούμεθα ὅτι ταῦτα, λέγω δὴ τὸ νεφέλιον καὶ τὸ ἐναιώρημα, παχέα εἰσί, τὸ δὲ χύμα λεπτόν ἐστι καὶ ὑδατῶδες, καὶ διὰ τοῦτο εὐχερῶς εἰσκρίνονται καὶ χρώννυσιν αὐτό· τὸ δὲ νεφέλιον καὶ τὸ ἐναιώρημα παχέα εἰσί, καὶ διὰ τοῦτο οὐ διεισέρχονται ἐν αὐτοῖς καὶ χρώννυσιν αὐτά.

VII

II 22 [12: 209,3 **A.** = **II 142,1 L.**] Θανατωδέστερα δὲ τῶν οὔρων τά τε δυσώδεα καὶ ὑδατώδη καὶ μέλανα καὶ παχέα.

Ἐντεῦθεν ἐπὶ ἑτέρας διαφορὰς θανατωδῶν οὔρων τρέπεται· καὶ λέγει τρεῖς συζυγίας θανατωδεστάτων οὔρων, ὧν πρώτη ἐστὶν αὕτη· φησὶν ὅτι θανατωδέστατα τῶν οὔρων εἰσὶ τά τε λευκὰ καὶ ὑδατώδεα καὶ δυσώδη· δεύτερον δὲ τὰ παχέα καὶ μέλανα· τρίτον δὲ τὰ λιπαρὰ καὶ ἐλαιώδη. εἶτα λοιπὸν δέον ἐστὶ καὶ τὴν αἰτίαν ἑκάστου εἰπεῖν. τὸ λεπτὸν καὶ δυσῶδες οὖρον ἐνδείκνυται ἐσχάτην ἀπεψίαν καὶ ἄκραν καταβολὴν τῶν φυσικῶν δυνάμεων καὶ μεγίστην σηπεδόνα ἐν τῷ βάθει οὖσαν. τὸ δὲ λοιπὸν καὶ μέλαν οὖρον ἐνδείκνυται ἢ κατάψυξιν καὶ νέκρωσιν τοῦ ἐμφύτου θερμοῦ ἢ πυρώδη καὶ φλογώδη θερμότητα· δεῖ γὰρ εἰδέναι ὅτι τὰ μέλανα οὖρα ἢ ἐπὶ καταψύξει καὶ νεκρώσει τοῦ ἐμφύτου θερμοῦ καὶ τοῦ αἵματος καὶ τῶν χυμῶν ἀπονεκρουμένων ἢ ἐπὶ μεγίστῃ καὶ φλογώδει καὶ πυρώδει θερμότητι, ἐξυπεροπτῶσαν καὶ οἷον ἀποτεφρουμένην, τοῦ τε αἵματος καὶ τῶν χυμῶν, γίνεται. τὸ δὲ παχὺ οὖρον ἐνδείκνυται περιουσίαν καὶ πλεονασμὸν παχέων χυμῶν καὶ πνευμάτων συναναπλεκομένων αὐτοῖς. δεῖ δὲ εἰδέναι ὅτι τὸ λεπτὸν οὖρον καὶ
167 μέλαν ἀδύνατόν ἐστιν εὑρεθῆναι ἢ μέλαν καὶ δυσῶ|δες. ἀλλὰ ταῦτα τὰ οὖρα καθ' αὑτὰ μὲν καὶ ἰδίᾳ ὀλέθριά εἰσι, τουτέστι τὸ λευκὸν καὶ τὸ δυσῶδες μόνον· συμπεπλεγμένα δὲ ἔτι μᾶλλόν εἰσιν ὀλέθρια. τὸ δὲ λεπτὸν καὶ παχὺ

25 τὰ[II] – ἐλαιώδη] *de his mentionem non facit Hippocrates*

5 χύμα *coni.* **Dietz**: χρῶμα γ ἡ *om.* P 8 ἀνεχύνονται M: ἀναισχύνονται P: *corr.* V 13 τί] ὅτι M ἔχεται MP *(ε sscr. P)*: *corr.* V 27 φυσικῶν *scripsi*: ψυχικῶν γ 32 sq. ἐξυπεροπτῶσαν ... ἀποτεφρουμένην] *cf. supra, pp. 170,28; 172,8* 33 ἀποτεφρουμένη P 36 καὶ] ἢ P 38 λεπτὸν *scr.* *Nickel*: λευκὸν γ

flamed and burning heat of the highest intensity. They are named bran-like from their similarity to bran.

And some raise a problem, "If it is true that the reddish and yellowish become such because the blood and bile color them – the reddish color being imparted by the blood, the yellowish by the bile –, is there any reason why the sediment too is not colored, as the fluid is, to become reddish or yellowish, but remains white?" We say that humors of this kind are composed of fine particles and consequently they easily penetrate and make their way into the serous liquid, and they spread around in it and color it for this reason. The sediment, on the other hand, sinks downwards, and besides it is thick and the humors cannot get inside it to color it; hence it is found to be white.

And again they raise a problem, "What have you to say about the cloud and suspension sediments? These are contained (in urine) and come to the surface, and still we see that they also are white." To which we answer that these, cloud and suspension, are thick, while the fluid is thin and watery; hence (the humors) have no trouble in penetrating and coloring the fluid; but the cloud and suspension are thick and for this reason they do not penetrate them and color them.

VII

II 22 But the more deadly urines are the fetid, watery, black and dense.

At this point he turns to other varieties of deadly urines; and he gives three combinations of the most fatal urines, the first of which is this: he says that the most fatal of the urines are the white and watery and fetid; second, the dense and black, and third, the greasy and oily. The next thing we should do is to give the cause of each. The thin fetid urine means extreme indigestion, acute collapse of the natural faculties and severe putrefaction in the depths. The black urine, for its part, points to either cooling and mortification of the innate heat or a fiery and inflamed heat; for you should be aware that black urines are caused either by cooling and mortification of the innate heat, when both the blood and the humors are destroyed, or by a very intense, inflamed and fiery heat in the blood and humors which overheats and, so to speak, burns them to ashes. Dense urine means a superabundance and surplus of dense humors and gases mixed up together with them. Note that the thin urine and black cannot be found nor black and fetid. But these urines by themselves and on their own are deadly, that is, the white and the fetid individually; in combination, on the other hand, they are even more deadly. The thin and dense are not deadly on their own; for the

οὐκ ἔστι καθ' αὑτὰ ὀλέθρια· τὸ μὲν γὰρ λεπτὸν καὶ ὑδατῶδες, διότι ἐνδέχεται τῷ χρόνῳ ῥωσθῆναι τὰς φυσικὰς δυνάμεις καὶ πέψαι καὶ χυμῶσαι καὶ εἰς τὸ κατὰ φύσιν ἐλθεῖν καὶ μὴ εἶναι ὀλέθριον. ἀλλὰ καὶ τὸ παχὺ οὖρον, ἐπειδὴ παχεῖαν δηλοῖ τὴν ὕλην καὶ περιουσίαν πνευμάτων, χρόνιον μὲν δηλοῖ τὸ νόσημα, οὐ μὴν ὀλέθριον. ἄλλως τε δὲ ἐνδέχεται παχέα ἐκκριθῆναι οὖρα ἐν τῇ ἀκμῇ τῆς νόσου καὶ μὴ εἶναι ὀλέθρια, ἀλλ' ὑγιαστικά· δηλοῖ γὰρ ὅτι ἀποκαθαίρεται τὸ σῶμα δι' οὔρων, καὶ διὰ τοῦτο παχέα κενοῦνται τὰ οὖρα. ἢ οὐχ ὁρῶμεν καὶ ἄλλων παρὰ φύσιν ὑλῶν κενουμένων ἐν ταῖς παρακμαῖς ἐπὶ ἀπαλλαγῇ τῶν νοσημάτων; διὸ χολώδης ἔκκρισις πολλάκις γίνεται ἢ φλεγματώδης καὶ ἕλμινθες ἐκκρίνονται καὶ οὐκ εἰσιν ὀλέθρια, ἀλλ' ὑγιαστικά. παχὺ δὲ οὖρον ἀκουστέον τὸ ἄγαν παχύ. ἀλλὰ καὶ τὸ λιπαρὸν καὶ ἐλαιῶδες καὶ τὰ τοιαῦτα οὖρα ὀλέθριά εἰσι καὶ θανατώδη· δηλοῦσι γὰρ σηπεδόνα καὶ ἔκτηξιν τῆς πιμελῆς ὑπὸ φλογώδους θερμότητος γινομένην.

Αὗταί εἰσιν αἱ συζυγίαι τῶν οὔρων αἱ θανατώδεις, ὧν ἐνταῦθα μέμνηται Ἱπποκράτης. ἐφ' οἷς καὶ προσδιορισμοὺς τίθησι τέσσαρες τὸν ἀριθμόν. ὧν πρῶτός ἐστιν αὐτός, ὅτι ταῖς μὲν γυναιξὶ καὶ τοῖς ἀνδράσι τὰ μέλανα τῶν οὔρων κάκιστα, τοῖς δὲ παιδίοισι τὰ ὑδατώδη. φησὶν ὅτι ταῖς ἀκμαζούσαις γυναιξὶ καὶ ἀνδράσι τοῖς ἀκμάζουσι τὰ μέλανα τῶν οὔρων ὀλέθρια καὶ θανατώδη εἰσί, τοῖς δὲ παιδίοις τὰ λεπτὰ καὶ ὑδατώδη. διὰ τί; ἐπειδὴ ἐπὶ τῶν παίδων ἐν τῷ κατὰ φύσιν παχέα ἐκκρίνονται τὰ οὖρα διὰ τὴν ἀδηφαγίαν, ὅθεν τῷ πάχει καὶ μέλανα ὑποφαίνονται· ἐπὶ δὲ τῶν ἀκμαζόντων τὰ λεπτὰ καὶ ὀλίγην ἔχοντα τὴν ὑπόστασίν εἰσι κατὰ φύσιν διὰ τὴν περιουσίαν τῆς κατὰ ποιότητα θερμότητος, συμπέττουσαν καὶ
168 λεπτύνουσαν. ἐὰν οὖν ἐναλλὰξ γένηται καὶ | ἐπὶ τῶν παίδων λεπτὰ ἐκκριθῶσι καὶ ὑδατώδη, ἐπὶ δὲ τῶν ἀκμαζόντων τὰ μέλανα καὶ παχέα οὖρα, ἐπειδὴ ἐπὶ τὸ πάντῃ ἐναντίον τοῦ κατὰ φύσιν ἐξετράπησαν, διὰ τοῦτο ὀλέθριά εἰσιν.

Δεύτερον λέγει προσδιορισμὸν τοιοῦτον, ὅτι ⟨εἰ⟩ ἐπὶ τῶν νοσημάτων εὔφορός ἐστιν ὁ ἄνθρωπος καὶ εὔπνους καὶ εὔϋπνος καὶ ἄδιψος καὶ μηδεμιᾶς αἰσθάνεται δυσφορίας ἢ ἀνωμαλίας, ἐκκρίνει δὲ οὖρα λεπτὰ καὶ ὑδατώδη ἐπὶ πολὺν χρόνον, γίνωσκε ὅτι εἰς ἀπόστασιν τρέπεται τὸ νόσημα. δεῖ δὲ εἰδέναι ἐν τῷ καθόλου ὅτι τὰ νοσήματα ἢ χρόνιά εἰσιν ἢ ὀξέα, καὶ τὰ μὲν χρόνια ἐπὶ ψυχρᾷ καὶ παχείᾳ ὕλῃ γίνονται· διὰ τοῦτο καὶ χρονίζουσιν, ἀλλὰ τῷ μήκει τοῦ χρόνου καὶ αἱ δυνάμεις καταβάλλονται. τὰ δὲ ὀξέα ἐπὶ θερμῇ καὶ λεπτῇ ὕλῃ γίνονται, ὅθεν καὶ κατ' ἔκρουν ἐκκρίνονται διὰ χολεμεσίας καὶ ἐκταράξεως γαστρὸς καὶ δι' ἐμέτων καὶ ἱδρώτων καὶ τῶν τοιούτων. τὰ δὲ χρόνια οὐ κρίνονται, ἀλλὰ λύονται κατὰ διαφόρησιν καὶ σύμπεψιν. εἰ δὲ καὶ κρίνονται, κατὰ ἀπόστασιν κρίνονται· δεῖ γὰρ εἰδέναι ὅτι χρονίου ὑποκειμένου νοσήματος καὶ παχείας οὔσης τῆς ὕλης καὶ παχέων οὔρων ὀφειλόντων

20 ἐπειδὴ – 27] *cf.* Gal. In Hipp. Progn. comm. II 33: CMG V 9,2 pp. 286,23–287,15 28 λέγει] Hipp. Progn. 12: p. 209,5–7 A. = II p. 142,4–6 L. 38–198,11] *cf.* Gal. In Hipp. Progn. comm. II 34: CMG V 9,2 pp. 287,20–288,14

4 *post* δηλοῖ^II^ *iter.* τὴν ὕλην καὶ M 15 *ante* Ἱπποκράτης *add.* ὁ P 20 παιδίων V 21 ὑποφαίνεται M 26 τῷ παντὶ γ: *corr. Wk.* 28 εἰ *addidi* 29 ἄφορος P ἄπνους P καὶ εὔϋπνος *om.* M ἄϋπνος P 30 ἐκκρίνονται M δὲ] καὶ V: *om.* M 35 *fort.* κρίνονται *scribendum est*

thin is watery too, for which reason it is possible for the natural faculties to regain their strength with time and to digest and convert to humor and (for the urine) to return to normal and not to be deadly. And the dense urine means that the disease is chronic and not deadly, since it indicates dense matter and a superabundance of gases. Moreover, dense urines may be passed at the climax of the disease and indicate, not death, but recovery; for they show that the body is being cleaned out by means of the urines, and this is why the urines are passed dense. And is it not a fact that we see other abnormal matter also evacuated during the abatement which brings diseases to an end? So it frequently happens that there is a bilious or phlegmatic discharge and worms are passed, and they are not fatal, but salutary. By dense urine we should understand the overly dense. And the greasy and oily and the like are deadly and fatal urines; for they mean putrefaction and melting of fat caused by an inflamed heat.

These are the fatal urine combinations that Hippocrates mentions at this point. To them he appends four specifications, the first of which is as follows, in women and men the worst urines are the black, in children the watery. What he means is that for women and men in their prime black urines are deadly and fatal, but in children the thin and watery. Why? Because it is normal for children to pass dense urines, on account of over-eating, and hence with the density black (urines) too show up; for adults, on the other hand, the normal is thin urines with small sediments, since they have a superabundance of the quality of heat which concocts and refines. If, then, the situations are reversed and children pass thin and watery, adults black and dense urines, since they have changed to the exact opposite of normal, for this reason they are deadly.

For the second specification he says that, if in diseases the person is in good spirits, is breathing easily and sleeping well, has no thirst, feels no discomfort or irregularity and passes thin and watery urines over a long period, this will tell you that the disease is turning to abscess. Now, one should be aware in general that diseases are either chronic or acute; the chronic are caused by cold and dense matter, which is why they are protracted, and because of the length of time the faculties too are overthrown. The acute are produced by hot and thin matter, and hence they are removed by discharge, whether by bringing up bile or by bowel disturbance or vomiting or sweating and the like. The chronic, on the other hand, do not come to crisis; they are relieved by dissipation and concoction. But if they do come to a crisis, it is by abscess; for note that in a chronic illness, where the matter is dense and dense urines ought to

ἐκκρίνεσθαι, ἐὰν λεπτὰ καὶ ὑδατώδη ἐκκρίνονται τὰ οὖρα, δηλοῖ ὅτι ἀλλαχοῦ πέμπεται ἡ ὕλη καὶ ἐνδομυχεῖ εἰς ἕτερον μόριον ἀσθενὲς γινόμενον, ὅπερ δι' οἰκείαν ἀσθένειαν ὑποδέξασθαι μὲν δύναται, ἀπωθῆσαι δὲ καὶ ἀποδιῶξαι οὐ δύναται· ἀλλὰ λοιπὸν ἐκεῖσε στέγεται καὶ ἐμφωλεύει ἡ τοιαύτη ὕλη, ὥστε τῷ χρόνῳ ἐξ ἀνάγκης ἀποστάσεις γενέσθαι. αἱ δὲ ἀποστάσεις ἐπὶ μὲν τῶν ἄγαν χρονίων νοσημάτων, ἡνίκα καὶ ψυχρά ἐστιν ἡ ὕλη καὶ παχεῖα, ἀπὸ τοῦ διαφράγματος ἐπὶ τὰ κάτω γίνονται, διὸ ἐπὶ τὸν ὀμφαλὸν καὶ τὴν ὀσφὺν καὶ τοὺς λαγόνας καὶ βουβῶνας καὶ τοῖς τοιούτοις· ἐπὶ δὲ τῶν μὴ οὕτως χρονιζόντων ἐπὶ τὰ ἄνω αἱ ἀποστάσεις γίνονται, ἤγουν ἐν τοῖς
169 παρισθμίοις καὶ παρωτίσι καὶ μασχάλαις καὶ τοῖς τοιούτοις. εἰ δὲ | μέσως πως, μέσως καὶ αἱ ἀποστάσεις γίνονται, ποτὲ μὲν ἄνω, ποτὲ δὲ κάτω.

Τρίτος προσδιορισμός ἐστιν, ὅτι ἐπὶ τῶν οὔρων παρὰ φύσιν ἐστὶ τὸ νεφελῶδες πάχος ἐν τῇ ὑποστάσει θεωρούμενον καὶ τὸ ἐναιώρημα, ἧττον δέ ἐστι παρὰ φύσιν· ἡ δὲ ὑπόστασις ὁμωνύμως τῷ γένει κατὰ φύσιν ἐστί. χειρίστη δὲ πασῶν τὸ νεφελῶδές ἐστιν, ἐπειδὴ πλείω ἐνδείκνυται ἀπεψίαν καὶ περιουσίαν πνευμάτων· διὰ τοῦτο καὶ πλέον μετεωρίζεται· ἧττον δὲ χείριστόν ἐστι τὸ ἐναιώρημα. ἐπειδὴ δὲ τῶν οὔρων τὰ μὲν οὐδ' ὅλως ἔχουσι πάχος ἐμφερόμενον ἐν αὐτοῖς, ἀλλ' ἀδιάκριτόν ἐστι, τούτου οὖν τοῦ μὴ ἔχοντος πάχος, τουτέστιν ὑπόστασιν, κάλλιόν ἐστι τὸ νεφελῶδες· τὸ γὰρ μὴ ἔχον τι πάχος οὖρον ἐν ἑαυτῷ χείριστόν ἐστι καὶ κάκιστον· δηλοῖ γὰρ ὅτι ἀλλαχοῦ ἀπασχολεῖται ἡ ὕλη καὶ ἐκεῖσε ἀποσκήπτει.

Τέταρτος προσδιορισμός ἐστιν, ἐν ᾧ φησιν ὅτι τὰ μέλανα καὶ δυσώδη οὖρα οὐ πάντως τοῦ παντὸς σώματος ἐνδείκνυται τὸ πάθος, ἀλλά τινος μορίου, ἡνίκα τυχὸν ἕλκος ἐστὶ περὶ τοὺς νεφροὺς ἢ τοὺς οὐρητῆρας ἢ τὴν κύστιν· τὸ τηνικαῦτα γὰρ δυσῶδες ἐκκρίνεται τὸ οὖρον διὰ τὸ πύον. καὶ μὴ παραλογισθῇς ἐπὶ τούτῳ ὅτι, ἐπειδὴ δυσῶδες ἐξεκρίθη, πάντως καὶ ὀλέθριον· ἰδοὺ γὰρ ἐνδέχεταί ποτε ἐκκριθῆναι δυσῶδες οὖρον καὶ μὴ εἶναι θανάσιμον, καθὼς καὶ αὐτὸς λέγει· μὴ ἐξαπατάτω δέ σε, ἤν τι καὶ αὐτὴ ἡ κύστις νόσημα ἔχουσα τοιαῦτα οὖρα ἀποδιδῷ· οὐ γὰρ τοῦ ὅλου σώματος σημεῖόν ἐστιν, ἀλλ' αὐτῆς καθ' ἑαυτήν.

Δεύτερόν ἐστιν, ἐν ᾧ περὶ ἐμέτου διαλέγεται. ὁ δὲ ἔμετος πολλὰς ἔχει διαφοράς, ἀλλὰ πρότερον περὶ τοῦ κατὰ φύσιν ἐμέτου διαλέγεται. κατὰ φύσιν δὲ ἔμετός ἐστιν ὁ ἄνευ βλάβης τῶν ἐνεργειῶν γινόμενος. καί φησιν ὅτι κατὰ φύσιν ἔμετός ἐστιν ὁ ἐξ ἐπιμιξίας χολῆς καὶ φλέγματος γινόμενος, ἵνα
170 συμπλακῶσι· τὸ μὲν γὰρ | φλέγμα ἐκ τῶν περισσῶν ἀπεψιῶν ἀθροίζεται ἐν τῷ στομίῳ τῆς γαστρός, ἡ δὲ χολὴ νῦν τίκτεται ἀπὸ τοῦ ὀξέου πυρετοῦ — ἐπὶ γὰρ ὀξέων νοσημάτων γυμνάζει τὸν λόγον —, ἐπειδὴ ἀβιάστως γίνεται καὶ ἀβλαβῶς· ἡ μὲν γὰρ χολὴ λεπτύνει καὶ διαχεῖ τὸ φλέγμα, ἐπειδὴ καὶ ἐχέκολλόν ἐστι· τὸ δὲ φλέγμα τῇ οἰκείᾳ ὑγρότητι καταπραΰνει τὸ δηκτικὸν

28 μὴ – 30] Hipp. Progn. 12: p. 210,1–3 A. = II p. 142,12–15 L. 33 φησιν] Hipp. Progn. 13: p. 210,4 A. = II p. 142,16 L.

2 γενόμενον V 4 ὥστε *coni. Dietz*: ὅπερ γ 5 ἀποστάσεις[I]] ἀπόστασις (ὑπό- P) PV: *corr.* M 7 ὀφθαλμὸν V 8 τοῖς τοιούτοις] *cf. lin. 10; debebat* τὰ τοιαῦτα 18 ἀδιάκριτά V 26 τοῦτο γ: *correxi* 29 αὕτη γ: *corr. Dietz* τοιαῦτα οὖρα] *sic nullus test. Hipp.* 33 *post* ἄνευ *add.* δὲ P 34 *post* γινόμενος *add.* καὶ φησὶν ὅτι κατὰ φύσιν ἔμετός ἐστιν ὁ τοιοῦτος M

be passed, if thin and watery urines are eliminated, it means that the matter is being sent elsewhere and lurks in some other weakened part which, because of its own weakness, is able to admit but unable to eject and get rid of it; and finally this matter is concealed and lurks there, so that through time abscesses form of necessity. Now abscesses in very chronic diseases, where the matter is both cold and dense, form from the diaphragm to the lower parts, therefore in the navel, the loins, the flanks, the groin, etc.; in those that are not so chronic the abscesses develop in the upper parts, namely in the tonsils, the parotid glands, the arm-pits and the like. In the moderately (chronic) the abscesses too are moderate, forming sometimes above, sometimes below.

The third specification is that in urines the cloudy thickness observed in the sediment is abnormal, and so is the suspended matter, though it is less abnormal; while the sediment – with the same name as the class – is normal. Worst of all is the cloud, for it means greater indigestion and superabundance of gases, which is why it also rises more; the suspension is less than the worst. Since, however, some urines have no thickness at all contained in them, but are unseparated, a cloudy (urine), then, is better than one which has no thickness, that is, sediment. For the urine without any thickness in itself is the worst and most unfavorable; for it shows that the matter is busy in another place whither it has determined.

The fourth specification is where he says that black and fetid urines do not invariably mean that the whole body is affected, only a part of it, for example, when there is an ulcer on the kidneys or the urinal ducts or the bladder; for in these cases the urine is passed fetid because of the pus. But do not be misled by this into thinking that, since it is passed fetid, it is necessarily deadly. For urine sometimes can be passed fetid without meaning death, just as he himself says, B u t y o u s h o u l d n o t b e d e c e i v e d i f t h e b l a d d e r i t s e l f, b e i n g a f f e c t e d, g i v e s o f f s u c h u r i n e s; f o r i t i s n o t a s i g n f o r t h e w h o l e b o d y, b u t f o r t h e b l a d d e r o n i t s o w n.

The second chapter is where he discusses vomiting. Now vomit has many varieties, but first he deals with the normal vomit. And normal vomit is that which occurs without injury to the functions. He says that normal vomit is that which comes from a mixture of bile and phlegm, when the two are combined; the phlegm gathers at the orifice of the stomach from excessive indigestions, while the bile in this case is the product of the acute fever – for the discussion is concerned with acute diseases –, since it is produced without violence and damage; for the bile refines the phlegm and makes it fusible, since it is also glutinous, while the phlegm moderates the sting of the bile with its own moisture.

τῆς χολῆς.

Ὁ δὲ παρὰ φύσιν ἔμετος πολλὰς ἔχει διαφοράς· ἐὰν γὰρ ἰδίως καὶ χωρὶς ἐμεθῇ χολὴ ἢ φλέγμα, παρὰ φύσιν ἐστίν. εἰ μὲν χολὴ ξανθὴ ἐμεθῇ, τῇ δήξει καὶ τῇ ἀνίᾳ βλάπτει τὰ μόρια, δι' ὧν παρέρχεται. αὕτη δὲ ἡ ξανθὴ χολὴ παχυνομένη ⟨ἢ⟩ λεκιθώδης γίνεται ἢ ὀρώδης ὑγρότης συναναμίσγει καὶ ἴσχει ἐπιμιξίαν τῇ ξανθῇ χολῇ καὶ ὠχρὰ γίνεται χολή. ἑκάτερα δὲ κακά ἐστιν ἐμούμενα διὰ τὸ πάχος. τί γάρ; ὅτι τῇ οἰκείᾳ θερμότητι τὸ λεπτὸν διαφορεῖται καὶ παχύνεται, καὶ παχυνομένου δυσχερὴς γίνεται ὁ ἔμετος καὶ μετὰ σπαραγμοῦ, ὡς πολλάκις τῇ βίᾳ καὶ τῷ σπαραγμῷ καὶ αἵματος γίνεσθαι ἔμετον. ὁμοίως καὶ τὸ φλέγμα, διά τε τὸ ψυχρὸν αὐτὸ εἶναι καὶ διὰ τὸ ἐχέκολλον· πρῶτον μὲν ψύχει τὰ μόρια, δι' ὧνπερ παρέρχεται· λοιπὸν δὲ καὶ ⟨διὰ⟩ τὸ ἐχέκολλον μετὰ βίας τινὸς καὶ συντάσεως ὁ ἔμετος γίνεται. παρὰ φύσιν ἔμετοί εἰσι καὶ κάκιστοι, ἐὰν πρασοειδὴς ἐμεθῇ χολή, ἀλλὰ καὶ πελιὰ ἢ μέλανα ἐμούμενα κάκιστά εἰσιν. οὐ μὴν ἀλλὰ καὶ τὰ δυσώδη κάκιστά εἰσι. ταῦτα δὲ καὶ ἰδίᾳ καὶ χωρὶς ἐμούμενα κάκιστά εἰσιν, ἀλλὰ καὶ ἐὰν συμπεπλεγμένα ἅμα ἐμεθῶσι, παγκάκιστά εἰσι· δηλοῦσι γὰρ ποικίλην κακοχυμίαν καὶ ποικίλην διάθεσιν οὖσαν ἐν τῷ σώματι· τὰ γὰρ μέλανα ἐμούμενα καὶ πελιὰ ἐνδείκνυνται ἢ ψῦξιν οὖσαν ἐν τῷ βάθει ἢ φλόγωσιν ἐξυπεροπτῶσαν τοὺς χυμούς· τὰ δὲ δυσώδη ἐνδείκνυνται μεγίστην σηπεδόνα. ἀλλὰ καὶ ἡ πρασώδης χολὴ ἐμουμένη κακίστη ἐστίν· αὕτη δὲ καὶ ἐν γαστρὶ γεννᾶται καὶ ἐν ταῖς φλεψί, καὶ καθ' ἑκάτερον διχῶς· ἢ γὰρ ἐπὶ ζέσει φλογώδει θερμότητος οὔσης ἐν τῇ γαστρὶ πρασώδης γίνεται χολή, εἴτε διὰ τὰς προ⟨σ⟩φερομένας |
171 τροφὰς τοιαύτας οὔσας καὶ ἀπεπτουμένας, κράμβας φημὶ καὶ σεῦτλα, πρασώδης γεννᾶται χολή· ὁμοίως καὶ εἰς τὰς φλέβας· ἢ διὰ ζέσιν ὑπερβάλλουσαν ἐν αὐταῖς πρασώδης γεννᾶται χολὴ καὶ ἀντικαταρρεῖ εἰς γαστέρα καὶ οὕτως ἐμεῖται, ἢ διὰ τοιοῦτον περίττωμα ἀθροισθὲν ἐν αὐταῖς, κραμβῶν φημὶ καὶ σεύτλων καὶ τῶν τοιούτων, πρασώδης γεννᾶται χολή. ἑκάτεροι οἱ τοιοῦτοι χυμοὶ κάκιστοί εἰσιν.

II 23 [12: 209,9 A.=II 142,8 L.] Σκοπεῖν δὲ χρὴ τῶν οὔρων ⟨ἐν οἷσιν⟩ αἱ νεφέλαι, εἴτε κάτω ἔωσιν εἴτε ἄνω

Δεῖ δὲ εἰδέναι ὅτι ὁ Ἱπποκράτης ποτὲ καὶ τὴν ὑπόστασιν καὶ τὴν νεφέλην καταχρηστικῶς ὑπόστασιν καλεῖ, ὅπερ καὶ νῦν πεποίηκεν· ἔφη γὰρ ἐν οἷς αἱ νεφέλαι, εἴτε ἄνω εἴτε κάτω ὦσιν· ἰδοὺ καταχρηστικῶς εἴτε ἄνω εἴτε κάτω ὑπόστασιν καλεῖ καὶ τὴν νεφέλην καὶ τὴν ὑπόστασιν. καί φησιν ὅτι ἀπὸ τῶν ὑποστάσεων δεῖ ποιεῖσθαι τὴν σημείωσιν· αἱ γὰρ ὑποστάσεις ἀγαθαί εἰσι καὶ ὑγιαστικαί· τὸ γὰρ νεφέλιον καὶ τὸ ἐναιώρημα

21–28] *cf.* Gal. In Hipp. Progn. comm. II 39: CMG V 9,2 p. 292,16–22 31 sq.] *cf.* Gal. In Hipp. Progn. comm. II 36: CMG V 9,2 p. 289,1–3

3 ξανθὴ χολὴ V 5 ἢ^{I} *addidi* 6 ἐπιμιξίας M καὶ *scripsi*: ἢ γ δὲ *om.* M 6 sq. ἐστιν κακὰ M 8 παχυνομένων γ: *correxi* 12 διὰ *sec. Dietz addidi* γίνεται ὁ ἔμετος P 13 ἐμεθῇ] ἔμετος ἡ V 14 ἢ] καὶ M 15 καὶ^{I} *om.* M 22 προφερομένας MP: *corr.* V 25 αὐταῖς] ταῖς M 26 καὶ *om.* V κράμβαις γ: *correxi* 27 γενᾶ V: γεννὰ P: γενᾶται *in* γενὰ *mut.* M: *corr. Dietz* 29 sq. ἐν οἷσιν *ex Hipp. addidi (cf. lin. 33)* 30 εἴτε . . . εἴτε] *sic nullus test. Hipp.* 33 εἴτε ἄνω *post* ὦσιν *trsp.* P ὦσιν] εἰσὶν V 34 εἴτε^{II}] καὶ PV: *corr.* M

And there are many varieties of abnormal vomit; for if bile or phlegm is brought up separately and on its own, it is abnormal. If yellow bile is vomited it injures the parts through which it passes by its sting and irritation. And when this yellow bile thickens, either it becomes like egg yolk or a serous fluid combines and mixes with the yellow bile and the bile becomes pale yellow. Each of these, when vomited, is bad because of the thickness. Why? Because the fine part is dissipated by the (bile's) own heat and thickens, and when it thickens vomiting becomes difficult and is accompanied by retching, which frequently results in throwing up blood because of the forcing and retching. Phlegm acts in a similar way, being both cold and glutinous; first, the parts through which it passes it leaves cold, and secondly, its glutinous nature causes the vomiting to be somewhat forced and strained. Vomits are abnormal and very bad if leek-green bile is thrown up, and livid or black vomits also are extremely bad. Fetid vomits, too, are extremely dangerous. And when these are brought up separately and individually they are very bad, but if they are vomited together in combination they are altogether the worst; for they indicate the presence in the body of multiple unwholesome humors and a variety of conditions; if black and livid are vomited they point to either coldness deep inside or a burning heat that overheats the humors, while the fetid mean serious putrefaction. And throwing up leek-green bile also is very bad; this type (of bile) is produced both in the stomach and in the veins, and in each place in one of two ways: for bile turns leek-green either due to a seething and inflamed heat in the stomach or bile is produced leek-green because foods of that kind have been consumed and not digested, for example cabbage and beet; similarly in the veins, bile is made leek-green either due to an excessive seething heat in them and runs back into the stomach and is vomited with this color, or bile is produced leek-green because a residue of this kind has collected there, namely (the residue) of cabbage and beet and the like. And each of these types of humor is very bad.

II 23 Those urines with clouds should be examined to see whether they are down or up

Note that Hippocrates sometimes uses the word sediment loosely to designate both the sediment (proper) and the cloud, which is what he has done here; he said with clouds, whether they are up or down; you see how he loosely calls the cloud and sediment (proper) the up or down sediment. And he tells us that we should take the symptoms from the sediments, since these are good and indicative of health, while the

παρὰ φύσιν εἰσίν, ἐπειδὴ συναναπεπλεγμέναι εἰσὶ μετὰ πνευμάτων παχέων, καὶ διὰ τοῦτο μετεωρίζονται.

Εἶτα καὶ ἀποροῦσιν ὅτι «Καὶ πῶς ἀνωτέρω ἐπὶ τῶν ἀκμαζόντων ἔλεγεν ὅτι, ἡνίκα αὐχμηρὸν καὶ κατάξηρόν ἐστι τὸ σῶμα, νεφέλιον ἢ ἐναιώρημα ὑφίσταται ἐν τοῖς οὔροις, ἅτινα καὶ κατὰ φύσιν εἰσί, πῶς οὖν λέγει ἐνταῦθα ὅτι παρὰ φύσιν εἰσί;» καὶ λέγομεν ὅτι πᾶσαι αἱ ἡλικίαι πάντως παχυμερεστέραις τροφαῖς κέχρηνται· διὰ οὖν τὴν παχυμερίαν τῶν τροφῶν πάντως ὑπόστασιν ἴσχουσι τὰ οὖρα. ὁ οὖν Ἱπποκράτης πρὸς τοῦτο ἀφεωρακὼς κατὰ φύσιν λέγει εἶναι τὴν ὑπόστασιν, καὶ διὰ τοῦτο ἐπαινεῖ τὴν τοιαύτην σημείωσιν ὡς ἀσφαλῆ οὖσαν.

VIII

II 24 [14: 210,12 A.=II 144,9 L.] Πτύελον δὲ χρὴ ἐπὶ πᾶσι τοῖσιν ἀλγήμασι τοῖσι περὶ τὸν πνεύμονά τε καὶ τὰς πλευρὰς ταχέως ἀναπτύεσθαι καὶ εὐπετέως

Ἐντεῦθεν ἐπὶ τῶν κενουμένων παρὰ φύσιν εἰς σημείωσιν ἐτράπη ὁ Ἱπποκράτης, καὶ σημειοῦται τὸ πτύελον καὶ πτύσμα· τὸ αὐτὸ δέ ἐστιν· οὐδὲ γὰρ ὥς τινες ὑπέλαβον, ὅτι τὸ μὲν πτύελόν ἐστι τὸ κατὰ φύσιν, πτύσμα
172 δὲ τὸ | παρὰ φύσιν, ἐπειδὴ αὐτὸς ἀδιόριστον καὶ πτύελον καὶ πτύσμα τὸ αὐτὸ καλεῖ. σημειοῦται οὖν τινα πάθη ἀπὸ τοῦ πτυέλου, πλευρῖτιν λέγω καὶ περιπνευμονίαν· ταῦτα γὰρ τὰ πάθη ἀπὸ τοῦ πτυέλου διαγινώσκονται. τί δέ ἐστι πλευρῖτις ἴσμεν καὶ νῦν εἰρήσεται. πλευρῖτις τοίνυν ἐστὶν φλεγμονὴ τοῦ τὰς πλευρὰς ὑπεζωκότος ὑμένος ἀπὸ χολωδεστέρου αἵματος γινομένη. περιπνευμονία δέ ἐστι φλεγμονὴ τοῦ πνεύμονος ἀπὸ φλεγματικωτέρου αἵματος γινομένη.

Καὶ ἀποροῦσί τινες ὅτι «Εἰ πᾶν μόριον, ἐξ οὗ τρέφεται, ἐκ τούτου καὶ ἐπηρεάζεται, ἔδει τὸν πνεύμονα ἀπὸ χολωδεστέρου αἵματος ἐπηρεάζεσθαι καὶ τὴν φλεγμονὴν γίνεσθαι ἐκ ταύτης καὶ μὴ ἀπὸ φλεγματώδους αἵματος. ὁμοίως καὶ ἡ πλευρῖτις, ὑπὸ φλεγματικωτέρου αἵματος ἔδει βλάπτεσθαι, ὡς νευρώδης οὖσα, καὶ τὴν φλεγμονὴν συνίστασθαι καὶ μὴ ἀπὸ χολωδεστέρου αἵματος.» καὶ λέγομεν ὅτι οὐ πάντα τὰ μόρια ἐξ οὗ τρέφονται πάντως καὶ βλάπτονται, ὥσπερ ἐνταῦθα ἐπὶ τῆς φλεγμονῆς· ὁ γὰρ πνεύμων μανός ἐστι καὶ ἀραιός, ἡ δὲ χολὴ ὡς λεπτομερὴς διεξέρχεται καὶ ἀπορρέει καὶ οὐ στέγεται καὶ τὸ τηνικαῦτα οὐκ ἐμφράττεται καὶ οὐ ποιεῖ φλεγμονήν. διὰ δὲ τὸ φλέγμα γίνεται ἡ περιπνευμονία, ἐπειδὴ παχύς ἐστιν οὗτος ὁ χυμὸς καὶ ὡς παχὺς ἐμφράττεται καὶ ποιεῖ τὴν περιπνευμονίαν.

Καὶ ἴσως ἐρεῖ τις· «Καὶ πόθεν φλέγμα εὑρίσκεται ἐν τῷ πνεύμονι, εἴ γε ἀπὸ χολωδεστέρου αἵματος τρέφεται;» καὶ λέγομεν ὅτι ἢ ἀπὸ τῆς κεφαλῆς ἀντικαταρρεῖ φλέγμα καὶ φέρεται ἐπὶ τὸν πνεύμονα ἢ ἐκ τῶν παρακειμένων μορίων φέρεται φλέγμα ἐπὶ τὸν πνεύμονα καὶ ἐμφράττεται καὶ

15 κινουμένων V   17 οὐδὲ] οὐ P   18 διόριστον P   19 τινα *scr. Dietz*: τί γ   20 περιπνεύμονα γ: *correxi*   23 περιπνευμονία] περιπνεύμονος γ: *correxi*   25 καί^II *om.* V   27 ταύτης] *sc.* τῆς χολῆς   28 ἡ πλευρῖτις] *sensu* ὁ ὑπεζωκώς? *(cf. infra, p. 204,2)*   33 οὐ *om.* M   34 περιπνευμονή P: περιπνεύμονος V: *corr.* M   35 περιπνευμονή P: περιπνεύμονος V: *corr.* M

cloud and suspension are abnormal, being charged with dense gases, and for this reason they are suspended.

Then the following problem is raised: "How is it that earlier, when speaking of those in their prime, he said that if the body is parched and very dry, a cloud or suspension will appear in the urines and these are normal; how can he state at this point, then, that they are abnormal?" Our reply is that all the age groups necessarily consume foods that are fairly coarse; because of the coarseness of the foods, then, the urines invariably contain a sediment. It is with this in mind, then, that Hippocrates calls the sediment normal, and he regards such a symptom as salutary for this reason.

VIII

II 24 In all cases of pains around the lungs and sides the spit should be brought up quickly and easily

Hippocrates has now passed on to the symptoms of abnormal evacuations, and he gives the signs of spit and sputum; these two are the same and it is not the case, as some have supposed, that spit is the normal and sputum the abnormal (evacuation), since (Hippocrates) himself uses both spit and sputum without distinction to refer to the same thing. He gives from spit, then, the symptoms for certain affections, namely pleurisy and pneumonia; for these affections are diagnosed from the spit. We already know what pleurisy is, but we shall now repeat it. Pleurisy is inflammation of the membrane lining the ribs produced by blood that is on the bilious side. Pneumonia, on the other hand, is inflammation of the lungs caused by blood that is on the phlegmatic side.

And some raise a problem, "If every part is also abused by that which nourishes it, the lungs ought to be abused by rather bilious blood and the inflammation should come from this (bile) and not from phlegmatic blood. Similarly, in the case of pleurisy, it (the membrane), being sinewy, ought to be damaged by rather phlegmatic blood and the inflammation should be produced by this and not by rather bilious blood." We say that not all parts are necessarily damaged by their nutrient, just as here in the case of inflammation (of the lungs); for the lung is loose and open in texture, while the bile, being composed of fine particles, penetrates, flows off and is not held; consequently it is not blocked in and does not produce inflammation. Phlegm, however, creates pneumonia, because this is a dense humor; being dense it is blocked inside and produces the pneumonia.

And someone may ask, "And how is it the phlegm is found in the lung, if it is true that it is nourished by blood that is on the bilious side?" Our answer is that phlegm either flows back down from the head and is conveyed to the lung or phlegm is brought from the surrounding parts to

ποιεῖ φλεγμονὴν κατὰ τὸν αὐτὸν τρόπον.

Καὶ ἐπὶ τῆς πλευρίτιδος ἔστιν εἰπεῖν ὅτι, κἂν ἀπὸ φλεγματικωτέρου αἵματος τρέφεται ὡς νευρώδης, ἀλλ' ὅμως ἀπὸ χολωδεστέρου αἵματος βλάπτεται· ἐπειδὴ γὰρ νευρώδης ἐστὶν ὁ ὑπεζωκώς, οὐ διεισέρχεται τὸ
173 φλέγμα, | ὥστε ποιῆσαι ἔμφραξιν καὶ ποιῆσαι φλεγμονήν, ἀλλ' ἡ χολὴ λεπτομερὴς οὖσα διεισέρχεται καὶ διεισδύνει καὶ στέγεται καὶ ἐμφράττεται καὶ ποιεῖ τὴν φλεγμονήν.

Ἀλλ' ἴσως ἀπορήσει τις ὅτι «Καὶ πόθεν ἡ χολὴ ἐν τῷ ὑπεζωκότι;» καὶ λέγομεν ὅτι ἢ ἀπὸ τῶν παρακειμένων μορίων φέρεται ἐκεῖσε χολὴ καὶ ποιεῖ τὴν φλεγμονὴν ἢ ὅτι ὑπόκειται προπεπονθὼς ὁ ὑπεζωκώς· καὶ τὸ τηνικαῦτα ἐπειδὴ πέπονθεν, ἀπεπτεῖται τὸ λόγῳ τροφῆς φερόμενον ἐν αὐτῷ, καὶ οὐ μόνον φλέγμα γεννᾶται, ἀλλὰ καὶ χολή, καὶ ποιεῖ τὴν φλεγμονήν. ἢ εἰπὲ ὅτι «Ἐν παντὶ μορίῳ διάφορος τίκτεται κακοχυμία· ἐνδέχεται οὖν ἀθροισθῆναι χολώδη ὕλην ἐν τῷ ὑπεζωκότι καὶ ἐμφραγῆναι καὶ ποιῆσαι φλεγμονήν, ὁμοίως καὶ ἐν τῷ πνεύμονι γεννηθῆναι φλέγμα καὶ ἐμφραγῆναι καὶ ποιῆσαι φλεγμονήν.»

Τούτων οὕτως ἐχόντων σημειοῦται τὸ πτύελον ἀπὸ πέντε τινῶν. πρῶτον μὲν ἀπὸ τοῦ καιροῦ, δεύτερον ἀπὸ τοῦ τρόπου τῆς ἀναγωγῆς, τρίτον ἀπὸ τῆς κράσεως ὧν ἐπιδέχεται χρωμάτων, τέταρτον ἀπὸ τῆς συστάσεως καὶ πέμπτον ἀπὸ τοῦ σχήματος.

Καὶ ἀρκτέον ἀπὸ τοῦ πρώτου· σημειοῦται τοίνυν τὸ πτύελον ἀπὸ τοῦ καιροῦ λέγων οὕτως, ὅτι ἄριστόν ἐστι τὸ πτύελον τὸ ταχέως ἀναπτυόμενον. τὸ δὲ ταχέως διττόν ἐστι· δηλοῖ γὰρ τὸν χρόνον, τουτέστι τὴν ἀρχήν, τοῦ νοσήματος, κατὰ τὸ εἰρημένον ἐν Ἀφορισμοῖς, «πτύελον ἢν αὐτίκα ἐπιφαίνηται, βραχύνει καὶ τὰ λοιπά»· ἢ τὸ ταχέως δηλοῖ τὸ συντόμως ἅμα τῇ βήξει τοῦ κάμνοντος ἀναγόμενον καὶ ἀποπτυόμενον. ὅθεν καὶ ἡμεῖς οὕτως λέγομεν, ὅτι τάχιστα ἀναπτύει καὶ εὐανάγωγά εἰσι τὰ ἀναπτυόμενα. πλὴν δεῖ εἰδέναι ὅτι κατὰ τοῦ πρώτου ἁρμόζει ἡ ἀπὸ τοῦ καιροῦ σημείωσις, λέγω δὴ κατὰ τοῦ ἐν τῇ ἀρχῇ τῆς νόσου, ἐπεί τοι τὸ εὐθέως ἀναπτύεσθαι τοῦ δευτέρου ἐστὶ σημαινομένου, λέγω δὴ τοῦ ἀπὸ τοῦ τρόπου τῆς ἀναγωγῆς.

⟨Ἀπὸ δὲ τοῦ τρόπου τῆς ἀναγωγῆς,⟩ ὅτι τὰ ἀναγόμενα εὐπετῆ θέλει εἶναι καὶ ῥᾳδίως ἀνάγεσθαι τὸ πτύελον. καὶ ἔστιν ἀγαθόν· δηλοῖ γὰρ εὐεπήκοον τὴν ὕλην καὶ ἀνωδυνίαν. |

174 Ἀπὸ δὲ τῆς συστάσεως, δεῖ μήτε παχεῖαν καὶ γλίσχραν εἶναι τὴν ὕλην

23–31] *cf.* Gal. In Hipp. Progn. comm. II 43: CMG V 9,2 pp. 293,15–295,10 24 ἐν Ἀφορισμοῖς] Hipp. Aph. I 12: IV p. 464,18sq. L. *cf.* Gal. In Hipp. Progn. comm. II 43: CMG V 9,2 p. 295,2sq. 35–206,5] *cf.* Gal. In Hipp. Progn. comm. II 43: CMG V 9,2 p. 294,2–7

1 *ante* φλεγμονὴν *add.* τὴν γ 2 τῆς πλευρίτιδος] *cf. supra, p. 202,28 app. crit.* εἰπεῖν] ἰδεῖν L ὅτι *om.* L 3 *post* τρέφεται *add.* ὁ ὑπεζωκὼς γ; *sed cf. supra, p. 202,28–30* 8 ἀπορήσει] καὶ ἐνταῦθα ἐρεῖ γ 11 τὸ] τῷ LM 14 οὖν] γὰρ γ 15 sq. ὁμοίως – φλεγμονήν *om.* L 20 καὶ *om.* γ 22 τὸ[I] *om.* γ 25 *post* ἐπιφαίνηται *habet* ἀρχομένου *Hipp.* 26 τοῦ κάμνοντος *om.* γ ἀναγόμενον] ἀνάγοιτο μὴ L 27 λέγομεν οὕτως γ 30 τὸ] τοῦ γ ἀνατρέπεσθαι γ 31 τοῦ *om.* L τρόπου] πρώτου γ 32 Ἀπὸ – ἀναγωγῆς *addidi* 33 τὸ – ἀγαθόν *om.* L 35 *post* παχεῖαν *add.* εἶναι L

the lung, where it is blocked inside and causes inflammation in the same way.

For pleurisy one can say that, even though it (the membrane), being sinewy, is nourished by blood that is on the phlegmatic side, nevertheless it is damaged by rather bilious blood; for, since the lining (membrane) is sinewy, the phlegm cannot penetrate so as to create a stoppage and produce inflammation, but the bile, being composed of fine particles, does make its way through, penetrates, is held inside and blocked up and creates inflammation.

But someone may raise this difficulty: "How can you explain the bile in the lining (membrane)?" We say that either the bile is conveyed there from the parts roundabout and causes inflammation or that the lining was affected beforehand; in the latter case, since (the part) was affected, the matter conveyed for nutriment in it is not concocted and not only is phlegm produced, but bile as well, and it creates the inflammation. Or you may say that "Different unwholesome humors are produced in each part; it is possible, then, for bilious matter to gather in the lining, be blocked up and create inflammation, in the same way that phlegm, too, can develop in the lung, be blocked up and produce inflammation."

Following this discussion he gives the symptoms of spit from five things. First from time, second from mode of expectoration, third from the blend of colors which it receives, fourth from the consistency, and fifth from the shape.

To begin with the first, he gives the symptoms of spit from time in the following words, that the best spit is that which is brought up q u i c k l y. Now q u i c k l y has a double sense; for it indicates the time, that is the beginning, of the disease, as is said in the Aphorisms, "If spit appears at the beginning, it shortens etc."; or q u i c k l y means that the spit is brought up and expectorated straightaway when the patient coughs. Hence we express it like this, that he spits very quickly and the expectorated matter is brought up easily. However, it must be noted that the symptom based on time goes with the first meaning, namely that of the beginning of the disease, since to spit straightaway belongs to the second meaning, in other words, to mode of expectoration.

From the mode of expectoration: he says that the sputum should be dislodged easily and the spit brought up without trouble. And this is a good sign, since it means that the matter is giving way readily and there is no pain.

From consistency: the matter should be neither thick and viscous

μήτε λεπτὴν καὶ ὑδατώδη· τὰ γὰρ παχέα καὶ γλίσχρα ἔχουσι τὸ ἐχέκολλον καὶ δυσαπόσπαστον καὶ οὐκ ἀνάγονται· εἶτα λοιπὸν μὴ ἀναγόμενα φέρονται ἐπὶ τοὺς σήραγγας τῆς τραχείας ἀρτηρίας καὶ τῆς ἀρτηριώδους φλεβὸς καὶ ἐμφράττει αὐτούς· καὶ ἐντεῦθεν οὐ γίνεται ἡ πάροδος τοῦ πνεύματος, ἀλλὰ πνιγμωδῶς κινδυνεύουσι. τὰ δὲ λεπτὰ καὶ ὑδατώδη ἐν τῇ ἀνόδῳ ἀντιπερισχίζονται, καὶ ἔνθεν κἀκεῖθεν ἀντικαταρρεῖ, καὶ οὐκ ἀνάγεταί τι ἐξ αὐτῶν, ἀλλὰ μόνον κοπιᾷ ἡ δύναμις ἀκαίρως. δεῖ γὰρ εἰδέναι ὅτι πρῶτον μὲν ἡ δύναμις τῶν μεσοπλευρίων μυῶν ἢ ὅλου τοῦ θώρακος συμβάλλεται εἰς τὴν ἀναγωγήν, εἶτα τὸ πνεῦμα. τί γάρ; ὅτι ἐν τῇ συστολῇ τοῦ θώρακος ἐκθλίβεται, εἶτα ἐν τῇ ἐξωθήσει τοῦ πνεύματος τὰ ἀποκρουόμενα ἀκοντίζονται δίκην βολίστρας καὶ οὕτως ἀποπτύονται. ἀλλὰ δεῖ μέσως πως εἶναι κατὰ σύστασιν τοῦ παχέος καὶ γλίσχρου καὶ τοῦ λεπτοῦ καὶ ὑδατώδους, ἵνα τὸ πνεῦμα ἐκπεμπόμενον προσκροῦον καταστερεωθῇ αὐτὸ καὶ ἐκπέμπῃ τὴν ὕλην.

Ἀπὸ δὲ τῆς κράσεως τῶν ἐπιμιγνυμένων χρωμάτων, δεῖ πᾶσι τοῖς ἀναγομένοις χυμοῖς, λέγω δὴ καὶ τῇ ξανθῇ χολῇ καὶ τῇ μελαίνῃ καὶ τοῖς πελιδνοῖς, συναναμεμίχθαι φλέγμα, εἰ μέλλει ἀγαθὸν εἶναι, ἵνα τὸ φλέγμα τῇ οἰκείᾳ ὑγρότητι ἐπιτέγξῃ καὶ κολάσῃ τὸ δηκτικὸν καὶ δακνῶδες αὐτῶν. χείριστα δέ εἰσι καὶ τὰ ποικίλα καὶ ἄκρατα ἀναγόμενα· δηλοῖ γὰρ πλείστην κακοχυμίαν οὖσαν ἐν τῷ σώματι καὶ διαφόρους τὰς διαθέσεις, ἅτινα καὶ ὀλέθριά εἰσι. τὰ δὲ μὴ ποικίλα, ἀλλὰ καὶ κεκραμένα ὄντα, οὔκ εἰσι κακά. ἐν οὖν τοῖς ἀναγομένοις κρεῖττόν ἐστι τὸ αἷμα καὶ τὸ φλέγμα ἀνάγεσθαι. διὰ τί; ἐπειδὴ οὗτοι οἱ χυμοὶ ἀδήκτως καὶ ἀβιάστως ἀνάγονται, ἐπειδὴ πραεῖς εἰσιν· οὐδὲ γὰρ ἔχουσι τὸ δηκτικόν. ἡ δὲ ξανθὴ χολὴ καὶ ὁ μελαγχολικὸς κενούμενα ἄκρατα, εἴτε καθ' αὑτὰ εἴτε καὶ συμπεπλεγμένα ἀλλήλοις,
175 κακά εἰσιν· ἡ μὲν γὰρ ξανθὴ | χολὴ ἐν τῷ ἀνάγεσθαι δάκνει καὶ ἀνιᾷ καὶ ἑλκοῖ τοὺς τόπους ἐκείνους τῇ οἰκείᾳ δριμύτητι· ἔστιν ὅτε δὲ καὶ πυρετοὺς ὀξεῖς ἐξάπτει. ὁ δὲ μελαγχολικός, παχὺς ὢν καὶ γεώδης, δηλοῖ εἰς μῆκος χρόνου ἐκταθήσεσθαι τὸ νόσημα, ὥστε τῷ μήκει μὴ αὐταρκέσαι τὴν δύναμιν καὶ ἐπιστῆναι τὸν κίνδυνον. ἀλλὰ δεῖ αὐτὰ κεκρᾶσθαι, καθ' ἣν καὶ αὐτὸς λέγει, συμμεμιγμένον τε φαίνεσθαι τὸ ξανθὸν ἰσχυρῶς τῷ πτυέλῳ. καὶ αὐτὸς μὲν ἐπὶ τῆς χολῆς ἔφη ὅτι δεῖ τὴν χολὴν συναναμεμίχθαι τῷ φλέγματι· σὺ δὲ καὶ ἐπὶ παντὸς χυμοῦ εἰπὲ ὅτι «Δεῖ συναναμεμίχθαι αὐτοῖς φλέγμα, ὥστε κολάζεσθαι αὐτοὺς ὑπὸ τῆς ὑγρότητος τοῦ φλέγματος.»

Ἀπὸ δὲ τοῦ σχήματος, ὅτι τὰ στρογγύλα ἀναγόμενα κάκιστά εἰσι· δηλοῖ γὰρ πάχος φλέγματος καὶ μεγίστην φλόγωσιν ἐν τῷ βάθει οὖσαν· περιφρύσσεται γὰρ πανταχόθεν τὸ φλέγμα καὶ ἐν τῷ ἀνάγεσθαι προσπταῖον τῇδε κἀκεῖσε καὶ περιφερόμενον καταθραύονται τὰ ἄκρα πανταχόθεν, καὶ τὸ τηνικαῦτα στρογγύλα ἀποπτύονται. ἢ εἰπὲ ὅτι «Ἡ θερ-

32 ἔφη] *cf.* Hipp. Progn. 13: p. 210,4 A. = II p. 142,16 L.

2 *post* δυσαπόσπαστον *add.* τὸ δυσεκμόχλευτον γ   ἀνάγοντα γ   ἀναγομένων γ   6 ἀντικαταρέει γ   8 συμβάλλονται *codd.*: *correxi*   11 δὴ L   13 ἐκπέμπει γ: ἐμπέμπῃ L: *correxi*   17 μέλλοι PV(M?)   τὸ φλέγμα *post* ὑγρότητι *(lin. 18) trsp.* γ   19 ἐστι γ   23 ἐπειδή[I]] ἐπεὶ γ   25 ἐμούμενα γ   ἄλλοις L   27 τύπους L   ἔστι δὲ ὅτε γ   28 ἀνάπτει γ   29 ἀνταρκέσαι *coni. Wk.*   30 δὴ LMP: *corr.* V   αὐτὸς] αὐτὸ L   33 φλέγματι] αἵματι L

nor thin and watery; for thick and viscous sputa are glutinous, difficult to dislodge and are not brought up; then not being brought up they are conveyed to the passages of the trachea and arterial vein and block these; and as a result there is no passage for the air and they are in danger of suffocating. The thin and watery, on the other hand, disintegrate on the way up and run back again from all sides; no part of them is expectorated and the only result is a prematurely exhausted faculty. For bear in mind that it is the faculty of the intercostal muscles or of the whole thorax which in the first place contributes to expectoration, then the air. Why? Because in the contraction of the thorax (the matter) is squeezed out, then in the expulsion of the air the dislodged matter is ejected just as from a catapult and is discharged in this way. But in consistency they should be intermediate between thick and viscous, and thin and watery, in order for the expelled air to have sufficient power to eject the matter when it makes contact with it.

From the blend of mixed colors: each of the expectorated humors, namely yellow, black and livid bile, if it is to be good, should have an admixture of phlegm, in order to have its sting and pungency diluted and checked by the phlegm's own fluid. The worst sputa are the variegated and unblended; for they indicate the presence in the body of a very large number of unwholesome humors and a variety of disorders, and they are also deadly. Those which are both non-variegated and blended are not bad. It is a better sign, then, when blood and phlegm are brought up in the sputa. Why? Because these humors are expectorated without force or damage, since they are mild, having no pungency. But if yellow and black bile are discharged unblended, either separately or combined, they are bad; for the yellow bile, in being brought up, stings, irritates and ulcerates those parts by means of its pungency and sometimes also touches off acute fevers. And the black, being thick and earthy, means that the disease will be extended for a long time, with the result that the power (of the body) does not hold out due to the length of time and danger presents itself. But they should be blended, just as (Hippocrates) himself says, and the spit should have a strong admixture of yellow. He also said about the bile that it should be mixed with phlegm; but you may say for every humor that "Phlegm should be mixed with them, so that they are tempered by the phlegm's fluid."

From the shape: (he says) that the rounded sputa are very bad, since they mean that the phlegm is thick and there is intense burning heat deep inside; for the phlegm is scorched all over and, colliding on every side and traveling around, when it is being brought up, its extremities on all sides are knocked off, and then (the sputa) are expectorated round. Or say that "The heat scorches the outside of the phlegm,

μότης περιφρύσσει τὰ πέριξ τοῦ φλέγματος, παχέος αὐτοῦ ὄντος, καὶ ἐν τῇ ἀναγωγῇ περιφερόμενον τῇδε κἀκεῖσε σφαιροῖ αὐτό.»

Οὕτως σημειωσάμενος ἀπὸ τῶν πέντε τὰ κατὰ φύσιν πτύελα σημειοῦται καὶ τὰ παρὰ φύσιν. καὶ λέγει ὅτι πάντα τἀναντία τούτοις κάκιστά εἰσι καὶ ὀλέθρια. καὶ ἄρχεται ἀπὸ τοῦ καιροῦ, καί φησιν ὅτι κάκιστά εἰσι τὰ μὴ ἐν τῇ ἀρχῇ ἀναπτυόμενα, ἀλλ' ἐν τῇ παρακμῇ· δηλοῖ γὰρ ἀσθένειαν καὶ καταβολὴν τῶν δυνάμεων καὶ μὴ ὑπείκουσαν τὴν ὕλην καὶ δηλοῖ ὅτι τῇ ἀσθενείᾳ μήποτε οὐκ ἰσχύσῃ ἡ δύναμις ἐκταθῆναι μέχρι τῆς κρίσεως καὶ ἐν τῷ μέσῳ ἀποκάμῃ.

Ἀλλὰ καὶ ἀπὸ τοῦ τρόπου τῆς ἀναγωγῆς, λέγει ὅτι τὰ βραδέως καὶ δυσχερῶς ἀναγόμενα κάκιστά ἐστιν· ἐνταῦθα γὰρ οὐχ ὑπείκει ἡ ὕλη, ἥτις δηλοῖ μεγίστην ὀδύνην τῶν περὶ τὸν θώρακα μορίων. |

176 Ἀλλὰ καὶ κατὰ σύστασιν, κάκιστά ἐστι καὶ τὸ παχὺ καὶ τὸ γλίσχρον καὶ τὸ λεπτὸν καὶ ὑδατῶδες.

Εἶτα μέμνηται καὶ τῶν κακίστων χρωμάτων. καὶ λέγει ὅτι τὸ χλωρὸν ἀναπτυόμενον δηλοῖ μεγίστην ζέσιν οὖσαν ἐν τῷ πνεύμονι. δεῖ γὰρ εἰδέναι ὅτι τὸ ὀρῶδες τοῦ αἵματος ἐξυπεροπτούμενον, ἡ ξανθὴ γίνεται χολή· εἶτα ταύτῃ τῇ ξανθῇ χολῇ ἐπιμίγνυται τὸ ὀρῶδες ὑγρόν, καὶ γίνεται ἡ ὠχρὰ χολή· καὶ πάλιν ἐὰν μεγίστη ἐστὶν ἡ ζέσις καὶ ὑπερκαυθῇ ἡ ὠχρὰ χολή, τίκτεται ἡ ἰώδης. περὶ ταύτης τῆς ἰώδους χολῆς ὁ λόγος τῷ Ἱπποκράτει· ταύτην γὰρ ἐκάλεσε χλωράν. ἀλλὰ καὶ τὰ μέλανα ἀναπτυόμενα κάκιστά ἐστιν. ὁ δὲ μελαγχολικὸς γίνεται χυμὸς ἢ τῆς ξανθῆς χολῆς ὑπεροπτουμένης, καθ' ἣν καὶ μέλαινα χολὴ ὀνομάζεται· γίνεται μελαγχολικὸς καὶ ἐκ τοῦ τρυγώδους τοῦ αἵματος ἐξυπεροπτουμένου, ὅστις καὶ κυρίως ἐστὶ μελαγχολικός. ἐὰν οὖν μέλανα ἀναπτύωνται, κάκιστά ἐστι· μεγίστην γὰρ ζέσιν δηλοῖ. ἔστι δ' ὅτε ποτὲ ἐνδέχεται μέλανα τῇ ψύξει γενέσθαι τῷ λόγῳ τῆς νεκρώσεως. ἀλλὰ καὶ τὸ ἀφρῶδες πτύελον παγκάκιστόν ἐστι. γίνεται δὲ ὑπὸ φλεγματικῆς οὐσίας καὶ ἀερώδους. τί γάρ; ὅτι ἡ θερμότης καταλεπτύνει καὶ καταθραύει εἰς λεπτὰ μόρια τὴν οὐσίαν τοῦ φλέγματος· ἐν γοῦν τῇ κινήσει πάντως τίκτονται πνεύματα καὶ γίνονται πομφόλυγγες ἐπὶ ἁδρομερεστέρᾳ καταθραύσει τοῦ φλέγματος· εἶτα ἡνίκα διαρραγῶσιν αἱ πομφόλυγγες, γίνεται ἀφρός.

Δεύτερόν ἐστι κεφάλαιον, ἐν ᾧ περὶ κορύζης καὶ πταρμοῦ διαλέγεται. κόρυζα δέ ἐστιν ἄπεπτος καὶ παχεῖα φερομένη ὕλη ἀπὸ τοῦ ἐγκεφάλου πρὸς τοὺς μυκτῆρας ἐμφράττουσα αὐτούς, ὥσπερ καὶ κατάρρους ἐστί, φερόμενον δι' ὑπερῴας ἐκεῖνο τὸ ὑγρόν. ὁ δὲ πταρμὸς γίνεται πνευμάτων τινῶν παχέων ἀπὸ τῆς κεφαλῆς καταφερομένων ἐπὶ τοὺς μυκτῆρας καὶ ποιούντων ἦχον μέγαν. ὁ οὖν Ἱπποκράτης φησὶν ὅτι ταῦτα τὰ συμπτώματα κακά

16–20] *cf.* Gal. In Hipp. Progn. comm. II 47: CMG V 9,2 p. 297,11–15 27–32] *cf.* Gal. In Hipp. Progn. comm. II 47: CMG V 9,2 pp. 297,20–298,26

2 σφαιρεοῖ MV: σφερέει P 4 ἐναντία τούτοις πάντη γ 5 ἐστὶ PV 7 καὶ δηλοῖ] δηλοῖ γὰρ γ 8 ἰσχύσει γ 11 *ante* ἐνταῦθα *add.* καὶ γ εἴκει L 13 κάκιστά *om.* L 17 ῥοῶδες L 20 ἡ *om.* γ 23 μέλανα LM 25 ἀναπτύονται γ 26 ποτὲ *post* ἐνδέχεται *trsp.* γ 28 καὶ *om.* L 34 ὕλη φερομένη γ 35 πρὸς τοὺς μυκτῆρας *om.* γ *ante* ἐμφράττουσα *add.* καὶ γ 36 τὸ ὑγρὸν ἐκεῖνο γ

it being thick, and makes it globular as it travels around from side to side on the way up."

Having thus given the symptoms of normal spits from the five points he gives also the symptoms of the abnormal. He says that all the opposite (spits) are very bad and deadly. He begins with time and he tells us that those brought up, not at the beginning, but during the abatement, are extremely bad; for they mean weakness and collapse of the faculties and resistance by the matter, and they show that the (body's) power is perhaps not able from weakness to hold out till the crisis, but has become exhausted halfway.

From the mode of expectoration: he says that those which are brought up slowly and with difficulty are very bad; for in such cases the matter does not let go and this indicates severe pain in the parts around the thorax.

In consistency, the thick and viscous and the thin and watery are extremely bad.

Next he discusses the very bad colors. He says that green sputum means intense seething heat in the lung. For it should be noted that when blood serum is overheated the result is yellow bile; then the serous fluid mixes with this yellow bile and pale-yellow bile develops; and again if the seething heat is very intense and the pale-yellow bile is overheated, the verdigris (bile) is produced. It is about this verdigris bile that Hippocrates is speaking now; for this is the one he means by green. But the black sputa also are very bad. Now black bile develops either when the yellow is overheated, which also explains why it is called black; or black bile arises when the thick (non-serous) part of the blood is overheated, which is black bile in the strict sense of the word. If black sputa, then, are brought up, they are extremely bad; for they point to a very strong seething heat. But it is sometimes also possible for black sputa to result from the cold due to mortification. Frothy spit, too, is a very bad symptom. It is produced by phlegmatic and gaseous matter. Why? Because the heat refines and breaks up into fine particles the phlegm's substance; this action, then, inevitably produces gases and bubbles appear as the thicker parts of the phlegm disintegrate; then when the bubbles burst, foam develops.

The second chapter is where he discusses coryza and sneezing. Now coryza is undigested and thick matter which travels from the brain to the nostrils and blocks them, as catarrh is too, that fluid being borne by way of the palate. And sneezing occurs when certain dense gases descend from the head to the nostrils and make a loud noise. Hippocrates, then, says

177 εἰσιν ἐπὶ τῆς περιπνευμονίας· δηλοῦσι γὰρ ὅτι | πλείστη ἐστὶ ἡ κακοχυμία ἐν τῷ πνεύμονι καὶ τοσαύτη ἐστὶν ὥστε ἠδυνήϑη πέμψαι ἀτμοὺς ἐπὶ τὴν κεφαλὴν καὶ παχυνϑῆναι καὶ ἀντικαταρρεῦσαι καὶ ποιῆσαι ταῦτα τὰ συμπτώματα. κακὰ δέ εἰσι τὰ συμπτώματα ταῦτα ἐπὶ τῆς περιπνευμονίας καὶ ὡς σημεῖον, καϑ' ὃν εἰρήκαμεν τρόπον, καὶ ὡς αἴτιον, ὅτι ἐν κινήσει ϑεωροῦνται. ἡ δὲ τοιαύτη κίνησις σύντασίς ἐστι τῆς ἀποκριτικῆς τοῦ ἐγκεφάλου δυνάμεως· εἶτα διαλανϑάνει μοῖρά τις καὶ φέρεται ἐπὶ τὸν πνεύμονα καὶ κακοηϑεστέραν τὴν περιπνευμονίαν ἐργάζεται. δεῖ γὰρ εἰδέναι ὅτι μάλιστα κακόν ἐστι σύμπτωμα ὁ κατάρρους ἤπερ ἡ κόρυζα καὶ ὁ πταρμός· ὁ μὲν γὰρ κατάρρους, αὐτόϑεν δι' ὑπερῴας φέρεται ἡ ὕλη καὶ διαλανϑάνει καὶ φέρεται ἐπὶ τὴν τραχεῖαν ἀρτηρίαν καὶ οὕτως ἐπὶ τὸν πνεύμονα καὶ ἐπιτείνει ἐπὶ τὸ κακὸν τὴν περιπνευμονίαν· ἐπὶ δὲ τοῦ πταρμοῦ καὶ τῆς κορύζης ἔξω φέρεται ἡ ὕλη διὰ τῶν μυκτήρων, καὶ διὰ τοῦτο ἧττόν εἰσι κακά. καὶ πῶς οὐκ ἐμνημόνευσε τοῦ κατάρρου ὁ Ἱπποκράτης; λέγομεν ὅτι συμπεριέλαβε τῇ κορύζῃ καὶ τὸν κατάρρουν.

Ἰστέον δὲ ὅτι τὰ συμπτώματα ταῦτα ἢ ἐξ ἀρχῆς συνεισβάλλουσι μετὰ τῆς περιπνευμονίας ἢ τελευταῖον ἐπιγίνονται. καὶ εἰ μὲν ἐξ ἀρχῆς συνεισβάλλουσι τὰ πάϑη ταῦτα, δηλοῦσι πολλὴν οὖσαν τὴν κακοχυμίαν· εἰ δὲ τελευταῖον ἐπιγένωνται, τί δηλοῦσιν; ὅτι τοσαύτη ἐστὶν ἡ κακοχυμία ὅτι καὶ ἀτμοὺς ἔπεμψεν ἐπὶ τὴν κεφαλὴν καὶ παχυνϑὲν καὶ ἀντικαταρρεῦσαν ἐποίησε τὰ πάϑη ταῦτα. καὶ χείριστόν ἐστιν, εἰ τελευταῖον ἐπιγένωνται. τί γάρ; ὅτι τῷ μήκει πάντως ἠσϑένησαν αἱ δυνάμεις καὶ οὐκ ἐξαρκοῦσι καὶ ἐντεῦϑεν ἐπιγίνεται ὁ κίνδυνος.

Δεῖ δὲ καὶ τοῦτο εἰδέναι, ὅτι τὰ πάϑη ταῦτα, λέγω δὴ ὁ κατάρρους καὶ ἡ κόρυζα καὶ ὁ πταρμός, ἐπὶ ἄλλων τινῶν νοσημάτων οὔκ εἰσι κακά, ἀλλὰ καὶ ὠφέλιμα καὶ αἴτια σωτηρίας. τί γάρ; ὅτι ἑτέροις πυρεκτικοῖς νοσήμασιν ἐπιγινόμενοι ἐν τῇ παρακμῇ δηλοῦσιν ὅτι ἐρρώσϑη ἡ δύναμις καὶ ἐπεγερϑεῖσα διὰ τῶν φυσικῶν ἐκροῶν ἀπεδίωξε τὴν ὕλην καὶ ὅσον οὔπω λύεται τὸ νόσημα. |

178 Ταῦτα εἰρηκὼς λέγει ὅτι κάκιστόν ἐστι καὶ ἐν τοῖς περιπνευμονικοῖς καὶ ἐν τοῖς πλευριτικοῖς, ἐὰν ἡ ξανϑὴ χολὴ παρὰ μέρος ἐμεϑῇ, καὶ τὸ αἷμα δὲ ὁμοίως. τί γάρ; ὅτι φλεγμονὴ ὑπόκειται· ἐν δὲ τῇ φλεγμονῇ πάντως καὶ χολή ἐστι καὶ αἷμα· κάλλιον οὖν ἐστιν, εἰ συμμιγῆ καὶ κεκραμένα ἀναπτύονται· δηλοῦσι γὰρ ὅτι ἐρρώσϑη ἡ δύναμις καὶ ἴσχυσεν, ὥστε μῖξαι αὐτὰ αἱ κεράσαι, ἀλλὰ καὶ τὴν ὕλην λεπτυνϑεῖσαν, ὥστε καὶ τῇ λεπτομερείᾳ ιεισελϑ εῖν ἐν ἑαυτοῖς καὶ ἀνακερασϑῆναι.

8–14 κακά] *cf.* Gal. In Hipp. Progn. comm. II 49: CMG V 9,2 p. 300,5–9

1 ἡ *om.* L 3 sq. ταῦτα – εἰσι *om.* γ 7 δυνάμεως *om.* γ 9 κάκιστόν γ εἴπερ γ 10 ὁ μὲν . . . ἡ ὕλη] *cf. supra, pp. 158,19; 188,34 sq.* 12 πταρμοῦ *scripsi*: κατάρρου *codd.* 14 λέγομεν *post* κατάρρου *trsp.* γ 18 πάϑη ταῦτα] παϑήματα L 19 ἐπιγίνονται L τί *om.* L 20 *fort.* παχυνϑέντων καὶ ἀντικαταρρευσάντων *scribendum est (cf. lin. 3)* 21 χειρίστη γ 25 οὔκ *om.* L 31 ἐμεϑῇ *post* χολὴ *trsp.* γ 33 ἐστι *post* αἷμα *trsp.* γ εἰ] ἵνα γ 36 διεισελϑῆναι γ αὐτοῖς L διακερασϑῆναι L

that these are dangerous symptoms in pneumonia, being indications of a very large quantity of unwholesome humors in the lung, large enough to have been able to transmit vapors to the head, which became dense, flowed back down and produced these symptoms. And in cases of pneumonia these symptoms are bad both as a sign, in the way we have described, and as a cause, in so far as they are regarded as a movement. Such a movement is a strain on the brain's excretory faculty; then a certain amount (of matter) escapes, travels to the lung and makes the pneumonia more malignant. And note that catarrh is a worse symptom than coryza and sneezing; for in the case of catarrh the matter is conveyed directly along the palate, and it escapes, goes into the trachea and from there to the lung, where it exacerbates the pneumonia; but in the case of sneezing and coryza the matter is carried out through the nostrils, and consequently they are not as bad. But why did Hippocrates not mention catarrh? We say that he included catarrh in coryza.

It should be noted that these symptoms either come on together at the beginning along with the pneumonia or they develop at the end. If these affections come on together from the beginning, they mean a great quantity of unwholesome humors; if they supervene at the end, what do they show? That the unwholesome humors were extensive enough to send to the head vapors which thickened and flowed back down to cause these affections. It is much worse when they appear at the end. Why? Because due to the length (of time) the faculties have inevitably weakened, they are not strong enough (for their work) and hence the danger sets in.

Note also that in certain other diseases these affections, namely catarrh, coryza and sneezing, are not bad, but both beneficial and conducive to health. Why? Because, appearing during abatement in other fever diseases, they mean that the power has recovered, has been roused to action and has expelled the matter by natural discharges, and the disease is all but cured.

After this he says that it is a very bad sign in both pneumonia and pleurisy cases, if yellow bile is brought up on its own; and the same applies to blood. Why? Because there is inflammation; and with inflammation there is always bile and blood; it is better, then, if they are expectorated mixed together and blended; for they show that the power has recovered and is strong enough to mix and blend the two; it also means that the matter has been refined, so that they penetrated each other and combined thanks to the small particles.

IX

II 25 [14: 211,13 A. = II 146,12 L.] Πάντα δὲ τὰ πτύελα πονηρά ἐστιν, ὁκόσα ἂν τὴν ὀδύνην μὴ παύῃ, κάκιστα δὲ τὰ μέλανα, ὡς διαγέγραπται καὶ τὰ ἑξῆς.

Ἔτι περὶ τοῦ πτυέλου διαλεγόμενος ὁ Ἱπποκράτης φλεγμονὴν τοῦ ὑπεζωκότος ὑποτίθεται καὶ ὡς ἐπὶ πλευρίτιδι γυμνάζει τὸν λόγον. καί φησιν ὅτι αὕτη ἡ πλευρῖτις ἢ κατ' ἔκρουν ἐστί, τουτέστι διὰ πτυέλων διαφορεῖται καὶ ἀνακαθαίρεται καὶ οὕτως παύεται, ἢ τῷ χρόνῳ εἰς ἐμπύημα μεθίσταται. αὕτη δὲ ἡ κατ' ἔκρουν φλεγμονὴ τοῦ ὑπεζωκότος, ἤγουν ἡ κατ' ἔκρουν πλευρῖτις, διττή ἐστιν· ἢ γὰρ λόγῳ κρίσεως γίνεται ἢ λόγῳ συμπτώματος. καὶ πόθεν ὀφείλομεν γνῶναι, εἴτε λόγῳ κρίσεως γίνεται εἴτε λόγῳ συμπτώματος; εἰ μὲν λόγῳ κρίσεως γίνεται, μετὰ τὸ ἀναπτυσθῆναι τὸ πτύελον ῥᾳστώνη ἕπεται τῆς ὀδύνης· πρὸς τούτοις δὲ καὶ εὐφορία ἐπακολουθήσει. εἰ δέ γε ἐπὶ τοῖς ἀναπτυομένοις μὴ ἐπιγένηται ῥᾳστώνη, ἔσο γινώσκων ὅτι λόγῳ συμπτώματος γέγονεν ὁ κατ' ἔκρουν πτύελος, ὅπερ κάκιστόν ἐστιν. ἀλλ' ἐπειδὴ τὸ κακὸν πλάτος ἔχει — ἔστι γὰρ ὑφειμένον κακόν, ἔστι καὶ ἐπιτεταμένον —, δεῖ ἡμᾶς ἐπεξελθεῖν ἕκαστα. εἰ μὲν γὰρ ὕφαιμα ὦσιν, ἐπ' ἔλαττόν εἰσι κακά· εἰ δὲ μέλανα ἢ πελιδνὰ ὦσιν, ἐπιτεταμένως εἰσὶ κακά. εἰ δὲ μηδὲν ἀναπτύεται, ἢ καὶ ἀναπτυόμενα ἐλάχιστα πάνυ καὶ ὀλίγα ἀναπτύεται, καὶ ἐπὶ τούτοις τοῖς ἀναπτυομένοις μηδόλως παύσηται τὰ τῆς ὀδύνης, εἶτα καὶ φλεβοτομίᾳ χρωμένων ἡμῶν καὶ καθάρσει
179 ἢ καὶ πυ|ρίαις μὴ ὑποχαλάσῃ τὰ τῆς ὀδύνης, ἔσο γινώσκων ὅτι εἰς ἐμπύημα μεθίσταται ἡ τοιαύτη πλευρῖτις.

Ἐπειδὴ δὲ περὶ ἐμπυήματος ἡμῖν ὁ λόγος, εἰς τρία περικλείσωμεν τὴν ὅλην πραγματείαν. καὶ ἐν μὲν τῷ πρώτῳ κεφαλαίῳ ζητήσωμεν, πόθεν ὀφείλομεν γνῶναι, πότε ἄρχεται γίνεσθαι ἡ πυοποίησις· ἐν δὲ τῷ δευτέρῳ ζητήσωμεν, ἐν ποίῳ καιρῷ ἡ ῥῆξις γίνεται τῆς πυοποιήσεως· ἐν δὲ τῷ τρίτῳ ζητήσωμεν, ποία ἐστὶν ἀγαθὴ πυοποίησις καὶ ποία κακίστη.

Καὶ ἀρκτέον ἀπὸ τοῦ πρώτου. τὴν ἀρχὴν τῆς πυοποιήσεως γινώσκομεν, ἡνίκα ἄλογον ῥῖγος ἐπιγίνεται· ἄλογον δὲ ῥῖγός ἐστιν, ἡνίκα μὴ περιοδίζει, ἀλλ' ἀτάκτως εἰσβάλλει. εἶτα ἐπὶ τῷ ῥίγει ἐὰν καὶ πυρετὸς ἐπακολουθήσῃ καὶ μηκέτι αἰσθάνηται ὀδύνης, ἀλλὰ βάρους τινὸς συναίσθησις ἐγγίνηται αὐτῷ, ἐὰν ταῦτα οὕτως διαφανῶσιν, ἔσο γινώσκων ὅτι ἡ ἀρχὴ τῆς πυοποιήσεώς ἐστιν. εἶτα λοιπὸν δεῖ ἡμᾶς ζητῆσαι, διὰ τί γίνονται ταῦτα. καὶ τὸ μὲν ἄλογον ῥῖγος γίνεται τῷ λόγῳ τῆς πυοποιήσεως· ἀτμῶν τινων δριμέων ἢ ποιότητος φερομένων ἐπὶ τὰ παρακείμενα μόρια, καὶ δάκνοντα καὶ ἀνιῶντα ταῦτα, γίνονται τὰ ἄλογα ῥίγη. οὕτως γὰρ καὶ

31–214,11] *cf.* Gal. In Hipp. Progn. comm. II 58: CMG V 9,2 pp. 309,15–310,4

6 ἐπὶ *om.* γ *post* πλευρίτιδι *add. et del.* καὶ L διαγυμνάζει MP *(e corr.)*: ἀναγυμνάζει V 11 εἴτε[II]] ἢ γ 14 ἐπὶ] ἐν L; *sed cf. lin. 20* 17 *post* ἔστι *add.* δὲ γ ἑκάστῳ γ 18 sq. εἰ — κακά *om.* γ 19 ἀναπτυόμενον γ 22 *ante* μὴ *add.* καὶ γ ἔσῃ, *ut vid.*, L 24 περικλείσομεν γ 25–28 ζητήσομεν *ter* γ *(lin. 27 PV)* 30 ἐστιν] ἐπιγίνεται L 31 περιοδίζῃ γ 32 αἰσθάνεται PV 33 γίνεται γ 36 φερομένης L 37 ταῦτα *om.* γ

IX

II 25 All sputa which do not stop the pain are bad, and the worst are the black, as we have described, etc.

Still on the subject of spit, Hippocrates proposes inflammation of the membrane lining (the ribs) and discusses the case of pleurisy. This pleurisy, he says, is either discharged, that is, is dissipated by spits and is cleared out and cured in this way, or it turns to empyema through time. And this discharging inflammation of the lining, or discharging pleurisy, is of two kinds; for it takes the form of either a crisis or a symptom. And how are we to know whether it has the form of a crisis or of a symptom? If it acts like a crisis, expectoration will bring relief from the pain; and, in addition, a sense of well-being will result. But if expectoration does not bring relief, you may conclude that the sputum discharge has the character of a symptom, which is very bad. However, since there are degrees of badness – for there is the slightly bad and the extremely bad –, we must examine each. If (the sputa) are shot with blood, they are slightly bad; if black or livid, they are extremely bad. On the other hand, if nothing is brought up or, even in the event of expectoration, a very slight and negligible amount is brought up, and the pain does not cease at all with these expectorations, and then after we employ venesection and purging and even heat treatment, the pain does not subside, you may conclude that such a case of pleurisy is turning to empyema.

And since we are speaking of empyema, let us cover the whole topic under three headings. And under the first heading let us examine how we are to know when suppuration begins; under the second let us inquire at what time rupture of the suppuration takes place; and under the third let us examine which is the best suppuration and which the worst.

Beginning with the first, we can tell that suppuration is starting, when unpredictable shivering develops; and shivering is unpredictable when it does not come in periods but attacks irregularly. Then if the shivering is followed by fever and the patient no longer feels pain, but experiences a sensation of heaviness, if these things occur in this way, you will know that it is the beginning of suppuration. Next we should examine the reasons for these developments. Unpredictable shivering is caused by the suppuration; for when pungent vapors or a (pungent) quality are transmitted to the surrounding parts they sting and irritate them, and unpredictable shiverings develop. It is like what we said also

ἐπὶ τοῦ ῥίγους ἐλέγομεν, ὅτι γίνεται τὸ ῥῖγος ἀτμῶν τινων δριμέων πεμπομένων ἐπὶ τὰ αἰσθητικὰ καὶ κινητικὰ μόρια καὶ ἐπὶ τὴν ἐπιφάνειαν, καὶ δακνόντων αὐτὰ καὶ ἀνιώντων γίνεται ῥῖγος. ὁ δὲ πυρετὸς ἐπακολουθεῖ τῷ λόγῳ τῆς ἀνίας· ὑποστέλλεται τὸ ἔμφυτον θερμὸν ἐπὶ τὸ βάθος, καὶ τῇ ὑποστολῇ διπλασιαζόμενον τὸ ἔμφυτον θερμὸν ὁμοτίμως ἐκθάλπει τὸ πᾶν σῶμα, καὶ γίνεται ὁ πυρετός· λοιπὸν δὲ ὅτι ἐξαναλίσκονται καὶ διαφοροῦνται οἱ ἀτμοὶ δριμεῖς, καὶ τὸ τηνικαῦτα ἐπιγίνεται ὁ πυρετός. τοῦ δὲ βάρους ἡ συναίσθησις γίνεται τρόπῳ τοιούτῳ· τὸ πρότερον καταμεμερισμένον ὑγρὸν εἰς διαφόρους χώρας τοῦ φλεγμαίνοντος μορίου ἐν τῇ πυο-
180 ποιήσει εἰς ἕνα καὶ τὸν αὐτὸν τόπον ἀθροίζεται τοῦ | φλεγμαίνοντος μορίου, καὶ τὸ τηνικαῦτα βάρους γίνεται συναίσθησις. οὕτως γοῦν καὶ ἐν ταῖς χειρουργίαις ἡμῶν χρωμένων ἐν ταῖς ἀποστάσεσιν, ἅμα τῇ διαιρέσει ἀθρόα γίνεται ἡ διέξοδος καὶ ἔκκρισις τοῦ πύου, ὡς εἰς ἕνα τόπον ἀθροισθὲν τὸ πύον· ἡνίκα δὲ θελήσωμεν ὠμοχειρούργητον ποιῆσαι τὴν χειρουργίαν ἐπὶ τῶν ἀποστημάτων, οὐ γίνεται ἀθρόα ἡ ἔκκρισις, ἀλλ' ὀλίγιστον ὑγρὸν καὶ λεπτὸν καὶ ὕφαιμον ἢ καὶ ἰχωρῶδες ἐκκρίνεται διὰ τὸ τέως καταμεμερισμένον εἶναι τὸ ὑγρὸν εἰς διαφόρους χώρας τοῦ φλεγμαίνοντος μορίου.

Δεύτερον δέ ἐστι κεφάλαιον, ἐν ᾧ δεῖ ἡμᾶς εἰπεῖν τὸν χρόνον, ἐν ᾧ αἱ ῥήξεις γίνονται τῶν πυοποιήσεων. καί φησιν ὅτι ἐν τῇ ἑβδόμῃ αἱ ῥήξεις γίνονται – ὅπερ σπανίως τοῦτο ὤφθη γινόμενον –, ἢ ἐν τῇ εἰκοστῇ ἢ τῇ τριακοστῇ· τὰ δὲ ἐν τῇ ἑξακοστῇ ἡμέρᾳ ῥήγνυνται, τὰ δὲ καὶ ἐπέκεινα. δεῖ δὲ εἰδέναι ὅτι αἱ πυοποιήσεις καθόλου δύο εἰσίν, ἡ μὲν ἀπὸ τοῦ πεπονθότος μορίου λαμβανομένη, ἡ δὲ ἀπὸ τῆς ὕλης, ἅτινα τῷ καιρῷ ἀφίστανται ἀπ' ἀλλήλων. καὶ ἀπὸ μὲν τοῦ πεπονθότος μορίου· ἐὰν θερμότερον καὶ ὑγρότερον καὶ σαρκωδέστερόν ἐστι τὸ πεπονθὸς τῇ φλεγμονῇ μόριον, τάχιστα γίνεται ἡ πυοποίησις· εἰ δὲ ψυχρότερόν ἐστι τὸ μόριον καὶ νευρωδέστερον, χρονία. ἀπὸ δὲ τῆς ὕλης· εἰ μὲν θερμή ἐστιν ἡ ὕλη καὶ χολώδης, ταχεῖα γίνεται ἡ πυοποίησις καὶ ἡ ῥῆξις· εἰ δὲ ψυχρά ἐστιν ἡ ὕλη καὶ φλεγματικωτέρα, χρονιωτέρα γίνεται ἡ πυοποίησις καὶ ἡ ῥῆξις. καὶ ἁπλῶς εἰπεῖν, ἐὰν πάντα θερμὰ συνδράμωσιν, ἥ τε ὥρα καὶ ἡ χώρα καὶ τὸ κατάστημα καὶ ἡ ἡλικία, καὶ ἐὰν ἡ δύναμις ἔρρωται καὶ τὸ μόριον κύριόν ἐστι, ταχίστη γίνεται ἡ πυοποίησις· εἰ δὲ τἀναντία ψυχρὰ συνέλθωσι καὶ ἡ δύναμις ἀσθενὴς καὶ ἄκυρον μόριον, βραδεῖα γίνεται ἡ πυοποίησις καὶ ἡ ῥῆξις.

Τρίτον κεφάλαιόν ἐστιν, ἐν ᾧ δεῖ ζητῆσαι, ποῖαι ἀγαθαί εἰσι πυοποιή-
181 σεις καὶ ποῖαι κάκισται. ταῦτα δὲ | διαγινώσκομεν ἀπὸ ἕξ τινων· πρῶτον μὲν ἀπὸ τῆς εὐπνοίας ἢ δυσπνοίας, δεύτερον ἀπὸ τῆς εὐφορίας ἢ δυσφορίας, τρίτον ἀπὸ τοῦ εὐπετῶς ἀνάγεσθαι τὸ πτύελον ἢ δυσχερῶς, τέταρτον ἀπὸ τοῦ ἄδιψον εἶναι τὸν κάμνοντα ἢ ἔκδιψον, πέμπτον ἀπὸ τοῦ ὁμαλῶς κεκρᾶσθαι τὸ σῶμα ἢ ἀνωμάλως, ἕκτον ἀπὸ τοῦ κατὰ φύσιν ἢ παρὰ φύσιν

1 ἐλέγομεν] *in alio commentario, ut vid.*

2 ἐπὶ[II] *om.* γ 6 ὁ *om.* γ πυρετός] ὑδερετός L 7 δριμεῖς ἀτμοὶ γ ὁ *om.* L 8 τρόπῳ] λόγῳ γ 10 τόπον *post* ἀθροίζεται *trsp.* γ 11 ἐν] ἐπὶ γ 14 θελήσομεν γ 16 καὶ[III] *om.* γ 18 εἰπεῖν ἡμᾶς γ 21 ῥηγνύμενα L 25 μόριον *post* πεπονθὸς *trsp.* γ 27 τάχιστα γ 29 καὶ ἡ ῥῆξις *om.* γ 30 ὥρα *om.*, δύναμις *supra lin. ins.* L 34 ἐστιν *om.* γ 39 ἢ παρὰ φύσιν *om.* L

about (simple) shivering, that it develops when pungent vapors are communicated to the sensory and motor parts and to the surface (of the body), and when they sting and irritate them shivering develops. The fever follows by reason of the irritation; for the innate heat draws itself together to the deep interior and, doubling in intensity by its contraction, the innate heat warms up the entire body to the same degree and fever develops; and finally because the pungent vapors are consumed and dissipated the fever then supervenes. The sensation of heaviness develops in the following way: the fluid which was formerly distributed to various areas of the inflamed part is collected, during suppuration, into one and the same place of the inflamed part and then there develops a sensation of weight. It is the same when we employ surgery for abscesses, immediately on opening there is a copious discharge and outflow of pus, since it has gathered in one place; but when we decide to perform premature surgery on abscesses, there is not a copious outflow, rather a very small amount of fluid is passed off which is thin and bloody or even serous, due to the fact that at the start the fluid is distributed over different areas of the inflamed part.

Under the second heading we must give the time when ruptures of suppurations occur. (Hippocrates) says that the ruptures occur on the seventh day – something which has rarely been seen to happen – or on the twentieth or thirtieth; and some break on the sixtieth day and others even later. It should be noted that in general there are two types of suppuration, the one based on the affected part and the other on the matter, which are separated from each other by time. Depending on the affected part: if the inflamed part is fairly warm, fluid and fleshy, the suppuration forms very quickly; but if the part is on the cold and sinewy side, it takes a long time to suppurate. Depending on the matter: if the matter is warm and bilious, the suppuration and rupture occur quickly; if the matter is cold and on the phlegmatic side, suppuration and rupture take place more slowly. And to speak in a general way, if all (the concomitant factors) are warm, namely the season, the region, the weather and the age, and if the (body's) power is strong and the part an important one, then the suppuration will form very quickly; but if, on the contrary, the circumstances are cold, and the power is weak and the part unimportant, suppuration and rupture will come about slowly.

Under the third heading we must inquire about which suppurations are good and which worst. And these are distinguished by six means; first by good or bad breathing, second by euphoria or malaise, third by easy or difficult expectoration, fourth by the presence or absence of thirst in the patient, fifth by even or uneven body temperament, sixth

εἶναι τὰ διαχωρήματα. πρὸς δὲ τούτοις δεῖ σκοπεῖν τὸ ἀναγόμενον. καὶ εἰ μὲν πύον ἐστὶ καθαρόν, γίνωσκε ὅτι καλόν ἐστιν· εἰ δὲ μετὰ τοῦ πύου συμμεμιγμένον ἐστὶ χολῶδές τι ἢ ὠχρόν, γίνωσκε ὅτι ὀλεθρία ἐστὶν ἡ πυοποίησις. εἰ δὲ σὺν τούτοις εἴη μεμιγμένα πελιδνὰ ἢ μέλανα, γίνωσκε ὅτι ὀλεθριώτατός ἐστιν ἡ πυοποίησις. εἰ δὲ ὑπόπυρρά εἰσι καὶ ὑπόξανθα ταῦτα, μέσης εἰσὶ τάξεως· σὺν τοῖς ἓξ ἐκείνοις τοῖς ἀγαθοῖς ἐπιφαινόμενα ἀγαθά εἰσιν· εἰ δὲ σὺν τοῖς ἓξ τοῖς κακίστοις ἐπιφανῇ τὸ ὑπέρυθρον καὶ ὑπόξανθον, κακόν ἐστι. δεῖ δὲ εἰδέναι ὅτι ⟨ἔστιν⟩ ἐκ τῶν ἓξ τῶν κακίστων καὶ τὸν καιρὸν τοῦ θανάτου γνῶναι. εἰ μὲν τὰ ἓξ κακὰ ὁμοτίμως συνέλθωσιν, ἔσο γινώσκων ὅτι ὑπόγυός ἐστιν ὁ θάνατος· εἰ δέ γε ὀλιγώτερα συνέλθωσι κακὰ σημεῖα, δύο τυχὸν ἢ τρία, γίνωσκε ὅτι τοσοῦτον ἀφέστηκεν ὁ θάνατος.

Καὶ τὸ μὲν εὐπετέως ἀνάγεσθαι τὰ πτύελα ἀγαθόν ἐστιν, ἐπειδὴ δηλοῖ ὅτι ἐλεπτύνθη ἡ ὕλη καὶ ὑπήκοός ἐστιν ἀλλὰ καὶ τὴν ἀποκριτικὴν δύναμιν ἐρρωμένην οὖσαν. ἀλλὰ καὶ ἡ εὐφορία ἀγαθόν ἐστι· δηλοῖ γὰρ καλῶς διακεῖσθαι τὴν ζωτικὴν δύναμιν, ἀλλὰ καὶ τὰς ψυχικὰς διαθέσεις καλῶς διαγούσας, καθ' ἣν κινεῖται ὁ θώραξ. ἀλλὰ καὶ ἡ ἀνωδυνία ἀγαθόν ἐστι· δηλοῖ γὰρ ὅτι οὐκ ἔστι μεγάλη ἡ φλεγμονὴ οὐδὲ πολλὴ ἡ κακοχυμία. ἀλλὰ καὶ τὸ ὁμαλῶς κεκρᾶσθαι τὸ ὅλον σῶμα ἀγαθόν ἐστι· δηλοῖ γὰρ ἐρρωμένον ὂν τὸ ἔμφυτον θερμόν, καθὸ ἀκτινοειδῶς πᾶσι τοῖς μορίοις ὁμοτίμως ἐλλάμπει. κακὸν δέ ἐστι τὸ ἀνωμάλως κεκρᾶσθαι, τυχὸν τὰ ἄκρα κατεψυγμένα ἔχειν, τὸ δὲ βάθος διακαίεσθαι· δηλοῖ γὰρ ὅτι ἐλάχιστόν ἐστι
182 τὸ ἔμφυτον θερμὸν καὶ μεγίστην τὴν φλεγμονὴν οὖσαν | ἐν τῷ βάθει, καθ' ἣν τὸ ἔμφυτον θερμὸν συνάξαν ἑαυτὸ ἐπὶ τὸ βάθος συνένευσε. καὶ διὰ τοῦτο τὰ ἄκρα ψυχρά εἰσι διὰ τὸ μὴ ἐλλάμπεσθαι αὐτὰ ὑπὸ τοῦ ἐμφύτου θερμοῦ. ἀγαθόν ἐστι καὶ τὸ μὴ διψᾶν τὸν ἄνθρωπον, ἐπειδὴ δηλοῖ ὅτι οὐκ ἔστι ζέσις τοσαύτη οὐδὲ κακοχυμία, ὥστε ποιῆσαι δίψαν.

Καὶ ἀποροῦσιν ὅτι «Καὶ πῶς ἐνδέχεται πλευρίτιδος ὑποκειμένης καὶ φλεγμονῆς ἀξιολόγου καὶ πυρετοῦ ὀξέος; ὅπου γὰρ πλευρῖτις, καὶ πυρετὸς ὀξὺς σύνεστιν· ὅπου δὲ πυρετὸς ὀξύς, πάντως καὶ δίψος ἐπιγίνεται· καὶ πῶς λέγει ὅτι δίψος μὴ ἔχειν;» καὶ λέγομεν ὅτι δεῖ προσθεῖναι τὸ 'κάρτα', ἵνα τυχὸν οὕτως ἔχῃ· 'καὶ δίψαν μὴ ἔχειν κάρτα'· δηλοῖ γὰρ ὅτι οὐ πάνυ παρενοχλεῖ ἡ ζέσις καὶ ἡ κακοχυμία, ἐπεί τοί γε ἐπ' ἔλαττον πάντως διψῶσιν. ἀγαθὸν δέ ἐστι καὶ τὸ τὰ οὖρα καὶ τὰ διαχωρήματα κατὰ φύσιν ἐκκρίνεσθαι· δηλοῖ γὰρ ῥώμην καὶ ἰσχὺν τῆς πεπτικῆς δυνάμεως.

II 26 [15: 213,4 A. = II 150,2 L.] Πνεῦμα μέγα καὶ πυκνὸν εἶναι, τὴν ὀδύνην μὴ πεπαῦσθαι καὶ τὰ ἑξῆς.

Ἐνταῦθα τὰ κακὰ καὶ ὀλέθρια ἀπαριθμεῖται ὁ Ἱπποκράτης. καί φησιν ὅτι πάντα τὰ ἐναντία κακά ἐστιν· ἀλλὰ καὶ πνεῦμα μέγα τὴν

30 δίψος – ἔχειν] Hipp. Progn. 15: p. 212,11 A. = II p. 148,12 L.

1 ἐπισκοπεῖν γ   3 τι *post* συμμεμιγμένον *trsp.* γ   4 εἴη μεμιγμένα *om.* γ *ante* πελιδνὰ *add.* ἢ γ   6 τοῖς ἀγαθοῖς ἐκείνοις τοῖς ἓξ γ   8 ἔστιν *sec. Dietz addidi*   10 γε *om.* γ   13 δηλοῦσι(ν) MP   16 *ante* ἀγαθόν *add.* τυχὸν L   17 ἐστι *om.* γ   23 ἑαυτῷ *codd.*: *correxi*   26 ζέσις – δίψαν] κακοχυμία ὥστε ποιῆσαι δίψαν οὐδὲ ζέσις L   τοιαύτη γ: *correxi*   27 ὑποκειμένου γ   32 πάνυ L   34 δηλοῦσι γ

by normal or abnormal excrements. In addition, the evacuated matter should be examined. If the pus is pure, conclude that this is good; if the pus has a bilious or pale yellow admixture, you should know that the suppuration is deadly. And if together with these there is mixed livid or black matter, conclude that the suppuration is extremely deadly. But if these (mixtures) are reddish and yellowish, they are intermediate; in conjunction with the six favorable signs they are good; but if the reddish and yellowish appears along with the six worst symptoms, it is bad. And note that it is possible to predict also the time of death from the six unfavorable symptoms. If the six bad signs are present together to the same degree, know that death is imminent; but if fewer bad symptoms occur together, e.g. two or three, conclude that death is just so far away.

To bring up spits easily is a good sign, since it shows that the matter has been refined and is yielding and also that the excretory faculty is strong. And euphoria is good, because it shows that both the vital faculty and the psychic dispositions, by which thorax movement is determined, are doing well. And absence of pain is favorable, being a sign that the inflammation is not serious and that the quantity of unwholesome humors is not great. An even temperament throughout the body is favorable; for it shows that the innate heat is strong, which enables it to radiate evenly to all the parts. But an uneven temperament, for example when the extremities are cold and the deep interior very hot, is bad; for it means that the innate heat is very scarce and that there is extensive inflammation in the depths, which has forced the heat to gather itself up and converge there. And the reason why the extremities are cold is that they are not being irradiated by the innate heat. Absence of thirst in the patient is good, because it means that there is not a seething heat or unwholesome humors powerful enough to create thirst.

And the problem is raised: "How is this possible in a case of pleurisy with serious inflammation and acute fever? For where there is pleurisy, there is also acute fever along with it; and where there is acute fever, thirst inevitably occurs; so how can he say not to be thirsty?" We say that the word 'very' should be added to make the text read 'not to be very thirsty'; this shows that the patients are not being overly troubled by the seething heat and unwholesome humors, even though they inevitably experience a slight thirst. And it is a good sign when normal urines and excrements are passed, since it means that the digestive faculty is strong and effective.

II 26 If the air is deep and fast, the pain has not stopped etc.

Here Hippocrates enumerates the unfavorable and deadly signs. And he says that all the opposite (of those discussed above) are bad.

ἀναπνοὴν ἐκάλεσεν ὁ Ἱπποκράτης· κακὸν οὖν ἐστιν ἐπὶ τῶν πλευριτικῶν μεγάλην τὴν ἀναπνοὴν εἶναι, ἐπειδὴ ἐνδείκνυται πολλὴν τὴν ζέσιν καὶ τὴν κακοχυμίαν καὶ δυσκρασίαν.

Καὶ ἀποροῦσιν ὅτι «Πῶς ἐνδέχεται ἐπὶ τῆς πλευρίτιδος μεγάλην γίνεσθαι τὴν ἀναπνοήν, εἴ γε φλεγμονή ἐστι τοῦ ὑπεζωκότος ὑμένος καὶ ὀδύνη σύνεστιν, ὥστε μὴ δύνασθαι μέγα διασταλῆναι τὸν θώρακα;» καὶ λέγομεν ὅτι περὶ τῆς φλεγμονῆς διαλεγόμενος καὶ περὶ ἐμπυήματος αὐτῷ ὁ λόγος γέγονε. περὶ τὸν καιρὸν οὖν τῆς ῥήξεως ἐλθὸν ἐνδέχεται ῥαγῆναι τὸ ἐμπύημα καὶ εἰς τὰ κενὰ τοῦ θώρακος ἐκχυθῆναι καὶ τὸ τηνικαῦτα μηδενὸς παρεμποδίζοντος μεγάλην γενέσθαι τὴν ἀναπνοήν.

Ἰστέον δὲ ὅτι ἐγὼ οὐ δέχομαι τὸ πύον μετὰ τοῦ ξανθοῦ καὶ ἐρυθροῦ
183 ἀνάγεσθαι μέσης | εἶναι τάξεως καὶ μετὰ τῶν ἓξ ἐκείνων ἀγαθῶν ἀγαθὸν εἶναι, ⟨καὶ⟩ ἐὰν οὕτως ἐκκριθῇ τὸ πύον, συμμεμιγμένον ἔχον ξανθὸν ἢ ἐρυθρόν, εἶναι αὐτὸ κατὰ φύσιν. ἐγὼ δὲ οὐ δέχομαι τοῦτο κατὰ φύσιν εἶναι· ἡ γὰρ δύναμις ἡ πάντα ἐκεῖνα δυνηθεῖσα ἀγαθὰ ἀποτελέσαι ἠδύνατο καὶ τὸ πύον συμπέψαι καὶ ὁλοκάθαρον ποιῆσαι καὶ μὴ ἔχειν συμμιγὲς χολῶδες ἢ ἐρυθρόν· τοῦτο οὖν οὐκ ἔστι κατὰ φύσιν, ἀλλὰ παρὰ φύσιν καὶ ὀλέθριον, τὸ συμμεμιγμένον μετὰ τοῦ πύου εἶναι ξανθὸν ἢ ἐρυθρὸν καὶ οὕτως ἀνάγεσθαι. ἐνδέχεται δὲ καὶ τοῦτο λέγειν τὸν Ἱπποκράτην, ὅτι μετὰ τὸ ἀνάγειν ξανθὸν ἢ ἐρυθρὸν πρότερον, ἐπανάγει τὸ πύον μετέπειτα· δηλοῖ γὰρ ἐρρῶσθαι τὴν ἀλλοιωτικὴν δύναμιν, καὶ ἔστιν ἀγαθὸν σημεῖον τοῦτο.

II 27 [15: 213,14 A. = II 150,15 L.] Αἱ δὲ ἄλλαι ἐκπυήσιες αἱ πλεῖσται ῥήγνυνται αἱ μὲν εἰκοσταῖαι, αἱ δὲ τριηκοσταῖαι, αἱ δὲ τεσσαρακονθήμεροι, αἱ δὲ πρὸς τὰς ἑξήκοντα ἡμέρας ἀφικνέονται.

Δεῖ εἰδέναι ὅτι πᾶσαι αἱ κενώσεις αἱ ἐν ταῖς κρισίμοις ἡμέραις γινόμεναι ἀγαθαί εἰσι καὶ σωτήριαι. ἄλλας δὲ ἐκπυήσεις καλεῖ τὰς ἐν τοῖς τυχοῦσι μορίοις γινομένας ἀποστάσεις καὶ ταύτας λέγει ῥήγνυσθαι. καὶ λέγομεν ὅτι ἄλλας ἐκπυήσεις λέγει οὐκ ἐν τοῖς τυχοῦσι μορίοις γινομένας ἀποστάσεις, ἀλλὰ περὶ τῆς πλευρίτιδος καὶ τῆς περιπνευμονίας αὐτῷ ὁ λόγος, οὐ κατὰ τόπον οὖν διαφερόντως ἐχούσας ἀποστάσεις, ἀλλὰ κατὰ τὴν ὕλην διαφερούσας, λέγω δὴ τὰς ἐπὶ ψυχροτέρᾳ ὕλῃ καὶ παχυτέρᾳ γινομένας· ἐν αἷς ἐπάγει καὶ τὰς κρισίμους ἡμέρας καί φησιν ὅτι αἱ μὲν ἐν τῇ εἰκοστῇ ἡμέρᾳ ῥήγνυνται, αἱ δὲ ἐν τῇ τριακοστῇ, αἱ δὲ ἐν τῇ τεσσαρακοστῇ, αἱ δὲ ἐν τῇ ἑξηκοστῇ, αἱ δὲ καὶ ἐπέκεινα.

II 28 [16: 214,4 A. = II 152,1 L.] Λογιζόμενον ἀπὸ τῆς ἡμέρης

27 sq.] *cf.* Gal. In Hipp. Progn. comm. II 57: CMG V 9,2 p. 308,8—10

8 ἐλθὼν L 12 μέσως MV εἰσὶ γ ἀγαθῶν *om.* PV ἀγαθὸν *om.* LM; *sed cf. supra, p. 216,6* 13 καὶ *add. Nickel* 20 ἐπανάγει] ἐπανάγειν γ 23 εἰκοσταὶ γ τριακοσταῖαι L: τριειкοσταὶ γ: *sec. Hipp. correxi* 24 τεσσαρακοσταῖαι L 29 ἐμπυήσεις γ 30 τῆς^{II} *om.* γ 32 τὴν . . . γινομένας L: τὴν . . . γινομένην γ: *corr. Dietz* 34 αἱ^{1} – τριακοστῇ *om.* γ 34 sq. αἱ^{III} – ἑξηκοστῇ *om.* L

Deep air is Hippocrates' way of saying breathing; it is bad in pleurisy cases, then, if the breathing is deep, since this means that the seething heat, the unwholesome humors and the distemper are serious.

And the problem is posed: "How can the breathing be deep in pleurisy, in view of the fact that there is inflammation of the lining membrane and pain, so that it is not possible for the thorax to expand much?" We say that in his discussion of inflammation the subject of empyema has also arisen for him. And empyema, then, when its time for rupture has come, can break and be poured into the empty parts of the thorax, and in that event the breathing can become deep, since there is no impediment.

But note that I do not accept that the pus discharged with yellow and red matter is intermediate, and that it is favorable in conjunction with those six good symptoms, and that if the pus is eliminated in this way, having an admixture of yellow or red, it is normal. I do not accept this as normal; for if the power (of the body) was strong enough to produce all those good symptoms, it could also have concocted the pus and made it completely pure without any bilious or red admixture; this, then, is not normal, but abnormal and deadly, namely for the pus to have an admixture of yellow or red and to be brought up in this way. What Hippocrates may be referring to is this, that after the yellow or red matter is evacuated first, the pus is brought up later; and this is a good sign, because it means that the converting faculty is strong.

II 27 Most of the other suppurations break, some on the twentieth day, some on the thirtieth, some on the fortieth, while others go on to the sixtieth.

Note that all evacuations on critical days are good and salutary. By other suppurations he means abscesses in any of the (other) parts of the body, and these are the ones which he says rupture. But we say that by other suppurations he does not refer to abscesses in any of the (other) parts; rather, being on the subject of pleurisy and pneumonia, (he means) abscesses then, which differ not in location but according to the matter, namely those which develop from fairly cold and thick matter; and for these also he supplies the critical days saying some break on the twentieth, some on the thirtieth, some on the fortieth, some on the sixtieth, others still later.

II 28 Counting from the day on which the patient first

ἧς τὸ πρῶτον ἐπύρεξεν ὁ ἄνθρωπος καὶ τὰ ἑξῆς.

Τί βούλεται καλεῖν ἀπὸ τῆς πρώτης ἡμέρας; ἆρα ἀφ' ἧς ἡμέρας ἐπύρεξεν ὁ ἄνθρωπος; καὶ λέγομεν ὅτι ἐκείνη ἡ ἀρχὴ τοῦ ὅλου νοσήματός
184 ἐστιν· ἐνταῦθα δὲ λέ|γει πρῶτον ἐπύρεξεν ὁ ἄνθρωπος, τουτέστιν ἀφ' ἧς ἡμέρας τὰ ἄλογα ῥίγη γεγόνασι καὶ οἱ πυρετοὶ οἱ ἄλογοι· ἔσο γινώσκων ὅτι ἀπ' ἐκείνης τῆς ἡμέρας ἡ ἀρχὴ τῆς πυοποιήσεως γέγονεν, ἤγουν τοῦ ἐμπυήματος.

II 29 [16: 214,9 A. = II 152,6 L.] Εἰ δὲ εἴη τὸ ἐμπύημα ἐπὶ θάτερα μόνον, στρέφειν τε καὶ καταμανθάνειν χρή

Δεῖ εἰδέναι ὅτι δύο ὑμένες διαφράττουσι τὸν θώρακα ἀρχόμενοι ἀπὸ τοῦ στέρνου καὶ ἀφικνοῦνται μέχρι τῆς ῥάχεως, ὡς γίνεσθαι δύο κοιλίας ἐν τῷ θώρακι καὶ διείργεσθαι ἀπ' ἀλλήλων, ὥστε μὴ ἐπικοινωνεῖν ἑκάτερον θατέρου, ἀλλ' ἀποκεχωρηκότας ἀπ' ἀλλήλων, ὡς μὴ δύνασθαι μεθίεσθαί τι ἀπὸ τῆς δεξιᾶς κοιλίας ἐπὶ τὴν ἀριστερὰν μήτε ἀπὸ τῆς ἀριστερᾶς ἐπὶ τὴν δεξιάν. ὅθεν τῆς μιᾶς πασχούσης κοιλίας τοῦ θώρακος ἡ λεγομένη ἡμιφωνία γίνεται, τῶν δὲ δύο πασχουσῶν ἡ ἀφωνία. μέσον δὲ ἐντέτακται ὁ πνεύμων. λέγει οὖν ἡμῖν ὁ Ἱπποκράτης σημεῖα, πόθεν ὀφείλομεν γνῶναι, ποία ἐστὶ κοιλία, ἐν ᾗ τὸ ἀπόστημα ἐρράγη. καί φησιν ὅτι τοσοῦτον μέσως τέτακται ὁ πνεύμων ὅτι ἐπὶ τῆς περιπνευμονίας εἰς ἀμφοτέρας τὰς κοιλίας ἐκχεῖται τοῦ θώρακος τὸ πύον. ὅθεν οὐδὲ συμβάλλονται ἡμῖν τὰ νῦν σημεῖα πρὸς διάγνωσιν ἐπὶ τῆς περιπνευμονίας. ἀλλὰ συμβάλλονται ἡμῖν, εἴτε ἐν τῇ δεξιᾷ πλευρᾷ συσταίη τὸ ἀπόστημα καὶ ἐκχυθῇ τὸ πύον εἴτε ἐπὶ τῆς ἀριστερᾶς πλευρᾶς. καί φησιν ὅτι ἐκ δύο τινῶν διαγινώσκομεν, εἴτε εἰς τὴν δεξιὰν κοιλίαν ἐστὶ τὸ πύον εἴτε εἰς τὴν ἀριστεράν, ἔκ τε τῆς παρὰ φύσιν ἡμῖν θερμότητος καὶ ἐκ τῆς τοῦ βάρους ἐφολκῆς ἐπὶ τῆς κατακλίσεως. καὶ ἀπὸ μὲν τῆς θερμότητος οὕτως· ἐκεῖνο τὸ μέρος τῆς πλευρᾶς, ἔνθα τὸ πύον ἐστί, δυσκρατότερόν ἐστιν καὶ θερμότερον ὑποπίπτει σοι τοῦ ἑτέρου πλευροῦ. ἀπὸ δὲ τῆς συναισθήσεως καὶ ἐφολκῆς τοῦ βάρους οὕτως· ὅτι εἰ μὲν ἐν τῇ δεξιᾷ κοιλίᾳ ἐστὶ τὸ πύον, ἀνάκλινον τὸν κάμνοντα ἐπὶ τὴν ἀριστερὰν πλευράν· καὶ ἐὰν αἴσθηται
185 ὁ | κάμνων βάρους καὶ ὀδύνης ἐν τῷ ὑπερκειμένῳ, γίνωσκε ὅτι ἐν τῇ δεξιᾷ κοιλίᾳ ἐστὶ τὸ πύον· εἰ δὲ τοὐναντίον ἀνακλίνῃς ἐπὶ τὸ δεξιὸν πλευρὸν καὶ αἴσθηται βάρους καὶ ὀδύνης ἐν τῷ ὑπερκειμένῳ μέρει, γίνωσκε ὅτι ἐν τῇ ἀριστερᾷ κοιλίᾳ ἐστὶ τὸ πύον.

2–7] *cf.* Gal. In Hipp. Progn. comm. II 58: CMG V 9,2 p. 309,22–25 10–15] *cf.* Gal. In Hipp. Progn. comm. II 59: CMG V 9,2 pp. 310,17–311,2 23 φησιν] Hipp. Progn. 16: p. 214,10–13 A. = II p. 152,8–12 L. ἐκ – 33] *cf.* Gal. In Hipp. Progn. comm. II 59: CMG V 9,2 p. 311,6–11

1 ὁ ἄνθρωπος ἐπύρεξεν *Hipp.* 18 μέσος *codd.*: *correxi* 19 sq. τοῦ θώρακος ἐκχεῖται γ 21 ἐπὶ] ἐκ L 23 διαγινώσκεις γ 24 ἡμῖν *om.* γ; *sed cf. supra, p. 144,34* 25 *post* ἐφολκῆς *add.* καὶ L 26 πύον] μέρος L 27 αἰσθήσεως L 29 *ante* ἀριστερὰν *add.* δεξιὰν L 31 ἀνακλίνεις *codd.*: *corr. Dietz*

succumbed to fever, etc.

What does he want to convey by from the first day? Is it from the day when the patient succumbed to fever? We say that this is the beginning of the entire disease; but he says here the patient first succumbed to fever, that is, from the day on which the unpredictable shiverings and irregular fevers developed; so you may conclude that the beginning of the suppuration, that is, of the empyema, was on that day.

II 29 But if the empyema is on one side only, you should turn (the patient) and find out

Note that two membranes divide the thorax, beginning from the breastbone and reaching to the spine, so that there are two cavities in the thorax and they are separated from one another; consequently neither communicates with the other, but they are cut off from one another, so that it is not possible for anything to be transferred from the right cavity to the left or from the left to the right. This explains why, when one of the thorax cavities is affected, so-called semivoicelessness results and (complete) voicelessness when both are diseased. And the lung is situated in the center. Hippocrates, then, gives us symptoms that should enable us to know in which cavity the abscess has erupted. He says that the lung occupies such a central position that in pneumonia the pus spills into both cavities of the thorax. Consequently, the present symptoms have nothing to offer for diagnosis in the case of pneumonia. But they do help us (to decide) whether the abscess has formed and the pus has spilled in the right or left side. He says that there are two ways of telling whether the pus is in the right or left cavity, from the presence of abnormal heat and from the pull of the weight in the reclining position. From the heat as follows: you will find that part of the side, where the pus is, to have a greater distemper and to be warmer than the other side. From the pull and sensation of weight thus: if the pus is in the right cavity, have the patient lean on his left side; if the patient feels a weight and pain in the upper part, conclude that the pus is in the right cavity; but if, conversely, you recline him on the right side and he feels weight and pain in the upper part, this will tell you that the pus is in the left cavity.

X

II 30 [17: 215,1 A. = II 152,13 L.] Τοὺς δὲ σύμπαντας ἐμπύους γινώσκειν χρὴ τοῖσδε τοῖς σημείοισιν καὶ τὰ ἑξῆς.

Ἐπειδὴ προσεχῶς περὶ ἐμπυημάτων διελέγετο, πάλιν ἐπαναλαμβάνει περὶ τῶν ἐμπυημάτων καὶ παραδίδωσιν ἡμῖν σημεῖα δηλωτικά, πόθεν ὀφείλομεν γνῶναι τοὺς ἐμπύους. καὶ τοῦτο ποιεῖ διὰ δέκα σημείων. ἐμπύημα δὲ λέγεται, ἡνίκα ἐν οἱῳδήποτε μορίῳ τοῦ σώματος ἀπὸ φλεγμονῆς ἢ ἀποστήματος ῥαγέντος ἀθροισθῇ ἀθρόον πύον, κἂν ἐν γαστροκνήμῃ κἂν ἐν μηρῷ κἂν ἐν μασχάλῃ κἂν ἐν βραχίονι καὶ τοῖς τοιούτοις. οἱ δὲ ἔμπυοι, εἰ μὲν ἀνενεχθῇ τὸ πύον καὶ ἀνακαθαρθῶσι, περισῴζονται· εἰ δὲ μή, εἰς φθίσιν μεθίστανται καὶ ἀπόλλυνται.

Σημειοῦται οὖν τοὺς ἐμπύους διὰ δέκα τινῶν δηλωτικῶν σημείων. ὧν πρῶτον σημεῖόν ἐστι τοῦτο· οἱ τοιοῦτοι ἀείσε πυρέττουσι λεπτὸν καὶ βραχὺν πυρετὸν οἷον ἑκτικόν· ἐν δὲ ταῖς νυξὶν αὔξεται καὶ ἐπιτείνεται αὐτοῖς ἡ τοῦ πυρετοῦ θερμασία, οὐ διὰ τὴν φύσιν τῆς νυκτός, ἀλλὰ κατὰ συμβεβηκός· διὰ γὰρ τὴν ἔκτηξιν κατεξηραμμένα αὐτοῖς ἐστι τὰ μόρια πάντα καὶ οἷον ἀποτεφρωμένα· ἡνίκα οὖν πίωσιν, ἐξ αὐτοῦ τοῦ πόματος τοῦ ὑγροῦ ἐπιτέγγονταί τινα μόρια – οὐδὲ γὰρ πάντα – καὶ ἄρχονται ἀτμίζειν, καὶ διαλάμπεται αὐτοῖς ἡ θερμότης, ἐπεὶ τὸ τέως ἐν τῇ γαστρί ἐστι τὸ πόμα· εἶτα μετὰ τὸ τραφῆναι αὐτούς, ἡνίκα ἀνενεχθῇ ἡ ὅλη τροφὴ ἐν τῷ ἥπατι καὶ πεφθῇ καὶ ἐξαιματωθῇ καὶ πάλιν ἐν ταῖς φλεψὶν ἀνενεχθῇ καὶ διανεμηθῇ ἐπὶ τὸ πᾶν σῶμα καὶ πάντα ὁμοτίμως μετασχῶσι τῆς τροφῆς καὶ προστεθῇ
186 αὐτοῖς, | ὡς ἂν ἐπιτεγγόμενα ὁμοτίμως, ἀτμίζουσι δριμεῖς τινας ἀτμοὺς τῷ λόγῳ τῆς ξηρότητος, καὶ οὕτως διαφαίνεται αὐτῶν ἡ θερμασία. τοῦτο δὲ τὸ ἔργον ἐν ταῖς νυξὶ μάλιστα ἐπιτελεῖται, ἐπειδὴ ἐν ταῖς νυξὶν αἱ φυσικαὶ δυνάμεις δραστικῶς ἐνεργοῦσι καὶ αἱ πέψεις κατὰ λόγον γίνονται, ἡ χυλοποίησις, ἡ ἐξαιμάτωσις, ἡ ἀνάδοσις, ἡ πρόσθεσις, ἡ πρόσφυσις καὶ ἡ ἐξομοίωσις. ὥσπερ καὶ ἐπὶ τῆς τιτάνου, ξηρᾶς αὐτῆς οὔσης, ἐγκατακεκρυμμένην ἔχει τὴν ἐν αὐτῇ θερμότητα· ὅθεν καὶ ἁπτομένης αὐτῆς, ξηρᾶς οὔσης, οὐδὲν βλαπτόμεθα· ἡνίκα μέντοι προστεθῇ αὐτῇ ἐπιτηδεία ὕλη, λέγω δὴ ὕδωρ, τότε δημοσιεύεται αὐτῆς ἡ θερμότης, ὡς μηδὲ δύνασθαι αὐτῆς ἄνευ βλάβης ἅψασθαί τις.

Δεύτερον σημεῖόν ἐστιν, οἱ τοιοῦτοι συνεχῶς ἱδροῦσι, καὶ σχεδὸν ἀείσε νενοτισμένον εὑρίσκεται αὐτῶν τὸ σῶμα. τοῦτο δὲ γίνεται ἀσθενούσης τῆς καθεκτικῆς δυνάμεως καὶ μὴ ἰσχυούσης κατασχεῖν τὴν τροφήν, ὥστε καὶ ἀλλοιωθῆναι καὶ πεφθῆναι, ἀλλ' ἐξ αὐτῆς τῆς ἀπεπτουμένης τροφῆς δια-

9–15] *cf.* Gal. In Hipp. Progn. comm. II 60: CMG V 9,2 p. 312,2–6   28–32] *cf.* Gal. In Hipp. Progn. comm. II 60: CMG V 9,2 p. 312,9–12

3 σημείοις γ   καὶ τὰ ἑξῆς *om.* γ   5 τῶν *om.* γ   8 *post* κἂν^I *add.* γὰρ L   9 *post* τοῖς *add.* ἑτέροις γ   17 τοῦ ὑγροῦ πόματος γ   19 τὸ^I] τῷ γ   20 στραφῆναι PV   ὅλη *om.* γ   22 sq. μετασχῶσι – ὁμοτίμως *om.* L   23 ἀτμίζωσι L   τινας δριμεῖς γ   24 ἀτμοὺς] αὐτοὺς L   27 ἡ πρόσφυσις ἡ πρόσθεσις γ   καὶ *om.* γ   28 τιτάνου *ex* τάνου *corr.* M: τάνου PV: τετάνου L   30 αὐτὸ L   31 sq. αὐτῆς ... τις] τις ... αὐτῆς γ   33 ἐστιν *om.* L   34 εὑρίσκεται *post* σῶμα *trsp.* γ   35 καὶ^II *om.* γ   36 *ante* ἐξ αὐτῆς *add.* ἐξ αὐτὸ καὶ γ

X

II 30 All empyema cases should be recognized by the following symptoms, etc.

Since he has just been discussing empyema, he takes up the same subject again and gives us visible signs by which we ought to recognize cases of empyema. And he does this by means of ten signs. And empyema is the name given to the condition in which a mass of pus from inflammation or erupted abscess gathers in any part of the body, whether it be in the calf of the leg, the thigh, the armpit, the arm, or the like. And the empyema subjects survive, if the pus is carried off and they are cleared out; otherwise the condition turns to phthisis and they die.

He identifies empyema subjects, then, by means of ten visible signs. The first is as follows: these cases are subject to a constant slight and low fever like a hectic; at night the heat of the fever heightens and intensifies, not because of the nature of the night, but as an accidental consequence; for due to the wasting all the parts are dried up and, in a manner of speaking, burned to ashes; so when a drink is taken the fluid of the drink itself wets certain parts – but not all – and they begin to steam and the heat becomes evident in them; this is because the drink is in the stomach first; then after they have been nourished, when all the nutriment is conveyed to the liver and undergoes coction and conversion to blood and again is carried in the veins and distributed throughout the body and all the parts have equally shared the nutriment and it has been applied to them, since they are moistened to the same degree they give off certain pungent vapors on account of the dryness and thus the heat in them becomes visible. This work is performed chiefly at night, since at night the natural faculties are very active and the digestions take place according to plan, namely conversion to chyle, blood formation, distribution, application, adhesion and assimilation. We see the same thing also in the case of lime: as long as it is dry it keeps its heat latent, so that it is quite harmless to touch in a dry state; however, when the right substance is applied, namely water, the heat in it manifests itself, so that it can no longer be handled without injury.

The second sign is that such cases sweat constantly and their bodies are nearly always wet. The cause of this is a weak retentive faculty which is unable to hold the nutriment so that it can be converted and digested, but a portion of the undigested nutriment itself escapes and is conveyed

διδράσκει τι μέρος καὶ φέρεται ἐπὶ τὴν ἐπιφάνειαν καὶ ποιεῖ τοὺς ἱδρῶτας.

Τρίτον σημεῖόν ἐστιν, ὅτι πρόθυμοί εἰσι τοῦ βήττειν. τοῦτο δὲ ποιοῦσιν, ἵνα ἀπαλλαγῶσι τῆς ἐνοχλήσεως τῆς ἐκ τῆς κακοχυμίας καὶ τοῦ βάρους· οὐδὲν δὲ εὐεργετοῦσι, κἂν βήττωσιν· οὐδὲ γὰρ ἀναφέρεται ἀξιόλογόν τι· εἰ γὰρ ἀνήγετο, εἶχον ἂν ἀποκαθαίρεσθαι καὶ περισῴζεσθαι. τοῦτο δὲ γίνεται διὰ τρεῖς αἰτίας· ἢ γὰρ διὰ τὸ εἶναι τὴν ὕλην παχεῖαν καὶ γλίσχραν, ὑπὸ τῆς θερμότητος οὕτως κατασκευασθείσης, ἢ διὰ τὸ στεγανὸν καὶ πυκνὸν τοῦ περιέχοντος ὑμένος τὸν πνεύμονα, μὴ διεισερχόμενον ὥστε φέρεσθαι τὸ πύον ἐπὶ τὰ βρόγχια τοῦ πνεύμονος καὶ οὕτως ἐκκρίνεσθαι, ἢ διὰ τὴν ἀσθένειαν τῆς ἀποκριτικῆς δυνάμεως μὴ ἰσχυούσης ῥοίζῳ τὴν ἐκπομπὴν τοῦ πνεύματος
187 ποιῆσαι, ὥστε ἀπω|θῆσαί τι μέρος τῆς ὕλης. διὰ ταύτας τὰς τρεῖς αἰτίας οὐκ ἀνάγεται ἐπὶ τῶν ἐμπυημάτων τι ἀξιόλογον· ὀλίγιστον δὲ πάνυ ἀναπτύουσι μηδὲν εὐεργετούμενοι.

Τέταρτον σημεῖόν ἐστι, κοιλαίνονται αὐτῶν οἱ ὀφθαλμοί, καθάπερ καὶ πάντα τὰ μόρια ἰσχναίνονται ἐπὶ τῶν ὁπωσοῦν χρονίων νοσημάτων τά τε ὑγρὰ καὶ στερεά· τῷ γὰρ μήκει τοῦ χρόνου ἐκτήκονται καὶ δαπανῶνται καὶ ἰσχναίνονται. οὐ μόνον τὰ ὑγρὰ καὶ στερεὰ καταξηραινόμενα δαπανῶνται καὶ σηπεδόνα ὑπομένουσιν, ἀλλὰ πολλῷ μᾶλλον πρότερον τὰ πνεύματα ἐκδαπανῶνται καὶ διαφοροῦνται διὰ τὸ λεπτομερὲς καὶ κοῦφον· ἐπειδὴ οὖν οἱ ὀφθαλμοὶ ἔξογκοι γίνονται ὑπὸ πνευμάτων μάλιστα, ἐπὶ δὲ τῇ ἐκτήξει διαφοροῦνται τὰ πνεύματα, εἰκότως κοιλαίνονται αὐτῶν οἱ ὀφθαλμοί.

Πέμπτον σημεῖον τοῦτο, ὅτι ἐρυθραίνονται αὐτῶν τὰ μῆλα τοῦ προσώπου, διχῶς· ἢ γὰρ τῇ βήξει ἢ τῇ κακοχυμίᾳ. τῇ μὲν βήξει, ἐπειδὴ σύντονος κίνησίς ἐστιν ἡ βήξ· τῇ οὖν κινήσει θάλπεται τὸ πρόσωπον καὶ τὰ περὶ τὴν κεφαλήν, καὶ τῇ θάλψει φέρονται αἱματικοὶ χυμοὶ περὶ τὰ μῆλα τοῦ προσώπου, ἐπειδὴ σαρκωδέστερά εἰσιν αὐτὰ παρὰ πάντα τὰ μόρια τοῦ προσώπου, καὶ ἐρυθραίνονται. ἢ ἐκ τῆς κακοχυμίας ἀτμοὶ δριμεῖς ἀναπέμπονται περὶ τὴν κεφαλὴν καὶ τὸ πρόσωπον· καὶ ἐπειδὴ σαρκώδη εἰσὶ τὰ μῆλα, ἐκεῖσε διαφαίνεται τὸ ἐρύθημα. ἐν τοῖς ἄλλοις δὲ μορίοις οὐ διαφαίνεται, ἐπειδὴ ὀστώδη εἰσὶ φύσει.

Ἕκτον σημεῖόν ἐστιν, ὅτι γρυποῦνται αὐτῶν οἱ ὄνυχες διὰ τὴν δαπάνην καὶ ἔκτηξιν τῶν ὑποκειμένων σαρκῶν τοῖς ὄνυξι· τούτων γὰρ δαπανωμένων, καθὸ μὲν ἐπίκεινται τῷ ὀστῷ τῆς σκυταλίδος, κυρτοῦνται οἱ ὄνυχες, καθὸ δὲ τὰ παρ' ἑκάτερα μέρη τῶν ὑποκειμένων σαρκῶν δαπανηθέντα ἐπὶ τὰ ἐντὸς κοιλαίνονται καὶ διεισέρχονται καὶ γρυποῦνται οἱ ὄνυχες. τὸ γὰρ τοιοῦτον σχῆμα τῶν ὀνύχων γρύπωσις ὀνομάζεται. |

188 Ἕβδομόν ἐστιν σημεῖον, τὸ ἐπὶ αὐτῶν θερμοὺς εἶναι τοὺς δακτύλους τῆς χειρός, ὑπεναντίως τοῖς χρονίοις νοσήμασιν· ἐπὶ γὰρ τῶν χρονίων νοσημάτων τῷ χρόνῳ ἀσθενοῦν τὸ ἔμφυτον θερμόν, ψύχονται οἱ δάκτυλοι, ἐπειδὴ τῇ ἀσθενείᾳ οὐκ ἐπεκτείνεται οὐδὲ ἐλλάμπει τὸ ἔμφυτον θερμόν, καὶ διὰ τοῦτο

2–11] *cf.* Gal. In Hipp. Progn. comm. II 60: CMG V 9,2 p. 312,20–25

4 οὐδὲν δὲ] ὁ δὲ οὐδὲν γ εὐεργετῶσι *codd.*: *corr. Dietz* βήττουσιν *codd.*: *corr. Dietz* οὐδὲ] οὐδὲν MV τι *om.* γ 7 κατασκευασθείσης] *sc.* τῆς ὕλης 8 διεισερχομένου γ 9 βρογχία *codd.*: *correxi* 14 αὐτῶν *om.* L 16 ἐκτήκεται . . . δαπανᾶται γ 31 τρυποῦνται L 32 γὰρ] οὖν γ 33 κυσταλίδος MP 34 δαπανηθέντων *codd.*: *correxi* 35 γρυποῦνται] γίνονται γρυποὶ γ 36 γρύπω γ

to the surface and produces the sweats.

The third sign is that they are eager to cough. They do this to get rid of the annoyance caused by the unwholesome humors and the weight; but coughing brings them no relief, since they cannot get up any matter worth mentioning; if they did, they would be cleaned out and recover. And this happens for three reasons: because the matter is thick and viscous, having been rendered that way by the heat; or because the pus, due to the imperviousness and compactness of the membrane surrounding the lung, does not penetrate so as to reach the bronchial tubes of the lung and to be thus discharged; or, due to weakness, the excretory faculty is not able to force out a stream of air strong enough to dislodge part of the matter. For these three reasons empyema patients cannot bring up any appreciable amount of matter; they do expectorate a minute quantity, but without any benefit.

The fourth sign is that their eyes become sunken, just as in any kind of chronic disease all the parts, both fluid and solid, shrivel; for due to the length of time they are consumed, waste away and wither. It is not only the fluids and solids which are consumed and decompose when dried up, the pneumas are much more subject to consumption and dissipation, being rarefied and light; since it is particularly the pneumas, then, which keep the eyes filled out and pneumas are dissipated by consumption, it is only to be expected that their eyes sink.

The fifth sign is this, that their cheeks become red, and in two ways: either because of the coughing or because of the unwholesome humors. From the coughing, since coughing is a vehement movement; the movement heats up the face and the head area, the heat causes bloody humors to go to the cheeks, these being more fleshy than any other part of the face, and so they turn red. From the unwholesome humors, because they send pungent vapors up around the head and face; and since the cheeks are fleshy the red shows through in them. But it is not visible in the other parts, because they are bony by nature.

The sixth sign is that their fingernails become crooked because the flesh underneath is consumed and wastes away; for when this (flesh) is consumed, in so far as it lies on top of the finger-bone, the nails bulge, while to the extent that the parts of the underlying flesh on either side are consumed, the nails sink inwards and penetrate the whole way and become hooked. For such a form of the nails is called hooking.

The seventh sign is that their fingers are hot, being the opposite of what happens in chronic diseases; for in chronic diseases the innate heat weakens through time and the fingers become cold, since, due to the weakness, the innate heat cannot reach (the fingers) to radiate them and

ψυχρὰ εὑρίσκονται τὰ ἄκρα. ἐν μέντοι τοῖς ἐμπύοις θερμοὶ εὑρίσκονται οἱ δάκτυλοι, οὐ δι' ὅλου, ἀλλ' αἱ ἄκραι τῶν δακτύλων, ἐπειδὴ ἐκεῖνα τὰ μέρη τῶν δακτύλων σαρκωδέστερά εἰσι. τὸ οὖν θερμόν, ὡς ἐν σαρκωδεστέροις τόποις ὑπαρχόντων αὐτῶν, διὰ τὴν ἰκμάδα ἐκεῖσε συνελαύνεται τὸ θερμόν. ἡ γὰρ ἰκμὰς τροφή ἐστιν τῆς θερμότητος· καὶ διὰ τοῦτο θερμὰ εὑρίσκονται τὰ ἄκρα τῶν δακτύλων. ἢ τοῦτο· ὅτι εὐκίνητοί εἰσιν οἱ δάκτυλοι καὶ ὡς εὐκίνητοι τῇ κινήσει θάλπονται· ἢ ὅτι τὰ πέρατα τῶν φλεβῶν καὶ ἀρτηριῶν ἐκεῖσε ἀποπερατοῦνται· τὰ οὖν πνεύματα τῇ κινήσει ἐκεῖσε συναπελαύνονται, καὶ διὰ τοῦτο θερμοὶ εὑρίσκονται οἱ δάκτυλοι.

Ὄγδοόν ἐστι σημεῖον, ὅτι οἱ πόδες οἰδαίνουσι χρονιζόντων αὐτῶν, ἐπειδὴ πόρρω ἀφίστανται οἱ πόδες καὶ ἀμοιροῦσι τοῦ ἐμφύτου θερμοῦ· τούτου οὖν ἀμοιροῦντες, τὸ λόγῳ τροφῆς ἐκεῖσε φερόμενον οὐ πέττεται καὶ ἀπεπτούμενον εἰς ὑγρότητά τινα καὶ εἰς πνεύματα ἀναλύεται, καὶ ἀθροιζόμενον ἐν τοῖς ποσὶν οἰδαίνονται.

Ἔννατον σημεῖόν ἐστιν, ὅτι οἱ τοιοῦτοι ἀνόρεκτοί εἰσι· διὰ γὰρ τὴν ἀσθένειαν τῆς ὀρεκτικῆς δυνάμεως οὐκ ὀρέγονται, τῷ λόγῳ τῆς κακοχυμίας βλαπτομένη.

Δέκατόν ἐστι σημεῖον, ὅτι φλύκταιναι αὐτοῖς γίνονται δι' ὅλου τοῦ σώματος. γίνονται δὲ ἐκ τῆς κακοχυμίας αὐτοῖς ἐκριπτομένων ἀτμῶν τινων δριμέων· καὶ τὰ μὲν ἐν βάθει μόρια διεξέρχονται· ἐπειδὴ δὲ στεγανὸν καὶ πυκνόν ἐστι τὸ δέρμα, στέγονται ἐκεῖσε καὶ γίνονται αἱ φλύκταιναι. ἢ τοῦτο·
189 ὅτι ἡ συνεκτικὴ ὑγρότης ἐκπί|πτει καὶ ἐκπίπτουσα τὸ δέρμα οὐ διεξέρχεται, ἀλλὰ στέγεται καὶ ὑμενοῦται τὸ δέρμα καὶ γίνονται αἱ φλύκταιναι.

Δυνατὸν δέ ἐστι πρὸς τούτοις καὶ ἄλλα σημεῖα ἐφευρεῖν, ἅτινά ἐστι ταῦτα· τριχορροοῦσι, γαστρόρροια αὐτοῖς γίνεται, καὶ δυσώδη εἰσὶ τὰ ἀναπτυόμενα.

Καὶ τριχορροοῦσι μὲν ἢ ὅτι ἐκ τῆς κακοχυμίας ἀτμοὶ δριμεῖς ἀναπέμπονται περὶ τὴν κεφαλὴν καὶ ἐκριζοῦσι τὰς τρίχας, ἢ ὅτι τῇ ἀτροφίᾳ καὶ τῇ ἰσχνάνσει ξηραίνεται αὐτῶν τὸ δέρμα τῆς κεφαλῆς, καὶ ἐπὶ τῇ ξηρότητι στεγανὸν γίνεται καὶ οὐ διεξέρχεται λιγνὺς διὰ τοῦ δέρματος, καὶ τὸ τηνικαῦτα τριχορροοῦσι.

Γαστρόρροια δὲ αὐτοῖς γίνεται ἀσθενουσῶν τῶν φυσικῶν δυνάμεων, ἐκ τῆς κακοχυμίας μετασχοῦσαι, καὶ τὰ οἰκεῖα ἔργα οὐ δύνανται ποιῆσαι.

Δυσώδη δέ εἰσι τὰ ἀναπτυόμενα διὰ τὴν τοῦ πύου γένεσιν· τὸ γὰρ πύον ἐνδείκνυται ὅτι μεγάλην ἔχει σηπεδόνα. ἐκ τούτων οὖν τῶν τριῶν διαγινώσκομεν τοὺς ἐμπυϊκούς.

Εἴρηται δὲ ἡμῖν μικρὸν ἔμπροσθεν, πόθεν ὀφείλομεν διαγινώσκειν, πότε ἄρχεται γίνεσθαι ἡ πυοποίησις, ἤγουν πότε ἄρχεται εἰς πυοποίησιν

18–23] *cf.* Gal. In Hipp. Progn. comm. II 60: CMG V 9,2 p. 313,19–26 37 Εἴρηται] *supra*, p. 212, 29–34

1 εὑρίσκονται ψυχρὰ γ 5 ὑγρότητος L 5 sq. θερμοὶ . . . οἱ ἄκροι γ 7 τῶν ἀρτηριῶν καὶ τῶν φλεβῶν γ 8 ἐκεῖσε^{II} *om.* γ 10 αὐτῶν χρονιζόντων οἰδαίνουσι γ 11 τοῦ ἐμφύτου *om.* L 12 τὸ] τῷ MP ἐκεῖσε *om.* γ 13 ἀπεπτούμενα γ 15 ἐστι σημεῖον γ 17 βλαπτόμενοι L; *sed cf. lin. 32 sq.* 19 αὐτῆς L 20 δὲ *om.* γ 23 ὑμενοῦσι γ 28 περὶ] ἐπὶ γ 29 ἰσχνότητι γ 37 πρόσθεν γ 38 ἄρχεται^{II}] ἄρχεσθαι L

so the extremities are found to be cold. In empyema cases, on the other hand, you will find the fingers hot; but they will not be hot all over, only at the tips, these parts of the fingers being more fleshy. The heat, then, since the fingertips are fleshier parts, is driven there for the moisture; for the moisture is the food of the heat; this explains why you will find the fingertips hot. Or (you could say) this: that the fingers are agile and being agile they become hot with movement; or that the ends of the veins and arteries terminate there; the gases, then, are driven off there by movement, and hence the fingers are found hot.

The eighth sign is that the feet swell as the condition becomes prolonged, since the feet are distant from, and deprived of, the innate heat; being deprived of this, then, the matter conveyed to them for nutriment is not digested, and undigested it breaks up into a fluid and gases, and collected in the feet it produces swelling.

The ninth sign is that such patients have no appetite; for, on account of the weakness of the appetitive faculty which has been damaged by the unhealthy humors, they do not desire (food).

The tenth sign is that blisters form in them throughout the body. And they are formed in them by certain pungent vapors discharged from the unwholesome humors; these (vapors) make their way out through the inner parts; but since the skin is impervious and compact, they are held in there and the blisters develop. Another explanation: the maintenance fluid is discharged and, being discharged, it does not penetrate the skin, but is retained and the skin forms a film and blisters develop.

In addition to these one can find still other signs, such as these: shedding hair, diarrhoea and fetid sputa.

And they shed hair either because the unwholesome humors send pungent vapors up around the head which uproot the hairs, or atrophy and wasting dry the scalp and with the dryness it becomes impervious and smoke does not get out through the skin and then they shed hair.

Diarrhoea develops in them because the natural faculties have been weakened by association with the unwholesome humors and are not able to perform their proper functions.

The expectorations are made foul-smelling by pus formation, since pus means serious putrefaction. Empyema cases, then, can be diagnosed from these three signs.

We described a little earlier how we ought to distinguish when suppuration starts or, in other words, when the abscess begins to turn to

τρέπεσθαι τὸ ἀπόστημα. ὅπερ διαγινώσκομεν ἐκ τοῦ ἀλόγου ῥίγους καὶ τοῦ ἑπομένου πυρετοῦ καὶ ἐκ τοῦ βάρους τῆς συναισθήσεως καὶ τῆς δυσπνοίας. καὶ ταῦτα μὲν ἀναμνήσεως χάριν προείρηται. ἐφ' οἷς παραδίδωσιν ἡμῖν σημεῖα ῥήξεως γινομένης, πόθεν ὀφείλομεν γνῶναι, εἰ ταχέως ἡ ῥῆξις γίνεται τοῦ ἀποστήματος ἢ βραδέως. καί φησιν ἐκ τεσσάρων τινῶν σημείων τοῦτο γινώσκομεν, ἀπό τε τῆς ὀδύνης καὶ τῆς βηχὸς καὶ τοῦ σιελισμοῦ καὶ τῆς δυσπνοίας. εἰ μὲν γὰρ ταῦτα πάντα συνεχῶς ἐπιγίνονται καὶ σφοδρῶς καὶ
190 συντεταμένως, γί|νωσκε ὅτι ταχέως ἡ ῥῆξις τοῦ ἀποστήματος γίνεται· εἰ δέ γε μήτε συνεχῶς γίνωνται ταῦτα μήτε σφοδρῶς μήτε συντεταμένως, γίνωσκε ὅτι βραδέως γίνεται ἡ ῥῆξις.

Καὶ τίς ἡ αἰτία τούτων; εἰ μὲν ἐπιτεταμένη γίνεται ἡ ὀδύνη, τῇ ἀνίᾳ καὶ τῇ δήξει τῇ ἀπὸ τοῦ πύου ἰχώρων τινῶν δριμέων καὶ ἀνιαρῶν δακνόντων τὸν περιέχοντα ὑμένα τὸν πνεύμονα καὶ κινδυνεύοντα διαρραγῆναι κατὰ τὴν αὐτοῦ συνέχειαν· αἰσθητικώτατος δέ ἐστι πάνυ, καὶ διὰ τοῦτο συντεταμένη ἡ ὀδύνη γίνεται. ⟨ὁ δὲ σιελισμὸς γίνεται⟩ ὑγρότητός τινος ἐκ τοῦ πύου διηθουμένης καὶ φερομένης ἐπὶ λάρυγγα καὶ τραχεῖαν ἀρτηρίαν καὶ φάρυγγα καὶ ἐπιγλωττίδα καὶ γλῶσσαν· καὶ γίνεται ὁ σιελισμὸς ἀείσε ἀναπτύοντες τὸ ὑγρὸν ἐκεῖνο. ἡ δὲ βὴξ γίνεται τοῦ πνεύματος διεξερχομένου καὶ ἐπιπίπτοντος τοῦ ὑγροῦ, ὡς ἐν ἀσυνηθεστέροις τόποις εὑρισκομένου, καὶ τῇ προσκρούσει γίνεται ἡ βήξ· οὐδὲν γάρ ἐστιν ἡ βὴξ ἢ μάχη ὑγροῦ καὶ πνεύματος. ἡ δὲ δύσπνοια γίνεται, ἢ ὅτι ὀδύνης ἐπιτεταμένης οὔσης οὐ δύναται μέγα διασταλῆναι ὁ θώραξ ἢ ὅτι ὑπόκειται φλεγμονὴ ἐν τῷ θώρακι καὶ μοῖραν ἐναπολαμβάνει τῆς εὐρυχωρίας τοῦ θώρακος, ἐν ᾧ ὤφειλε τὸ πνεῦμα ἐμφιλοχωρῆσαι εἰσερχόμενον· τούτου οὖν ἐναποληφθέντος ἐξ ἀνάγκης ἡ δύσπνοια γίνεται.

Πρὸς τούτοις δὲ καὶ ἕτερα σημεῖα πέντε παραδίδωσι, δι' ὧν ὀφείλομεν γινώσκειν, πότε ἐστὶν ἀγαθὴ ἡ ῥῆξις καὶ πότε κακίστη. εἰσὶ δὲ ταῦτα ἀπὸ τοῦ πυρετοῦ, ἀπὸ τῆς ὀδύνης, ἀπὸ τοῦ δίψους, ἀπὸ τῆς ὀρέξεως καὶ ἀπὸ τοῦ ἀναγομένου πύου. εἰ μὲν γὰρ ἐπ' ἀγαθῷ ἡ ῥῆξις γίνεται, εὐθέως ἐν αὐτῇ τῇ ἡμέρᾳ, ἐν ᾗ ἡ ῥῆξις γένηται, ἀπύρετοι σχεδὸν γίνονται, ἀλλὰ καὶ ἀνώδυνοι καὶ ἄδιψοι καὶ εὐόρεκτοι. ἀλλὰ καὶ τὸ ἀναπτυόμενον δεῖ λευκὸν εἶναι καὶ συνεστηκὸς καὶ λεῖον καὶ ὁμαλὸν καὶ μὴ μετέχειν δυσωδίας. εἰ δὲ μετὰ τὸ ῥαγῆναι τὴν ῥῆξιν μὴ παύσηται ὁ πυρετός, ἀλλὰ καὶ ἐπιγένηται,
191 καὶ ἡ ὀδύνη ἐπιταθῇ καὶ τὸ δίψος καὶ πάντῃ ἀνόρεκτοι | μείνωσι καὶ τὸ ἀναπτυόμενον πύον πολλῆς μετέχει δυσωδίας καὶ πολυποίκιλόν ἐστι καὶ

3–5 παραδίδωσιν ... φησιν] Hipp. Progn. 17: pp. 215,12–216,4 A. = II pp. 154,10–156,2 L. 26 παραδίδωσι] Hipp. Progn. 17: p. 216,5–14 A. = II p. 156,2–13 L.

2 *post* βάρους *add.* καὶ L συνθέσεως γ 5 τινῶν *om.* γ 8 ἡ *ante* ταχέως *trsp.* γ 9 γίνονται PV(M?) μήτε σφοδρῶς *om.* L 10 γενήσεται γ ἡ ῥῆξις *post* ὅτι *trsp.* γ 12 τῇ^II] τοῦ γ δριμέων καὶ ἀνιαρῶν *om.* L δακόντων L 13 τὸν πνεύμονα *scripsi*: τὸ πύον *codd.* ῥαγῆναι L 14 αὐτοῦ *om.* L 15 ἡ *om.* MV ὁ – γίνεται *addidi* 18 συνεξερχομένου L 19 εὑρισκομέν *(ambig.)* M: εὑρισκομένη P: εὑρισκόμενον L: *corr.* V 22 ὅτι *om.* L φλεγμονὴ ὑπόκειται γ 24 ἐναπολειφθέντος *codd.*: *correxi* 26 πέντε σημεῖα γ 29 γίνεται *post* ἀγαθῷ *trsp.* γ 30 τῇ *om.* L ἀπύρεκτοι γ 32 μὴ *om.* L

suppuration. It is diagnosed from the unpredictable shivering, from the fever which follows, from the sensation of weight and from the difficult breathing. And these have been mentioned as preliminaries, in order to refresh the memory. Next he gives us signs for the occurrence of rupture which enable us to tell whether the abscess will erupt quickly or slowly. He says that we will know this from four signs: the pain, coughing, sputum and difficult breathing. For if all these are constantly present in a severe and intense form, you will know that the abscess is going to break quickly; but if they are not present continually and are not severe or intense, you may conclude that the eruption will come slowly.

What is the cause of these? If the pain becomes intense it results from the sting and irritation of the pus, when certain pungent and mordant serous fluids sting the membrane surrounding the lung and it is in danger of having its continuity ruptured; it is an extremely sensitive part and this is why the pain becomes intense. The sputum develops because a certain fluid oozes from the pus and is conveyed to the larynx, trachea, pharynx, epiglottis and tongue; and constant expectoration of this fluid produces the sputum. The coughing is caused by a clash between the emerging air and the fluid, it (the fluid) being encountered in rather unaccustomed areas, and the collision produces a cough; you see, coughing is simply a struggle between fluid and air. Difficult breathing results either from the inability of the thorax to expand much due to intense pain, or from the presence of inflammation in the thorax which takes over part of its free space, the space which is the natural receptacle and habitat of the air; this, then, being taken over, difficult breathing is inevitable.

In addition to these he gives five other signs which enable us to distinguish when a rupture is good and when it is very bad. They are based on the fever, pain, thirst, appetite and pus discharged. For, if the rupture is for the good, straightaway on the day the rupture occurs they become almost free of fever and without pain or thirst and have a good appetite. And the expectorated matter should be white, solid, smooth, uniform and not foul-smelling. On the other hand, if after the rupture has broken, the fever does not end but reappears, and the pain and thirst intensify, and complete lack of appetite continues, and the expectorated pus is very fetid, variegated and partakes of a variety of unwholesome

διαφόρου[ς] μετέχει κακοχυμίας, γίνωσκε ὅτι ἐπὶ κακῷ γέγονεν ἡ ῥῆξις· ὅσον γὰρ οὔπω ἀπόλλυται ὁ ἄνθρωπος. εἰ δέ γε τὰ μὲν γένωνται, τὰ δὲ μὴ γένωνται, πρὸς τὴν ἐπικράτειαν οὕτως δεῖ καὶ προσδέχεσθαι.

XI

II 31 [18: 218,5 A. = II 160,7 L.] Αἱ δὲ ἀποστάσιες αἱ εἰς τὰ σκέλεα ἐν τῇσι περιπνευμονίῃσι

Διαλεχθεὶς περὶ τῶν ἐμπυημάτων, ταὐτὸν δὲ εἰπεῖν περὶ φλεγμονῆς τοῦ ὑπεζωκότος τῆς εἰς πύον μεταβαλλούσης καὶ ῥαγείσης καὶ τοῦ πύου ἐκχυθέντος μεταξὺ θώρακός τε καὶ πνεύμονος, ἔτι γε μὴν καὶ περὶ τῆς γινομένης φθίσεως ἐπὶ τοῖς πάθεσι θώρακός τε καὶ πνεύμονος, νῦν βούλεται εἰπεῖν καὶ περὶ τῶν ἀποστάσεων τῶν γινομένων ἐν ταῖς περιπνευμονίαις. ἡ γὰρ φλεγμονὴ τοῦ πνεύμονος οὐ πάντως εἰς πυοποίησιν τρέπεται οὐδὲ πάντως εἰς ἐμπύημα ἀποκαθίσταται, ἀλλ' ἔστιν ὅτε εἰς ἀπόστασιν τρέπεται τῆς ὕλης εἰς ἕτερα μετατιθεμένης μόρια. τὸ σύμπαν οὖν τοῦ λόγου ἐστὶ διαλαβεῖν περὶ τῶν ἐν τοῖς περιπνευμονικοῖς γινομένων ἀποστημάτων. διμερὴς δὲ ἡ τοιαύτη σκέψις. καὶ ἐν μὲν τῷ πρώτῳ μέρει σημεῖά τινα παραδίδωσιν ὁ συγγραφεύς, οἷς τισι χρώμενοι διαγινώσκομεν, εἰ ὅλως μελέτη ἐστὶ τῇ φύσει τῆς περιπνευμονίας ὑποκειμένης ἀπόστασιν ἐργάσασθαι. τὸ δὲ δεύτερον μέρος τοῦ λόγου, τὸ γνωρίσαι ἡμῖν, ἐν ποίοις μέρεσι προσδοκᾶται ἡ ἀπόστασις.

Καὶ ἀρκτέον ἀπὸ τοῦ πρώτου μέρους τοῦ λόγου· δεῖ τὴν ὕλην ὠμὴν εἶναι καὶ ἄπεπτον καὶ τὸ νόσημα οὐκ ὀλέθριον, ἀλλὰ καὶ τὴν δύναμιν ἐπ' ἔλαττον· εἰ γὰρ πεπεμμένη ἐστὶν ἡ ὕλη, εἰς ἀπόστασιν οὐ τρέπεται ἡ περιπνευμονία, ἀλλ' ἢ κατ' ἔκρουν ἐκκρίνεται ἡ ὕλη ἢ κατὰ σύμπεψιν κατὰ μικρὸν τῷ χρόνῳ διαφορεῖται καὶ πέττεται ἡ ὕλη, καὶ οὕτως ἀπαλλάσσονται. τὸ δὲ νόσημα οὐ δεῖ ὀλέθριον εἶναι, ἐπειδὴ προφθάνει ὁ θάνατος
192 τὴν ἀπό|στασιν. πρὸς τούτοις δὲ δεῖ καὶ πυρετὸν συνεχῆ εἶναι καὶ βραχὺν καὶ ἐπίμονον, ἀλλὰ καὶ ὀδύνην ἐπιτεταμένην καὶ μόνιμον, καὶ ὁ σιελισμὸς μὴ ἐκχωρέῃ, τουτέστι μὴ ἀναπτύωσί τι, ἐπειδὴ ἀλλαχόσε ἡ ὕλη ἀπασχολεῖται, καὶ χολῶδες οὐκ ἐκχωρέουσι διὰ γαστρός. ἐὰν οὖν ταῦτα πάντα συνέλθωσι, γίνωσκε ὅτι εἰς ἀπόστασιν τρέπεται ἡ περιπνευμονία. εἰ δέ γε παύηται ὁ πυρετός, ἀλλὰ καὶ ἡ ὀδύνη παύσηται, ἀπόστασις οὐ γενήσεται, ἐπειδὴ δηλοῖ μηδεμίαν μοχθηρίαν παρενοχλοῦσαν. ἀλλὰ καὶ σιελισμὸς ἐὰν γένηται, εἰς ἀπόστασιν οὐ τρέπεται ἡ περιπνευμονία, ἐπειδὴ διὰ τοῦ πτυέλου κενοῦται ἡ ὕλη καὶ ἀνακαθαίρεται ἡ περιπνευμονία. ἀλλὰ καὶ χολωδῶν ἐκκρινομένων διαχωρημάτων οὐδ' οὕτως εἰς ἀπόστασιν τρέπεται ἡ πε-

10 νῦν – 232,22] *cf.* Gal. In Hipp. Progn. comm. II 65: CMG V 9,2 pp. 316,15–318,23 16 παραδίδωσιν] Hipp. Progn. 18: p. 217,6–11 A. = II pp. 158,5–160,3 L.

1 διαφόρους *codd.*: *correxi* 7 εἶπε γ 8 τῆς] τῇ γ 11 περιπ νεύμονος γ 15 τοῖς] τῆς, *ut vid.*, V: τῇ M περιπνεύμονι γ: πνευμονικοῖς L: *correxi* ἀποστάσεων M: ἀποστάσεως PV 18 τῇ φύσει *om.* L πνευμ ονίας L 21 τοῦ λόγου *om.* γ *post* λόγου *iter. ex lin. 19 sq.* τὸ γνω ρίσαι – ἀπόστασις L 24 ἢ[II] *om.* L 25 σμικρὸν γ 26 οὐ δεῖ *om.* L ἐπειδὴ] ἐπείτοι γε γ 27 καὶ[II] *om.* γ 30 χολώδη γ ἐκχορεύουσι γ οὖν *om.* L 34 sq. ἐπειδὴ – περιπνευμονία *om.* L

humors, this will tell you that the rupture has occurred for the bad; for the patient is on the verge of death. However, if some of the signs occur and others not, you should base your expectations on whichever prevails.

XI

II 31 Abscesses to the legs in pneumonia

Having talked about empyemas, that is to say, about the inflammation of the lining (membrane) which has turned to pus and has ruptured, with the pus being discharged between the thorax and lung, and further about the phthisis which occurs in affections of the thorax and lung, he now wants to take up also the subject of abscesses in pneumonia cases. For inflammation of the lung does not always turn to suppuration nor does it invariably develop into empyema, but it sometimes turns to abscession, when the matter transfers to other parts. The whole discussion, then, is devoted to the abscesses which form in pneumonia cases. This inquiry has two parts. In the first part our author gives us some signs which help us to decide if nature intends to form an abscess at all from the underlying pneumonia. And in the second (he tells us) how to recognize in which parts the abscession can be expected.

To begin with the first part of the discussion, the matter should be crude and undigested, the disease not deadly, and the power on the weak side; for if the matter is digested, the pneumonia does not turn to abscess; instead, the matter either is evacuated by discharge or, concocting, the matter is gradually dissipated and digested through time, and thus they are cured. The disease should not be deadly, since (in that case) death anticipates the abscession. As well, there should be a constant and protracted slight fever and a severe persistent pain, and the spit should not discharge, that is, they should not expectorate anything, since the matter is occupied elsewhere, nor should there be a bilious discharge through the stomach. If, then, all these are present together, conclude that the pneumonia will turn to abscess. But if the fever stops and the pain also ends, abscession will not occur, since it shows that there is no distress troubling (the body). And if there is spit, the pneumonia does not turn to abscession, since by means of the spit the matter is evacuated and the pneumonia is cleared out. And even when bilious excrements are passed, the pneumonia does not turn to abscession, since the matter is

ριπνευμονία, ἐπειδὴ λεπτὴ καὶ θερμή ἐστιν ἡ ὕλη. ἐπὶ δὲ τῶν χρονίων νοσημάτων παχεῖαν δεῖ εἶναι τὴν ὕλην καὶ ὠμὴν καὶ ψυχράν, ἐν ᾧτινι χρόνῳ καὶ ἡ ἀπόστασις γίνεται, καθὸ καὶ αὐτὸς κατὰ λέξιν ᾐνίξατο εἰπὼν ἀδιάκριτοι αἱ ὑποχωρήσιες. ἀδιακρίτους δὲ ὑποχωρήσεις καλεῖ ἐνταῦθα τὰ λεπτὰ καὶ ὑδατώδη καὶ ὠμὰ ὑποχωρήματα καὶ μηδεμίαν ἔχοντα ἐπιμιξίαν χολώδους ὕλης. ἡ τοιαύτη ὑποχώρησις καὶ ὠμὴν ἐνδείκνυται τὴν ὕλην καὶ παχεῖαν, ἥτις πολλοῦ χρόνου δεῖται ὥστε πεφθῆναι, ἐν ᾧτινι χρόνῳ, ὡς εἴρηται, ἡ ἀπόστασις γίνεται. ὡς γὰρ διαφόρως μεμαθήκαμεν, τὰ ὀξέα τῶν νοσημάτων κατ' ἔκρουν κενουμένης τῆς ὕλης λύονται· τὰ δὲ χρόνια τῶν νοσημάτων ὡς ἐπίπαν κατ' ἀπόσκηψιν καὶ ἀπόστασιν τρέπονται καὶ οὕτως λύονται, εἰ μή τι ἄρα διὰ ῥώμην δυνάμεώς τινα τῶν νοσημάτων κατὰ σύμπεψιν ἀπαλλαγῶσι κατὰ μικρὸν συμπεττομένης τῆς ὕλης καὶ οὕτως παυομένων. ὅθεν ἀμέλει καὶ πέψεως ἡμῖν σημεῖα παραδίδωσιν ἐπὶ τῆς περιπνευμονίας λέγων οὕτως, ὅτι ἐὰν περιπνευμονίας ὑποκειμένης καὶ πεπεμμένη ἐστὶν ἡ ὕλη καὶ τὰ οὖρα πολλὰ ἐκκρίνονται καὶ παχέα καὶ τὴν ὑπόστασιν πολλὴν ἴσχει· ἐνδείκνυται γὰρ ὅτι ἡ περιπνευμονία οὐ
193 τρέπεται | εἰς ἀπόστασιν, ἐπειδὴ κατ' ἔκρουν ἐκκρίνεται ἡ ὕλη διὰ τῶν οὔρων. ἡ δὲ τοιαύτη ἔκκρισις τῶν οὔρων ἰσχὺν καὶ ῥώμην τῆς δυνάμεως ἐνδείκνυται, καθ' ἣν ἰσχύσασα τὴν μὲν ὕλην ἐξέκρινε, τὸ δὲ ἐγκαταλιμπανόμενον πέττει καὶ αὐτό, καὶ οὕτως ἀπαλλάσσονται τῆς περιπνευμονίας. εἰ δέ γε τοὐναντίον ὀλίγον ἐκκριθῇ τὸ οὖρον καὶ λεπτὸν καὶ ὑπόστασιν μὴ ἔχον, σχεδὸν παντὶ τρόπῳ εἰς ἀπόστασιν τρέπεται ἡ περιπνευμονία.

Ἐν δὲ τῷ δευτέρῳ μέρει τοῦ λόγου παραδίδωσιν ἡμῖν σημείωσιν, καθ' ἣν ὀφείλομεν διαγνῶναι, εἴτε ἐν τοῖς ἄνωθεν καὶ ὑπερκειμένοις μορίοις τοῦ θώρακος αἱ ἀποστάσεις γίνονται ἐπὶ τῇ περιπνευμονίᾳ εἴτε ἐν τοῖς κάτω καὶ ὑποκειμένοις. καί φησιν ὅτι, ἐὰν ἄνευ προφάσεως γένηται ἀθρόον δύσπνοια ἐπὶ τῇ περιπνευμονίᾳ καὶ γενομένη δοκῇ ὑποχαλᾶν καὶ οἷον ὑφειμένη γίνεσθαι καὶ μειοῦσθαι, εἶτα πάλιν ἐπιταθῇ ἡ δύσπνοια, γίνωσκε ὅτι ἐν τοῖς ἄνωθεν καὶ ὑπερκειμένοις μορίοις, τυχὸν περὶ τὴν κεφαλήν, ἡ ῥοπὴ τῶν χυμῶν καὶ τῆς ὕλης γέγονε, καὶ ἐκεῖσε περὶ τὴν κεφαλὴν αἱ ἀποστάσεις γίνονται. εἰ δέ γε μηδὲν τούτων εἴη παρενοχλοῦν, ἀλλὰ ζέσις καὶ φλόγωσίς τις περὶ τὸ στέρνον καὶ τὸ διάφραγμα — ἥντινα φλόγωσιν σύνηθες τῷ Ἱπποκράτει φλέγμα καλεῖν, καὶ νῦν οὕτως κατὰ τὴν λέξιν

4 ἀδιάκριτοι αἱ ὑποχωρήσιες] Hipp. Progn. 18: p. 217,8 A. = II p. 158,8 L. 8 εἴρηται] *supra*, linn. 2 sq. μεμαθήκαμεν] *e.g. supra*, p. 196,34–36 *cf.* Gal. In Hipp. Progn. comm. II 65: CMG V 9,2 p. 318,7sq. 23 παραδίδωσιν] Hipp. Progn. 18: pp. 217,11–218,4 A. = II p. 160,3–7 L. 26 ἐὰν – 234,3] *cf.* Gal. In Hipp. Progn. comm. II 66: CMG V 9,2 p. 319,5–16 32 sq. ἥντινα – καλεῖν] *cf.* Gal. Gloss. Hipp.: XIX p. 151,16sq. K.

1 θερμὴ καὶ λεπτή γ 3 *post* εἰπὼν *add.* ὅτι γ 4 ἀδιάκριτοι] ἄκρητοι (-ιτ-) *aut* εὔκριτοι *codd. Hipp.* ὑποχωρήσιες] ὑποχωρήσεις L δὲ *om.* MP 9 *post* οσημάτων *add.* ἢ L τὰ δὲ – 11 λύονται *om.* γ 12 σμικρὸν γ 13 παυομένης γ: παυόμενον L: *correxi* 14 περιπνευμονίας[I]] περιπνεύμονος PV 16 περιπνεύμονος γ 17 εἰς] εἰ μὴ γ *post* ἀπόστασιν *add.* πολλὴν ἴσχει *(ex lin. 16)* γ 20 περιπνευμόνου M, *in* περιπνευμονίας *corr.* P 22 ἀπόστασιν] ἀπόσκηψιν V: ἀπόσκεψιν P: ἀπόσηψιν M; *cf. supra, lin. 10* 24 καθ' ἣν] καθὼς L 25 γίνεται L 27 δοκεῖ *codd.*: *corr. Dietz*

thin and warm. In chronic diseases, on the other hand, the matter should be thick, crude and cold, during which time the abscess forms, just as (Hippocrates) hints in the text when he says stools unseparated. By unseparated stools here he means the thin, watery and crude excrements having no admixture of bilious matter. Such a stool shows that the matter is crude and thick and this needs a long time to be concocted; and it is during this time, as we have said, that the abscess forms. For, as we have learned on different occasions, acute diseases are cured when the matter is evacuated by discharge, while the chronic are mainly ended by turning to determination or abscession, except that some diseases, on account of the strength of the (body's) power, are removed by concoction, when the matter is concocted little by little and they end in this way. And so it is that he gives us signs of coction in pneumonia as follows: if in a case of pneumonia the matter is digested and copious and thick urines are passed which have a lot of sediment. For this indicates that the pneumonia will not turn to abscess, the matter being eliminated by discharge of the urines. And such discharge of urines means vigor and strength of the (body's) power, fortified by which it discharged the matter and digests even the remainder and in this way they are cured of the pneumonia. But, conversely, if little and thin urine is passed without a sediment, the pneumonia almost certainly turns to abscession.

In the second part of the discussion he gives us signs which enable us to diagnose whether the abscesses in pneumonia will form in the upper and superior parts of the thorax or in the lower and inferior. He says that if in pneumonia difficult breathing develops suddenly for no reason, then seems to ease off, become milder and lessen, and then difficult breathing intensifies again, conclude that the humors and matter have inclined to the upper and superior parts, that is, around the head, and that the abscesses will form there around the head. However, if none of these is causing annoyance, but a seething and burning heat around the breastbone and diaphragm – Hippocrates has the habit of calling this burning heat "phlegm", and he has done so in the present text, calling the burning

ἐκάλεσε τὴν φλόγωσιν φλέγμα –, ἐὰν ὀδύνη ἐστὶν ἐν τοῖς τόποις ἐκείνοις καὶ σκληρία, γίνωσκε ὅτι ἐν τοῖς ὑποκειμένοις μορίοις αἱ ἀποστάσεις γίνονται.

Τίθησι δὲ καὶ προσδιορισμοὺς ἀναγκαίους. ὧν πρῶτον λέγει τοιοῦτον, ὅτι βέλτιόν ἐστι τὰς ἀποστάσεις ἐπὶ τὰ κάτω καὶ ἐν τοῖς σκέλεσι γίνεσθαι μᾶλλον ἤπερ ἐν τοῖς ὑπερκειμένοις μορίοις. καὶ δήλη ἡ αἰτία· τοσοῦτον γὰρ ἀκινδυνότερόν ἐστι τὸ ἐν τοῖς σκέλεσι γίνεσθαι τὰς ἀποστάσεις, ὅσον καὶ ἀκυρότερά εἰσι τῶν ὑπερκειμένων διὰ τὸ πόρρω ἀφεστάναι αὐτῶν.

Δεύτερον προσδιορισμὸν λέγει, ὅτι αὗται αἱ ἀποστάσεις αἱ ἐν τοῖς
194 σκέλεσι γινόμεναι, κάλλιόν ἐστι συριγ|γοῦσθαι αὐτάς· εἰ γὰρ συριγγωθῶσιν, ὡς μονοειδῆ ἔχουσαι τὴν ἐπιρροὴν τῆς ὕλης, ἐκεῖθεν ἀπορρεῖ καὶ ἐκκρίνεται καὶ οὐ κατασπείρεται εἰς διάφορα μόρια ἡ ὕλη ἐκείνη ὥστε βλάψαι αὐτά, ὡς ἂν ἐκεῖθεν διὰ τῶν συριγγωθέντων ἀποστημάτων τῆς ὕλης ἐκκρινομένης καὶ ἀπορρεούσης. ἄλλως τε δὲ καὶ διὰ τῶν συρίγγων αὐτῶν, τῇ ἀεννάῳ φορᾷ τῆς ὕλης καὶ τῇ ἀεὶ κενώσει, ἀποκενοῦται πᾶσα ἡ ὕλη καὶ ἀνακαθαίρεται ἡ περιπνευμονία.

Τρίτον προσδιορισμόν φησι τοιοῦτον, ὅτι αὗται αἱ ἀποστάσεις τὴν μὲν περιπνευμονίαν ἀπαλλάσσουσι προδήλως, ἔστι δ' ὅτε, ἐὰν φανῶσι πέψεως σημεῖα ἐν τοῖς κενουμένοις, καὶ αὗται αἱ ἀποστάσεις τάχιστα λύονται καὶ ἀποπαύονται. εἰ μὲν γὰρ ἐν τοῖς ἀναπτυομένοις σιελισμοῖς φανῶσι πέψεως σημεῖα καὶ συμπεπεμμένα ἐστί, γίνωσκε ὅτι ἀπαλλάσσονται αἱ ἀποστάσεις. εἰ δέ γε πρὸς τούτοις καὶ ἐν τοῖς οὔροις φανῇ χρηστὴ ὑπόστασις, γίνωσκε ὅτι ἐπὶ ἀπαλλαγῇ εἰσιν αἱ ἀποστάσεις καὶ ὅσον οὔπω ἀποπαύονται καὶ διαφοροῦνται. εἰ δέ γε μὴ φανῶσιν ἐν τούτοις πέψεως σημεῖα μήτε ἐν τοῖς πτυέλοις μήτε ἐν τοῖς οὔροις, ἀλλὰ τὰ τῆς ἀπεψίας καὶ τῆς ὠμότητος ἐπικρατεῖ σημεῖα, γίνωσκε ὅτι εἰς χρόνον ἐκταθήσονται αἱ ἀποστάσεις. ὅθεν τῷ χρόνῳ καὶ χωλοῦνται αὐτῶν τὰ ἄρθρα, κατὰ δύο αἰτίας· ἢ γὰρ διὰ τὴν εὐρύτητα ἐκεῖσε φέρονται οἱ χυμοὶ καὶ ἡ ὕλη, ὥστε περιέχεσθαι αὐτούς, καὶ τὸ τηνικαῦτα χωλεύουσιν διὰ τὴν εὐρύτητα ὑποδεχόμενα· διὰ δὲ τὴν κίνησιν, ἐπὶ τῇ ἐπιτεταμένῃ κινήσει θάλπονται τὰ ἄρθρα, καὶ τῇ θάλψει ἐκεῖσε συρρέουσιν οἱ χυμοὶ καὶ ἡ ὕλη, καὶ ἐπὶ τούτῳ χωλοῦνται αὐτῶν τὰ ἄρθρα.

Λέγει καὶ τέταρτον προσδιορισμὸν τοιοῦτον, ὅτι κακόν ἐστιν, ἐάν, γενομένων τῶν ἀποστάσεων, ἐξαίφνης ἀφανεῖς γένωνται, ἣν μὴ ὁ πυρετὸς παύσηται· δηλοῖ γὰρ ὅτι ἐν τῷ βάθει ἔρρευσεν ἡ ὕλη καὶ ἐν τοῖς κυριω-|
195 τέροις μορίοις καὶ ἔστιν ἐπικίνδυνον. εἰ δέ γε παύσηται ὁ πυρετός, παύεται δὲ οὕτως, ἀφανῶν γενομένων τῶν ἀποστάσεων· ἀφανεῖς δὲ γίνονται ῥωσθείσης τῆς δυνάμεως καὶ ἰσχυσάσης. σὺν τούτοις δὲ ⟨εἰ⟩ εἴη καὶ ἡ ὥρα

1 φλέγμα] Hipp. Progn. 18: p. 218,1 A. = II p. 160,4 L. 37–236,3] *cf.* Gal. In Hipp. Progn. comm. II 68: CMG V 9,2 p. 322,1–5

6 ὑποκειμένοις γ 8 αὐτά γ 14 δὲ καὶ] δὲ M: καὶ P: *om.* V 20 ἀποπαύονται *scripsi (cf. lin. 24)*: ἀπολύονται *codd.* *post* γὰρ *add.* τοῖς L σιελισμὸν L 21 ἐστί *om.* γ 26 τῆς *om.* γ ἐπικρατεῖ] ἐπιφαίνονται L εἰς] εἰ L 27 χολοῦνται *codd.*: *corr. Dietz* 28 ἢ] εἰ γ αἱ ὕλαι L 29 χολεύουσιν *codd.*: *corr. Dietz* 31 τοῦτο L 34 ἀφανὴς γένηται L 38 εἰ *addidi*: εἰ ᾖ *coni. Dietz* ἡ *om.* L

heat "phlegm"–, (and) if there is pain and hardness in those areas, it means that the abscesses will form in the lower parts.

He adds also necessary qualifications. For the first he says that abscesses to the lower parts and in the legs are better than those in the upper parts. The reason is obvious; abscesses in the legs are that much less dangerous, to the extent that these parts are less important than the upper on account of their being far distant from them.

He mentions a second qualification, that it is better when these leg abscesses form fistulas. For if they develop into fistulas, since they have only one way for the matter to flow, that matter runs off from there and is discharged, and is not spread to different parts to damage them, since it is discharged and flows off from there by means of the abscessions which have formed fistulas. Moreover, through the fistulas themselves, by the constant flow of the matter and the continual evacuation, all the matter is eliminated and the pneumonia is cleared out.

The third qualification is this, that these abscesses obviously get rid of the pneumonia, but sometimes, if signs of digestion appear in the excreta, then these abscesses are quickly cured and come to an end. For if signs of digestion appear in the expectorated spits and they are concocted, it means that the abscesses will end. And if in addition to this a useful sediment shows up in the urines, it will tell you that the abscesses are being cured and will very soon end and dissipate. However, if signs of digestion do not appear in these, neither in the sputa nor in the urines, but those of indigestion and crudity predominate, you may conclude that the abscesses are going to be protracted. Whence through time their limbs also are made lame, for two reasons; either because, due to the breadth, the humors and matter are conveyed there, so that they are retained, and then (the limbs) become lame by admitting them because of the breadth; (or it happens) on account of the movement; for with intense movement the limbs become hot, and due to the heat the humors and matter flow together there, and from this their limbs become lame.

He gives this fourth qualification, that it is a bad sign if, after they have formed, the abscesses suddenly disappear without the fever stopping; for it means that the matter has flowed into the deep interior and to the more important parts, which is dangerous. But if the fever stops, it does so upon the disappearance of the abscesses; and these disappear when the power has become strong and vigorous. Along with this if the season is

θερινὴ καὶ ἡ ἡλικία ἀκμαστικὴ καὶ τὸ χωρίον θερμὸν καὶ τὰ ἐπιβαλλόμενα καὶ τὰ ἐπιβληθέντα βοηθήματα εἴη θερμά, πεπαίνεται ἡ ὕλη ἐν τοῖς ἀποστήμασι καὶ διαφορεῖται. σὺν τούτοις δὲ καὶ ὁ πυρετὸς ἀποπαύεται, καὶ ἐπ' ἀγαθῷ τρόπῳ ἀφανεῖς γίνονται αἱ ἀποστάσεις, ἐὰν ὁ πυρετὸς παυθῇ.

II 32 [18: 219,3 A. = II 162,4 L.] Τῶν δὲ ἐμπυημάτων τῶν ἐκ τῶν περιπνευμονικῶν οἱ γεραίτεροι μᾶλλον ἀπόλλυνται, ἐκ δὲ τῶν ἄλλων ἐμπυημάτων οἱ νεώτεροι μᾶλλον ἀποθνήσκουσι καὶ τὰ ἑξῆς.

Εἰκότως οἱ γέροντες ἀπόλλυνται ἐν ταῖς περιπνευμονίαις, οἱ δὲ νεώτεροι περισῴζονται ἤπερ ἀπόλλυνται, ἐπειδὴ ἀσθενεῖς ἔχουσι τὰς δυνάμεις, ὧν τινων χρείαν ἔχουσιν· ἀσθενῶν γὰρ ὑποκειμένων τῶν δυνάμεων καὶ περιπνευμονίας οὔσης οὐκ ἀνακαθαίρονται, ἀλλ' οὕτως ἀπόλλυνται οἱ γέροντες. οἱ δὲ νεώτεροι ἤγουν οἱ ἀκμάζοντες ἐρρωμένας ἔχουσι τὰς δυνάμεις καὶ τῇ ῥώμῃ ἀναπτύουσι, καὶ ἀνακαθαίρεται αὐτῶν ἡ περιπνευμονία, καὶ περισῴζονται. ἐπὶ δὲ τῶν ἄλλων ἐμπυημάτων καὶ ἀποστάσεων τῶν ἐν τοῖς παρισθμίοις καὶ παρωτίσι συνισταμένων οἱ ἀκμάζοντες μᾶλλον ἀπόλλυνται, οἱ δὲ γέροντες περισῴζονται. καὶ τίς ἡ αἰτία; ὅτι ἐπὶ μὲν τῶν ἀκμαζόντων ἐπὶ θερμῇ ὕλῃ καὶ χολώδει ταῦτα γίνονται· ἀλλὰ καὶ τὰς αἰσθήσεις περιττὰς ἔχουσι καὶ μεγίστας ὀδύνας ὑπομένουσι· διά τε οὖν τὸ θερμὸν τῆς ὕλης καὶ τὸ περιττὸν τῆς αἰσθήσεως καὶ διὰ τὰς μεγίστας ὀδύνας μὴ φέροντες ἀπόλλυνται· προφθάνει γὰρ ὁ θάνατος τὴν πυοποίησιν. ἐπὶ δὲ τῶν γερόντων οὐ γίνονται ἐπὶ θερμῇ ὕλῃ ταῦτα τὰ πάθη, ἀλλ' οὐδὲ
196 ἠκριβω|μένας ἔχουσι τὰς αἰσθήσεις, ἀλλ' οὐδὲ μέγισται ὀδύναι γίνονται ἐπ' αὐτῶν, καὶ τὸ τηνικαῦτα περισῴζονται. ἐπεὶ οὖν ταῦτα εἴρηται, ἐν οἷς σὺν θεῷ καὶ τὸ δεύτερον τμῆμα πεπλήρωται.

15–24] *cf.* Gal. In Hipp. Progn. comm. II 69: CMG V 9,2 p. 323,12–22

2 τὰ *om.* γ εἴη] ὦσι γ 5 ἐμπύων *Hipp.* 7 ἐκ] ἐπὶ γ μᾶλλον ἀποθνήσκουσι *om.* γ 11 τινων *om.* γ 14 ἐναποπτύουσι L 16 καὶ] ἐν γ 18 θερμῆς ὕλης καὶ χολώδη L 21 ἀπόλλυσθαι L 24 τὸ *om.* L 24 sq. ἐπεὶ — πεπλήρωται *om.* L 25 *cum verbo* πεπλήρωται *des.* V

summery, the (patient's) age prime, the region warm and the present and former applied remedies hot, the matter is concocted in the abscesses and dissipates. In addition the fever also stops, and the abscesses disappear in a healthy manner, if the fever stops.

> **II 32** In cases of empyema which develop out of pneumonia the older patients are more likely to die, but in other kinds of empyema the younger succumb more easily, etc.

It stands to reason that the old die in pneumonia cases, while the younger survive (rather) than die, since the faculties of which they have need are weak (in the old); for when the faculties are weak and pneumonia is present, the old are not cleared out, but die in this state. The younger or those in their prime, on the other hand, have strong faculties and thanks to this strength they expectorate and their pneumonia is cleared out and they survive. However, in other types of empyema and in abscessions of the tonsils and parotid glands those in their prime are more liable to succumb, while the old survive. What is the reason for this? It is that in people of prime age these conditions are produced by hot and bilious matter; and they have over-sharp senses and are subject to very intense pains; because of the heat of the matter, then, and the over-sharpness of their sensation and their inability to bear very intense pains, they die; for death anticipates the suppuration. In the old, on the other hand, these affections are not caused by hot matter, nor do (the old) have sharpened senses nor do they experience very intense pains, and so they survive. These words, then, with God's help, bring the second section to an end.

ΑΡΧΗ ΣΥΝ ΘΕΩΙ ΤΟΥ ΤΡΙΤΟΥ ΤΜΗΜΑΤΟΣ

I

III 1 [19: 219,6 A. = II 164,4 L.] Αἱ δὲ ξὺν πυρετῷ ὀδύναι γινόμεναι περὶ τὴν ὀσφύν τε καὶ τὰ κάτω χωρία καὶ τὰ ἑξῆς.

Ἐντεῦθεν ἄρχεται τοῦ τρίτου τμήματος ὁ Ἱπποκράτης· καί φησιν· «Ὁκόσοισιν αἱ ὀδύναι ἤγουν αἱ ἀποστάσεις ἀπὸ τῶν κάτω ἐπὶ τὰ ἄνω γίνωνται, κάκισταί εἰσι»· δηλοῖ γὰρ ὅτι ἀπὸ τῶν ἀκυροτέρων μορίων ἐπὶ τὰ κυριώτερα μετέστη ἡ ὕλη. πλὴν οὐ πάντως ὀλέθριαι, ἀλλὰ δεῖ συνελθεῖν καὶ τὰ ἄλλα σημεῖα, οἷον ἐάν ἐστιν ὀξὺς πυρετὸς καὶ δύσπνοια καὶ παραφροσύνη καὶ σφοδρὰ ὀδύνη ἀπὸ τῶν κάτω χωρίων ἐπὶ τὰ ἄνω σύνεστι· τότε ὀλέθριαί εἰσιν αἱ τοιαῦται μεταστάσεις τῆς ὕλης. εἰ δὲ μηδὲν τούτων συνέλθῃ, γίνωσκε ὅτι αἱ ἀποστάσεις εἰς πυοποίησιν τρέπονται.

Καὶ ταῦτα εἰρηκώς φησιν ὅτι κάκιστόν ἐστι τὸ φλεγμαίνειν τὴν κύστιν, ἐπειδὴ ἡ κύστις νευρώδης ἐστί, καὶ διὰ τοῦτο μέγισται γίνονται αἱ ὀδύναι, διὰ τὸ περιττὸν τῆς αἰσθήσεως τῶν νεύρων. πλὴν δὲ ὡς νευρώδης ἡ κύστις
197 καὶ τὸν ἐγκέφαλον εἰς συμπάθειαν ἄγει, ἀλλὰ καὶ | σπασμοὺς ἐπιφέρει διὰ τὸ νευρῶδες. πρὸς τούτοις δὲ καὶ ἐποχὴ οὔρων καὶ διαχωρημάτων γίνεται. ἡ δὲ ἐποχὴ τοῦ οὔρου καὶ τοῦ διαχωρήματος κατὰ δύο αἰτίας γίνεται, ἢ γὰρ δι' ὀργανικὴν βλάβην ἢ δι' ἐπιτεταμένην ὀδύνην. καὶ ὀργανικῶς μὲν οὕτως. φλεγμαίνοντος τοῦ τραχήλου τῆς κύστεως ἀποστενοῦται ὁ οὐρητικὸς πόρος τῆς κύστεως, καὶ τὸ τηνικαῦτα ἐπέχεται τὸ οὖρον. εἶτα ἐπίκειται ὁ τράχηλος τῆς κύστεως καὶ αὐτὴ ἡ κύστις τῷ ἐντέρῳ, λέγω δὴ τῷ ἀπευθυσμένῳ· ἐπὶ τῇ φλεγμονῇ ἐπικείμενα ἐναπολαμβάνει τὴν διέξοδον τῆς κόπρου καὶ οὐ συγχωρεῖ διεξελθεῖν τὴν κόπρον· καὶ ἐντεῦθεν ἡ ἐποχὴ γίνεται τῆς κόπρου ὀργανικῶς. διὰ δὲ ἐπιτεταμένην ὀδύνην οὕτως· ἐπειδὴ νευρώδης ἐστὶν ἡ κύστις, ἐπὶ τῇ φλεγμονῇ μεγίστας ὑφίσταται ὀδύνας· ἐπὶ οὖν τῇ σφοδρᾷ ὀδύνῃ ἡ φύσις συννεύει ὡς ἐπὶ τὴν οἰκείαν ἀρχὴν καὶ ἐπὶ τὸ βάθος καὶ οὐκ ἐπιτίθεται ταῖς οἰκείαις ἐνεργείαις· αἱ γὰρ φυσικαὶ ἐνέργειαι ἐν ἐπιτεταμένῃ κινήσει ἐπιτελοῦνται, ἡ δὲ κίνησις ἐπιτείνει τὸν ῥευματισμὸν καὶ τὰς ὀδύνας· ἡ οὖν φύσις, ἵνα μὴ ἐπιταθῇ ἡ ὀδύνη, οὐκ ἐπιτίθεται, ὡς εἴρηται, ταῖς οἰκείαις ἐνεργείαις, τυχὸν τὴν ἀπο-

13–240,5] *cf.* Gal. In Hipp. Progn. comm. III 2: CMG V 9,2 pp. 325,19–326,2
φησιν] Hipp. Progn. 19: p. 220,1–4 A. = II p. 166,1–5 L.

1 ΑΡΧΗ – ΘΕΩΙ] περὶ MP 6 αἱ^{II} *om.* MP 7 γινόμεναι L 8 ὀλέθρια MP 17 καὶ^{II} *om.* L 22 τῇ κύστει MP τῶν ἐντέρων L 23 ἐπικείμενον L: *ambig.* P: *corr.* M τῇ διεξόδῳ *codd.*: *correxi* 24 ἐντεῦθεν καὶ L 30 τὰς ὀδύνας] τὴν ὀδύνην MP 31 ὡς – οἰκείαις] ταῖς εἰρηκείαις L

THE BEGINNING, WITH GOD'S HELP, OF THE THIRD SECTION

I

III 1 Pains around the loins and the lower parts when there is fever etc.

Hippocrates begins here the third section with the words "When the pains, i.e. the abscesses, go from the lower to the upper parts, they are very dangerous"; for this shows that the matter has transferred from the less important to the more important parts. However, they are not always deadly, but it is necessary for the other symptoms to occur together, that is, if there is acute fever, difficult breathing, delirium and severe pain from the lower to the upper regions; in these circumstances such relocations of the matter are deadly. But if none of these occurs, conclude that the abscesses will turn to suppuration.

Having said these things he tells us that inflammation of the bladder is very serious, the bladder being a nervy organ, and for this reason the pains are very intense, the sensitivity of the nerves being excessive. But the bladder, being nervy, also causes the brain to be sympathetically affected, and it induces spasms as well on account of its nervy nature. In addition to these retention of urines and excrements occurs. And retention of urine and excrement occurs for two reasons, either from organic damage or from intense pain. Organically as follows: when the neck of the bladder is inflamed, the urinary passage of the bladder narrows and in that case the urine is retained. Then, the neck of the bladder and the bladder itself lie on the intestine, I mean the rectum; with inflammation (these parts) lying on top cut off the passage of the feces and do not allow the feces to pass out; and hence the retention of feces for an organic reason. Because of intense pain, as follows: since the bladder is nervy, it is subject to very intense pains during inflammation; because of the intense pain, then, nature converges on its own source and to the depths and does not apply itself to its proper functions; for the natural functions are carried out by means of intense movement, and the movement intensifies the flow (of matter) and the pains; nature, then, in order that the pain might not be intensified, does not apply itself, as was said, to its proper functions, namely the excretory faculty, so as to excrete;

κριτικὴν δύναμιν, ὥστε ἀποκρῖναι· καὶ τὸ τηνικαῦτα γίνεται ἡ ἐποχὴ τοῦ οὔρου καὶ τῆς κόπρου. ῥύεται δέ ποτε σπανίως τὴν φλεγμονὴν τῆς κύστεως οὔρου παχέος καὶ πολλοῦ καὶ πεπυοποιημένου ἀπούρησις· δηλοῖ γὰρ ὅτι ἐπέφθη ἡ ὕλη καὶ οἱ χυμοί, καὶ φέρονται ἐπὶ τὴν κοιλότητα τῆς κύστεως, καὶ σὺν τῷ οὔρῳ ἐκκρίνεται τὸ πύον καὶ οἱ χυμοί, καὶ οὕτως ἀνακαθαίρεται.

Δεύτερόν ἐστι κεφάλαιον, ἐν ᾧ περὶ κρισίμων ἡμερῶν διαλέγεται. ἐπειδὴ δὲ περὶ κρίσεως ἡμῖν ὁ λόγος, δεῖ ἡμᾶς πέντε τινὰ περὶ κρίσεως ζητῆσαι· πρῶτον, τί ἐστι κρίσις, δεύτερον, πόθεν ὠνομάσθη κρίσις, τρίτον,
198 ποσαχῶς τελειοῦνται αἱ κρίσεις, καὶ τέταρτον, κατὰ πόσους | τρόπους γίνονται αἱ κρίσεις, καὶ πέμπτον, ποῖαί εἰσιν αἱ κρίσιμοι ἡμέραι.

Καὶ ἀρκτέον ἀπὸ τοῦ πρώτου· τί ἐστι κρίσις; κρίσις ἐστὶν ὀξύρροπος καὶ ἀθρόα ἐν νόσῳ μεταβολή.

Δεύτερον, πόθεν ὠνόμασται κρίσις; ἐκ μεταφορᾶς τῶν ἐν δικαστηρίῳ κρινομένων· ὥσπερ γὰρ ἐκεῖσε ὁ καταδικαζόμενος ἐν μέσῳ ζωῆς καὶ θανάτου ἐστίν, οὕτως ἰδών τις νοσοῦντα καὶ ἐν δυσφορίᾳ διάγοντα ἔφη· «Ἐλέησον, οὗτος ὁ ἄνθρωπος κρίνεται μεταξὺ ζωῆς καὶ θανάτου.»

Τρίτον, ποσαχῶς τελειοῦνται αἱ κρίσεις; τετραχῶς· ἢ γὰρ ἐπὶ ἀπαλλαγῇ καὶ ὑγείᾳ τελειοῦνται αἱ κρίσεις ἢ ἐπὶ μεγίστῃ μεταβολῇ ἐπὶ τὸ βέλτιον. ἢ τοὐναντίον· ἢ γὰρ ἐπὶ ὄλεθρον καὶ θάνατον ἢ ἐπὶ μεγίστῃ μεταβολῇ ἐπὶ τὸ χεῖρον.

Τέταρτον, κατὰ πόσους τρόπους γίνονται αἱ κρίσεις; κατὰ δύο· ἢ γὰρ κατ' ἔκρουν κρίνονται τὰ νοσήματα ἢ κατ' ἀπόσκηψιν. ὤφθη δέ ποτε καὶ ὕπνος μακρὸς καὶ βαθὺς μεγίστην μεταβολὴν ἐπὶ τὸ βέλτιον ποιήσας, ὅπερ οὐδὲ κυρίως κρίσιν ὀνομάζουσι, διὰ τὸ σπανίως γίνεσθαι καὶ ἐπὶ μόνων τῶν παίδων ὤφθη γινόμενον.

Πέμπτον, ποῖαί εἰσιν αἱ κρίσιμοι ἡμέραι, ἐν αἷς κρίνονται τὰ νοσήματα; ἐκεῖναί εἰσιν αἱ κρίσιμοι ἡμέραι, ἐν αἷς ταῦτα συνέλθῃ, ἐν αἷς πλεῖσται γίνονται κρίσεις καὶ βέβαιοι καὶ τέλειαι συνέλθωσιν· ἐκείνας καλοῦμεν κρισίμους ἡμέρας. τούτων δὲ τῶν κρινουσῶν ἡμερῶν αἱ μὲν τετραδικῶς ἀριθμοῦνται, αἱ δὲ ἑβδομαδικῶς. καὶ ἰσχυρότεραι μέν εἰσιν αἱ ἑβδομαδικαὶ τῶν τετραδικῶν. τούτων δὲ τῶν ἑβδομαδικῶν αἱ μὲν κατὰ διέχειαν ἀριθμοῦνται, αἱ δὲ κατὰ συνέχειαν. καὶ αἱ μὲν | ἑβδομαδικαὶ περίοδοι τὰς δύο ἔχουσιν
199 ἑβδομάδας κατὰ διέχειαν, | τὴν δὲ τρίτην ἀεὶ κατὰ συνέχειαν· ἑπτὰ γὰρ

6 διαλέγεται] Hipp. Progn. 20: pp. 220,10–221,7 A. = II pp. 168,6–170,1 L. 11–14] *cf.* Gal. In Hipp. Progn. comm. III 6: CMG V 9,2 p. 329,3–5 17–20] *cf.* Gal. In Hipp. Progn. comm. III 6: CMG V 9,2 p. 329,5–7 21–25] *cf.* Gal. In Hipp. Progn. comm. III 6: CMG V 9,2 p. 329,10–14 26–29] *cf.* Gal. In Hipp. Progn. comm. III 6: CMG V 9,2 p. 329,14–16 29–242,6] *cf.* Gal. In Hipp. Progn. comm. III 6: CMG V 9,2 pp. 329,20–330,27

1 γίνεται *post* ἐποχὴ *trsp.* MP 4 καί[II] *om.* MP 5 ἀνακαθαίρενται L 9 γίνονται] τελειοῦνται L 10 αἱ[II] *om.* MP 11 *post* ἐστὶν *add.* ἡ MP 13 *post* ἐν *add.* τῶ L; *cf. supra, pp. 14 sq.* 16 Ἐλέησον] ἐλέ *(ambig.)* P: ἔλεγεν M κρίνεται *post* θανάτου *trsp.* MP 19 *exspectaveris* ὀλέθρῳ καὶ θανάτῳ 20 ἐπὶ τὸ χεῖρον *om.* MP 22 ποτε *om.* MP 23 βαθὺς] βραδὺς MP 26 *post* Πέμπτον *add.* ἐστὶ MP κρίσιμοι ἡμέραι] κρίσεις L 26 sq. κρίνονται – ἐν αἷς[I] *om.* MP 27 συνέλθοι MP 30–32 ἑβδομαδικ-] ἑβδοματικ- *quater* MP 31 δὲ] οὖν L 33 διέχειαν] συνέχειαν L

and then the retention of urine and feces occurs. On some rare occasions a copious discharge of thick purulent urine rids the bladder of the inflammation; for it indicates that the matter and the humors have been digested, and they are conveyed to the hollow of the bladder, and the pus and the humors are evacuated with urine, and thus (the inflammation) is cleared out.

The second chapter is where he discusses the critical days. And since we are on the subject of crisis, we must ask five questions concerning crisis; first, what is a crisis; second, from where has the name crisis come; third, in how many ways do crises turn out; fourth, in how many ways do crises take place, and fifth, which are the critical days.

Let us begin with the first: What is a crisis? A crisis is a vehement and rapid change in a disease.

Second, whence has the name crisis come? By a metaphor from defendants in court; for, just as there the accused is between life and death, so it was that somebody, on seeing a person sick and in distress, said: "Mercy! This person's life or death is being decided."

Third, in how many ways do crises turn out? In four; for crises result in a cure and health or in a significant change for the better. Or the opposite; either in destruction and death or a significant change for the worse.

Fourth, in how many ways do crises take place? In two; for diseases reach a crisis either by discharge or by determination (of the matter to another place). A long and deep sleep has sometimes been seen to make a very great change for the better, but this is not termed a crisis in the strict sense, because it occurs rarely and has been seen to happen in children only.

Fifth, which are the critical days, (the days) on which diseases reach a crisis? The critical days are those on which this happens, that the greatest number of crises occur which are genuine and complete; those we call critical days. And of these critical days some are reckoned in periods of four, others in periods of seven. And the sevens are more powerful than the fours. Of these periods of seven some are reckoned exclusively, others conjunctively. And the periods of seven have two sevens counted exclusively and the third always conjunctively; for seven and seven (make)

καὶ ἑπτά, ιδ', καὶ ἑπτὰ γίνονται εἴκοσι μία· ἀλλὰ τὴν εἰκοστὴν ἔχομεν κρίσιμον καὶ οὐ τὴν εἰκοστὴν πρώτην ὡς κατὰ συνέχειαν ταττομένης τῆς τρίτης ἑβδομάδος. αἱ δὲ τετραδικαὶ περίοδοι τὸ ἀνάπαλιν. αἱ μὲν δύο κατὰ συνέχειαν· εἰς γὰρ τὴν ἑβδόμην ἀπαρτίζουσιν ὡς τῆς τετάρτης τέλο⟨υ⟩ς οὔσης τῆς πρώτης τετράδος, ἀρχῆς δὲ πάλιν τῆς δευτέρας τετράδος. ἡ δὲ τρίτη τετρὰς κατὰ διέχειαν, ὅϑεν τὴν ἑνδεκάτην ἔχομεν κρίσιμον.

Ταῦτα εἰρηκὼς προσδιορισμοῖς κέχρηται ὁ Ἱπποκράτης πρὸς τὴν ἤδη λεχϑεῖσαν ὑπόϑεσιν ὑπ' αὐτοῦ. ὧν πρῶτον προσδιορισμὸν λέγει τοιοῦτον, ὅτι αὗται αἱ ἡμέραι κρίσιμοι ὀνομάζονται καί εἰσι διὰ τὸ πλείστας ἐν αὐταῖς γενέσϑαι κρίσεις καὶ βεβαίας αὐτὰς γενέσϑαι καὶ τελείας, ἐπὶ ἀπαλλαγῇ τῶν νοσημάτων. εἰσὶ δὲ καὶ ἕτεραι κρίσεις, ὧν οὐκ ἐμνημονεύσαμεν, αἵτινες καὶ παρεμπίπτουσαι ὀνομάζονται, ὥσπερ ἡ τρίτη καὶ ἡ πέμπτη καὶ ἡ ϑ' ἡμέρα. ἔστι δ' ὅτε καὶ ἡ ἕκτη ἡμέρα κρίνει, ἀλλ' ἐπὶ κακῷ· εἰ δέ γε ὁ κρινόμενος ἐν τῇ ἕκτῃ ἡμέρᾳ τὸν κίνδυνον φεύξει, πάντως ὑποτροπιᾷ καὶ νοσεῖ.

Λέγει καὶ δεύτερον προσδιορισμόν, ὅτι τίς ὁ παραλογισμὸς οὗτος, ὅτι ἐπὶ μὲν τῶν δύο τετράδων τὴν ἑβδόμην λέγομεν κρίσιμον καὶ οὐχὶ τὴν ὀγδόην καὶ ἐπὶ μὲν τῶν τριῶν ἑβδομάδων τὴν εἰκοστὴν καὶ οὐχὶ τὴν εἰκοστὴν πρώτην· λείπει γὰρ ἡμέρα ἐν ἑκάστῃ ὑποϑέσει. καὶ λέγει ὅτι οὐκ ἔστιν ἄπορος ὁ λόγος· οὐδὲ γὰρ ὁ ἐνιαυτός τε καὶ οἱ μῆνες ὅλῃσιν ἡμέρῃσιν πεφύκασιν ἀριϑμέεσϑαι ἀτρεκέως. τὸν γὰρ ἐνιαυτὸν τξε' ἡμέραις ἀριϑμούντων ἡμῶν πλείονας ἔχει· ἔχει γὰρ καὶ ἄλλο τέταρτον ἡμέρας καὶ ἑκατοστὸν μέρος, καϑ' ἣν καὶ τὸ βίσεξτον ἀπαντᾷ γίνεσϑαι. ὁμοίως δὲ καὶ ὁ μὴν οὐδὲ λ' ἡμερῶν ἐστιν οὐδὲ κϑ', ἀλλ' εἴκοσι ἐννέα ἥμισυ καὶ ἄλλο
200 μόριον, ὡς οἱ ἀστρονόμοι ἀριϑ|μοῦσιν. ἐὰν οὖν οὐδὲ ὁ ἐνιαυτὸς ὅλῃσιν ἡμέρῃσιν ἀριϑμεῖται οὔτε οἱ μῆνες, οὐδὲν ἄκαιρον καὶ ἡμᾶς τῇ μακρᾷ πείρᾳ καὶ τῇ τῶν παλαιῶν μαρτυρίᾳ τὴν ἑβδόμην λέγειν κρισίμην καὶ τὴν εἰκοστὴν καὶ μὴ ἀποσῴζειν ἀκριβῆ ἀπαρίϑμησιν.

Τρίτος προσδιορισμός ἐστιν, ἐν ᾧ φησιν ὅτι ἐπὶ τῶν ὀξέων νοσημάτων καὶ συνεχῶν πυρετῶν ἡμέρας ἀριϑμοῦμεν ἐπὶ τῶν κρίσεων· τυχὸν ἡ τετάρτη ἡμέρα ἐπίδηλός ἐστιν τῆς ἑβδόμης καὶ ἡ ζ' τῆς ἑνδεκάτης καὶ ἐφεξῆς ὡσαύτως. ἐπὶ δὲ τῶν περιοδικῶν νοσημάτων καὶ τῶν χρονίων οὐκέτι ἡμέρας ἀπαριϑμοῦμεν, ἀλλὰ περιόδους, τουτέστιν ἡ τετάρτη περίοδος ἐπίδηλός ἐστι τῆς ἑβδόμης περιόδου καὶ ἡ ἑβδόμη τῆς ἑνδεκάτης. καὶ ἰστέον ὅτι ἐπὶ τῶν ὀξέων νοσημάτων εὐϑέως ἐξ ἀρχῆς δυνατόν ἐστι τὴν ἔκβασιν προγνῶναι τοῦ νοσήματος, εἴτε ἐπὶ ἀγαϑῷ γενήσεται ἡ κρίσις εἴτε ἐπὶ

11–15] *cf.* Gal. In Hipp. Progn. comm. III 6: CMG V 9,2 pp. 330,28–331,2 20 sq.] Hipp. Progn. 20: p. 221,7sq. A. = II 170,1sq. L. 29 φησιν] Hipp. Progn. 20: p. 221,2–6 A. = II p. 168,11–16 L.

2 κρισίμην MP 4 τετάρτης *om.* L τέλος *codd.*: *sec. Dietz correxi* 5 ἀρχὴν L 8 ὃν L 10 γενέσϑαι *om.* MP τελείας *om.* L; *sed cf. supra, p. 240,28* 11 τοῦ νοσήματος MP 14 ἐν — ἡμέρᾳ] καὶ ἡ ἕκτη ἡμέρα MP 18 μὲν *om.* MP 20 τε *om.* MP 21 *ante* ἀτρεκέως *add.* οὐδὲν τουτέων *ex Hipp.* L ἀτρεκέως] *hic nullus test. Hipp.* ἡμέρας MP 23 βίσεξστον L 24 οὐδὲ^{II} — ἥμισυ] ἀλλ' οὐδὲ κϑ' MP 25 ἀριϑμοῦνται MP 31 *post* ἑβδόμης *add.* ἡμέρας MP 33 τουτέστιν — περίοδος *om.* MP 34 τῆς ἑβδόμης περιόδου] ἡ ἑβδόμη περίοδος MP 35 ὅτι — ὀξέων *om.* L 35 sq. προγνῶναι τὴν ἔκβασιν MP

14 and seven more give twenty-one; but we have the critical day on the twentieth and not the twenty-first, since the third period of seven is reckoned conjunctively. And the periods of four contrariwise. Two (are counted) conjunctively; for they end on the seventh, since the fourth is the end of the first period of four and again the beginning of the second period. Then the third period of four (is reckoned) exclusively, whence we have the eleventh critical.

Having said this Hippocrates applies qualifications to the proposition already presented by him. For the first qualification he says that these days are called, and are, critical, because on them occurs the greatest number of crises which are both genuine and complete, resulting in a cure of the diseases. And there are other crises which we have not mentioned and which are called intercident (days), such as the third, the fifth and the 9th day. Sometimes the sixth also brings a crisis, but for the bad; and even if the one who has a crisis on the sixth escapes the danger, he always suffers a relapse and falls ill (again).

He gives also a second qualification, (asking) what is this false calculation, that from two periods of four days we call the seventh day critical and not the eighth, and in the case of three periods of seven days (we call) the twentieth critical and not the twenty-first; for there is a day missing in each case. And he says that the argument is not in difficulty, for neither the year nor the months can be calculated in whole days exactly. For while we count the year as 365 days, it has more; for it has another quarter day plus a hundreth part, which also accounts for the occurrence of the leap year. In the same way the month consists of neither 30 nor 29 days, but twenty-nine and a half plus a fraction, as the astronomers count. If, then, neither the year nor the months are calculated in whole days, it should be nothing strange if we, relying on long experience and the testimony of the ancients, call the seventh and the twentieth critical at the expense of precise arithmetic.

The third qualification is where he says that in acute diseases and continuous fevers we calculate days for the crisis; that is, the fourth day is indicative of the seventh, the 7th of the eleventh and so on like that. But in periodic and chronic diseases we no longer count days, but periods, i.e. the fourth period is indicative of the seventh period and the seventh of the eleventh. And note that in acute diseases it is possible to predict the outcome of the disease right from the start, whether the crisis will

κακῷ. ἐπὶ δὲ τῶν χρονίων νοσημάτων ἀδύνατόν ἐστιν εὐθέως ἐξ ἀρχῆς προγνῶναι τὴν ἔκβασιν τοῦ νοσήματος, ὁποία ἔσται. καὶ τίς ἡ αἰτία ὅτι ἐπὶ τῶν ὀξέων νοσημάτων ἐξ ἀρχῆς γινώσκομεν τὴν ἔκβασιν, ἐπὶ δὲ τῶν χρονίων οὔ; καὶ λέγομεν ὅτι ἐπὶ τῶν ὀξέων νοσημάτων εὐθὺς ἐξ ἀρχῆς ἡ φύσις καὶ τὰ αἴτια εἰσβάλλουσιν, ὡς ἔχουσιν ἰσχύν, καὶ οὕτως ἀγωνίζονται, ἐπειδὴ ὀξεῖά ἐστιν ἡ κίνησις. καὶ εἰ μὲν διαφανῶσι πέψεως σημεῖα ἐξ ἀρχῆς, 〈. . .〉, γίνωσκε ὅτι τὰ αἴτια ἴσχυσαν καὶ ἐπὶ κακῷ γίνεται ἡ κρίσις. ἐπὶ δὲ τῶν χρονίων νοσημάτων ἀδύνατόν ἐστιν ἐξ ἀρχῆς προγνῶναι τὴν ἔκβασιν τοῦ νοσήματος, ἐπειδὴ τὰ χρόνια νοσήματα ἐπὶ ψυχροτέρᾳ ὕλῃ καὶ παχυτέρᾳ γίνονται καὶ τὸ τηνικαῦτα βραχεῖα πάνυ γίνεται ἡ κίνησις, ἐπειδὴ οὐδέν ἐστι τὸ κατεπεῖγον· ἀλλὰ χλιαρῶς καὶ βραχέως εἰσβάλλει καὶ ἡ φύσις καὶ ἡ ὕλη, διότι συμμετρεῖ ἑαυτὴν ἡ φύσις· καὶ τὸ τηνικαῦτα ἀδύνατόν ἐστιν ἐξ ἀρχῆς προγνῶναι τὴν ἔκβασιν ἐπὶ τῶν χρονίων νοσημάτων,
201 εἴτε ἀγαθὴ γενήσεται εἴτε κακὴ καὶ ὀλέθριος. καὶ ἔστι τούτου παρά|δειγμα τοιοῦτον ἐπὶ τῶν ἐκτός· ἡνίκα δύο παλαισταὶ ἀγωνίζονται πρὸς ἑαυτούς, εἰ μὲν ὁ ἕτερος κατισχύει τοῦ ἑτέρου, εὐθέως ἐξ ἀρχῆς διαγινώσκομεν ὅτι οὗτος ἰσχυρότερός ἐστι καὶ νικῆσαι ἔχει, ὥσπερ ἐπὶ τῶν ὀξέων νοσημάτων. εἰ δὲ οἱ δύο ἀγωνισταὶ ἰσοσθενῶς ἔχουσι τὴν ἰσχύν, ἀδύνατόν ἐστιν εὐθέως ἐξ ἀρχῆς εἰπεῖν τὴν ἔκβασιν, ποῖος ἔχει νικῆσαι. οὕτως ἔχει καὶ ἐπὶ τῶν χρονίων νοσημάτων· οἷον γὰρ ἰσοσθενὲς ἔχουσι τὴν προσβολὴν καὶ ἡ φύσις καὶ τὰ αἴτια, καὶ διὰ τοῦτο ἀδύνατόν ἐστιν εὐθέως ἐξ ἀρχῆς προειπεῖν τι περὶ τῆς ἐκβάσεως. πλὴν ὁ Ἱπποκράτης πρὸς παραμυθίαν τοῦ λόγου λέγει ὅτι ἐπιστήμων καὶ ἀκριβὴς ἰατρὸς ἐπιστάμενος τὰς ἡμέρας τῶν κρίσεων, ποῖαί εἰσιν ἐπίδηλοι καὶ ποῖαι θεωρηταί, οὐ μὴν ἀλλὰ καὶ τὰς ἀνταποδόσεις ὁ γινώσκων τῶν περιόδων, ποῖαί εἰσιν ἐπίδηλοι, ὅτι ἡ τετάρτη περίοδος ἐπίδηλός ἐστι τῆς ἑβδόμης, ἐκ τούτων προγινώσκει καὶ τὴν ἔκβασιν τῶν χρονίων νοσημάτων· ὡς γὰρ αὐτὸς λέγει ὅτι οὐ λήσῃ ὅπῃ τρέψηται τὸ νόσημα.

Τέταρτος προσδιορισμός ἐστιν, ἐν ᾧ φησιν ὅτι ὡσαύτως καὶ ἐπὶ τῶν κυουσῶν γυναικῶν τὴν ἀπαρίθμησιν ποιεῖται τῶν ἡμερῶν ἐπὶ τῶν κρίσεων εὐθὺς ἐξ ἀρχῆς. τί γάρ; ὅτι αἱ πλεῖσται τῶν γυναικῶν μετὰ τὴν γένναν ἐν τῇ τρίτῃ ἡμέρᾳ πυρέττουσιν. οὐ δεῖ οὖν ἀπὸ τῆς τρίτης ἡμέρας τὴν ἀρχὴν ἀριθμεῖν τοῦ νοσήματος, ἀλλ᾽ ἐξ ἀρχῆς ἀφ᾽ ἧς ἔτεκεν ἡ γυνή, ἐπειδὴ προϋπῆρχε τὸ αἴτιον· οὐδὲ γὰρ τῇ τρίτῃ ἡμέρᾳ ἠθροίσθη, ἀλλ᾽ ὡς εἴρηται, ἦν πρὸ τούτου καὶ οὐ διεφαίνετο, ἐπειδὴ ἡ φύσις ἐπὶ τὴν δημιουργίαν τοῦ

15–28] *cf.* Gal. In Hipp. Progn. comm. III 11: CMG V 9,2 pp. 336,19–337,8 27 sq. οὐ – νόσημα] Hipp. Progn. 20: pp. 221,14–222,1 A. = II p. 170,9 L. *item cit. infra*, p. 288,27sq. 29 φησιν] Hipp. Progn. 20: p. 222,9sq. A. = II p. 172,2–4 L.

1 *post* νοσημάτων *add.* τοῦτο MP 4 εὐθέως MP *post* φύσις *add.* ἀγωνίζεται L 5 εἰσβάλλουσιν *post* ἰσχύν *trsp.* MP ἰσχύος L 6 *lacunam indicavi; suppleas fere* γίνωσκε ὅτι ἡ φύσις ἴσχυσε καὶ ἐπ᾽ ἀγαθῷ γίνεται ἡ κρίσις. εἰ δὲ μὴ διαφανῶσι πέψεως σημεῖα ἐξ ἀρχῆς 10 βραχέα MP 12 καί^{II} – 14 ὀλέθριος *om.* L 15 τοιοῦτον *post* ἐκτός *trsp.* MP 19 ἔχει^{II} *om.* L 22 τι *om.* L 24 *post* εἰσιν *add.* αἱ κρίσιμοι καὶ L 27 sq. λήσει . . . τρέψεται *Hipp.; sed cf. infra, p. 288,27sq.* 27 ὅπερ MP 31 εὐθέως MP 32 τρίτῃ] ἕκτῃ L 33 ἀριθμεῖν *ante* ἀρχὴν *(lin. 32) trsp.* MP τοῦ νοσήματος *ante* ἡμέρας *(lin. 32) trsp.* L 34 τῇ *om.* MP 35 καὶ] ἀλλ᾽ MP

take place for the good or for the bad. But in chronic diseases it is not possible to predict right from the beginning what kind the outcome of the disease will be. And what is the reason that in acute diseases we know the outcome from the start, but not in chronic diseases? We say that in acute diseases nature and the causes attack (each other) right from the start, since they have strength, and they join battle in this way, since the movement is fast. And if signs of digestion show through from the beginning, . . ., conclude that the causes have prevailed and the crisis will be for the bad. In chronic diseases, on the other hand, it is impossible to predict the outcome of the disease from the start, since chronic diseases develop from matter which is on the cold and thick side, and hence the movement is very slow, since there is nothing pressing; rather, nature and the matter attack (each other) halfheartedly and slowly, since nature paces itself; and so it is impossible in chronic diseases to predict from the beginning the outcome, whether it will be good or bad and deadly. And for an illustration of this in the external world we have the following: when two wrestlers contend with each other, if one overpowers the other, right from the start we can see that this one is stronger and will win, just as in the case of acute diseases. But if the two contenders are equally matched in strength, it is impossible right from the start to give the outcome, (and to say) which will win. This is also the case in chronic diseases; for nature and the causes are equally strong in attack and for this reason it is impossible to predict anything about the outcome right from the start. However, Hippocrates with a view to alleviating the account says that the skilled and precise doctor by knowing the days of crises, which are indicative and which are to be watched, and in addition by knowing the correlations of the periods, which are indicative – that the fourth period is indicative of the seventh –, from these he will prognose even the outcome of chronic diseases; for as he himself says, the direction that the disease takes will not escape him.

The fourth qualification is where he says that also in the case of women who have given birth he makes the calculation of the critical days in the same way, right from the start. Why? Because the majority of women after delivery develop fever on the third day. The beginning of the disease should not be reckoned from the third day for that reason, but from the beginning (the day) on which the woman gave birth, since the cause was there beforehand; for it did not form on the third day, but existed before this, as was said, and did not show up, since nature was pre-

ἐμβρύου ἐναπησχολεῖτο. ὅταν οὖν ἀπετέχθη τὸ ἔμβρυον, καὶ διὰ τῆς λοχικῆς καθάρσεως ὀφειλούσης κενωθῆναι ἐκείνην τὴν ὕλην κινηθεῖσα ἀνῆψε τὸν πυρετόν. δεῖ οὖν ἐξ ἀρχῆς ἀφ' ἧς ἡμέρας ἔτεκεν ἡ γυνὴ τὴν ἀπαρίθμησιν ποιεῖσθαι τοῦ νοσήματος, ἐπειδὴ προῆν ἡ ὕλη, καὶ μὴ ἀπὸ τῆς τρίτης ἡμέρας ἀφ' ἧς ὁ πυρετὸς ἀνήφθη. |

202 III 2 [20: 220,11 A. = II 168,8 L.] Οἵ τε γὰρ εὐηθέστατοι τῶν πυρετῶν καὶ ἐπὶ σημείων ἀσφαλεστάτων βεβῶτες τεταρταῖοι παύονται ἢ πρόσθεν· οἱ δὲ κακοηθέστατοι καὶ ἐπὶ σημείων δεινοτάτων βεβῶτες τεταρταῖοι κτείνουσιν ἢ πρόσθεν.

Ἰστέον ὅτι ὁ Ἱπποκράτης οἶδε τὴν τρίτην ἡμέραν κρίνουσαν· ἔφη γὰρ οἵ τε γὰρ εὐηθέστατοι τῶν πυρετῶν καὶ ἐπὶ σημείων ἀσφαλεστάτων βεβῶτες τεταρταῖοι παύονται ἢ πρόσθεν· ἔμπροσθεν δὲ τῆς τετάρτης ἡμέρας ἡ τρίτη ἐστίν· ἡ γὰρ δευτέρα παρὰ πᾶσιν ὡμολόγηται ὅτι οὐδέποτε κρίνει· οὐκοῦν περὶ τῆς τρίτης ἡμέρας νῦν λέγει ὁ Ἱπποκράτης. σκόπει δὲ ὅτι ἐνταῦθα τὸ εὐηθέστατοι τῶν πυρετῶν ἐπὶ ἀγαθῷ ἔλαβεν ἀντὶ τοῦ ἁπλούστατοι, ὑπεναντίως τοῖς Ἀττικοῖς· οἱ γὰρ Ἀττικοὶ πάντως τὸ εὔηθες ἐπὶ κακῷ λαμβάνουσιν. οὕτω γοῦν εὐήθεις ἀνθρώπους καλοῦσιν ἀντὶ τοῦ τυχὸν ὅτι δυσχερεῖς εἰσιν οὗτοι οἱ ἄνθρωποι· σπανίως δέ ποτε τὸ εὔηθες ἐπὶ ἀγαθῷ λαμβάνουσιν. ὁ μέντοι Ἱπποκράτης ἐπὶ ἀγαθῷ τὸ εὔηθες τέθεικεν. καὶ ὅτι ἐπὶ καλῷ καὶ ἐπὶ ἀγαθῷ ἔλαβε, δηλοῖ τὸ ἀντιτάξαι αὐτὸν οἱ δὲ κακοηθέστατοι τῶν πυρετῶν καὶ ἐπὶ σημείων δεινοτάτων ἐντὸς τῆς τετάρτης ἡμέρας κτείνουσιν ἢ πρόσθεν, τυχὸν ἐν τῇ τρίτῃ ἡμέρᾳ. ἀσφαλέστατα δὲ σημεῖα καὶ βέβαια καὶ ἀγαθὰ λέγει ἐπὶ τῶν ἁπλουστάτων καὶ εὐηθεστάτων πυρετῶν ταῦτα· τὸ εὔπνουν εἶναι τὸν ἄνθρωπον, τὸ εὐόρεκτον εἶναι, τὸ πέττειν καλῶς καὶ δεόντως, τὸ ὑπνοῦν εἰς νύκτα, τὸ στρέφεσθαι ῥᾳδίως ἔνθεν καὶ ἔνθεν. ἐὰν οὖν ταῦτα συνδράμωσιν ἐντὸς τῆς τετάρτης ἡμέρας ἢ ἐν τῇ τρίτῃ, παύονται οἱ πυρετοί. δεινότατα δὲ σημεῖα λέγει ἐπὶ τῶν κακοηθεστάτων πυρετῶν τὸ δύσπνουν εἶναι τὸν ἄνθρωπον, τὸ ἀνόρεκτον, τὸ μὴ καλῶς πέττειν, ἡ ἀγρυπνία, τὸ ὀδυνᾶσθαί τι τῶν ὑποχονδρίων, τὸ ἀλλοφάσσειν, τουτέστι τὸ ληρεῖν, καὶ τὰ τοιαῦτα. ἐὰν ταῦτα συνέλθωσιν ἐπὶ τῶν κακοηθεστάτων πυρετῶν, ἐντὸς τῆς τετάρτης ἀπόλλυνται ἢ πρόσθεν. |

203 III 3 [20: 221,8 A. = II 170,2 L.] Μετὰ δὲ ταῦτα ἐν τῷ αὐτέῳ

16–27] *cf.* Gal. In Hipp. Progn. comm. III 7: CMG V 9,2 pp. 331,23–333,4

1 ἀπησχολεῖτο MP ἐτέχθη MP λογικῆς *codd.*: *corr. Dietz* 2 *fort.* ἐκείνης τῆς ὕλης *scribendum est* 3 ἔτεκε(ν) ἡμέρας MP 4 πρώην *codd.*: *corr. Dietz* 8 *post* κακοηθέστατοι *add.* τῶν πυρετῶν MP *(cf. Hipp.)* 9 βεβῶτες] γινόμενοι *codd. Hipp. praeter* V 12 τε *om.* MP σήμείως L 14 *post* τρίτη *add.* ἡμέρα MP 16 *post* ἐνταῦθα *add.* ὅτι L 18 πάντες MP τὸ εὔηθες *om.* MP 21 ἐπὶ^{III} *om.* MP 22 *post* κακοηθέστατοι *add.* καὶ L 24 τετάρτη L 27 ῥαδίως στρέφεσθαι MP 28 ταῦτα *om.* L 29 λέγει] ἐστὶν MP 31 ἀλλοφυλάσσειν MP 32 *post* ληρεῖν *add.* τὸ ἄλλο ἀντ' ἄλλου φθέγγεσθαι L

occupied with creating the embryo. After the embryo, then, was brought forth, that matter which has to be cleared out in the child-birth discharge was activated and touched off the fever. It is necessary, then, to make the calculation of the disease from the beginning, (that is) from the day on which the woman gave birth, since the matter was present beforehand, and not from the third, the day on which the fever was touched off.

III 2 The fevers that are simplest and have the most favorable symptoms end by the fourth day or sooner; but the most malignant fevers with the most dangerous symptoms kill by the fourth day or sooner.

Note that Hippocrates knows that the third is a critical day; for he said, The fevers that are simplest and have the most favorable symptoms end by the fourth day or sooner; and the one before the fourth is the third day; for the second by universal agreement is never critical; therefore Hippocrates is speaking now about the third day. And note that here he took the simplest fevers in a good sense to mean the most straightforward, which is the opposite of Attic usage; for Attic writers invariably take "simple" in a pejorative sense. Thus they describe people as "simple" when they mean that they are difficult; and it is rarely that they take "simple" in a good sense. Hippocrates, however, has used the word "simple" in a good sense. And that he took it in a favorable and good sense is shown by his opposing statement, that the most malignant fevers with the most dangerous symptoms kill by the fourth day or sooner, that is, on the third day. By very safe, genuine and good signs in the most straightforward and simplest fevers he means the following: that the person breathes without difficulty, has a good appetite, digests well and in the proper way, sleeps at night, turns easily from place to place. If these, then, occur together by the fourth day or on the third, the fevers will stop. The most dangerous signs in the most malignant fevers he says are: if the person breathes with difficulty, has no appetite, does not digest well, has insomnia, has pain in a part of the hypochondria, is delirious, that is, raving, and so on. If these occur together in the most malignant fevers, they die by the fourth or sooner.

III 3 After these in the same way and by the same increase, etc.

τρόπῳ καὶ κατὰ τὴν αὐτὴν πρόσθεσιν καὶ τὰ ἑξῆς.

Τὸ λεγόμενόν ἐστι τοιοῦτον, ὅτι αἱ τρεῖς ἑβδομάδες τὴν εἰκοστὴν ἡμέραν ἀποτελοῦσι κρίσιμον τῶν δύο πρώτων ἑβδομάδων κατὰ διέχειαν ἀριθμουμένων, ὡς ποιεῖν τὴν τεσσαρεσκαιδεκάτην κρίσιμον· εἶτα ἡ τρίτη ἑβδομὰς κατὰ συνέχειαν ἀριθμουμένη τὴν εἰκάδα ποιεῖ κρίσιμον. εἰπὼν οὖν Μετὰ δὲ ταύτας ἐν τῷ αὐτῷ τρόπῳ καὶ κατὰ τὴν αὐτὴν πρόσθεσιν, φησὶν ὅτι δεῖ κατὰ τὸν αὐτὸν τρόπον ἀριθμεῖν, καὶ ἡ τεσσαρακοστὴ καὶ ἡ ἑξηκοστὴ καὶ ἡ ὀγδοηκοστὴ εὑρίσκονται κρίσιμοι. τριακοστὴν δὲ τετάρτην ἐμνημόνευσεν, ἵνα δείξῃ σοι ὅτι αἱ δύο πρῶται ἑβδομάδες κατὰ διέχειαν ἀριθμοῦνται, ἡ δὲ ἑτέρα κατὰ συνέχειαν ἀριθμουμένη, ἡ τεσσαρακοστὴ ἡμέρα ὑπαντᾷ κρίσιμος. ἰστέον δὲ ὅτι καὶ τετραδικῶς καὶ ἑβδομαδικῶς ἀριθμούμεναι αἱ περίοδοι τὴν εἰκοστὴν ἡμέραν ἀπαρτίζουσι κρίσιμον. καὶ μάλιστα ταῖς τετραδικαῖς προσέχομεν τὸν νοῦν μέχρι τῆς εἰκοστῆς ἡμέρας· ἀπὸ δὲ τῆς εἰκοστῆς οὐκέτι ταῖς τετραδικαῖς περιόδοις προσέχομεν τὸν νοῦν, ἀλλὰ ταῖς ἑβδομαδικαῖς. ὅθεν μετὰ τὴν εἰκοστὴν τριακάδα τετάρτην ἐμνημόνευσε. καὶ τίς ἡ αἰτία τούτου; καὶ λέγομεν ὅτι ἐπὶ τῶν ὀξέων νοσημάτων λεπτή ἐστιν ἡ ὕλη, καὶ ὡς λεπτὴ ἐντὸς τῆς τετάρτης πάντως τι πάσχει. καὶ διὰ τοῦτο τετραδικῶς ἀριθμοῦμεν μέχρι τῆς εἰκάδος. ἀπὸ δὲ τῆς εἰκοστῆς οὐκέτι τετραδικῶς, ἀλλ' ἑβδομαδικῶς ἀριθμοῦμεν, ἐπειδὴ ὅσον χρονίζει τὸ νόσημα, τοσοῦτον καὶ ἡ ὕλη νωθροτέρα καὶ παχυτέρα γίνεται, καὶ διὰ τοῦτο καὶ τὸ νόσημα χρονιώτερον γίνεται. καὶ ἑβδομαδικῶς μὲν ἀριθμοῦμεν μέχρι τῆς ὀγδοηκοστῆς ἡμέρας. ἀπὸ δὲ τῆς ὀγδοηκοστῆς οὐκέτι ἡμέρας ἀριθμοῦμεν, ἀλλὰ μῆνας, τέσσαρας καὶ ἑπτὰ καὶ ἕνδεκα καὶ δεκατέσσαρα. εἶτα λοιπὸν ἀπαριθμοῦμεν ἔτη, δ' καὶ ἑπτὰ καὶ ια' καὶ ιδ'. καὶ τοῦτο πολύς ἐστιν ὁ Ἱπποκράτης ἐν Ἀφορισμοῖς ἀποδεικνύων, ἐν οἷς φησιν ὅτι «Τῶν
204 ἐπιληπτικῶν τοῖσιν νέοισιν αἱ μεταβολαὶ τῶν ὡρέων καὶ τῶν ἡλι|κιῶν ἀπαλλάσσουσιν», ἀλλὰ καὶ ἐπὶ τῶν θηλέων ἐπὶ τῶν χρονίων νοσημάτων ἀπαλλάσσεσθαι αὐτὰς ἐν ταῖς τῶν καταμηνίων ῥήξεσιν· αἱ δὲ ῥήξεις ἐν τῷ τεσσαρεσκαιδεκάτῳ ἔτει γίνονται.

II

III 4 [21. 22: 222,11; 223,6 A. = II 172,5; 174,1 L.] Κεφαλῆς δὲ ὀδύναι ἰσχυραί τε καὶ ξυνεχέες σὺν πυρετῷ ξυνεχεῖ τε καὶ ἰσχυρῷ δεινὸν καὶ τὰ ἑξῆς.

25 ἐν Ἀφορισμοῖς] Hipp. Aph. II 45: IV p. 482,13sq. L. 27 sq.] *cf.* Hipp. Aph. III 28: IV p. 500,7sq. L.

1 καί^{I} *om.* MP κατὰ] μετὰ L πρόσθ *(ambig.)* M: πρόσθεν P 2 τοιοῦτόν ἐστιν MP 3 ἀποτελοῦνται MP 6 sq. ἐν – δεῖ *om.* MP 7 *ante* κατὰ *add.* καὶ MP σαρακοστὴ L (μ' MP): *corr. Dietz* 9 *post* δύο *add.* αἱ L 10 σαρακοστὴ MP 11 ἑβδοματικῶς MP 14 περιόδοις] ἡμέραις MP 15 μετὰ *sec. Dietz scripsi*: ἀπὸ *codd.* 17 πάντα MP 19 οὐκ ἔστι L 21 μὲν *om.* MP 24 *ante* καί^{IV} *add.* εἶτα L 25 ὅτι *om.* L 25 sq. τοῖς ἐπιληπτικοῖς MP 28 ῥήξεσιν] ῥήξεων MP 32 τε^{I} *om.* L ξυνεχεῖ – 33 δεινὸν] *hic nullus test. Hipp. (ex p. 223,6 sq. A. deprompta)* τε^{II} *om.* L

What is meant is this, that the three periods of seven make the twentieth day critical, when the first two sevens are calculated exclusively, so as to render the fourteenth critical; then the third period of seven reckoned conjunctively makes the twentieth critical. By saying, then, After these in the same way and by the same increase, he means that the calculation should be made in the same way, and the fortieth, the sixtieth and the eightieth will be found to be critical. And he mentioned the thirty-fourth, in order to show you that when the first two sevens are counted exclusively and the other is reckoned conjunctively, the fortieth day turns out critical. And note that the periods which make the twentieth day critical are reckoned by both fours and sevens. And up to the twentieth day we pay attention especially to the fours; after the twentieth we attend, no longer to the periods of four, but to the sevens. Hence he mentioned the thirty-fourth after the twentieth. And what is the reason for this? We say that in acute diseases the matter is thin and, because thin, it invariably undergoes some change by the fourth. And it is for this reason that we count in fours up to the twentieth. But after the twentieth we count, no longer in fours, but in sevens, since the longer the disease lasts, the heavier and thicker the matter becomes, and due to this the disease (in turn) becomes more chronic. And we count in sevens up to the eightieth day. But after the eightieth we count, no longer days, but months, four, seven, eleven, fourteen. Then finally we count years, 4, seven, 11, 14. And Hippocrates often points this out in the Aphorisms, where he says that "In young epileptics the changes of seasons and years bring cures", and that, in the case of women with chronic diseases, the monthly discharges cure them; and the discharges occur in the fourteenth year.

II

III 4 Constant severe headaches with a continuous and strong fever is a dangerous sign, etc.

Ἐνταῦθα ὀξὺ ὑποτίθεται νόσημα καὶ τὴν ὕλην διάφορα ἐπηρεάζουσαν μόρια. ἀλλὰ τὸ τέως τὴν κεφαλὴν ὑποτίθεται ἐπηρεαζομένην καὶ σημειοῦται κεφαλαλγίαν, οὐ τὴν ἐπὶ πνεύμασι γινομένην, αὕτη γὰρ τονώδης ἐστίν· ἀλλ' οὐδὲ τὴν ἐπὶ χολῇ γινομένην, αὕτη γὰρ δακνώδης ἐστίν· ἀλλ' οὐδὲ τὴν κατὰ συμπάθειαν τῶν μηνίγγων τὴν ἐπὶ φλεγμονῇ γινομένην, οὐδὲ γὰρ ὅλως μέμνηται φλεγμονῆς· ἀλλὰ κεφαλαλγίαν νῦν ὑποτίθεται τὴν ἐπὶ ἐμφράξει αἵματος καὶ πλήθει γινομένην· αὕτη γὰρ ἡ κεφαλαλγία χειρίστη ἐστὶ διὰ τὸ συνεχὲς καὶ ἐπίμονον τῆς ὀδύνης ἔνδον οὔσης τῶν ἀγγείων τῆς αἱματικῆς ὕλης. καὶ μάλιστα κακίστη ἐστὶν ἡ τοιαύτη κεφαλαλγία, εἰ καὶ ὀξύς ἐστιν ὁ πυρετός, διὰ τὸ κύριον τοῦ μορίου, πρωτίστου ὄντος· ἐγκέφαλος γάρ ἐστιν. καὶ ἀνέλπιστός ἐστιν ὁ κίνδυνος· εἰ γὰρ ἄνευ πυρετοῦ παγχάλεπός ἐστιν ἡ τοιαύτη κεφαλαλγία, πολλῷ μᾶλλον εἰ καὶ ὀξὺς πυρετὸς σύνεστιν.

Εἶτα καὶ σημεῖα λέγει ἐπὶ τῆς κεφαλαλγίας τῆς ἄνευ πυρετοῦ ὀξέος, ἐφ' ὧν ἀνέλπιστος ὁ θάνατος. καί φησιν ὅτι δύσπνους ἐάν ἐστιν ὁ ἄνθρωπος καὶ ἀνόρεκτος καὶ παραφροσύνη σύνεστιν αὐτῷ, ἔσο γινώσκων ὅτι πάντως ἀπόλλυται ὁ ἄνθρωπος. εἰ δέ γε τυχὸν εὔπνους ἐστὶν ὁ ἄνθρωπος καὶ εὐόρεκτος καὶ οὐ παραφρονεῖ, γίνωσκε ὅτι καὶ οὕτως οὐ πάντως περισῴζεται, διὰ τὸ κύριον τοῦ μορίου. εἰ δέ γε καὶ περισῴζεται, παραδίδωσιν ἡμῖν σημεῖα, ἐφ' ὧν λύεται τὸ νόσημα. καί φησιν ὅτι ἡ τοιαύτη κεφαλαλγία ἢ δι' ἐμπυημάτων ἢ δι' αἱμορραγίας. τί γάρ; ὅτι φέρεται δι' ὑπερῴας ἐπὶ θώρακα
205 καὶ πνεύ|μονα, καὶ δεύτερον πλοῦν ὁδεύουσα ἡ φύσις πυοποιεῖ τὴν τοιαύτην ὕλην καὶ εἰς ἐμπύημα μεθίστησι, καὶ τῷ χρόνῳ ἀναπτύεται καὶ ἀνακαθαίρεται, καὶ οὕτως περισῴζονται.

Εἶτα καὶ λέγει ἡμῖν σημεῖα, ἐφ' ὧν ὀφείλομεν γνῶναι, εἴτε δι' αἱμορραγίας ῥινῶν ἔχει γενέσθαι ἡ ἀπαλλαγὴ τῆς κεφαλαλγίας εἴτε δι' ἐμπυημάτων. καὶ παραδίδωσιν ἡμῖν σημεῖα τρία, ἀπὸ τοῦ τόπου, ἀπὸ τοῦ χρόνου καὶ ἀπὸ τῆς ἡλικίας.

Καὶ ἀπὸ τοῦ τόπου, εἰ ἔμφραξις γίνεται τῷ πλήθει τοῦ αἵματος, ἢ ἐντὸς τοῦ περικρανίου ὀστοῦ ἐν τοῖς ἀγγείοις ἢ ἐκτὸς τῆς κεφαλῆς. καὶ εἰ μὲν ἐντός ἐστιν ἡ ἔμφραξις, δεύτερον πλοῦν ὁδεύουσα ἡ φύσις εἰς τὰ παρακείμενα μόρια, τουτέστιν ἐν ταῖς μήνιγξι, πυοποιεῖ τὴν τοιαύτην ὕλην, καὶ διὰ ῥινῶν ἢ καὶ δι' ὤτων ἐκκρίνεται τὸ πύον, καὶ οὕτως περισῴζονται· ὠράθη γὰρ πολλάκις τοῦτο γινόμενον. ἢ φέρεται δι' ὑπερῴας ἐπὶ τὸν πνεύμονα καὶ εἰς ἐμπύημα μεθίστησι τὴν ὕλην, καὶ ἀνακαθαίρεται τὸ ἐμπύημα, καὶ περισῴζονται. εἰ δὲ ἐκτός ἐστιν, ἐπειδὴ καὶ μύες καὶ ἀξιόλογοι φλέβες εἰσί, δῆλον ὅτι καὶ θερμότεροί εἰσιν οἱ τόποι ἐκεῖνοι, καὶ δεῖ διὰ ῥινῶν προσδοκᾶν

3 κεφαλαλγίαν – 5 γινομένην] *cf.* Gal. De loc. aff. III 13: VIII pp. 205sq. K. 20 φησιν] Hipp. Progn. 21: pp. 222,12–223,1 A. = II p. 172,7–10 L. 27 παραδίδωσιν] Hipp. Progn. 21: p. 223,1–5 A. = II p. 172,10–15 L.

1 ἐπηρεάζουσι MP 2 ἐπηρεαζόμενον MP 3 τρομώδης L; *sed cf. Gal. De loc. aff. III 13: VIII 206,13 K.* 5 φλεγμονῆς M: φλεγμονὴν P 10 ὁ πυρετός] ὅπου MP 11 ἐστιν[I] *om.* MP 14 ἄνευ] *immo* μετὰ ὀξέος *ante* πυρετοῦ *trsp.* MP 15 ἐὰν δύσπνους MP 17 ἔμπνους L 18 οὗτος MP 20 ἢ] ἡ MP 21 ἢ δι' αἱμορραγίας *om.* MP θώρακος MP 22 καὶ[I] *om.* MP πνεῦμα MP 27 σημεῖα τρία] διὰ τριῶν σημείων MP *post* τόπου *add.* καὶ MP 29 Καὶ ἀπὸ] ἀπὸ μὲν MP γένηται MP 30 περικράνου MP 31 περικείμενα MP 37 δεῖ *om.* MP

Here he proposes an acute disease in which the matter attacks different parts. And first he supposes that the head is under attack and he gives the symptoms for headache, not that caused by gases, for it brings tension; nor the one caused by bile, for it is mordant; nor that which comes from a sympathetic affection of the (brain) membranes as a result of inflammation, for he does not mention inflammation at all; rather, he supposes here the headache produced by a superabundance and stoppage of blood; for this is a very serious headache, since the pain is constant and lasting, the bloody matter being inside the vessels (of the head). And this kind of headache is especially bad, if the fever is acute, on account of the importance of the part, which is the very first; for it is the brain. And there is no hope against the danger; for if such a headache is very serious without fever, it is much more so when there is acute fever present.

Next he gives signs for the headache without acute fever, which mean that death is inevitable. He says that if the person breathes with difficulty, has no appetite and is delirious, you may conclude that the person will certainly die. And even if, for example, the person breathes easily, has a good appetite and is not delirious, you must know that even in that case he does not always survive, on account of the importance of the part. But if he does survive, (Hippocrates) gives us signs which indicate that the disease will be cured. He says that such a headache (is cured) either through empyemas or through haemorrhage. Why? Because (the matter) is conveyed along the palate to the thorax and lung, and nature, using a second option, suppurates that matter and turns it to empyema, and in time it is expectorated and cleared out, and in this way they survive.

Next he gives us signs from which we ought to recognize whether the headache cure will come by nose haemorrhage or by empyemas. And he gives us three signs, based on the place, the time and the age.

From the place: if a stoppage is caused by the superabundance of blood, (it occurs) either in the vessels within the cranial bone or outside the head. And if the stoppage is inside, nature, using a second option, suppurates that matter in the surrounding parts, that is, in the membranes, and the pus is discharged through the nose or even through the ears, and in this way they survive; for this has often been seen to happen. Or, (nature) conveys the matter along the palate to the lung and turns it to empyema, and the empyema is cleared out and they survive. But if it (the stoppage) is outside, since there are muscles and important veins, it is obvious that those places are warmer, and one should expect

τὴν ῥύσιν τοῦ αἵματος, καὶ οὕτως παύεται ἡ τοιαύτη κεφαλαλγία.

Ἀπὸ δὲ τοῦ χρόνου, ἐὰν ὀξὺς ὁ πυρετὸς εἴη καὶ πάντα ὀξυκίνητά εἰσι, δίψος καὶ τὰ λοιπά, γίνωσκε ὅτι δι' αἱμορραγίας ἔχει λυθῆναι τάχιον ἡ κεφαλαλγία. εἰ δέ γε βληχρός ἐστιν ὁ πυρετὸς καὶ ὑφειμένα πάντα καὶ οὐδὲν κατεπείγει, γίνωσκε ὅτι χρονιωτέρα γίνεται ἡ ἀπαλλαγή.

Ἀπὸ δὲ τῆς ἡλικίας, ἐὰν θερμή ἐστιν ἡ ἡλικία, τυχὸν παιδικὴ ἢ ἀκμαστική, μετὰ καὶ τῶν ἄλλων συστοίχων, γίνωσκε ὅτι δι' αἱμορραγίας παύεται
206 τὸ νόσημα. εἰ δὲ | παρακμαστική ἐστιν ἡ ἡλικία καὶ γεροντική, γίνωσκε ὅτι δι' ἐμπυημάτων ἡ ἀπαλλαγὴ γίνεται τῆς κεφαλαλγίας.

Εἶτα καὶ γνωρίσματα ἡμῖν παραδίδωσι μελλούσης γίνεσθαι αἱμορραγίας διὰ ῥινῶν. καί φησιν ὅτι κνῶνται τὴν ῥῖνα, αἱ φλέβες αἱ ἐν τοῖς ὀφθαλμοῖς ἔνογκοι γίνονται, πυραυγῆ φαντάσματα ὁρῶσι πρὸ τῶν ὀφθαλμῶν καὶ τὰ τοιαῦτα.

Δεύτερον κεφάλαιόν ἐστιν, ἐν ᾧ ὑποτίθεται τὴν ὕλην τὴν δριμεῖαν καὶ διαβρωτικὴν οὐκέτι τὴν κεφαλὴν ἐπηρεάζουσαν, ἀλλὰ φερομένην εἰς τὸ ἀκουστικὸν νεῦρον καὶ ποιοῦσαν φλεγμονὴν χαλεπωτάτην. καὶ ἐπικίνδυνός ἐστιν ἡ τοιαύτη διάθεσις διά τε τὸ παρακεῖσθαι τὸν ἐγκέφαλον, τὴν τοιαύτην ἀρχήν, καὶ διὰ τὸ τὴν δευτέραν αἴσθησιν ἐπηρεαζομένην καὶ πάσχουσαν. τί γάρ; ὅτι καὶ ὀξὺς πυρετὸς συνεδρεύει καὶ σπασμὸς διὰ τὸν ἐγκέφαλον· ἀλλὰ καὶ παραφροσύνη γίνεται, καὶ διὰ τοῦτο χαλεπωτάτη καὶ ἐπικίνδυνός ἐστιν ἡ τοιαύτη διάθεσις. μάλιστα δὲ οἱ ἀκμάζοντες περιτυγχάνοντες τῇ τοιαύτῃ διαθέσει ἀπόλλυνται ἤπερ οἱ γέροντες. καὶ ἡ αἰτία δήλη ἐστίν· οἱ γὰρ ἀκμάζοντες μᾶλλον ἀπόλλυνται διὰ τὸ περιττὸν τῆς αἰσθήσεως· μεγάλας γὰρ ὑφίστανται καὶ σφακελώδεις καὶ σφοδροτέρας τὰς ὀδύνας καὶ μὴ ὑποφέροντες ἀπόλλυνται. περισῴζονται δὲ οἱ γέροντες, ἐπειδὴ οὐκ ἔχουσιν οὕτως ἠκριβωμένην τὴν αἴσθησιν, ἀλλ' ἀσθενῆ καὶ ἀδρανῆ, καὶ οὐχ οὕτως μεγάλας καὶ σφακελώδεις ὑφίστανται τὰς ὀδύνας. εἰ δέ γε συμβαίη ποτὲ τὸν δεύτερον πλοῦν ὁδεῦσαι τὴν φύσιν καὶ πυοποιῆσαι τὴν ὕλην, μᾶλλον οἱ ἀκμάζοντες περισῴζονται, ἐὰν ὑπενέγκωσι τὰς ἐν τῷ μέσῳ τῆς πυοποιήσεως ὀδύνας, ἤπερ οἱ γέροντες, ἐπειδὴ τοῖς ἀκμάζουσι καὶ πλούσιόν ἐστι τὸ ἔμφυτον θερμὸν καὶ ἡ δύναμις ἐρρωμενεστέρα ἐστί, καὶ τὸ τηνικαῦτα ὅλη ὡς ὅλη μεταβάλλεται καὶ πέττεται ἡ ὕλη καὶ διαφορεῖται τῇ περιουσίᾳ τοῦ θερμοῦ καὶ τῇ ῥώμῃ τῆς δυνάμεως. οἱ δὲ γέροντες ἀπόλλυνται μᾶλλον,
207 ἐπειδὴ οὐκ ἔστι περιουσία θερμοῦ ἐν αὐτοῖς, ἀλλ' ἀμυδρά ἐστι καὶ | ἀνίσχυρος, ἀλλὰ καὶ ἡ δύναμις ἀσθενεστέρα ἐστὶν ἐπ' αὐτῶν, καὶ τὸ τηνικαῦτα οὐ πέττεται οὐδὲ διαφορεῖται ἡ ὕλη, ὅθεν τῷ μήκει τοῦ χρόνου καὶ ὑποτροπιασμοὺς ὑπομένουσι καὶ οὕτως ἀπόλλυνται.

Τρίτον κεφάλαιόν ἐστιν, ἐν ᾧ ὑποτίθεται τὴν δριμεῖαν καὶ διαβρωτικὴν

14 ὑποτίθεται] Hipp. Progn. 22: pp. 223,6–224,5 A. = II p. 174,1–13 L. 38 ὑποτίθεται] Hipp. Progn. 23: pp. 224,6–226,2 A. = II pp. 174,4–178,9 L.

2 εἴη *post* ὀξὺς *trsp.* MP 3 παυθῆναι MP *ante* τάχιον *add.* καὶ MP 5 γίνεται *post* ἀπαλλαγή *trsp.* MP 14 ἐστι(ν) κεφάλαιον MP 17 τὸ *om.* MP παρακεῖσθαι *post* ἐγκέφαλον *trsp.* MP τοιαύτην] *fort.* πρώτην *scribendum est* 18 ἐπηρεαζόμενον MP πάσχουσι MP 22 εἴπερ MP 27 τὸν *om.* MP 34 ἀμαυρά MP

the flow of blood through the nose and thus this kind of headache comes to an end.

From the time: if the fever is acute and all (the symptoms) are vehement, thirst and the rest, conclude that the headache must be terminated fairly quickly by haemorrhage. But if the fever is slight and all (the symptoms) are subdued and nothing is pressing, conclude that the cure will be fairly tardy.

From the age: if the age is a warm one, namely the child or the prime age, and the other concomitant circumstances (are warm) also, conclude that the disease will end by haemorrhage. But if the age is past prime or old age, you will know that the headache's cure will come through empyemas.

Then he gives us indications for impending nasal haemorrhage. He says that they scratch the nose, the veins in the eyes become swollen, they see fiery flashes before the eyes and suchlike.

The second chapter is where he supposes that the pungent and corrosive matter no longer attacks the head, but is conveyed to the acoustic nerve and produces very serious inflammation. And such a condition is dangerous both because the brain, the principal part, is situated nearby and because the second sense is under attack and is affected. Why? Because acute fever and spasm are present together on account of the brain; delirium also occurs, and for this reason such a condition is very serious and dangerous. Those in their prime, on succumbing to such a condition, are much more likely to die than the old. And the reason is obvious; for, those in their prime are more likely to die because of their excessive sensitivity; for they are subject to intense, mortifying and rather violent pains, and, unable to bear these, they die. The old, on the other hand, survive, since their sensation does not have that much keenness, but is weak and ineffective, and they are not subject to such intense and mortifying pains. But if it sometimes happens that nature, taking a second option, suppurates the matter, those in their prime, if subjected to the pains in the midst of suppuration, are more liable to survive than the old, for in those of prime age the innate heat is plentiful and the power (of the body) is stronger, and so the matter as a whole is all converted and digested, and it is dissipated thanks to the superabundance of the heat and the strength of the power. The old, on the other hand, are more liable to die, since the heat in them is not superabundant, but feeble and powerless, and the power in them is rather weak, and hence the matter is neither digested nor dissipated, so that with the length of time they suffer relapses and thus die.

The third chapter is where he supposes that the pungent and corro-

ὕλην φερομένην ἐπὶ φάρυγγα καὶ λάρυγγα. καὶ φάρυγξ ἐστὶν ἡ ἔνδον ἀχάνεια τοῦ στόματος, ἡνίκα ἐπὶ τὰ κάτω πιλοῦντες τὴν γλῶσσαν ὁρῶμεν αὐτὴν καὶ ψαύομεν, ᾗτινι ἀποπερατοῦνται καὶ οἱ δύο πόροι, ὅ τε τοῦ οἰσοφάγου καὶ ὁ τοῦ λάρυγγος. ⟨καὶ εἰ⟩ ἐκεῖ ἐνεχθῇ ἡ ὕλη, χαλεπώτατόν ἐστι, μάλιστα συνεδρευόντων καὶ τῶν χαλεπῶν συμπτωμάτων, λέγω δὴ ὀξὺς πυρετός, δύσπνοια, δυσκαταποσία καὶ τὰ τοιαῦτα, ἐπειδὴ καὶ ἡ κατάποσις καὶ ἡ ἀναπνοὴ περὶ τὸ ζῆν ἡμῖν συμβάλλονται· τούτων δὲ βλαπτομένων ἀνέλπιστός ἐστιν ἡ ζωή.

Εἶτα καὶ διορίζει ἑκάτερον καὶ λέγει ἰδίᾳ καὶ χωρὶς τῆς τε λάρυγγος καὶ τῆς φάρυγγος πάθη. καὶ ὑποτίθεται ὁ Ἱπποκράτης τὴν ὕλην τὴν δριμεῖαν καὶ διαβρωτικὴν ἐπὶ φάρυγγα ἐνεχθεῖσαν καὶ καταλέγει τρεῖς διαφορὰς κυνάγχης ὁμωνύμως τῷ γένει, ἀμφοτέροις τοῖς πάθεσι κοινὰς πάσας. οἱ μέντοι ἐξηγηταὶ ὑπὸ διαίρεσιν ἀνάγοντες τὸν λόγον τέσσαρας διαφορὰς λέγουσι κυνάγχης καὶ ἑκάστῃ ἰδίᾳ καὶ χωρὶς ὀνόματα ἐπιτιθέασι· φασὶ γὰρ ὅτι αὕτη ἡ δριμεῖα ὕλη φερομένη ἐπὶ λάρυγγα ἢ εἰς τοὺς ἔνδον μύας τοῦ λάρυγγος φέρεται ἢ εἰς τοὺς ἐκτός. καὶ εἰ μὲν εἰς τοὺς ἔνδον, ποιεῖ φλεγμονήν, ἥντινα φλεγμονὴν καὶ οἱ ἐξηγηταὶ καὶ ὁ Ἱπποκράτης κυνάγχην ὀνομάζουσιν, ἥτις φλεγμονὴ οὔτε τῇ ὁράσει ὑποπίπτει οὔτε τῇ ἁφῇ· ἔνδον γάρ ἐστιν ἡ φλεγμονή, καὶ διὰ τοῦτο κακίστη ἐστὶ καὶ ἐπικίνδυνος· τῆς γὰρ φλεγμονῆς εἰς τοὺς ἔνδον μύας γινομένης μεγίστη γίνεται ἡ ὀδύνη καὶ σφακελώδης, ἀλλὰ καὶ ἡ κατάποσις ἐμποδίζεται καὶ δυσχερὴς γίνεται, ἀλλὰ καὶ δύσπνοια παρακολουθεῖ, καὶ κινδυνεύουσι πνιγμωδῶς. |

208 Εἰ δέ γε εἰς τοὺς ἔξωθεν μύας ἐνεχθῇ ἡ ὕλη καὶ ἡ φλεγμονὴ εἰς αὐτὰ συσταίη, εἰς τὰ περὶ τὸν τράχηλον καὶ αὐχένα χωρία, καλοῦσιν οἱ ἐξηγηταὶ τὴν τοιαύτην διάθεσιν παρακυνάγχην, ἥτις οὐδέ ἐστι χαλεπὴ ὥσπερ ἡ πρώτη· ἡ μὲν γὰρ ὀδύνη σύνεστι διὰ τὴν φλεγμονήν, ἀλλ' ὑφειμένη, ἀλλ' οὐδὲ ἡ κατάποσις κωλύεται οὕτως, ἀλλ' οὐδὲ δύσπνοια παρακολουθεῖ, ἐπειδὴ ἔξω ἐστὶν ἡ φλεγμονή. εἰ μέντοι χρονίζει, καὶ οὗτοι ἀπόλλυνται.

Εἶτα ὑποτίθεται φερομένην τὴν ὕλην ἐπὶ φάρυγγα. καὶ ἐνταῦθα ἢ εἰς τοὺς ἔνδον μύας τῆς φάρυγγος φέρεται ἡ ὕλη ἢ εἰς τοὺς ἐκτός. καὶ εἰ μὲν εἰς τοὺς ἔνδον, οὐ γίνεται ὄγκος φλεγμονώδης, ἀλλ' ὄγκος ἐρυσιπελατώδης ἔχων ἔρευθος ὡς ἀπὸ χολωδεστέρου καὶ λεπτοτέρου αἵματος γινομένου τοῦ ῥευματισμοῦ, ὅντινα ἐρυσιπελατώδη ὄγκον συνάγχην ὀνομάζουσιν οἱ ἐξηγηταὶ ἰδίως, ἥτις οὐδέ ἐστιν ἐπικίνδυνος ὥσπερ αἱ πρῶται διαθέσεις. αὕτη δὲ ἡ διάθεσις καὶ ὁρᾶται ἀνοιγομένου τοῦ στόματος, οὐκ ἔστι δὲ

1–4] *cf.* Gal. In Hipp. Progn. comm. III 21: CMG V 9,2 p. 348,7–10 10 Ἱπποκράτης] Hipp. Progn. 23: pp. 224,6–225,6 A. = II pp. 174,14–178,2 L. 12–256,7] *cf.* Gal. De loc. aff. IV 6: VIII pp. 248sq. K. In Hipp. Aph. comm. IV 34: XVII B p. 706 K. 29 ὑποτίθεται] Hipp. Progn. 23: pp. 225,6–226,2 A. = II p. 178,2–9 L.

3 ᾗτινι] ἢ ἔνθα MP 4 ὁ *om.* MP *post* λάρυγγος *fort. excidit descriptio huius partis* καὶ εἰ *addidi; cf. infra, lin. 23*: ἐὰν *coni. Dietz* 7 συμβάλλουσι L 12 ἀμφότερα τὰ πάθη *codd.*: *correxi* κοινῶς *codd.*: *corr. Wk.* 14 κυνάγχης] δυσπνοίας L ὀνόματι M: ὀνόματος P 15 sq. ἢ . . . ἢ] καὶ . . . καὶ MP 20 ἡ *om.* L; *cf. supra, pp. 14sq.* 24 ἐξηγηταὶ *post* διάθεσιν *(lin. 25) trsp.* MP 26 συνέστη L 32 ὡς *om.* MP τοῦ γινομένου *codd.*: *trsp. Dietz* 35 δὲ[I] *om.* MP

sive matter is conveyed to the pharynx and larynx. The pharynx is the inner cavity of the mouth, which we see and touch when we press the tongue down, where the two passages of the esophagus and larynx terminate. And if the matter is brought there, it is very serious, especially when the dangerous symptoms too are present together, I mean acute fever, difficult breathing, difficult swallowing and the like, since both swallowing and respiration contribute to our life; and when these are damaged, there is no hope for life.

Next he distinguishes each and gives separately and apart the affections of larynx and pharynx. And Hippocrates supposes that the pungent and corrosive matter has been conveyed into the pharynx, and he lists three varieties of cynanche, all having the same name as the class and being common to both affections. The commentators, however, submitting the account to division, give four varieties of cynanche and apply names to each separately and individually; for they say that this pungent matter conveyed to the larynx is brought either to the inner muscles of the larynx or to the outer. And if to the inner, it creates inflammation, which inflammation the commentators and Hippocrates both designate cynanche, and it is subject to neither sight nor touch; for the inflammation is inside, and for this reason it is very bad and dangerous; for when the inflammation is in the inner muscles, the pain becomes very intense and mortifying, and swallowing is impeded and becomes difficult, and difficulty in breathing follows and they are in danger of suffocating.

If, on the other hand, the matter is conveyed to the external muscles and the inflammation occurs in these, (that is) in the parts around the throat and neck, the commentators call such a condition paracynanche; it is not as dangerous as the first; for while pain is present on account of the inflammation, it is subdued; neither is the swallowing impeded in the same way, nor does difficult breathing result, since the inflammation is external. However, if the condition becomes chronic, these (patients) too die.

Then he supposes that the matter is conveyed to the pharynx. And here the matter is brought either to the inner muscles of the pharynx or to the outer. And if to the inner, there develops, not an inflamed swelling, but an erysipelatoid swelling with a red color, since the flux comes from blood that is on the bilious and thin side; this erysipelatoid swelling has been given the separate name of synanche by the commentators and it is not as dangerous as the first conditions. And this condition is visible when the mouth is open, but it is not dangerous, since they do

ἐπικίνδυνος, ἐπειδὴ οὐδὲ οὕτως ὀδυνῶνται σφοδρῶς, οὔτε μὴν δύσπνοια παρακολουθεῖ, ἀλλ' οὐδὲ δυσχεραίνουσι περὶ τὴν κατάποσιν, εἰ μὴ ἐπ' ὀλίγον τι.

Εἰ δέ γε ὡς ἐλαχίστη τις μοῖρα τῆς ὕλης ἔλθῃ εἰς τοὺς ἔνδον μύας τοῦ φάρυγγος καὶ ποιήσῃ σμικρὸν ἔρευθος, τὸ δὲ πλεῖστον τῆς ὕλης ἐνεχθῇ εἰς τοὺς ἔξω μύας, λέγεται τὸ πάθος παρασυνάγχη, ἥτις περὶ τὸν τράχηλον καὶ τὸν αὐχένα συνίσταται, ἥτις καὶ σαφῶς ὁρᾶται. αὕτη δὲ ἡ διάθεσις ἀκινδυνοτέρα πασῶν ἐστιν, ἐπειδὴ οὐδὲ παρεμποδίζεται τῇ καταπόσει, οὔτε μὴν ὀδύνη παρακολουθεῖ, ἀλλ' οὐδὲ δύσπνοια ἕπεται, ἐπειδὴ ἐκτός ἐστιν ἡ φλεγμονή· καὶ διὰ τοῦτο ἀκινδυνοτέρα ἐστίν, εἰ μή τι ὅτι, ὥς φησιν Ἱπποκράτης, ἐξαίφνης ἀφανὴς γένηται ἡ τοιαύτη φλεγμονή· ἐὰν γὰρ ἐξαίφνης ἀφανὴς γένηται, δηλοῖ ὅτι ἐγκαταλιποῦσα ἡ ὕλη τὰ ἀκυρότερα μόρια καὶ τὰ ἐπιπολῆς, ἐπὶ τὸ βάθος καὶ ἐπὶ τὰ κυριώτερα μόρια ἔρρευσεν ἡ
209 ὕλη. καὶ ὅσον οὔπω κίνδυνος ἕπεται ἀπειλῆς καὶ | θανάτου, εἰ μὴ ἄρα ὅτι μετὰ τὸ ἐξαίφνης ἀφανῆ γενέσθαι τὴν φλεγμονὴν ἢ πύου πλήθους ἀναγωγὴ γένηται ἢ πτυέλου πλῆθος ἐκκριθῇ, καὶ οὕτως κενωθεῖσα ἡ ὕλη, ἐλευθερωθῶσι τοῦ κινδύνου.

III 5 [21: 223,4 A. = II 172,13 L.] Τοῖσι δὲ νεωτέροισι πέντε καὶ τριήκοντα ἐτέων

Ἰστέον ὅτι ὁ Ἱπποκράτης τὴν ἀκμαστικὴν ἡλικίαν μέχρι τοῦ λε' χρόνου εἶναι λέγει. πλὴν ὁ Ἱπποκράτης τὸ ὡς ἐπίπαν θεωρήσας εἶπε τοῦτο, ἐπεί τοί γε ἡ κρᾶσίς ἐστιν ἡ ἐπιτιθεῖσα τοὺς ὅρους ταῖς ἡλικίαις· πολλοὶ μὲν γὰρ θερμοὶ ὄντες τὴν κρᾶσιν καὶ μέχρι τῶν μ' ἐτῶν καὶ πεντήκοντα ἤκμασαν κατὰ τὴν ἡλικίαν, ἄλλοι δὲ ψυχροὶ ὄντες τῇ κράσει μέχρι τῶν τριάκοντα ἐτῶν ἤκμασαν.

III 6 [22: 223,7 A. = II 174,2 L.] Παραφρονῆσαι γὰρ κίνδυνος τὸν ἄνθρωπον καὶ ἀπολέσθαι.

Ἐπιχειροῦσί τινες καὶ ὅσον ἐκ τοῦ νῦν λεγομένου καὶ λέγουσιν ἐν ἐγκεφάλῳ εἶναι τὸ ἡγεμονικόν, ὡς καὶ τῷ Γαληνῷ δοκεῖ. ἐὰν γὰρ πυοποιουμένης τῆς ὕλης ἐν τῇ ἀκοῇ παραφροσύνη ἐπακολουθῇ, διὰ τὸ ἐπιπαρακεῖσθαι τὸν ἐγκέφαλον· ἡ δὲ παραφροσύνη βλάβη ἐστὶ τῶν ἡγεμονικῶν ἐνεργειῶν· οὐκοῦν ἐν ἐγκεφάλῳ ἐστὶ τὸ ἡγεμονικόν. ὁ δὲ νέος ἐξηγητὴς λέγει ὅτι οὐ διὰ

11 Ἱπποκράτης] Hipp. Progn. 23: p. 225,6 A. = II p. 178,2sq. L. 29 τῷ Γαληνῷ δοκεῖ] *v. e. g.* Gal. In Hipp. Progn. comm. II 6: CMG V 9,2 p. 266,13sq. De plac. Hipp. et Plat. VI 3,7: CMG V 4,1,2 p. 374,11–13 De usu part. IX 4: II p. 13 Helmr. = III p. 700 K. 32 ὁ – ἐξηγητὴς] *v. supra*, pp. 13; 126,1 Steph. Comm. in Hipp. Aph.: Escor. Σ. II. 10 fol. 69^v

1 μὴν *om.* L; *sed cf. lin. 9* 4 ὡς *om.* MP τοῦ] τῆς MP; *sed cf. supra, p. 254,4* 5 ποιήσει *codd.*: *corr. Dietz* μικρὸν MP 8 παρέμποδος γίνεται τῆς καταπόσεως MP 10 *post* τοῦτο *add.* καὶ MP τι ὅτι] ὅτι P: τι L: *suppl.* M; *cf. lin. 14* 14 ἄρα] τι MP 15 μετὰ *om.* L τὴν φλεγμονὴν] τὸν ὄγκον L πλῆθος *codd.*: *correxi* 17 τὸν κίνδυνον M: τῶν κινδύνων P 18 δὲ *non hab. Hipp.* νεωτέροις MP 19 τριάκοντα L 20 *ante* τὴν *add.* καὶ MP 22 ἐπιτιθεῖσα *ex* ἐπιτεθεῖσα, *ut vid.*, *corr.* L: ἐπιτεθεῖσα MP 30 ἐπίκεισθαι MP

not have such severe pains, nor does difficult breathing result, nor do they have difficulty in swallowing, unless to a small degree.

But if only a very minute amount of the matter enters the inner muscles of the pharynx and produces a slight redness, while the greatest part of the matter is conveyed to the external muscles, the affection is termed parasynanche and it is found around the throat and neck and is clearly visible. This condition is less dangerous than any of the others, since there is no impediment to swallowing, nor does pain result, nor does difficult breathing follow, seeing that the inflammation is outside; and for this reason it is less dangerous, unless, as Hippocrates says, such inflammation suddenly becomes invisible; for if it suddenly becomes invisible, it means that the matter, leaving the less important parts and the surface area, has flowed to the deep interior and to the more important parts. And there follows immediately the danger of a threat and death, unless the sudden disappearance of the inflammation is followed by either a copious discharge of pus or a copious excretion of spit, and, the matter having been evacuated in this way, they are freed from the danger.

III 5 Those younger than thirty-five years

Note that Hippocrates says that the prime age goes to the 35th year. However, Hippocrates said this as a general observation, since in fact it is the temperament which sets the limits for the ages; for many people with warm temperaments have been in their prime up to 40 and fifty years of age, while others with cold temperaments have flourished up to the age of thirty.

III 6 For there is a danger that the person will become delirious and die.

Some, basing themselves on the present text, try to claim that the governing principle is in the brain, which is also the opinion of Galen. For if, (they argue,) the matter having been suppurated in the ear, delirium results, it is because the brain is situated above nearby; and delirium is damage to the governing functions; therefore the governing principle is in the brain. But the new commentator says that the delirium

τὸν ἐγκέφαλον γέγονεν ἡ παραφροσύνη, ἀλλὰ διὰ τὸν πυρετόν· ἔφη γὰρ ὅτι ὀξὺς πυρετὸς σύνεστιν· ὁ δὲ πυρετὸς ἀπὸ καρδίας ὁρμᾶται· διὰ δὲ τὸν πυρετὸν ἡ παραφροσύνη γίνεται· οὐκοῦν ἐν καρδίᾳ ἐστὶ τὸ ἡγεμονικόν.

III

III 7 [23: 226,3 A. = II 178,9 L.] Οἱ δὲ γαργαρεῶνες ἐπικίνδυνοι καὶ ἀποτέμνεσθαι καὶ ἀποσχάζεσθαι καὶ ἀποκαίεσθαι, ἔστ' ἂν ἐρυθροί τ' ἔωσι καὶ μεγάλοι.

Νῦν διαλέγεται ὁ Ἱπποκράτης περὶ τοῦ γαργαρεῶνος καὶ σημειοῦται καὶ τὰ ἐν αὐτῷ συνιστάμενα πάθη καὶ συμπλέκει τῷ σημειωτικῷ λόγῳ καὶ
210 θεραπευτικὴν | θεωρίαν. ἐπειδὴ οὖν πρόκειται αὐτῷ περὶ γαργαρεῶνος διαλεχθῆναι, πέντε τινὰ περὶ τοῦ γαργαρεῶνος ζητήσωμεν· πρῶτον τὴν οὐσίαν αὐτοῦ, δεύτερον τὴν χρείαν, τρίτον τὴν ἐνέργειαν, τέταρτον τὰ πάθη τὰ συνιστάμενα ἐν αὐτῷ καὶ πέμπτον τὰς θεραπείας.

Καὶ ἀρκτέον ἀπὸ τοῦ πρώτου. τίς ἡ οὐσία τοῦ γαργαρεῶνος; σαρκώδης ἐστί· κατά τινας δὲ ἁπλῆ ἐστι σὰρξ ἐκ τῆς πρώτης πήξεως τοῦ αἵματος.

Ἡ δὲ ἐνέργειά ἐστι τοῦ γαργαρεῶνος τὸ δίκην πλήκτρου τὸ ἐκπνεόμενον πνεῦμα ἀπὸ θώρακος τυγχάνειν καὶ ἀποτελεῖν τὴν φωνήν. τί γάρ; ὅτι τοῦ πνεύματος ἀπωθουμένου ἀπὸ θώρακος, δίκην πλήκτρου προσκροῦον ἐν τῷ γαργαρεῶνι μορφοῦται καὶ οἷον εἰδοποιεῖται καὶ ῥυθμίζεται καὶ ποιεῖ τὴν ἀπήχησιν τῆς φωνῆς.

Ἡ δὲ χρεία διάφορός ἐστι. τί γάρ; ὅτι χρειώδης ἐστὶν ὁ γαργαρεὼν πρὸς τὰς ἀκρατεῖς καὶ ἀκολάστους καὶ ἀμέτρους τοῦ ἀέρος εἰσπνοάς, τυχὸν ὅτε θερμὸς εἰσπνεῖται ἄγαν ἀὴρ ἢ ψυχρός, τούτων ὁ γαργαρεὼν κολάζει τὴν ἀμετρίαν τοῦ ἀέρος καὶ ἄκρατον ἐν τῇ εἰσπνοῇ καὶ ἐν συμμετρίᾳ ἄγει, καὶ οὐκέτι πληκτικὸς εὑρίσκεται ὁ εἰσπνεόμενος ἀὴρ τῆς τραχείας ἀρτηρίας καὶ τοῦ πνεύμονος καὶ τῆς καρδίας. ἀλλὰ καὶ καθ' ἕτερον τρόπον χρειώδης ἐστὶν ὁ γαργαρεών. τί γάρ; ὅτι ἀκαθάρτου εἰσπνεομένου τοῦ ἀέρος, τυχὸν μετὰ κονιορτοῦ ἢ καπνοῦ ἢ ἄλλως ἀκαθάρτου αὐτοῦ εἰσπνεομένου, ἀποκαθαίρεται δίκην ἠθμοῦ τὸ ἀκάθαρτον καὶ καθαρὰν τὴν εἰσπνοὴν τοῦ ἀέρος ποιεῖται.

Τὰ δὲ πάθη τὰ συνιστάμενα ἐν αὐτῷ διάφορά εἰσι· πάσχει γὰρ καὶ ὁμοιομερῆ πάθη, πάσχει καὶ ὀργανικά. καὶ ὁμοιομερῆ μὲν πάσχει πάσας τὰς δυσκρασίας, ἡνίκα θερμαίνεται ἢ ψύχεται ἢ ξηραίνεται ἢ ὑγραίνεται, ἢ κατὰ συζυγίαν ἑκάστην δυσκρασίαν πάσχει, τυχὸν θερμαίνεται καὶ ὑγραίνεται ἢ

16 Ἡ – πλήκτρου] *cf.* Gal. De usu part. VII 5: I p. 382 Helmr. = III p. 526 K. 21 sq. ὅτι – εἰσπνοάς] *cf.* [Gal.] Introd. s. med. 11: XIV p. 713 K. Gal. De usu part. XI 11: II p. 145 Helmr. = III p. 888 K.

1 ὅτι *om.* L 2 ὥρμηται MP 3 ἡ *om.* L 6 καί^I *om.* L καὶ ἀποσκάζεσθαι *(sic) post* ἀποκαίεσθαι *trsp.* L ἀποσκάζεσθαι *codd.*: *corr. Dietz; cf. infra, p. 260,27* 8 περὶ *scripsi*: ἀπὸ *codd.* 11 ζητήσομεν MP 15 ἐστι σὰρξ] σάρξ ἐστιν MP πρώτης *om.* L τοῦ *om.* MP 16 θωρακεῶνος L 18 ἐξωθουμένου MP προσκρούων MP 22 πνοὰς L 23 ὅτι *codd.*: *corr. Dietz* 24 τὸ ἄμετρον MP 26 πνεύματος L καί^II *om.* L 27 τοῦ *om.* L 29 ἠθμοῦ *coni. Kollesch*: ἰσθμοῦ *codd.* 34 καὶ ὑγραίνεται *om.* L ἢ – 260,1 ξηραίνεται *om.* MP

occurred, not on account of the brain, but because of the fever; for (Hippocrates) said that there is acute fever present; the fever originates in the heart; the delirium develops on account of the fever; therefore the governing principle is in the heart.

III

III 7 Uvulas are dangerous to remove, to lance and to cauterize, as long as they are red and enlarged.

Now Hippocrates discusses the uvula; he gives the symptoms for the affections which develop in it and he joins to the discussion of symptoms a therapeutic exposition as well. Since, then, it is his proposal to discuss the uvula, let us ask five things concerning the uvula; first, its substance, second the use, third the function, fourth the affections which develop in it, and fifth the treatments.

And let us begin with the first. What is the substance of the uvula? (It is composed of) a flesh-like substance; but according to some it consists of simple flesh from the first solidification of the blood.

The function of the uvula is to meet the air exhaled from the thorax, like a plectrum, and to create the voice. Why? Because when the air is forced out of the thorax it knocks against the uvula, as against a plectrum, is given a shape and, so to say, a form and articulation, and it produces the resonance of voice.

Its use is varied. Why? Because the uvula is useful for the immoderate, uncontrolled and unbalanced inhalations of air, that is, when air is inhaled too hot or too cold, in these cases the uvula checks the imbalance and intemperance of the air during the inhalation and produces a balance, and (then) the trachea, lungs and heart are no longer stricken by the inhaled air. But the uvula is also useful in another way. Why? Because when the air is inhaled unclean, e.g. with dust or smoke or some other impurity, it cleans out the impurity, like a strainer, and makes the inhaled air pure.

The affections which arise in it are of different kinds; for it is subject to both homogeneous and organic affections. And as homogeneous affections it suffers all the distempers, when it becomes warm or cold or dry or moist, or it suffers each distemper in combination, i.e. it be-

211 θερμαίνεται καὶ ξηραίνεται, | καὶ τὰς λοιπάς. ἀλλὰ καὶ ὀργανικὰ πάθη πάσχει, παντοῖον τυχὸν ὄγκον. ὁ μέντοι Ἱπποκράτης ὀλίγων παθῶν ἐνταῦθα μέμνηται· φησὶ γὰρ ὅτι ὁ γαργαρεὼν ἢ ἰσχναίνεται καὶ ταπεινοῦται καὶ λέγεται ἱμάς, ὅπερ ἐστὶ λῶρος, ἢ ὅλως ὀγκοῦται καὶ φλεγμαίνει δίκην κίονος καὶ λέγεται κιονίς, ἢ κατωφερὴς γίνεται ὁ ῥευματισμὸς τῆς ὕλης, καὶ τὸ κάτω μέρος φλεγμαίνει καὶ λέγεται σταφυλή, ἐοικυῖα τῇ ῥαγὶ τῆς σταφυλῆς. κακὰ δέ ἐστι τὰ πάθη ταῦτα, ἐπειδὴ μεγάλους καὶ τοὺς κινδύνους ἐπιφέρουσι κατὰ δύο τρόπους. τί γάρ; ὅτι πρῶτον μὲν κωλύεται ἡ κατάποσις καὶ ἡ ἀναπνοή. λοιπὸν δὲ καὶ κατ' ἄλλον τρόπον εἰσὶ τὰ πάθη ταῦτα κακά, ὅτι κατὰ τὸ συνεχὲς μεταδίδοται τῷ ἐγκεφάλῳ τὸ πάθος καὶ ποιεῖ παραφροσύνας καὶ σπασμούς.

Λοιπὸν δὲ ἡ θεραπεία ζητείσθω. καί φησιν ὅτι, ἐὰν ὅλως φλεγμαίνῃ ὁ γαργαρεὼν καὶ λέγεται κιονίς, καὶ ἐπίφοβός ἐστιν ἡ θεραπεία, οὔτε τομῇ χρεὼν ἐστι χρήσασθαι, οὔτε δὲ καύσει, διὰ δύο αἰτίας. ἐπειδὴ γὰρ εὐαίσθητός ἐστιν ὁ γαργαρεὼν διὰ τὸ πλησιάζειν τὸν ἐγκέφαλον, διὰ τοῦτο μεγάλαι ἐπιγίνονται ὀδύναι καὶ ἐπὶ τῇ τομῇ καὶ ἐπὶ τῇ καύσει. ⟨. . .⟩ ἀλλὰ δέον τοῖς στυπτικοῖς καὶ ἀποκρουστικοῖς χρήσασθαι βοηθήμασιν, ἅτινά ἐστι τὸ ὑδροροσᾶτον ἢ τὸ ἀφέψημα τὸ ἀπὸ τῆς φακῆς καὶ ξυλοκεράτων καὶ ἀκάνθης Αἰγυπτίας καὶ στυπτηρίας καὶ τῶν τοιούτων. εἰ δὲ ἐπὶ τὰ κάτω ὁ ῥευματισμὸς τῆς ὕλης γένηται, ὥστε γενέσθαι σταφυλήν, τότε ἀδεῶς χρῆσθαι καὶ τῇ τομῇ καὶ τῇ καύσει, μὴ ἐκ βάθους καὶ ἄνωθεν, ἐπεί τοί γε ἄφωνος γίνεται ὁ ἄνθρωπος, ἐπειδὴ αὐτό ἐστι τὸ μορφοῦν τὴν φωνήν, ἀλλὰ δεῖ κάτω, ἐν ᾧ ἐστιν ἡ φλεγμονή, τῇ τομῇ χρήσασθαι καὶ τῇ καύσει. πλὴν δέον προσέχειν τὴν φλεγμονήν· εἰ μὲν γὰρ μετά τινος νομώδους ἢ σήψεώς ἐστιν ἡ φλεγμονή, τότε δεῖ ἀποτέμνειν ἢ καίειν, καὶ λοιπὸν κατὰ τὸ ἄνω μέρος τὸ ἐναπομένον
212 τοῖς εἰρημένοις στυπτικοῖς καὶ ἀπο|κρουστικοῖς δέον χρήσασθαι. εἰ δέ γε μηδὲν τούτων σύνεστιν, ἀλλὰ φλεγμονὴ μόνη, τότε δεῖ κατασχάζειν καὶ τέμνειν· τὸ τηνικαῦτα γὰρ διὰ τῶν τομῶν ἐκκενοῦται ἡ ὕλη καὶ ὑγιάζονται ἐπὶ τῇ κενώσει. πλὴν τοῦτο δεῖ σε ποιεῖν καὶ προκαθαίρειν δέον ἐστὶν ὑπηλάτῳ τὴν γαστέρα καὶ κενοῦν αὐτὴν καὶ ἀρρευμάτιστον ποιεῖν τὸν τόπον καὶ εἶθ' οὕτως καίειν ἢ τέμνειν τὴν σταφυλὴν καὶ χρῆσθαι τοῖς προειρημένοις βοηθήμασι. πλὴν δεῖ σε καὶ τοῦτο γινώσκειν, ὡς πολλάκις μεγάλη ἐστὶν ἡ φλεγμονή, ὥστε πνιγμὸν ποιῆσαι, καὶ τὸ τηνικαῦτα οὐ δεῖ ἐγχειρεῖν τῇ θεραπείᾳ, ἐπειδὴ οὐ περιγίνονται τοῦ πάθους, ἀλλὰ πνιγμωδῶς ἀπόλλυνται. δέον οὖν ἐστιν ἐκφυγεῖν τὴν θεραπείαν καὶ μὴ ἐγχειρεῖν διὰ τὸ ἄμεμπτον καὶ ἀνέγκλητον φυλάξαι τὴν τέχνην.

18 sq.] *cf.* Gal. De sect. ad eos qui introd. 8: I p. 91 K.

1 τὰ λοιπὰ MP   1 sq. πάσχει πάθη MP   2 παντοίων MP: παντοίως L: *correxi*   3 ὁ *om.* MP   6 ῥογῇ (*i. e.* ῥωγὶ) MP   8 *post* ἡ *add.* τε MP   9 καὶ^{II} *supra lin. ins.* L: *om.* P   *ante* εἰσὶ *add.* καὶ L   κακά *post* τρόπον *trsp.* MP   12 φλεγμαίνει MP   13 καὶ^{II} *om.* MP   15 διὰ τὸ πλησιάζειν] διπλασιάζειν MP   16 *lacunam indicavi; possis supplere fere* ἀλλὰ καὶ διὰ τὸ ἀφορήτους γίνεσθαι αἱμορραγίας οὐ δεῖ χρῆσθαι τῇ τομῇ ἢ τῇ καύσει (*cf. infra, p. 264,33 sq.*)   δέον] δεόντως L   17 χρῆσθαι MP   22 δεῖ] δὴ MP   24 ἡ φλεγμονή *om.* MP   25 καὶ λοιπὸν *om.* L   ἀπομένον MP   28 τὸ *om.* L   ἀποκενοῦται MP   30 εὑρεμάτιστον MP   34 περιτίνονται L

comes warm and moist or warm and dry, and the rest. It also suffers organic affections, in other words, every kind of swelling. Hippocrates, however, mentions few affections here; for he says that the uvula becomes attenuated and shrinks and is called *himas*, i.e. thong, or it becomes completely swollen and is inflamed like a pillar (*kiōn*) and is called *kionis*, or the flow of matter tends downwards and the bottom part becomes inflamed and is called *staphylē*, resembling the berry of the grape (*staphylē*). And these affections are bad, for they bring on serious dangers also in two ways. Why? Because in the first place swallowing and breathing are impeded. And then these affections are bad in another way, because due to the contiguity the affection is transmitted to the brain and produces delirium and spasms.

Finally let us ask about the treatment. He says that if the uvula is totally inflamed and is called *kionis*, then the treatment is risky and one should not employ either cutting or cautery for two reasons. For since the uvula is highly sensitive on account of the proximity of the brain, for this reason intense pains occur with both cutting and cautery. . . . , but it is necessary to use astringent and dispelling remedies, such as rosewater or decoctions from lentils and Ceratonia Siliqua and Acacia Aegyptica and alum and the like. But if the flow of matter is to the bottom, so that *staphylē* develops, then freely use both cutting and cautery, not deep inside and on top, since (that way) the person becomes voiceless, seeing that it is this (part) which gives shape to the voice, but the cutting and cautery should be employed below, where the inflammation is. But one must pay attention to the inflammation; for if the inflammation is accompanied by some spreading (ulceration?) or putrefaction, then it is necessary to cut away or burn, and afterwards on the top part that remains the aforementioned astringent and dispelling remedies should be used. However, if none of these is present, but only the inflammation, then one should lance and cut; for then the matter is emptied out through the incisions and health is restored upon the evacuation. However, it is necessary for you to do this: you must first clean the bowels with a purgative and empty them and make the place free from flux, and then burn or cut the *staphylē* and use the aforementioned remedies. But you should also know this, that frequently the inflammation is extensive enough to cause suffocation, and in that case one should not attempt treatment, since they do not survive the affection, but die by suffocation. It is necessary, then, to shun and not attempt the treatment, in order to keep the art free from blame and censure.

Δεύτερόν ἐστι κεφάλαιον, ἐν ᾧ ἐπαναλαμβάνεται περὶ τῶν ἤδη λεχθέντων ἀποστημάτων. ἀλλὰ πρὸ τούτου περὶ τῶν ἐξ ὑποστροφῆς γινομένων νοσημάτων κεφαλαιωδῶς διαλέγεται. καί φησιν ὅτι, ⟨εἰ οἱ⟩ πυρετοὶ ἀθρόως παύονται μὴ φανέντων τῶν λυτηρίων σημείων μηδὲ ἐν κρισίμοις ἡμέραις γινομένων ἢ καὶ γενομένων ἀτελῶς καὶ ἐλλιπῶς, τυχὸν οὔρου πλήθους κένωσις ἢ γαστρόρροια ἢ αἱμορραγία, ἀλλ' οὕτως ἀνεπαισθήτως ἀθρόως ἐπαύθησαν οἱ πυρετοί, τότε γίνωσκε ὅτι τὰ τοιαῦτα νοσήματα φιλυπόστροφά εἰσι κατὰ τὸ εἰρημένον τῷ Ἱπποκράτει· «Τὰ γὰρ ἀσήμως ῥαστωνήσαντα φιλυπόστροφά εἰσιν». εἰ δὲ φανέντων τῶν λυτηρίων σημείων καὶ ἐν κρισίμοις ἡμέραις αὐτῶν φανέντων, τότε ἀσφαλὴς καὶ βεβαία γίνεται ἡ ἀπαλλαγὴ τοῦ νοσήματος.

Τούτων οὕτως προλεχθέντων διαλέγεται περὶ τῶν ἄνωθεν αὐτῷ λεχθεισῶν ἀποστάσεων. ἀλλὰ πρὸ τούτου δέον ἐστὶν διαιρέσει τινὶ ἐπιμνησθῆναι, ἥντινα διαφόρως εἰρήκαμεν. ἔστι δὲ αὕτη· τῶν νοσημάτων τὰ μέν εἰσιν ὀξέα, τὰ δὲ χρόνια· τὰ δὲ χρόνια νοσήματα διαφόρως γίνονται· ἢ γὰρ
213 δυσλύτως ἔχει τὸ μόριον τῷ πάθει, ὥσπερ | περιπνευμονία καὶ ἕλκωσις εἰς τὴν κύστιν καὶ νεφρῖτις καὶ τὰ τοιαῦτα, χρόνια ἐνδείκνυται τὰ νοσήματα, ἢ διὰ τὸ ὠμὴν καὶ παχεῖαν καὶ γλίσχραν εἶναι τὴν ὕλην χρόνια γίνονται τὰ νοσήματα, ἢ διά τι περιστατικόν, τυχὸν διὰ λύπην ἐπίμονον καὶ συνεχῆ καὶ φροντίδα ὁμοίως ἐπίμονον, χρόνια γίνονται τὰ νοσήματα· ἐπὶ γὰρ τῶν τοιούτων παθῶν, διὰ τὸ ἀπασχολεῖσθαι τὴν φύσιν, οὐ συμπέττει τὴν ὕλην, καὶ τὸ τηνικαῦτα χρόνια γίνονται τὰ νοσήματα. τὰ δὲ ὀξέα νοσήματα ἐπὶ θερμῇ καὶ λεπτῇ καὶ χολώδει ὕλῃ γίνονται. ἐὰν οὖν ἀποστάσεις ἐπὶ τῶν παθῶν γίνωνται, τῷ τρόπῳ τούτῳ· ἐὰν γὰρ λεπτή ἐστιν ἡ ὕλη καὶ θερμὴ καὶ ἡ δύναμις ἐρρωμένη, τότε καὶ πάντως κατ' ἔκρουν κενοῦται ἡ ὕλη διὰ τῶν φυσικῶν ὑπονόμων καὶ κριτικῶς παύεται τὸ νόσημα. εἰ δέ γε ὠμή ἐστιν ἡ ὕλη καὶ παχεῖα καὶ γλίσχρα καὶ ψυχρά, ὑπόκειται δὲ καὶ ἀσθενὴς ἡ δύναμις καὶ καταβεβλημένη, οἱ τοιοῦτοι φθείρονται καὶ ἀπόλλυνται. εἰ δέ γέ ποτε σπανίως περισῴζονται χρόνῳ τινὶ κατακερματιζομένης τῆς ὕλης καὶ εἰς λεπτὰ καταθραυομένης καὶ οἷον συμπεττομένης ἀπό τινος συστοίχου, ὥρας θερμῆς ἢ ἡλικίας ἢ καταστήματος θερμοῦ γινομένου, λύεται τὸ νόσημα δι' οὔρων τυχὸν κατὰ σμικρὸν συμπεττομένης, σπανίως δὲ διὰ γαστρός· καὶ οὕτως λύεται τὸ νόσημα καὶ περισῴζονται. εἰ δὲ ὠμῆς καὶ παχείας καὶ γλίσχρας οὔσης τῆς ὕλης καὶ ἔρρωται ἡ δύναμις, τότε ἡ φύσις δεύτερον

1–3 ἐπαναλαμβάνεται ... διαλέγεται ... φησιν] Hipp. Progn. 24: pp. 226,12–227,2 A. = II p. 180,6–13 L. 8 τὸ – Ἱπποκράτει] *immo Galenus, v.* In Hipp. Progn. comm. III 27: CMG V 9,2 p. 352,15 14 διαφόρως εἰρήκαμεν] *e. g. supra,* p. 196,32–36

3 εἰ οἱ *addidi* 5 ἢ καὶ γενομένων *om.* L πλήθους *coni. Dietz*: πλῆθος *codd.* 9 τῶν *om.* MP 12 αὐτῷ] αὐτῶν MP 13 *exspectaveris* διαιρέσεώς τινος 14 *post* αὕτη *add.* ὅτι MP 15 ὀξέα εἰσί MP ἢ] *fort.* εἰ *scribendum est* 16 ἕλκος L 17 ἢ – 19 νοσήματα *om.* L 18 καὶ γλίσχραν *om.* M; *sed cf. infra, linn. 27.33 sq.* γίνονται] ἐνδείκνυται M 20 καὶ *om.* MP 22 τὰ[I] *om.* L 23 ἀποστασίαι MP 24 γίνονται MP γὰρ] οὖν MP 25 *post* τότε *add.* πάντη τε MP *post* πάντως *add.* καὶ L 27 ἡ ὕλη *om.* MP 32 κατὰ – γαστρός *om.* L 33 περισώζεται P: διὰ γαστρὸς δὲ σπανίως L 34 γλίσχρου *codd.*: *corr. Kollesch*

The second chapter is where he takes up again the subject of abscesses, which have been discussed already. But before this he discusses in a summary fashion the diseases which arise from recurrence. And he says that if the fevers stop all of a sudden, when the salutary signs have not appeared and have not occurred on critical days or, even if they did occur, have done so in an incomplete and imperfect way – I mean a copious evacuation of urine or diarrhoea or haemorrhage –, but the fevers stopped all of a sudden in this way without being perceived, then you will know that such diseases are likely to recur, in accordance with what Hippocrates says, "For those that ease off without indication are likely to recur". But if (they stop all of a sudden) after the salutary signs have appeared and when they have appeared on critical days, then the cure from the disease is safe and sure.

Following these preliminaries he talks about the abscesses discussed by him earlier. But before this it is necessary to recall a division which we have mentioned on various occasions. It is this: of diseases some are acute, some are chronic; chronic diseases arise in different ways; for the part has difficulty in shaking off the affection, as happens in pneumonia and ulceration on the bladder and nephritis and the like, (and this) shows the diseases to be chronic, or diseases become chronic because the matter is crude and thick and viscous, or diseases become chronic on account of some circumstantial factor, such as lasting and constant grief and equally long worry; for in such affections nature, being fully occupied, does not concoct the matter and then the diseases become chronic. Acute diseases, on the other hand, arise from warm and thin and bilious matter. If, then, abscessions occur in the affections, (they do so) in the following way; for if the matter is thin and warm and the power strong, then the matter is invariably emptied by discharge through the natural channels and the disease is ended by way of a crisis. But if the matter is crude and thick and viscous and cold, and the power weak and overthrown, such patients are destroyed and die. But if, as happens on rare occasions, they survive for a time because the matter has been divided and broken up into fine pieces and more or less concocted by one of the concomitant circumstances, warm season or age or hot weather, the disease is cured through urines for example, when (the matter) has been slightly concocted, and on rare occasions through the bowels; and in this way the disease is cured and they survive. But if, when the matter is crude and thick and viscous, the power is strong, then nature,

πλοῦν ὁδεύουσα ἀποδιώκει τὴν ὕλην ἀπὸ τῶν κυριωτέρων μορίων ἐπὶ τὰ ἀκυρότερα μόρια καὶ εἰς ἀπόστασιν τρέπεται τὸ νόσημα. καὶ εἰ μὲν ἐπ' ἔλαττόν ἐστι ἐρρωμένη ἡ δύναμις, ἐπὶ τὰ παρακείμενα πέμπει τὴν ὕλην, τυχὸν ἐπὶ τὰ παρίσθμια. εἰ δὲ ἐπὶ πλέον ἔρρωται, ἐπὶ τὰ ἄκρα ἀποδιώκει τὴν ὕλην, καὶ οὕτως γίνονται αἱ ἀποστάσεις. εἰ δέ γε λεπτῆς οὔσης τῆς
214 ὕλης καὶ θερμῆς, ἀσθενής τε ἡ δύναμις, τότε μὴ ἰσχύουσα ἡ φύ|σις ἀπωθῆσαι ἐπὶ τοὺς φυσικοὺς ὑπονόμους τὴν ὕλην ἐξ ἀνάγκης διὰ τὴν οἰκείαν ἀσθένειαν ἐπὶ τὰ παρακείμενα μόρια πέμπει τὴν ὕλην, καὶ τότε πάλιν εἰς ἀπόστασιν τρέπεται τὸ νόσημα, οὐ διὰ τὴν ὕλην, ἀλλὰ διὰ τὴν ἀσθένειαν τῆς δυνάμεως.

Καὶ οἱ μὲν ἐξηγηταὶ ταῦτα καὶ μόνα ἡμῖν παραδιδοῦσιν. ὁ μέντοι Ἱπποκράτης ἀπὸ τῆς ἡλικίας λαμβάνει τὴν ἔνδειξιν καί φησιν ὅτι ἐπὶ τῶν ἀκμαζόντων ὡς ἐπίπαν αἱ ἀποστάσεις γίνονται, ἐπ' ἔλαττον δὲ ἐπὶ τῶν παρακμαζόντων, ἐπὶ δὲ τῶν γερόντων οὐδόλως γίνονται αἱ ἀποστάσεις. εἰ μὲν γὰρ ἀκμαστική ἐστιν ἡ ἡλικία καὶ θερμὴ καὶ λεπτὴ ἡ ὕλη, ἀσθενὴς δὲ ἡ δύναμις, εἰς ἀπόστασιν τρέπεται τὸ νόσημα. εἰ δὲ ἀκμαστικῆς οὔσης τῆς ἡλικίας ὠμὴ καὶ παχεῖα καὶ ψυχρὰ καὶ γλίσχρα ἐστὶν ἡ ὕλη, ἐρρωμένη δὲ ἡ δύναμις, πάλιν εἰς ἀπόστασιν τρέπεται τὸ νόσημα. ἐπὶ δὲ τῶν παρακμαζόντων ἐπ' ἔλαττον γίνονται αἱ ἀποστάσεις. τί γάρ; ὅτι ὠμὴ καὶ παχεῖα καὶ ψυχρά ἐστιν ἡ ὕλη ἐπ' αὐτῶν, ἐρρωμένη δὲ τὸ τέως ἡ δύναμις, καὶ διὰ τοῦτο εἰς ἀπόστασιν τρέπεται τὸ νόσημα. ἐπὶ μέντοι τῶν γερόντων ἀμφότερά εἰσι καὶ ὠμὴ καὶ ψυχρὰ καὶ παχεῖα ἡ ὕλη καὶ ἡ δύναμις ἀσθενής, καὶ τὸ τηνικαῦτα φθείρονται καὶ ἀπόλλυνται· ἀποστάσεις γὰρ αὐτοῖς οὐ γίνονται.

Ταῦτα εἰρηκὼς θεώρημα πάνυ ἀναγκαῖον καὶ ἀσφαλὲς ἐπάγει, καί φησιν ὅτι ἐπὶ πάντων τῶν ἀποστάσεων τῶν ἤδη λεχθεισῶν συνεχεῖς καὶ ἀδιάκοποί εἰσιν οἱ πυρετοί· εἰ δὲ μετὰ τὸ ἤδη προγενέσθαι χρόνῳ τινὶ τὴν συνέχειαν τῶν πυρετῶν διαδέξηται διάλειμμα, εἶτα μετὰ τὸ διάλειμμα ἐπιγένωνται πλανῆταί τινες πυρετοί, γίνωσκε ὅτι εἰς τεταρταῖον πυρετὸν τελευτᾷ.

III 8 [23: 226,5 A. = II 178,12 L.] Ἀλλὰ χρὴ τὰ τοιαῦτα τοῖσιν ἄλλοισι μηχανήμασι πειρᾶσθαι κατισχναίνειν

Τὸ λεγόμενον τοιοῦτόν ἐστιν, ὅτι ἐπὶ τῆς κιονίδος οὐ δεῖ χρῆσθαι τομῇ ἢ καύσει διὰ τὸ ἀφορήτους γίνεσθαι αἱμορραγίας, ἀλλὰ καὶ μεγίστας

12 Ἱπποκράτης] Hipp. Progn. 24: p. 227,2–11 A. = II pp. 180,13–182,7 L. 26 φησιν] Hipp. Progn. 24: p. 227,6sq. A. = II p. 182,1–3 L.

1 κυριωτέρων] ἀκυριοτέρων L τὰ *om.* L 2 μόρια *om.* MP ἀποστάσεις MP 5 ἀποστασίαι MP 8 προκείμενα MP τότε *om.* MP ἀποστασίαν MP 9 οὐ *om.* MP 11 παραδίδωσιν *(sic)* ἡμῖν MP παραδίδωσιν *codd.*: *sec. Dietz correxi* 14 αἱ *om.* MP 15 καὶ[I] – 17 ἡλικίας *om.* L 16 ἀποστασίαν MP: *correxi* 17 καὶ γλίσχρα *om.* L 18 ἀποστασίαν MP 20 ψυχρὰ καὶ παχεῖα MP τὸ τέως *om.* L 21 ἀποστασίαν MP 22 παχεῖα καὶ ψυχρὰ MP 23 ἀποστασία M: ἀπόστασις L 24 *ante* αὐτοῖς *add.* ἐν MP γίνεται L 25 πάνυ *om.* MP 26 πάντων] *sic codd.* 29 πλανίτες MP τέταρτον MP 34 γενέσθαι MP

using a second option, expels the matter from the more important to the less important parts and the disease turns to abscession. And if the power is slightly strong, (nature) sends the matter to the surrounding parts, e.g. to the tonsils; but if it has still more strength, it expels the matter to the extremities and thus the abscessions develop. If, on the other hand, when the matter is thin and warm, the power is weak, then nature, not having the strength to expel the matter to the natural channels, is obliged on account of its own weakness to send the matter to the surrounding parts, and then again the disease turns to abscession, not because of the matter, but because of the weakness of the power.

This is all that the commentators give us (on the subject). Hippocrates, however, bases his demonstration on age and says that in general abscessions occur in those of prime age, to a lesser extent in those past prime and abscessions do not occur at all in the old. For if the age is prime and the matter warm and thin and the power weak, the disease turns to abscession. If, on the other hand, the age being prime, the matter is crude and thick and cold and viscous, and the power is strong, again the disease turns to abscession. But abscessions occur to a lesser extent in those past prime. Why? Because in them the matter is crude and thick and cold, and the power is strong at first, and for this reason the disease turns to abscession. In the old, however, both (factors) are present, namely crude, cold and thick matter along with weak power, and so they are destroyed and die; for abscesses do not occur in them.

Having said this, he introduces a very necessary and reliable rule; he says that in all the abscessions already mentioned the fevers are continuous and unintermittent; and if, after the continuity of the fevers has been present already for a time, an interval should follow, and then (if), after the interval, irregular fevers should develop, you will know that the fever will end up a quartan.

III 8 But one must try to reduce these by the other means

The meaning is as follows, that in the case of *kionis* one should not use cutting or cautery, since they give rise to unbearable haemorrhages

215 ὀδύνας καὶ παραφροσύ|νας καὶ σπασμοὺς καὶ τὰ τοιαῦτα, ἀλλὰ δεῖ ἐπὶ τῆς τοιαύτης διαθέσεως, λέγω δὴ ἐπὶ τῆς κιονίδος, τοῖς ἄλλοις μηχανήμασι χρῆσθαι, τυχὸν τοῖς ἀποκρουστικοῖς καὶ τοῖς στύφουσι καὶ τοῖς συμπέττουσιν, ὁποῖά ἐστιν ἄκανθα Αἰγυπτία καὶ ὄμφαξ καὶ κηκὶς καὶ φακῆ καὶ στυπτηρία σχιστὴ καὶ ἕτερα πλεῖστα βοηθήματα πρὸς τὸ πάθος ἁρμόζοντα.

III 9 [23: 226,8 A. = II 180,2 L.] Ἐν τουτέῳ τῷ καιρῷ ἀσφαλὲς διαχειρίζειν

Καλῶς πάνυ καὶ θαυμασίως ἐχρήσατο τῇ λέξει εἰρηκὼς διαχειρίζειν· πλατυκωτέρως γὰρ τοῦτο πεποίηκε καὶ οὐκ εἶπεν «ἀσφαλὲς χειρουργεῖν». ἡ γὰρ χειρουργία, πᾶσα ἡ διὰ τῶν χειρῶν γινομένη ἐπιμέλεια τοῖς νοσοῦσι, χειρουργία ὀνομάζεται παρὰ τὸ τὴν χεῖρα ὀργᾶν. καὶ γὰρ τὸ διακαίειν χειρουργία ὀνομάζεται καὶ τὸ διαβρέχειν καὶ τὸ καταπλάττειν καὶ τὸ διατέμνειν, καὶ ἁπλῶς πάντα τὰ διὰ τῶν χειρῶν γενόμενα χειρουργία λέγεται. ἐπειδὴ οὖν τὸ πλεῖστον τῶν ἰδιωτῶν χειρουργίαν τὴν διὰ τοῦ σιδήρου τομὴν καὶ μόνην καλοῦσι, τοῦτο ἐκφυγὼν ὁ Ἱπποκράτης, ἵνα μὴ ἁπλῶς καὶ ὡς ἔτυχεν ὡς ὁμολογούμενον λαμβάνοντες οἱ ἄνθρωποι ἐκτέμνουσι τὴν σταφυλὴν ἢ τὴν κιονίδα, ἔφη πλατικῇ τῇ φωνῇ ἀσφαλὲς διαχειρίζειν. δεῖ γὰρ καὶ ἐπὶ τῆς σταφυλῆς τοῖς προρρηθεῖσι βοηθήμασι χρήσασθαι, καὶ ὅταν κατὰ τὸ κάτω μέρος ἔλθῃ ἡ ὕλη καὶ ἐκεῖσε γένηται ἡ φλεγμονή, τότε δεῖ χρήσασθαι τῇ κατασχάσει καὶ τῇ τομῇ.

III 10 [24: 226,14 A. = II 180,8 L.] Ὅστις δ' ἂν τῶν πυρετῶν μηκύνῃ περιεστηκῶς διακειμένου τἀνθρώπου, μήτε ὀδύνης ἐχούσης μήτε διὰ φλεγμονὴν καὶ τὰ ἑξῆς.

Φησὶν ὅτι, ἐὰν ὁ πυρετὸς ἐπίμονός ἐστι καὶ συνεχὴς ἄνευ ὀδύνης ὑποκειμένης ἐν τῷ βάθει καὶ ἄνευ φλεγμονῆς καὶ ἄνευ τινὸς ἄλλης προφάσεως, τότε γίνωσκε ὅτι εἰς ἀπόστασιν τρέπεται τὸ νόσημα μετὰ οἰδήματος. ἰστέον δὲ ὅτι πάντες οἱ παλαιοὶ πάντα ὄγκον οἴδημα ἐκάλουν, ἀλλὰ μετὰ προσδιορισμοῦ. προ⟨σ⟩διωρίζοντο γὰρ οὕτως· |
216 οἴδημα μετὰ ζέσεως, ὅπερ ἐδήλουν τὸ ἐρυσίπελας· οἴδημα ἐκάλουν ἐκεῖνον τὸν ὄγκον τὸν εἴκοντα τῇ ἁφῇ καὶ ἀνώδυνον, ὅπερ ἐστὶ τὸ κυρίως οἴδημα· οἴδημα ἐκάλουν καὶ τὸ σκληρὸν καὶ ἀντίτυπον, ὅπερ ἐστὶν ὁ σκίρρος. ἐνταῦθα μέντοι οἴδημα τὴν φλεγμονὴν ἐδήλωσεν ὁ Ἱπποκράτης.

27–28 ἐκάλουν] *cf. supra*, pp. 126,19; 184,21 sq.

3 τοῖς^III *om.* MP 4 κικὶς L: κικίδες MP: *correxi* 5 στυπτικὴ MP 7 *post* ἀσφαλὲς *add.* δὲ MP 9 *post* Καλῶς *add.* καὶ MP 12 *post* γὰρ *add.* καὶ MP 13 λέγεται MP διὰ τὸ βρέχειν MP τὸ^II *om.* L 14 γινόμενα MP 16 καλοῦμεν MP 17 λαμβάνουσιν L *fort.* ἐκτέμνωσι *scribendum est* 20 ὅτε MP γενήσεται MP 21 κατασχέσει MP 23 περιεστηκῶς] *cf. supra, p. 64,23; infra, p. 282,5* 24 μήτε διὰ φλεγμονὴν *om.* MP μήτε] *sic nullus test. Hipp.* 27 ὅτι *om.* MP 28 προδιορισμοῦ MP 29 προδιορίζοντο L: προδιορίζοντος MP: *corr. Wk.* 30 ἐκάλουν *om.* MP ἥκοντα MP: εἰκότα L: *corr. Dietz* 31 οἴδημα *semel scr.* MP 33 ἐκάλεσεν MP

as well as intense pains and delirium and spasms and the like, but in such a condition, I mean in *kionis*, the other remedies should be used, namely those which dispel and astringe and concoct, such as Acacia Aegyptica, sour-grape juice, oak-gall, lentil soup, alum schist and very many other remedies which are suitable for the affection.

III 9 At this time it is safe to undertake treatment

(Hippocrates) made a very good and admirable choice of words when he said undertake treatment; for he did this to give a broader meaning and he did not say "it is safe to employ surgery". For surgery, meaning every service done to the sick by means of the hands, is so called from the words "hand" and "active" (*cheir organ*). And cauterizing is called surgery, and so is soaking and poulticing and cutting, and simply all the things done by means of the hands are termed surgery. But since the majority of laymen use the word surgery only of cutting with the knife, Hippocrates avoided this and, in order that people might not take the word simply for granted in the ordinary sense and cut out a *staphylē* or *kionis*, he used the general word and said, it is safe to undertake treatment. For in the case of *staphylē* one should use the aforementioned remedies, and when the matter comes to the bottom part and the inflammation develops there, (only) then should incision and cutting be employed.

III 10 Whenever a fever is prolonged, while the patient is in a salutary state and no pain persists due either to inflammation, etc.

He says that if the fever is lasting and continuous without an underlying pain in the depths and without inflammation or any other cause, then conclude that the disease will turn to abscession with tumor. And note that all the ancients called every swelling a tumor, but with distinctions. For they distinguished as follows: tumor with seething heat, by which they meant erysipelas; tumor they called that swelling that yields to pressure and is painless, which is tumor in the strict sense; tumor they called also the hard and resistant, which is induration. Here, however, by tumor Hippocrates means inflammation.

III 11 [24: 227,2 A. = II 180,13 L.] Μᾶλλον δὲ γίνονται αἱ τοιαῦται ἀποστάσιες καὶ ἐν ἐλάσσονι χρόνῳ τοῖσι νεωτέροισι πέντε καὶ τριήκοντα ἐτέων.

Οὐ τοῦτο λέγει ὁ Ἱπποκράτης, ὅτι ὡς ἐπίπαν ἐπὶ τῶν ἀκμαστικῶν αἱ ἀποστάσεις μάλιστα γίνονται, ἐπὶ δὲ τῶν γερόντων οὐ γίνονται ὅλως ἀποστάσεις· ἀλλὰ λέγει ὅτι μάλιστα καὶ ὡς ἐπίπαν ἐπὶ τῶν ἀκμαζόντων γίνονται αἱ ἀποστάσεις διὰ τὸ πλούσιον τοῦ ἐμφύτου θερμοῦ. γίνονται δὲ καὶ ἐπὶ τῶν γερόντων, ἀλλὰ σπανίως διὰ τὴν ὀλιγότητα τοῦ θερμοῦ.

III 12 [24: 227,8 A. = II 182,4 L.] Καὶ ἐπιλαμβάνῃ πεπλανημένῳ τρόπῳ

Ἀπορία ἐνταῦθα ἀναφύεται, ἥτις ἐν διαφόροις ἀπορεῖται. ἔχει δὲ οὕτως· διὰ τί ἐπὶ μόνου τοῦ τεταρταίου προηγοῦνται πλανῆται, ἐπὶ δὲ τῶν ἄλλων πυρετῶν, τυχὸν τοῦ ἀφημερινοῦ ἢ ἐπὶ τοῦ τριταίου, οὔ; καὶ ἔστι πρώτη λύσις αὕτη, ὅτι διὰ τοῦτο ἐπὶ τῶν τεταρταίων προηγοῦνται πλανῆται, ἐπειδὴ ἐν διαφόροις τίκτεται μορίοις· καὶ ἐν μὲν τούτῳ τῷ μορίῳ ἀπὸ χολῆς ἔχει τὴν γένεσιν, ἐν ἑτέρῳ δὲ ἀπὸ φλέγματος, ἐν ἄλλῳ δὲ ἀπὸ τοῦ τρυγώδους τοῦ αἵματος, καὶ ἐπὶ τούτῳ, ἤγουν ἐπὶ τῆς ἐν ἑκάστῳ μορίῳ φερομένης καὶ ἐκπεμπομένης ὕλης, διάφοροι καὶ αἱ εἰσβολαὶ γίνονται. ὅταν μέντοι τύχωσι τὰ μέτρα τοῦ μελαγχολικοῦ, τότε ὁ τεταρταῖος τύπος ἐπικρατεῖ. καὶ τῷ λόγῳ τούτῳ προηγοῦνται πλανῆται. πιθανὴ δέ ἐστιν ἡ λύσις αὕτη, οὐ μὴν τὸ ἀληθὲς ἔχει. ὅσον γὰρ ἐπὶ τούτῳ, ἐὰν ἐν διαφόροις γεννᾶται ὁ μελαγχολικός, οὐκοῦν διάφοροι καὶ τεταρταῖοι γενήσονται,
217 πλέον δὲ δύο | ἤτοι τὸ πλεῖστον τρεῖς τεταρταῖοι γενήσονται, ἅτινα καὶ σπανίως γίνονται.

Ἕτεροι δὲ ἑτέραν λύσιν λέγουσιν ἀπὸ τῆς γεννήσεως τοῦ μελαγχολικοῦ ὁρμώμενοι, ὅτι οὗτος ὁ χυμὸς ἐκ τοῦ τρυγώδους τοῦ αἵματος γίνεται, καὶ ἐφ' ὅσον ἐν τῷ τέως τρύξ ἐστιν, ἀνάψει ἐφήμερον· γίνεται μελαγχολικὸς καὶ ἐκ τῆς ὑπεροπτηθείσης χολῆς, καὶ ἐφ' ὅσον τὸ τέως ἐστὶ χολή, τριταϊκὸν ποιεῖται τὸν κλόνον καὶ περίψυξιν· γίνεται μελαγχολικὸς καὶ ἀπὸ τοῦ ἀπογεωθέντος φλέγματος, ἀλλ' ἐφ' ὅσον φλέγμα ἐστίν, ἀφημερινὴν ποιήσει τὴν περίψυξιν. ὅταν μέντοι ἀναλάβωσι τὰ μέτρα τοῦ μελαγχολικοῦ, τότε τεταρταϊκὴν ποιοῦνται τὴν περίοδον. καὶ αὕτη δὲ τὸ πιθανὸν ἔχει μόνον. ὅσον γὰρ ἐπὶ τούτῳ ἔχει τις εἰπεῖν ὅτι «Ἴσως γενήσεται τύπος παροξυσμοῦ πρὸ τοῦ τεταρταίου. εἰ μὲν χολή ἐστιν ἡ ἐξυπερωπτημένη, τριταϊκὸν ποιεῖ τὸν παροξυσμὸν καὶ μόνον· εἰ δὲ φλέγμα, ἀφημερινόν. ἀλλὰ νῦν ὁρῶμεν ὅτι οἱ πλανῆται διάφοροι ἢ καὶ πολλοὶ εἰσβάλλουσι καὶ ἀτάκτως

1sq. αἱ τοιαῦται ἀποστάσιες *post* χρόνῳ *hab. Hipp.* 2 νεωτέροις L 3 τριάκοντα L ἐτέων *om.* MP 9 ἐπιλαμβάνειν L: ἐπιλαμβάνηται MP: *sec. Hipp. correxi* 10 *ante* τρόπῳ *add.* τῷ MP 13 τρίτου MP 16 ἑτέροις MP 17 τοῦ^{I} – αἵματος] αἵματος τρυγώδους L; *sed cf. infra, lin. 26; supra, p. 208,24* ἐπὶ^{II}] *fort.* ἀπὸ *scribendum est* 19 τέταρτος MP τόπος L 21 τοῦτο *codd.*: *correxi* 22 *post* οὐκοῦν *add.* εἰ L καὶ *ante* διάφοροι *trsp.* L 23 ἤτοι] εἴτε MP γίνονται MP 25 γενέσεως MP 27 ἐστιν – ἐφήμερον] ἀναφανεῖ ἐφήμερος L 28 ὑπεροπτήσεως τῆς χολῆς MP *ante* χολή *add.* ἡ MP 29 τὸν *om.* L ἀπὸ τοῦ *om.* MP 32 ποιεῖται MP 33 τοῦτο *codd.*: *correxi* ἴσος L 34 ὑπεροπτημένη MP 35 ποιήσεται MP 36 ἢ] εἰπεῖν L

III 11 Such abscesses occur more frequently and in a shorter time in those younger than thirty-five years.

Hippocrates is not saying this, that in general abscesses occur above all in those of prime age, but not at all in the old; rather he means that abscesses occur above all and in general in those of prime age on account of the wealth of innate heat. And they also occur in the old, but rarely, on account of the scarceness of the heat.

III 12 And attacks in an irregular way

A problem arises here which is raised in various works. It is this: why is it that only the quartan is preceded by irregulars, while other fevers, e.g. the quotidian and the tertian, are not? And this is the first solution, that the quartans are preceded by irregulars, since (the irregular) is produced in different parts; in one part it is generated from bile, in another from phlegm, in another from the thick (non-serous) part of the blood, and due to this, that is, due to the matter conveyed to and discharged from each part, the attacks also are different. However, when they achieve the proper proportion of the atrabilious (humor), then the quartan type prevails. And this is the reason why the irregulars precede. Now this solution is plausible, but it is not true. For on that basis (it can be argued) that, if the atrabilious (humor) is created in different parts, then the quartans too will be different, (that is) there will be for the most part two or at most three quartans, which rarely happens.

But others give a different solution basing themselves on the generation of the atrabilious (humor): that this humor comes from the thick part of the blood, and to the extent that it is thick at first, it touches off a quotidian; atrabilious (humor) also comes from overheated bile, and insofar as it is bile at first it produces tertian trembling and shivering; atrabilious (humor) is also produced from coarsened phlegm, and to the extent that it is phlegm it creates quotidian shivering. However, when they receive the proper proportion of the atrabilious (humor), then they produce the quartan period. And this solution has only plausibility. For on this basis one can say that "Perhaps a (set) type of paroxysm will occur before the quartan. If the overheated matter is bile, it creates the tertian paroxysm alone, while if it is phlegm, then a quotidian. But, as it is, we see that the irregulars which attack are

καὶ ἀλληνάλλως ὑπαντῶσιν οἱ παροξυσμοὶ ἐπὶ τῶν πλανήτων.» Διὸ λέγουσιν ἑτέραν λύσιν, ἥντινα δέον ἐστὶ πειθαρχῆσαι, ἀπὸ τῆς συστάσεως τοῦ χυμοῦ λαμβάνοντες τὴν λύσιν. φησὶ γὰρ ὅτι, ἐφ' ὅσον λεπτότερός ἐστιν ὁ μελαγχολικὸς χυμός, θερμότερος τέως ἐστὶ καὶ τὰ τῆς χολῆς ποιεῖ· καὶ ἑτοίμως διὰ τὴν λέπτυνσιν διεξέρχεται τὸ βάθος καὶ φέρεται ἐπὶ τὰ αἰσθητικὰ νεῦρα καὶ ποιεῖ τὸν κλόνον καὶ τὴν τριταϊκὴν περίψυξιν. ἐφ' ὅσον δὲ παχύς ἐστι, ψυχρὰς αὔρας πέμπει ἐπὶ τὰ αἰσθητικὰ νεῦρα καὶ περὶ τὴν ἐπιφάνειαν καὶ ποιεῖ περίψυξιν ἀφημερινήν. οὕτως γίνονται οἱ πλανῆται καὶ προηγοῦνται τῷ τεταρταίῳ. ὅταν μέντοι εἰδοποιηθῇ καὶ ἀποτελεσθῇ ὁ κυρίως μελαγχολικός, τότε λοιπὸν τεταρταϊκῶς παροξύνει· ὅθεν ἀμέλει τινὲς καὶ τέσσαρας μῆνας ἐτεταρτάϊσαν, ἕτεροι δὲ καὶ ἑπτὰ καὶ ἐννέα, ἄλλοι δὲ καὶ ἐνιαυτὸν καὶ δύο ἔτη, τινὲς δὲ καὶ ἐκινδύνευσαν. |

IV

218 **III 13** [24: 227,14 A. = II 182,9 L.] Ὅστις δ' ἂν ἐν πυρετῷ μὴ θανατώδει φῇ τὴν κεφαλὴν ἀλγέειν ἢ καὶ ὀρφνῶδές τι πρὸ τῶν ὀφθαλμῶν φαίνεσθαι καὶ τὰ ἑξῆς.

Ἰστέον ὅτι καὶ νῦν περὶ τῶν ὀξέων νοσημάτων διαλέγεται, σημειούμενος αὐτά, εἴτε δι' ἐμέτων εἴτε δι' αἱμορραγίας μέλλει γίνεσθαι ἡ κατ' ἔκρουν κρίσις. καὶ πρῶτον λέγει κοινὰ σημεῖα ἀμφοτέρων τῶν κενώσεων, ὅτι κοινῶς ἐπ' ἀμφοτέρων κεφαλαλγίαι γίνονται αὐτοῖς καὶ δυσφορία καὶ τάραχος τῶν ὀφθαλμῶν. λέγει δὲ καὶ ἴδια σημεῖα ἑκάστου. καὶ πρῶτον τῆς δι' ἐμέτων γινομένης κενώσεως λέγει, ὅτι ἐπὶ τῶν δι' ἐμέτων μελλόντων κενοῦσθαι κριτικῶς σὺν τοῖς ῥηθεῖσι σημείοις καὶ ὀρφνώδη τινὰ ὁρῶσι πρὸ τῶν ὀφθαλμῶν. ἐπὶ γὰρ τῶν ἐμέτων χολή ἐστι πάντως ἡ ἔχουσα ἐμεθῆναι, ἐπειδὴ ὀξὺ ὑπεθέμεθα νόσημα· ἐν οὖν τῇ τοιαύτῃ κινήσει φέρεταί τι μέρος τῆς τοιαύτης χολώδους ὕλης περὶ τὸν ἐγκέφαλον· ὁ οὖν ἐγκέφαλος δεχόμενος τὴν τοιαύτην χολώδη ὕλην δι' οἰκείαν ἰσχὺν καὶ ῥώμην δυνάμεως ἀποδιώκει αὐτὴν εἰς τὰ παρακείμενα μόρια, καὶ λοιπὸν μέρος τι τῆς ὕλης πέμπεται ἐπὶ τοὺς ὀφθαλμοὺς διὰ τοῦ ὀπτικοῦ νεύρου μολῦνον τὸ ὀπτικὸν πνεῦμα, καὶ τὸ τηνικαῦτα ὀρφνώδη ὁρῶσι πρὸ τῶν ὀφθαλμῶν. ὀρφνώδη δέ εἰσι τὰ μέλανα ὁρώμενα κατὰ φαντασίαν.

Καὶ μὴ ἀπορήσῃς ὅτι «Πῶς ἐπὶ τῇ ξανθῇ χολῇ ὀρφνώδη τινὰ μελάσματα ὁρῶσιν· ὤφειλον γὰρ ξανθὰ ὁρᾶν· ἡ γὰρ χολὴ ξανθή ἐστι· πῶς οὖν μέλανά τινα ὁρῶσιν;» οὐδὲ γὰρ ἀπορεῖ τις ἐπὶ τοῦ πυρὸς ὅτι πῶς τοῦ πυρὸς ἐρυθροῦ ὄντος μέλας ἐστὶν ὁ ἐξ αὐτοῦ γινόμενος καπνός. τί γάρ; ὅτι ἐκ τοῦ ξηρότερον εἶναι τὸ περίττωμα καὶ γεωδέστερον τὸν καπνὸν τοῦ πυρός, διὰ τοῦτο μέλας φαίνεται.

Γίνεται δὲ αὐτοῖς καὶ καρδιωγμὸς τρόπῳ τοιούτῳ· φερομένη ἡ χο-

1 πλανήτων] πλειόνων MP   2 ἕτεραν M: ἕτεροι P   3 *fort.* φασὶ *scribendum est*   4 χυμός *om.* MP   6 sq. καὶ^{I} – νεῦρα *om.* MP   8 ἀφημερινήν] ἄμφω MP   11 καὶ^{II} *om.* MP   12 ἐκινδύνευσαν] *an* ἐπέκεινα *scribendum est?*   20 δυσφορίαι MP   22 γινομένης *om.* L   ἐπὶ *om.* MP   23 κενοῦσθαι *om.* L   24 τῶ ἐμέτω L   25 ὀξὺν ὑποθέμενος (ὑπερθ. P) νόσον MP   26 χολώδους τοιαύτης L   27 αὐτήν] τὴν ὕλην L   36 εἶναι *post* περίττωμα *trsp.* MP   πυρός] ξηρὸς L

many and different and the paroxysms in irregulars occur without order or sequence."

For this reason another solution is given, which must be accepted; it is based on the composition of the humor. And it argues that, insofar as the atrabilious humor is fairly thin, it is on the warm side at first and produces bile; and on account of the thinness it readily passes through the deep interior, travels to the sensory nerves and produces trembling and tertian shivering. But insofar as it is thick, it sends cold vapors to the sensory nerves and around the surface and produces quotidian shivering. In this way the irregulars arise and precede the quartan. However, when the atrabilious (humor) proper is formed and fully shaped, then finally the fever has quartan paroxysms; this is why, for example, some people have had quartans for four months, and others for seven and nine, others for a year and two years, and some have been in danger (of death).

IV

III 13 Whenever someone in a fever that is not fatal says that his head aches or that a darkness appears before his eyes, etc.

Note that he is still on the subject of acute diseases, giving the signs for them (that tell) whether the crisis by discharge will take place through vomits or through haemorrhage. And first he gives signs common to both evacuations, (saying) that common to both in these cases are headaches, malaise and disturbance of the eyes. And he gives also the signs peculiar to each. First he gives those for the evacuation through vomits, that in those who are going to have a critical evacuation through vomits, along with the signs mentioned they see also certain dark things before the eyes. For in the case of vomits bile is always the matter which has to be brought up, since we are supposing the disease to be acute; in such a movement, then, a part of that bilious matter is conveyed around the brain; the brain, then, having admitted that bilious matter, by its own vigor and strength of power expels it to the surrounding parts, and finally a portion of the matter is transmitted to the eyes through the optic nerve, corrupting the optic pneuma, and so they see dark things before the eyes. Dark things are the black spots seen by imagination.

And do not raise the problem that "How is it that with yellow bile they see dark black spots; for they ought to see yellow things, the bile being yellow; how, then, do they see black?" For nobody asks in the case of fire how, the fire being red, the smoke coming from it is black. Why? Because the residue, the smoke, is drier and more earthy than the fire, and this is why it appears black.

They also develop heartburn, in the following way: when the bilious

λώδης ὕλη περὶ τὸν στόμαχον δάκνει αὐτόν, καὶ γίνεται ὀδύνη. οὐδὲν γάρ ἐστι καρδιαλγία ἢ δῆξις καὶ ἀνία καὶ ὀδύνη περὶ τὸν στόμαχον· καρδίαν γὰρ οἱ παλαιοὶ τὸν στόμαχον ἐκάλουν. οὐδέποτε γὰρ χολὴ ἀπὸ καρδίας
219 ἐμεῖται, ἀλλ' ἀπὸ τοῦ στομάχου καὶ | τῆς γαστρός. ἐπεὶ δὲ ἐν τῷ στομάχῳ ἀθροιζομένη ἡ χολὴ δῆξιν καὶ ἀνίαν καὶ περίτασιν ἀπεργάζεται, τὸ τηνικαῦτα τῇ δήξει καὶ τῇ ἀνίᾳ γίνεται αὐτοῖς συστολὴ καὶ περίψυξις τῶν ἄκρων μορίων καὶ ῥῖγος· ἐπὶ δὲ τῇ δήξει καὶ τῇ τάσει καὶ τῇ ἀνίᾳ συστέλλει ἡ φύσις ἑαυτὴν καὶ συννεύει ἐπὶ τὸ βάθος· καὶ τὸ τηνικαῦτα τῆς ἀπὸ τῆς φύσεως ἐλλάμψεως καὶ τοῦ ἐμφύτου θερμοῦ στερηθέντα περιψύχονται καὶ ῥιγῶσιν. ἀλλὰ καὶ τὰ ὑποχόνδρια αὐτῶν ἀνασπᾶσθαι δοκοῦσι καὶ ψυχρότερά εἰσιν ἐπὶ τῶν τοιούτων, τὰ δὲ ἄνω μέρη θερμότερα, ἐπειδὴ ἡ χολώδης ὕλη ἐπὶ τὰ ἄνω μόρια φερομένη, δῆλον καὶ ἡ φύσις μετὰ τῶν οἰκείων ὀχημάτων, αἵματος λέγω καὶ πνεύματος, ἐκεῖσε ὥρμηται. καὶ διὰ τοῦτο ὅσον ἐστέρηνται τῆς ἀπὸ τῆς φύσεως ἐπικουρίας, τὰ ὑποχόνδρια ψυχρότερά εἰσι, τὰ δὲ ἄνω ὡς ἐν ἀπολαύσει αὐτῆς τυγχάνοντα, λοιπὸν δὲ καὶ ἡ χολώδης ὕλη ἐκεῖσε ἤθροισται, διὰ τοῦτο θερμότερά εἰσι.

Πολλάκις δὲ αὐτὴ ἡ χολὴ παχυτέρα ἐστὶν καὶ διὰ τὴν παχύτητα οὐκ ἐμεῖται. τότε καὶ εὔκρατον παρέχομεν, ὥστε ἐμεθῆναι αὐτήν. τὸ γὰρ εὔκρατον κατακερματίζει αὐτὴν καὶ σύγχυσιν ἐν αὐτῇ ποιεῖται καὶ ἐπιπολάζειν αὐτὴν ἀπεργάζεται, καὶ οὕτως ἀπεμεῖται ἡ χολή. οὕτως γὰρ καὶ ἐπὶ τῶν ἔξω ἐπιτηδεύομεν ἐπὶ τῆς ἰλύος· ἡνίκα ἀγγεῖον βουλόμεθα καθᾶραι ἔχον τρυγίαν ἢ σωλῆνας ἔχοντας ἰλύν, ἐπιβάλλομεν ὕδωρ καὶ ἀνατινάσσομεν, καὶ συναναμίγνυται ἡ ἰλὺς τῷ ὕδατι, ὁμοίως καὶ ἡ τρύξ, καὶ οὕτως καθαίρομεν τὰ ἀγγεῖα καὶ τοὺς σωλῆνας. οὕτως οὖν καὶ ἐπὶ τῆς παχυτέρας χολῆς γίνεται· παρέχομεν τὸ εὔκρατον, καὶ ποιεῖ τὴν χύσιν καὶ λεπτύνει αὐτὴν καὶ εὔρουν ἀπεργάζεται, καὶ ὑπερπολάζουσα ἐμεῖται, καὶ παύονται τὰ συμπτώματα.

Καὶ ταῦτα μέν, ἐὰν ἔρρωται ἡ δύναμις. εἰ δὲ ἀσθενής ἐστιν ἡ δύναμις καὶ διὰ τὴν ἀσθένειαν μὴ ἐμῆται ἡ χολή, καὶ τροφὰς παρέχομεν, οὐ τὰς βαρυνούσας δέ, ἀλλὰ τὰς φαρμακώδεις, οἷον τυχὸν χυλὸν πτισάνης καὶ |
220 μελίκρατον καὶ οἶνον κεκραμένον· αἱ γὰρ τοιαῦται τροφαὶ ἔχουσι καὶ τὸ τρέφον καὶ τὰ φαρμάκου ποιεῖν. ἡ γὰρ πτισάνη καὶ τρέφει, ἀλλὰ καὶ ῥυπτική ἐστι. τὸ δὲ μελίκρατον καὶ αὐτὸ ἔχει τι καὶ τρόφιμον, ἀλλὰ καὶ τμητικὸν καὶ λεπτυντικόν. ὁ δὲ οἶνος καὶ τρέφει καὶ τονεῖ καὶ στύφει. καὶ διὰ τῶν τοιούτων

2 sq.] *cf.* Gal. In Hipp. Progn. comm. III 35: CMG V 9,2 p. 360,16sq. De plac. Hipp. et Plat. II 8,8: CMG V 4,1,2 p. 158,20sq. De sanit. tuenda VI 14,1: CMG V 4,2 p. 194,28–30

2 sq. καρδίαν – στόμαχον *om.* MP 8 *post* τηνικαῦτα *add.* χηρεύοντες MP τῆς *om.* MP 9 φύσεως] φυσικῆς *codd.*: *corr. Wk.* στερηθέντες MP 10 ἀλλὰ – δοκοῦσι *om.* MP 11 ψυχρότεροί P: *ambig.* M 12 ὕλη *om.* MP 13 πνεύματος] φλέγματος MP 14 φύσεως] φυσικῆς *codd.*: *corr. Wk.* 14 sq. ψυχρότερά εἰσι *om.* MP 15 ὡς *om.* L 17 δὲ] δὲ καὶ M: καὶ P 17 sq. καὶ – ἐμεῖται] ὥστε ἐμεθῆναι ἀδύνατον L 22 τρυγίας MP ἰλύν] ὑλὴν M: ὕλην LP: *corr. Dietz* 23 ἰλὺς *coni. Wk.*: ὕλη *codd.* 25 ποιεῖται MP φύσιν L 27 τὰ *om.* MP 28 sq. ἡ δύναμις καὶ *om.* MP 29 ἐμεῖται MP 30 δέ *om.* MP οἷον *om.* MP 32 *ante* τὰ *intelligendum* τὸ *monet Wk.* ῥιπτική L 34 τονοῖ *coni. Dietz*

matter is conveyed around the orifice of the stomach it stings it and pain occurs. For heartburn is nothing but stinging and irritation and pain around the orifice of the stomach; for the ancients used to call the orifice of the stomach heart (*kardia*). And bile is never vomited from the heart, but from the orifice of the stomach and the stomach (itself). Since the bile collected at the orifice of the stomach produces stinging and irritation and contraction, then because of the stinging and irritation there develops in them systole and chilling of the extreme parts and shivering; and with the stinging, tension and irritation nature contracts itself and converges on the deep interior; and in that event (the extremities), deprived of nature's radiation and the innate heat, become chilled and shiver. And their hypochondria seem to retract and they are colder in these cases, while the upper parts are warmer, since, the bilious matter being conveyed to the upper parts, it is clear that nature has rushed there along with its own vehicles, namely blood and pneuma. And for this reason, to the extent that they have been deprived of nature's help, the hypochondria are colder, while the upper parts, because they are enjoying nature's company and because the bilious matter has collected there, are warmer on this account.

Frequently the bile itself is on the thick side and due to the thickness it is not vomited. Then we give a lukewarm drink in order to have it vomited. For the lukewarm drink breaks it up, creates a mixture with it and makes it come to the surface and in this way the bile is vomited. And we employ the same means in the external world in the case of dirt; when we want to clean a vessel with sediment or pipes with mud, we throw water in them and shake; the mud is mixed up with the water, and the sediment likewise, and it is in this way that we clean vessels and pipes. In the case of fairly thick bile, then, the same thing happens; we give the lukewarm drink, it creates the mixture, refines the bile and makes it run easily; then, flowing upwards, it is vomited and the symptoms stop.

And this happens, if the power is strong. But if the power is weak and the bile is not vomited because of the weakness, then we administer nutriments, not the heavy ones, however, but the medicinal, such as water of barley gruel and hydromel and wine-mix; for nutriments such as these are able to act as both nourishment and drugs. For barley gruel nourishes and is also able to purge. Hydromel, too, has some nourishment and the power to dissolve and refine as well. Wine nourishes and strengthens and acts as an astringent. And the power becomes strong by means

τροφῶν ῥωννυμένη ἡ δύναμις ἐπιγίνεται καὶ ἀπεμεῖ τὴν χολώδη ὕλην, καὶ παύεται ἡ καρδιαλγία.

Ἔστι καὶ ἕτερον σημεῖον κατὰ τὸν Γαληνὸν ἐπὶ τῶν ἐμεῖν μελλόντων, τὸ κραδαίνεσθαι ἐπὶ τῶν τοιούτων τὸ κάτω χεῖλος, διὰ τὸν ὑμένα τὸν ὑπαλείφοντα ἀπὸ τοῦ στομάχου καὶ μέχρι τοῦ κάτω χείλους φέρεσθαι· τοῦ γὰρ στομάχου δακνομένου καὶ ἀνιωμένου δῆλον καὶ ὁ ὑμὴν οὗτος διὰ τὴν κοινωνίαν ἐξ ἀνάγκης κραδαίνεται ἐπὶ τῶν μελλόντων ἐμεῖν τὸ κάτω χεῖλος.

Τούτων δὲ οὕτως ἐχόντων παραδίδωσιν ἡμῖν καὶ τὰ σημεῖα τῆς δι' αἱμορραγίας γινομένης κριτικῶς κενώσεως. καί φησιν ὅτι σὺν τῇ κεφαλαλγίᾳ καὶ τῇ ταραχῇ καὶ συστροφῇ τῶν ὀφθαλμῶν, ἐπειδὴ ταῦτα κοινὰ ὑπῆρχον σημεῖα ἀμφοτέρων τῶν κενώσεων, ἐὰν μηκέτι ὁρῶσιν ὀρφνώδη [καὶ] τινὰ μελάσματα πρὸ τῶν ὀφθαλμῶν, ἀλλὰ μαρμαρυγάς τινας καὶ πυραυγῆ φαντάσματα ὁρῶσι, τότε γίνωσκε ὅτι δι' αἱμορραγίας γίνεται ἡ κένωσις. εἰ μὲν γὰρ λεπτοτάτη τις καὶ ἀτμώδης ποιότης τῆς ὕλης ἐνεχθῇ ἐπὶ τὰ ὀπτικὰ νεῦρα, τότε τὰ πυραυγῆ καὶ τὰς μαρμαρυγὰς καὶ τὰ μελάσματα ὁρῶσιν. εἰ δὲ ἐνεχθῇ παχυτέρα ὕλη ἐπὶ τοὺς ὀφθαλμούς, ἐναπολαμβάνει τοὺς πόρους τῶν ὀπτικῶν νεύρων, καὶ τότε οὐ δύναται διεξελθεῖν τὸ ὁρατικὸν πνεῦμα, καὶ παντελῆ ποιεῖται ἀορασίαν. εἰ δέ γε πρὸς τούτῳ κνῶνται τὸ ἄκρον τῆς ῥινός, ἔστι δὲ καὶ ἐρυθρὰ τὰ μῆλα τοῦ προσώπου, γίνωσκε ὅτι δι' αἱμορραγίας γίνεται ἡ κένωσις.

221 Ἐπὶ τούτων καὶ τὰ ὑποχόν|δρια ἀνασπῶνται. καὶ τοῦτο δὲ κοινὸν ὑπῆρχεν· ὁ μέντοι Ἱπποκράτης ὡς ἰδικὸν τέθεικεν αὐτὸ ἐπὶ τῶν αἱμορραγεῖν μελλόντων. ἁπλῶς οὖν καὶ ἐπὶ τούτων ἀνασπᾶται τὰ ὑποχόνδρια, τυχὸν ἄνευ ὀδύνης καὶ φλεγμονῆς. ἐὰν γὰρ ἁπτομένου σου τὰ ὑποχόνδρια ὦσι μαλθακὰ καὶ ὁμαλὰ καὶ μήτε ὀδύνη σύνεστι μήτε φλεγμονή, ἀλλ' ἀνασπῶνται, ἔσο γινώσκων δι' αἱμορραγίας γίνεσθαι τὴν κένωσιν.

Ἐκ τοῦ διανασπᾶσθαι τὰ ὑποχόνδρια καὶ τὸν τόπον ἤγουν διὰ ποίας ῥινὸς προγινώσκει ὁ Ἱπποκράτης τὴν αἱμορραγίαν γίνεσθαι. καί φησιν ὅτι, ἐὰν τὸ δεξιὸν ὑποχόνδριον ἀνασπᾶται, γίνωσκε ὅτι ἐκ τοῦ δεξιοῦ μέλλει γενέσθαι μέρους ἡ αἱμορραγία· εἰ δὲ τὸ ἀριστερόν, ἐκ τοῦ ἀριστεροῦ· εἰ δὲ τὰ ἀμφότερα ὑποχόνδρια ἀνασπῶνται, ἐξ ἀμφοτέρων τῶν ῥινῶν ἡ αἱμορραγία γίνεται. ἡ γὰρ φύσις, ἔστ' ἂν ἔρρωται καὶ ταῖς οἰκείαις δυνάμεσι κατὰ τὸν οἰκεῖον σκοπὸν κέχρηται, κατ' εὐθυωρίαν καὶ κατ' εὐθὺ τὰς ὕλας πέμπει

3 κατὰ τὸν Γαληνὸν] Gal. In Hipp. Progn. comm. III 35: CMG V 9,2 p. 361,1–10 10 φησιν] Hipp. Progn. 24: p. 229,1–6 A. = II pp. 184,12–186,3 L. 29 φησιν] Hipp. Progn. 24: p. 229,3sq. A. = II pp. 184,15–186,1 L.

1 ἐπιγίνεται] *fort.* ἐπεγείρεται *scribendum est; cf. infra, p. 276,28* 4 κραδάνεσθαι M: κραδάνασθαι P 6 ὁ ὑμὴν] οὐ μὴν L 7 κραδαίνεσθαι L ἐμεῖν μελλόντων MP 9 τὰ *om.* MP 11 καὶ τῇ ταραχῇ *om.* MP καὶ συστροφῇ] ἡ συστροφὴ MP 12 καὶ *seclusi; cf. supra, p. 270,32* 13 τινας] τινὰ L 14 κένωσις] κεφαλαλγία MP 18 καὶ *om.* MP ἐξελθεῖν MP 19 ποιεῖ MP πρὸ MP τοῦτο LP: τούτου M: *correxi* 19 sq. τὰ ἄκρονα M: *corr.* P; *cf. infra, p. 282,10*: *om.* L 21 κένωσις] κεφαλαλγία MP 23 *post* αὐτὸ *add.* καὶ MP 25 *post* ὑποχόνδρια *iter.* τυχὸν – φλεγμονῆς MP 26 ὁμαλὰ καὶ μαλθακὰ MP μήτε φλεγμονή *om.* MP 27 κένωσιν] κεφαλαλγίαν MP 31 γίνεσθαι MP

of such nutriments and vomits the bilious matter and the heartburn stops.

According to Galen there is also another sign for those who are going to vomit: the lower lip vibrates in these cases, on account of the lining membrane which goes from the orifice of the stomach as far as the lower lip; for when the stomach orifice is stung and irritated, it is obvious that this membrane, due to the communication, necessarily vibrates the lower lip of those who are going to vomit.

After this he gives us also the signs for the critical evacuation through haemorrhage. He says that if, along with the headache and the disturbance and contortion of the eyes – these being signs which are common to both evacuations –, they no longer see dark black spots before the eyes, but "stars" and flashing visions, then you will know that the evacuation will take place through haemorrhage. For if a very thin and rarefied quality of the matter is introduced to the optic nerves, they then see the flashes and the "stars" and the black spots. But if fairly thick matter is introduced to the eyes, it blocks the passages of the optic nerves, and then the optic pneuma is not able to pass through, and it causes complete loss of vision. And if in addition to this they scratch the tip of the nose, and the cheeks of the face are red, conclude that the evacuation will take place through haemorrhage.

In these cases the hypochondria are retracted as well. And this is common (to both), though Hippocrates makes it peculiar to those who are going to haemorrhage. In these cases, then, the hypochondria are retracted simply, that is, without pain and inflammation. For if, when you touch the hypochondria, they are soft and even and there is no pain present nor inflammation, but they are retracted, you will know that the evacuation will occur by haemorrhage.

From the retraction of the hypochondria Hippocrates prognoses also the place, that is, the nostril through which the haemorrhage will occur. And he says that if the right hypochondrium is retracted, conclude that the haemorrhage is going to occur from the right (nostril); and if the left, from the left; and if both hypochondria are retracted, the haemorrhage will be from both nostrils. For as long as nature is strong and uses its own faculties for its proper objective, it sends and expels the matters directly and straight, in the same way that an expert archer

καὶ ἀποδιώκει, ὥσπερ καὶ ἄριστος τοξότης κατ' εὐθὺ τοῦ σκοποῦ πέμπει τὸ βέλος καὶ μὴ δι' ἀφυΐαν τῆδε κἀκεῖσε περιάγεται.

III 14 [24: 228,1 A. = II 182,11 L.] Ἦν δὲ καὶ καρδιωγμὸς τουτέῳ προσγένηται, χολώδης ἔμετος παρέσται.

Ἐπειδὴ παράκειται ἡ καλουμένη ἀορτὴ τῷ στομάχῳ, μεταλαμβάνει τῆς δήξεως τῆς περὶ τὸν στόμαχον ἀθροιζομένης χολῆς. ἔστι δ' ὅτε ἀναγγέλλεται καὶ αὐτῇ τῇ καρδίᾳ, καὶ διὰ τοῦτο καρδίαν τὸν στόμαχον ὀνομάζουσιν ἐκ τοῦ μεταδίδοσθαι ἐκ τοῦ σύνεγγυς τὴν δῆξιν τῇ καρδίᾳ.

III 15 [24: 228,2 A. = II 182,13 L.] Ἦν δὲ καὶ ῥῖγος ἐπιλάβῃ καὶ τὰ κάτω τοῦ ὑποχονδρίου ψυχρὰ ᾖ καὶ τὰ ἑξῆς.

Ἰστέον ὅτι ἔστι ῥῖγος τὸ λόγῳ κρίσεως γινόμενον, ὅπερ αὐτὸς ἐν Ἀφορισμοῖς εἶπεν· «Ὑπὸ καύσου ἐχομένῳ ῥίγεος ἐπιγενομένου λύσις.» ἔστι ῥῖγος καὶ τὸ προηγούμενον τοῦ πυρετοῦ ὡς ἐν τριταίοις. ἔστι καὶ ῥῖγος
222 τὸ παρεμπῖπτον, τὸ | λόγῳ συμπτώματος γινόμενον. ἐνταῦθα δὲ ῥῖγος λέγει τὸ ἐπὶ τῇ δήξει τοῦ στομάχου γινόμενον· ἐπὶ γὰρ τῇ ἀθροίσει τῆς χολῆς ἐπὶ τὸν στόμαχον δάκνεται καὶ ἀνιᾶται, καὶ μεταλαμβάνει τῆς δήξεως ἡ ἀορτὴ καλουμένη ἀρτηρία, καὶ συστέλλεται τὸ ἔμφυτον θερμὸν καὶ συννεύει ὡς ἐπὶ τὴν οἰκείαν ἀρχὴν ἐπὶ τὸ βάθος, καὶ ἀμοιροῦντα τὰ ἐπιπολῆς μόρια τῆς ἐλλάμψεως τοῦ ἐμφύτου θερμοῦ περιψύχονται, καὶ γίνεται τὸ ῥῖγος.

III 16 [24: 228,3 A. = II 182,15 L.] Ἦν δέ τι καὶ πίῃ ἢ φάγῃ ὑπὸ τοῦτον τὸν χρόνον, κάρτα ταχέως ἐμέεται.

Παρακελεύεται οὖν ἡμῖν ἀναμιμνήσκεσθαι τῶν συμβεβηκότων, ὡς πολλάκις τὰ γινόμενα ὠφελήσαντα. τί γάρ; ὅτι οὐκ ἐμεῖται ἡ χολὴ ἢ διὰ πάχος ἢ δι' ἀσθένειαν τῆς δυνάμεως. καὶ δεῖ καί σε μιμεῖσθαι τοῖς πράγμασι καὶ χρήσασθαι, εἰ μὲν παχεῖά ἐστιν ἡ ὕλη καὶ διὰ τοῦτο οὐκ ἐμεῖται, τῷ εὐκράτῳ. εἰ δὲ ἀσθενής ἐστιν ἡ δύναμις, δεῖ σε καὶ τροφαῖς χρήσασθαι, ἔστι δ' ὅτε καὶ στερεωτέραις τροφαῖς χρήσασθαι, οἷά ἐστι μῆλα καὶ σταφυλαὶ καὶ σταφίδες καὶ ῥόοκοκκα. καὶ γὰρ ῥωννυμένη ἡ δύναμις ἐπεγείρεται καὶ ἀποδιώκει καὶ ἀπεμεῖ τὴν χολώδη ὕλην.

11–19] *cf.* Steph. Comm. in Hipp. Aph.: Escor. Σ. II. 10 fol. 89r–89v 11–14] *cf.* Ioann. Comm. in Hipp. De morb. pop. VI: 121d45–47 Pritchet Pall. Comm. in Hipp. De morb. pop. VI: II p. 22,11–17 Dietz 11sq. ἐν Ἀφορισμοῖς] Hipp. Aph. IV 58: IV p. 522,14 L.

1 τοῦ] σοῦ, *ut vid.*, L πέμπει *om.* L 3 δὲ *non hab. Hipp.* διωγμὸς MP 4 πάρεστιν MP 7 ὀνομάζομεν MP 8 *ante* ἐκ^II *add.* καὶ MP τῆς καρδίας L 9 ἐπιλάβοι MP 10 *post* κάτω *add.* μέρη MP ψυχρὰ ᾖ *om.* MP 11 ὅτι *om.* L τῶ LM: *corr.* P αὐτὸ L 14 τὸ^II] τῶ MP 18 ὡς *om.* MP ἀμοιροῦνται τὰ L: ἀμοιροῦντά M: ἀμοιροῦντ *(ambig.)* P: *correxi* 20 καὶ *om.* MP 21 κάρτα *om.* MP ταχείης L ἐμεῖται L 23 τὰ] αὐτὰ MP *post* ἐμεῖται *add.* καὶ L 24 δι' ἀσθένειαν] διὰ θέσεως P: διαθέσεως M πράγμασι] προσάρμασι *coni. Wk.* 25 χρήσεσθαι L ὕλη] χολὴ MP 26 εἰ] ἡ L τροφαῖς] εὐτροφῇ L 26sq. ἔστι – χρήσασθαι *om.* MP 29 ἐκδιώκει P: διώκει M

sends the arrow straight on target and it does not go a roundabout way due to a lack of natural ability (in him).

III 14 And if heartburn also develops in him, a bilious vomit is near.

Since the so-called aorta is situated near the orifice of the stomach, it contracts some of the stinging of the bile collected around the orifice of the stomach. And sometimes it is communicated even to the heart itself, and this is why they call the orifice of the stomach heart (*kardia*), because, being adjacent, it passes on the stinging to the heart.

III 15 And if a shivering as well supervenes and the parts below the hypochondrium are cold, etc.

Note that there is the shivering which takes the form of a crisis, which he himself mentioned in the Aphorisms, "In a case of causus a supervening shivering brings a cure." There is also the shivering which precedes fever, as in tertians. There is the intercident shivering as well, which takes the form of a symptom. But here by shivering he means the one which results from stinging of the stomach orifice; for the collection of bile at the orifice of the stomach stings and irritates it, and the artery known as the aorta contracts the sting, and the innate heat gathers itself together and converges on its own source in the deep interior, and the surface parts, having no share of the innate heat's radiation, become chilled and shivering develops.

III 16 And if he drinks or eats something around this time, he will vomit very quickly.

He is advising us, then, to recall the side-effects, since oftentimes what has happened (to the patient) is useful. Why? Because (if) the bile is not vomited, it is due to either thickness or weakness of the power. And you must follow exactly the circumstances and use lukewarm drink, if the matter is thick and is not vomited for this reason. But if the power is weak, you must use nutriments too, and sometimes you have to use fairly solid foods, such as apples, grapes, raisins and pomegranate seeds. For once the power has been strengthened, it is aroused and expels and vomits off the bilious matter.

III 17 [24: 228,5 A. = II 184,1 L.] Τουτέων δὲ οἷσι μὲν ἂν ὁ πόνος ἄρξηται τῇ πρώτῃ ἡμέρᾳ, τεταρταῖοι μάλιστα πιεζοῦνται καὶ πεμπταῖοι, ἐς δὲ τὴν ἑβδόμην ἀπαλλάσσονται.

Ἐνταῦθα ὁ Ἱπποκράτης πόνον τὴν κεφαλαλγίαν ἐκάλεσεν εἰπὼν ἣν ἄρξηται πονέειν, τυχὸν πονεῖν τὴν κεφαλήν. κεφαλαλγίαν δὲ ὑποτίθεται οὐ μὴν λόγῳ κρίσεως γινομένην – αὕτη γὰρ τὸ μέγιστον μίαν ἡμέραν ἐπικρατεῖ, ὡς αὐτός φησιν ὅτι «Ὁκόσοισι κρίσις γίνεται, τουτέοισιν ἡ νὺξ δύσφορος ἡ πρὸ τοῦ παροξυσμοῦ» –, ἀλλὰ κεφαλαλγίαν ὑποτίθεται τὴν λόγῳ συμπτώματος γινομένην, ἥτις ἕως τῆς ἑβδόμης παρεκτείνεται. τὸ δὲ
223 ἀληθὲς εἰπεῖν, ὅτι καὶ τῇ λόγῳ κρίσεως ἁρμόζει κεφα|λαλγίᾳ καὶ τῇ λόγῳ συμπτώματος. καὶ γὰρ λόγῳ συμπτώματός ἐστιν ἡ τοιαύτη κεφαλαλγία, ἐπειδὴ ἐξ ἀρχῆς ἀπὸ τῆς πρώτης ἡμέρας λέγει γίνεσθαι τὴν κεφαλαλγίαν, καὶ μάλιστα, ἐὰν ἐξ ἀρχῆς γενομένη ἐν τῇ τρίτῃ παύσηται, τότε καὶ λόγῳ συμπτώματός ἐστιν. ἀλλὰ ἐπέχει ἡ τοιαύτη κεφαλαλγία, ἐπειδὴ μέχρι τῆς κρίσεως συνεκτείνεται καὶ οὕτως ἀπαλλάσσονται. ὅτι δὲ μέχρι τῆς ἑβδόμης λέγει παρεκτείνεσθαι τὴν τοιαύτην κεφαλαλγίαν, αὐτὸς ἐπὶ λέξεώς φησιν ὅτι ὁκόσοισιν ἄρξηται ἡ κεφαλαλγία τῇ πρώτῃ ἡμέρᾳ, τεταρταῖοι πιεζοῦνται, ἐς δὲ τὴν ἑβδόμην ἀπαλλάσσονται, ἤγουν αὔξεται αὐτῶν ἡ κεφαλαλγία ἀπὸ τῆς πρώτης ἡμέρας, καὶ γίνεται προσθήκη ἕως τῆς τετάρτης, καὶ πιεζοῦνται καὶ κρατοῦνται καὶ οὐκέτι ἀναβιβασμὸν δέχονται, ἀλλὰ στάσις γίνεται καὶ ἀκμὴ μέχρι τῆς ἑβδόμης, καὶ οὕτως ἐν τῇ ἑβδόμῃ ἡμέρᾳ λύεται καὶ παύεται.

Εἶτα ἔφη· ὁκόσοι δὲ τῇ τρίτῃ ἄρξονται πονεῖν τὴν κεφαλὴν πεμπταῖοι πιεζοῦνται καὶ ἀπαλλάσσονται ἢ ἐνναταῖοι ἢ ἑνδεκαταῖοι. ὅθεν τινὲς λέγουσιν ὅτι «Ἀπροσφόρως τοῦτο εἴρηκεν· ἐὰν ἀπὸ τῆς τρίτης ἄρξωνται, τρεῖς καὶ ἑπτά, δέκα· οὐκοῦν ἐν τῇ δεκάτῃ ἔχουσιν ἀπαλλαγῆναι· καὶ πῶς ἔφη· ἢ τῇ θ′ ἢ τῇ ια′ ἀπαλλάσσονται;» καὶ λέγομεν ὅτι τοῦτο ἔφη, ἵνα δείξῃ τὴν δεκάτην μηδέποτε κρίνουσαν, ἀλλὰ τὴν ἑνδεκάτην ἢ τὴν θ′ κρινούσας. καὶ διὰ τί μὴ μόνης τῆς ια′ ἐμνημόνευσεν ἢ μόνης τῆς θ′, ἀλλὰ τῶν δύο ἐμνημόνευσεν; καὶ λέγομεν τοῦτο παρὰ τὴν σύστασιν τῆς ὕλης ἀπὸ θεωρίας εἴρηκε καὶ τὸν τόνον τῆς δυνάμεως· ἐὰν γὰρ λεπτή ἐστιν ἡ ὕλη καὶ ἐρρωμένη ἡ δύναμις, τῇ θ′ ἀπαλλάσσονται· εἰ δὲ παχυτέρα ἐστὶν ἡ ὕλη καὶ ἀσθενὴς ἡ δύναμις, ὡς ἂν πλείονος χρόνου δεομένη τῇ ἑνδεκάτῃ ἔφη παύσασθαι. καὶ διὰ τοῦτο ἀμφοτέρων ἐμνημόνευσεν.

Εἶτα λέγει· Οἳ δ᾽ ἂν ἄρξωνται πεμπταῖοι πονέεσθαι, τουτέοισι

7 αὐτός φησιν] Hipp. Aph. II 13: IV p. 472,11sq. L. 23 ἔφη] Hipp. Progn. 24: p. 228,6–8 A. = II p. 184,3–6 L. 35 λέγει] Hipp. Progn. 24: p. 228,8–10 A. = II p. 184,6–8 L.

3 εἰς L: εἰ M; *cf. infra, lin. 18* 5 πονεῖν] ποιεῖν *codd.*: *corr. Dietz* 7 ὡσαύτως MP 9 τῇ ἑβδόμῃ MP 11 *post* γὰρ *add.* καὶ MP 12 ἐπειδὴ – 14 κεφαλαλγία *om.* MP 14 ἐστιν *scripsi*: ἐπέχει L 17 ὅτι *om.* MP ἄρξηται ἡ] ἡ ἄρξηται τῇ L 18 πιέζονται MP ἐς] εἰ MP; *cf. supra, lin. 3* *post* ἤγουν *add.* ὅτι MP 19 καὶ *om.* MP 23 ὁκόσοισι L ποιεῖν LP: *corr.* M 25 ἄρξονται MP 26 τρὶς L 27 ια′] ι′ L ὅτι *om.* L 29 κρίνουσαν MP μόνης[I]] μόνον MP 30 παρὰ] περὶ MP 34 παύονται L ἐμνημόνευσεν] μνήμην ἐποιήσατο MP

III 17 In these cases, those who begin to have pain on the first day are most distressed on the fourth and fifth and they are cured on the seventh.

Here Hippocrates called the headache pain, saying begin to have pain, that is, pain in the head. And the headache he has in mind is not the one which takes the form of a crisis – for that one lasts one day at most, as he himself says, "For those who have a crisis the night before the paroxysm is uncomfortable"– rather he has in mind the headache which takes the form of a symptom, and this continues to the seventh day. But to tell the truth, it fits the headache both in the form of a crisis and in the form of a symptom. For such a headache has the form of a symptom, since he says that the headache develops at the beginning from the first day, and especially if, developing from the beginning, it should cease on the third, then it has the form of a symptom. But this kind of headache continues, since it extends to the crisis, and they are cured in this way. That he claims that such a headache extends to the seventh is shown by his own words in the text, Those who begin to have headache on the first day are distressed on the fourth and are cured on the seventh, in other words, their headache increases from the first day and there is an addition until the fourth, and they are distressed and are overcome, and they are subject to no more aggravation, but there is a stabilization and high point until the seventh, and in this way it is cured and ends on the seventh day.

Then he said, Those who begin to have pain in the head on the third are distressed on the fifth and are cured either on the ninth or on the eleventh. This has led some to say, "He has said this incorrectly; if they begin on the third day, three plus seven, ten; therefore they should be cured on the tenth; so how did he say that they are cured either on the 9th or on the 11th?" We reply that he said this, in order to show that the tenth is never critical, but the eleventh or the 9th are. And why did he not mention the 11th alone or the 9th alone, but he mentioned the two? We say that he did this taking into consideration the composition of the matter and the strength of (the body's) power; for if the matter is thin and the power strong, they are cured on the 9th; and if the matter is fairly thick and the power weak, he said that it ceases on the eleventh, since it needs more time. And this is why he mentioned both.

Then he says, Those who begin to have pain on the fifth,

τῇ ιδ' κρίνεται ἡ νοῦσος. καὶ πάλιν ἐνίστανταί τινες λέγοντες ὅτι «Ἐὰν|
224 ψηφίσῃς ἀπὸ τῆς πρώτης ἡμέρας πέντε καὶ ἑπτά, δώδεκα, εἰς τὴν ιβ' ἢ τὸ μέγιστον εἰς τὴν ιγ' κρίνεται ἡ νοῦσος· πῶς οὖν ἔφη ἐν τῇ ιδ' ἡμέρᾳ κρίνεσθαι τὸ νόσημα;» καὶ λέγομεν ὅτι τοῦτο εἴρηκεν, ἵνα δείξῃ μὴ εἶναι κρισίμους μήτε τὴν ιβ' μήτε τὴν ιγ', ἀλλὰ τὴν ιδ'. ἄλλως τε δὲ παχυτέραν ἔλαβε τὴν ὕλην καὶ ἐν τῷ μέσῳ δεηθῆναι μιᾶς καὶ δύο ἡμερῶν ἐν τῇ πέψει καὶ ἐν τῇ ιδ' ὑπαντῆσαι τὴν κρίσιν. καὶ διὰ τοῦτο τῆς ιδ' ἐμνημόνευσεν.

III 18 [24: 228,9 A. = II 184,7 L.] Καὶ τὰ ἄλλα κατὰ λόγον αὐτέοισι τῶν πρόσθεν γίγνηται, εἰς τὴν ιδ' κρίνεται ἡ νοῦσος

Λέγει ὅτι, ἐὰν τῇ ε' ἄρξωνται πονεῖν τὴν κεφαλὴν καὶ μηδὲν πλημμεληθῇ ὑπὸ τοῦ ἀρρώστου ἢ ἀμέλεια γένηται ὑπὸ τοῦ ἰατροῦ, τῇ ιδ' ἀπαλλάσσονται ἡμέρᾳ. τὰ δὲ ἄλλα κατὰ λόγον καλεῖ τὰ ἀνωτέρω εἰρημένα, ἵνα ἀρίστη γένηται ἡ κατάκλισις καὶ τὰ οὖρα καὶ τὰ διαχωρήματα καὶ ἵνα εὔπνους ἐστὶν ὁ ἄνθρωπος καὶ τὰ τοιαῦτα, ὡς ἀνωτέρω εἴρηται, κατὰ λόγον ὑπαντῆσαι, γίνωσκε ὅτι τῇ ιδ' κρίνεται ἡ νοῦσος καὶ ἀπαλλάσσονται.

III 19 [24: 228,10 A. = II 184,8 L.] Γίνεται δὲ τὰ τοιαῦτα τοῖσι μὲν ἀνδράσι καὶ τῇσι γυναιξί

Ταῦτα τὰ πάθη μάλιστα γίνονται, τυχὸν ὁ ἔμετος, τοῖς ἀνδράσι καὶ ταῖς γυναιξίν. εἰπὼν δὲ ἀνδράσι καὶ γυναιξὶ τὴν τελείαν ἡλικίαν ἐδήλωσεν, λέγω δὴ τὴν ἀκμαστικήν· ἐν γὰρ τῇ ἀκμαστικῇ ἡλικίᾳ ἀθροίζεται ἡ χολὴ καὶ διὰ τοῦτο ἐμεῖται. λέγει γὰρ καὶ ἀλλαχοῦ ὅτι «Οἱ ἀκμάζοντες τριταίοις ἁλίσκονται.»

III 20 [24: 228,12 A. = II 184,10 L.] Τοῖσι δὲ νεωτέροισι γίνεται μὲν καὶ τουτέοισι, μᾶλλον δὲ ἐν τοῖσι συνεχέσι πυρετοῖσι, καὶ μάλιστα ἐν τοῖσι γνησίοισι τριταίοισι.

Νεωτέρους, φησί, τοὺς μειρακιώδεις τῇ ἡλικίᾳ τυχὸν ἐκάλεσε. τοῖς
225 δὲ μειρακίοις οὐ γίνεται ἔμετος ὡς ἐπίπαν | χολῆς· εἰ δὲ καὶ γίνεται, σπανιάκις, ἐπειδὴ ἐπ' αὐτῶν χολὴ οὐκ ἀθροίζεται, ἀλλὰ τὸ αἷμα μάλιστα πλεονάζει. εἰ δὲ καὶ ἐμοῦσι, σπανίως ποτὲ ἐν τοῖς συνεχέσι πυρετοῖς —συνεχεῖς δὲ εἶπε τοὺς συνόχους — καὶ ἐν τοῖσι γνησίοισι τριταίοισι περιπίπτει, ἐπειδὴ ἐπὶ τούτων φλέγμα οὐκ ἀθροίζεται.

23 ἀλλαχοῦ] *locum non inveni; cf.* Hipp. De nat. hom. 15,5: CMG I 1,3 p. 204,15sq.

1 ια' MP ἐκρίνεται L 2 εἰς] εἰ L 3 κρίνεται] κρίνονται MP ἡ νοῦσος *om.* MP ἔφη *post* ἡμέρᾳ *trsp.* MP 6 καὶ^{I} *om.* MP 7 τοῦτο] τοῦ L τῆς] τὴν MP 11 τῇ] τὴν MP 12 γίνεται L 14 γένηται] ἐστὶν MP 15 *post* ἄνθρωπος *vel* τοιαῦτα *fort. lacuna statuenda est* 16 γίνωσκε *om.* MP 18 *post* δὲ *add.* καὶ L τὰ τοιαῦτα] ταῦτα *Hipp.* 19 τῇσι] τοῖσι L: ταῖς MP: *corr. Dietz* 21 γυναιξίν – καὶ *om.* L 28 ἐκάλεσε τυχόν MP 33 τούτοις MP

in these cases the disease comes to crisis on the 14th. And again some object saying that, "If you count from the first day five plus seven, twelve, the disease comes to crisis on the 12th or, at most, on the 13th; how, then, did he say that the disease comes to crisis on the 14th day?" We reply that he says this, in order to show that neither the 12th nor the 13th are critical, but the 14th is. Moreover, he assumed that the matter is on the thick side and needs one or two days in the middle during coction and the crisis falls on the 14th. So this is why he mentioned the 14th.

III 18 And when the rest of the symptoms mentioned before occur according to plan in them, the disease comes to crisis on the 14th

He says that, if on the 5th they begin to have pain in the head and the patient has not transgressed in anything and there has been no negligence by the doctor, they are cured on the 14th day. By the rest according to plan he means the symptoms mentioned earlier, that the reclining position be very good and the urines and feces, that the person be breathing easily and so on; (when these,) as was said above, occur according to plan, you will know that the disease reaches crisis on the 14th and they are cured.

III 19 These things occur in men and women

These affections, for example vomiting, occur for the most part in men and women. When he said men and women, he indicated the mature age, I mean the prime age; for bile collects in the prime age, and this is why it is vomited. For he says in another place also that "Those in their prime are seized by tertians."

III 20 And they occur in the younger also in tertians, but more often in the continuous fevers and especially in the genuine tertians.

By younger, he (the commentator) says, (Hippocrates) meant those in their youth. But in general vomiting of bile does not occur in youths; and if it does occur, it is a rare event, since bile does not collect in them, but it is blood which is especially abundant in them. And if they do vomit, it happens on rare occasions in the continuous fevers — by continuous he meant the unintermittent —, and in the genuine tertians, since phlegm does not collect in these.

III 21 [24: 229,1 A. = II 184,12 L.] Οἷσι δ' ἂν ἐν τοιούτῳ τρόπῳ πυρετῷ κεφαλὴν ἀλγέουσιν ἀντὶ μὲν τοῦ ὀρφνῶδές τι πρὸ τῶν ὀφθαλμῶν φαίνεσθαι

Ὅπερ λέγει τοιοῦτόν ἐστιν, ὅτι τοιούτῳ τρόπῳ, κατὰ τὸν αὐτὸν τρόπον, τυχὸν περιεστηκῶς ὄντος τοῦ νοσήματος, ὡς ἤδη καὶ ἐπὶ τῆς κατ' ἔκρουν δι' ἐμέτων κρίσεως, καὶ ἐνταῦθα καὶ ἐπὶ τῆς αἱμορραγίας περιεστηκότι νοσήματι ὑποτίθεται γίνεσθαι τὰ σημεῖα τῆς αἱμορραγίας, τυχὸν τὸ συνεῖναι τὴν κεφαλαλγίαν καὶ μηκέτι ὀρφνώδη ὁρᾶν πρὸ τῶν ὀφθαλμῶν, ἀλλὰ μαρμαρυγὰς καὶ λόφους ἀλεκτρυόνων καὶ πυραυγῆ τινα, ἀλλὰ καὶ τὸ ἀνασπᾶσθαι τὰ ὑποχόνδρια καὶ τὸ κνᾶσθαι τὸ ἄκρον τῆς ῥινὸς καὶ τὸ ἐρυθρὰ εἶναι τὰ μῆλα τοῦ προσώπου, τότε γίνωσκε ὅτι ἡ κατ' ἔκρουν κρίσις δι' αἱμορραγίας μέλλει γίνεσθαι. προστίθησι δὲ καὶ τοῦτο ἐνταῦθα, ὅτι, ὅτε μέμνηται ὁ Ἱπποκράτης [τῆς] διὰ χολῆς ἔμετον, οὐ τὴν ἄκρατον λέγει χολὴν ἐμεῖσθαι, ἀλλὰ τὴν συμμεμιγμένην μετὰ φλέγματος· τότε γὰρ ἄριστός ἐστιν ὁ ἔμετος. σπανίως δέ ποτε ἐὰν ἐμεθῇ ἄκρατος χολὴ ἅπαξ. ὁ δὲ ἐπίμονος ἔμετος τῆς ἀκράτου χολῆς μεγάλους τοὺς κινδύνους ἐπιφέρει· δήξεις γὰρ καὶ ἀνίας καὶ ἑλκώσεις ἀπεργάζεται δι' ὧν παροδεύει μορίων.

III 22 [24: 229,7 A. = II 186,4 L.] Τοῖσι δὲ πέντε καὶ τριάκοντα ἐτέων καὶ γεραιτέροισι

Φησὶν ὅτι τοῖς παρακμάζουσι τῇ ἡλικίᾳ ὁ ἔμετος τῆς χολῆς γίνεται, τοῖς δὲ γέρουσιν οὐδόλως. καὶ λέγομεν ὅτι ἡ παρακμαστικὴ ἡλικία οὐκ ἔστι γεννητικὴ χολῆς, ἀλλ' ἡ ἀκμαστική. καὶ λέγομεν ὅτι τὴν προθησαυ-
226 ρισθεῖσαν ἀπὸ τοῦ θέρους ἢ τοῦ θερινοῦ καταστήματος χολὴν ταύ|την ἐμοῦσι.

Γίνωσκε δὲ ὅτι τινὰ τῶν ἀντιγράφων ἔχει τοῖσι δὲ πέντε καὶ τριάκοντα, τινὰ δὲ τεσσαράκοντα ἔχει. καὶ διὰ μὲν τοῦ εἰπεῖν πέντε καὶ τριάκοντα τὸ πέρας τῆς ἀκμαστικῆς ἐδήλωσεν ἡλικίας, ἀρχὴν δὲ τῆς παρακμαστικῆς· διὰ δὲ τοῦ εἰπεῖν τεσσαράκοντα ἐτῶν τὸ πέρας τῆς παρακμαστικῆς ἐδήλωσεν, ἀρχὴν δὲ τῆς τῶν ὠμογερόντων ἡλικίας ἐμήνυσεν.

V

III 23 [24: 229,9 A. = II 186,6 L.] Τοῖσι δὲ παιδίοισι σπασμοὶ γίνονται

2 μὲν τοῦ] τοῦ μὲν L: μὲν M ὀρφνώδους MP 2 sq. τι — φαίνεσθαι *om.* MP 5 περιεστηκῶς] *cf. supra, pp. 64,23; 266,23* 13 τῆς *om.* M, *del. Dietz*: *fort.* τὸν *pro* τῆς *vel* τῆς δι' ἐμέτων χολῆς *scribendum est* ἐμέτων MP 14 ἄκραν MP 15 ἄριστόν L 17 δῆξιν MP 20 ἔτεσι *Hipp.* 22 λέγομεν] *fort.* λέγουσί τινες *vel sim. scribendum est* 25 ἐμοῦ MP 26 τριήκοντα MP; *sed cf. lin. 19* 28 τριήκοντα M (λ' P) 29 παρακμῆς MP σαράκοντα MP 30 ὁμογερόντων *codd.*: *correxi* ἐμνημόνευσεν L

III 21 Those with a headache in this type of fever who (experience) instead of the vision of something dark before the eyes

What he is saying is this, that in such a way, in the same manner, that is, the disease being one that can be survived – just as earlier in the case of the crisis by discharge through vomits, so here also for haemorrhage, he supposes that the signs of haemorrhage occur in a disease that can be survived –, (if) the headache is present and they no longer see dark things before the eyes, but "stars" and "cockscombs" and flashes, and the hypochondria are retracted and they scratch the tip of the nose and the cheeks of the face are red, then you will know that the crisis by discharge through haemorrhage is about to happen. And he adds this here also, that when Hippocrates mentions vomit through bile, he does not mean that the unmixed bile is vomited, but the one blended with phlegm; for then the vomit is best. If unmixed bile is vomited, it is seldom brought up just once. And persistent vomiting of unmixed bile brings on serious dangers; for it produces stings and irritations and ulcerations in the parts through which it makes its way.

III 22 In those who are thirty-five years and older

He says that the vomiting of bile occurs in those past prime, but not at all in the old. And we say that the post-prime age is not productive of bile, but the prime age is. And we say that it is the bile stored up from the summer or from summery weather which is vomited.

Note that some of the copies have In those who are thirty-five, while others have forty. By saying thirty-five he indicated the end of the prime age and the beginning of the post-prime. By saying forty years he indicated the end of the post-prime and marked the beginning of early old-age.

V

III 23 In children spasms occur

Ἐνταῦθα γενόμενος ὁ Γαληνὸς λέγει τὴν αἰτίαν καὶ μόνην, καθ' ἣν σπῶνται οἱ παῖδες, λέγων ὅτι σπῶνται οἱ παῖδες διὰ τὴν εὐπάθειαν τῶν νεύρων· εὐπαθῆ γάρ εἰσι τὰ νεῦρα ἐπ' αὐτῶν, καὶ ἑτοίμως τὸ τηνικαῦτα σπῶνται. ἡμεῖς δὲ λέγομεν ὅτι ἐνταῦθα τὸν σπασμὸν ἐμνημόνευσεν ὁ Ἱπποκράτης, ἐπεὶ ὁ σπασμὸς ὀξύ ἐστι πάθος· ἐνταῦθα δὲ περὶ ὀξέων νοσημάτων αὐτῷ ὁ λόγος. ἡ δὲ αἰτία, καθ' ἣν γίνεται ὁ σπασμὸς τοῖς παιδίοις, διάφορός ἐστι· γίνεται γὰρ αὐτοῖς ὁ σπασμὸς ἢ διὰ τὴν ἀσθένειαν τῶν ψυχικῶν δυνάμεων ἢ διὰ τὸ ἀδηφάγα εἶναι ἢ διὰ τὸ κλαυθμυρίζεσθαι αὐτά.

Καὶ διὰ μὲν τὴν ἀσθένειαν τῶν ψυχικῶν δυνάμεων οὕτως· τριττῶν γὰρ ὄντων κατὰ γένος ἡμῖν δυνάμεων, ψυχικῶν, ζωτικῶν, φυσικῶν, τὸ διττὸν μέρος καλῶς καὶ ἐρρωμένως διάκειται ἐν τοῖς παισίν, αἱ ζωτικαὶ καὶ φυσικαί. καὶ αἱ μὲν ζωτικαί, ὡς δηλοῖ ⟨τὸ⟩ πλούσιον εἶναι ἐπὶ τῶν παίδων τὸ ἔμφυτον θερμὸν κατὰ τὸ εἰρημένον ἐν Ἀφορισμοῖς· «Τοῖσι δὲ παιδίοισι πλεῖστόν ἐστι τὸ ἔμφυτον θερμόν.» ἀλλὰ καὶ αἱ φυσικαὶ δυνάμεις ἐρρωμέναι εἰσίν, ὡς δηλοῖ τὸ τρέφεσθαι καὶ αὐξάνειν. κατὰ μέντοι τὰς ψυχικὰς ἀρρώστως διάκεινται τὰ παιδία· οὐ γὰρ λογίζονται δεόντως, οὔτε μὴν εὐκίνητα κατὰ τὰς πράξεις εἰσὶ καὶ μάλιστα κατὰ τοὺς πρώτους καιρούς. διὰ οὖν τὸ ἀκίνητον εὐπαθῆ καὶ εὐεπηρέαστά εἰσι τὰ νεῦρα ἐπ' αὐτῶν, καὶ διὰ τοῦτο σπῶνται.

Ἀλλὰ καὶ διὰ τὸ ἀδηφάγα εἶναι πάλιν σπῶνται· ὑπὸ γὰρ τῆς ἀδηφα-
227 γίας καὶ τῆς ἀπεψίας ἀθροίζουσι | χυμοὺς παχεῖς καὶ γλίσχρους καὶ ψυχροὺς
καὶ ὠμούς, καθ' ἣν εἴωθε τὸ νευρῶδες γένος τρέφεσθαι, καὶ τὸ τηνικαῦτα διὰ τὸ πάχος ἐμφράττονται τὰ νεῦρα, καὶ οὕτως σπῶνται.

Ἀλλὰ καὶ διὰ τὸ κλαυθμυρίζεσθαι αὐτὰ σπῶνται· ἐν γὰρ τῷ κλαυθμυρίζειν κίνησις γίνεται τοῦ ἐγκεφάλου· τῇ οὖν κινήσει χύσις γίνεται τῶν πνευμάτων καὶ τῶν χυμῶν, καὶ φέρονται ἐπὶ τὰ νεῦρα οἱ χυμοὶ καὶ ἐμφράττουσιν αὐτά, καὶ οὕτως σπῶνται.

Σπασμὸν δὲ ἐνταῦθα οὐ τὸν ἐπὶ ξηρότητι λέγει γίνεσθαι ἐπὶ τῶν παίδων, ὅστις καὶ ἀνίατός ἐστιν, ἀλλὰ τὸν ἐπὶ πλήθει καὶ ἐμφράξει ὑποτίθεται σπασμόν, ὡς δηλοῖ τὸ ἐπάγειν αὐτὸν ἣν καὶ ἀγρυπνῶσιν. ἡ δὲ ἀγρυπνία ξηρότητα ἐντίθησι τῷ σώματι καὶ ἐπὶ ξηρότητι γίνεται. πρὸς ὃ ἔστιν εἰπεῖν ὅτι ἡ ἀγρυπνία οὐ μόνον ξηραίνει, ἀλλὰ καὶ ὑγραίνει. εἰ μὲν γὰρ ξηρὸν παραλάβῃ ἡ ἀγρυπνία τὸ σῶμα, τῇ διαφορήσει ἐπὶ πλέον ξηραίνει αὐτό· εἰ δὲ περιττωματικὸν καὶ ὑγρόν, χύσιν ποιεῖται αὐτῶν τῶν ὑγρῶν καὶ ὑγραίνει τὸ σῶμα ἡ ἀγρυπνία οὕτως καὶ φυλάττει. ὅτι δὲ περὶ τοῦ ἐπὶ πλήθει καὶ ἐμφράξει σπασμοῦ ὁ λόγος τῷ Ἱπποκράτει, δηλοῖ τὸ

1 Γαληνὸς] Gal. In Hipp. Progn. comm. III 39: CMG V 9,2 p. 365,4–8 9 τριττῶν – 18] *cf.* Gal. In Hipp. Progn. comm. III 39: CMG V 9,2 p. 365,5–8 13 ἐν Ἀφορισμοῖς] *cf.* Hipp. Aph. I 14: IV p. 466,8 L.

3 *post* ἑτοίμως *add.* τὰ νεῦρα MP τὸ τηνικαῦτα *post* σπῶνται *(lin. 4) trsp.* MP 4 τὸν σπασμὸν] τοῦ σπασμοῦ MP 5 ἐπειδὴ MP 6 *post* αἰτία *add.* τὸ MP 8 *ante* ψυχικῶν *add.* νεύρων L διάφαγα P: διαδήφαγα M 9 οὕτως *om.* L 10 ὄντων] *cf. supra, p. 68,26* 11 μέρος] γέρος L καὶ^{I} *om.* MP 12 δηλοῖ *om.* L τὸ^{I} *addidi* 16 εὐκίνητοι MP 17 τοῖς πρώτοις καιροῖς MP 17 sq. εὐκίνητον ἀπαθῆ L 19 Ἀλλὰ – σπῶνται *om.* M ἀδήφαγα P 20 τῆς *om.* MP χυμοὺς *post* ὠμούς *(lin. 21) trsp.* MP 23 Ἀλλὰ – 26 σπῶνται *om.* M 26 αὐτά *om.* P 27 λέγει *om.* MP 29 ἀγρυπνοῦσιν MP 30 ξηρότητι] ξηρότητα L 32 γὰρ *om.* MP ἔτι πλεῖον MP

At this point Galen gives only one reason why children are convulsed, saying that children are convulsed on account of the sensitivity of the nerves; for the nerves in them are sensitive and hence they are easily convulsed. But we say that Hippocrates mentioned spasm here, since spasm is an acute affection; and here his subject is acute diseases. And the cause of spasm in children is varied; for spasm occurs in them because of the weakness of the psychic faculties or because they are overeaters and because they wail.

And because of the weakness of the psychic faculties as follows: our faculties being three in kind, psychic, vital, natural, two of them are in good and strong condition in children, the vital and natural. And the vital, as is shown by the fact that there is a rich supply of innate heat in children, according to the saying in the Aphorisms, "Children have the most innate heat." And the natural faculties are strong too, as is shown by their nourishment and growth. However, with respect to the psychic (faculties), children are in weak condition; for they do not reason properly nor are they agile in their actions, especially in the early period. Because of the lack of agility, then, the nerves in them are sensitive and easily damaged and for this reason they are convulsed.

And again they are convulsed because they are overeaters; for due to the overeating and the indigestion they collect humors which are thick and viscous and cold and crude, by which the nerve class is usually nourished, and so, on account of the thickness, the nerves are blocked and thus they are convulsed.

And they are convulsed as well because they wail; for in wailing there occurs a movement of the brain; with the movement, then, a flow of gases and humors develops and the humors are conveyed to the nerves and block them and thus they are convulsed.

By spasm in children here he does not mean the one that develops from dryness, which is incurable, but he has in mind the spasm from overabundance and stoppage, as is shown by his going on to say and if they do not sleep. But (it is objected) insomnia causes dryness in the body, so (the spasm) arises from dryness. To this it can be said that insomnia not only dries, but moistens also. For if insomnia finds the body dry, it dries it more by dissipation; but (if it finds it) containing residues and fluids, it creates a flow of the fluids themselves and in this way insomnia moistens the body and keeps it (moist). And that Hippocrates is talking about the spasm from overabundance and stoppage is

ἐπάγειν αὐτὸν ἣν καὶ ἡ γαστὴρ ἐπέχεται· τοῦτο δὲ τὸ σημεῖον πληρώσεως. ἄλλως τε δὲ φύσει ἀδηφάγα ὄντα τὰ παιδία δίυγρά εἰσι καὶ διὰ τοῦτο τὸν ἐπὶ πλήθει ὑφίστανται σπασμόν.

Ἰστέον δὲ ὅτι, εἰ μὲν ἕν ἐστι τὸ σπασθὲν μόριον, μία ἔκφυσις πέπονθεν· εἰ δὲ διάφορά εἰσι τὰ μόρια τὰ σπασθέντα, διαφόρους δηλοῖ καὶ ἐκφύσεις πεπονθυίας· εἰ δὲ ὅλον τὸ σῶμα ἐσπάσθη, τότε δηλοῖ τὴν πρώτην ἀρχήν, λέγω δὴ τὸν ἐγκέφαλον, πεπονθυῖαν. δεῖ δὲ καὶ τοῦτο γινώσκειν, ὅτι γίνεται σπασμὸς καὶ διὰ φόβον. ἀλλ' οὗτος ὁ φόβος ἢ μέγιστός ἐστιν ἢ ὑφειμένος· καὶ εἰ μὲν μέγας ἐστὶ καὶ φοβερὸς ὁ φόβος, ὥστε ὑπερβαίνειν τὴν αἴσθησιν, ὥσπερ βροντὴ μεγίστη ἢ ἀστραπή, καὶ ἐκπλαγῇ ἡ αἴσθησις,
228 τότε καὶ ἀπόλλυνται οἱ ἐκ|φοβούμενοι· εἰ δὲ ὑφειμένος ἐστὶν ὁ φόβος, σπασμὸν ποιεῖται.

III 24 [24: 229,11 A. = II 186,9 L.] Καὶ τὸ χρῶμα μεταβάλλουσι χλωρὸν ἢ πελιδνόν

Ἰστέον δὲ ὅτι τὰ εἰρημένα τῷ Ἱπποκράτει περὶ τοῦ σπασμοῦ, τὰ μὲν αἰτίου λόγον ἐπέχουσιν, οἷον ἡ ἐποχὴ τῆς γαστρός, ἡ ἀγρυπνία, ἡ ἀδηφαγία καὶ ὁ κλαυθμυρισμός, τὰ δὲ σημείου, οἷον τὰ χρώματα. εἰ μὲν γὰρ χύσις γένηται τοῦ αἱματικοῦ χυμοῦ, τότε ἐρυθρὸν χρῶμα γίνεται· εἰ δὲ ὁ φλεγματικὸς χυμὸς χυθῇ, συναναμίγνυται τῷ αἵματι καὶ χλωρὸν ἀναδέχεται χρῶμα· εἰ δέ γε πιληθῇ καὶ ἀποσφιγ[γ]ῇ ὁ αἱματικὸς χυμός, ὑποπέλιον γίνεται χρῶμα· εἰ δὲ ἔτι πλέον πιληθῇ ὁ αἱματικὸς χυμὸς καὶ ἀποσφηνωθῇ, τότε μέλαν γίνεται χρῶμα.

III 25 [24: 229,15 A. = II 186,14 L.] Οἷά περ ἐπὶ τῇσι φρενίτισι γίνεται

Λέγει ὅτι ἐπὶ πληρώσει σπασμὸς τοῖς παιδίοις συμβαίνει γίνεσθαι τοῖς μέχρι ζ' ἐτῶν· τὰ δὲ πρεσβύτερα τῶν παίδων καὶ οἱ ἄνδρες, τουτέστιν ἡ μειρακιώδης καὶ ἀκμαστικὴ ἡλικία, τῷ ἐπὶ ξηρότητι σπασμῷ ὡς ἐπίπαν περιπίπτουσιν. εἰ δὲ ἐπὶ σπασμῷ τῷ ἐπὶ ξηρότητι ἐκεῖνα συμβῇ τὰ ὅμοια σημεῖα ἐπιγενέσθαι οἷά περ ἐπὶ τῶν φρενιτικῶν, οἷά εἰσι τὸ δοκεῖν κροκύδας ἐκλέγειν καὶ ἀνασπᾶν ἀπὸ τῶν ἱματίων καὶ καρφολογεῖν καὶ κατὰ τὸ συνεχὲς τὰς χεῖρας ἐπὶ τὸ πρόσωπον ἀπάγειν, ἐὰν ταῦτα ἐπιφανῶσιν ἐπὶ τῷ σπασμῷ τὰ σημεῖα τοῖς ἀνδράσι, τότε γίνωσκε ὅτι καὶ ἐπιληψίαις ἐπιπίπτουσι καὶ ἀποπληξίαις καὶ οὕτως ἀπόλλυνται.

III 26 [24: 230,2 A. = II 188,2 L.] Καὶ τῶν ἄλλων τεκμαίρεσθαι ξύμπασι τοῖς σημείοισιν, ὡς ἐφ' ἑκάστοισιν ἕκαστα διαγέγραπται

1 τὸ *om.* MP 2 ἀδήφαγα MP 6 τότε] λέγω L 9 ὑπεραίνει M: ὑπεραίρειν P 10 ἐκπληγῇ MP 13 μεταβάλλωσιν *Hipp.* 14 *ante* χλωρὸν *hab.* καὶ *Hipp.* πέλιον MP 15 δὲ *om.* MP 18 *ante* χρῶμα *add.* τὸ L 19 χυμὸς *om.* MP ἀναδέχεται] γίνεται L 20 ἀποσφιγγῇ *codd.*: *correxi*: ἀποσφιγχθῇ *coni. Dietz* 20 sq. ὑποπέλιον – χυμὸς *om.* MP 22 τότε] τὸ L 23 ἐπὶ] ἐν L; *sed cf. lin. 29* τοῖσι MP 24 γίνεται *om.* L 26 παιδίων MP 28 ὅμοια *om.* MP 29 οἷά^{II} *om.* MP 35 τοῖσι ξύμπασι *Hipp.*

shown by his going on to say and if the bowels stop; and this is the sign of repletion. Moreover, being overeaters by nature, children are very moist and for this reason they are subject to the spasm caused by overabundance.

And note that if a single part is convulsed, one outgrowth is affected; but if various parts are convulsed, it means that various outgrowths too are affected; and if the whole body is convulsed, then it shows that the first principle, I mean the brain, is affected. You should know this too, that spasm is produced also by fright. But this fright is either very great or mild; and if the fright is great and terrible, so as to exceed sensation, as in the case of very great thunder or lightning, and the wits are driven out, then the victims of fright die; but if the fright is mild, it produces spasm.

III 24 And they change their color to yellow or livid

Note that, of the things mentioned by Hippocrates concerning spasm, some have the form of a cause, namely bowel retention, insomnia, overeating and wailing, while some have the form of a sign, namely the colors. For if a flow of the bloody humor occurs, then the color becomes red; if the phlegmatic humor is made to flow, it mixes up with the blood and assumes a yellow color; and if the bloody humor is compressed and condensed, it becomes a dark-livid color; and if the bloody humor is compressed even more and is compacted, then it becomes a black color.

III 25 Such as occur in cases of phrenitis

He says that spasm from repletion happens in children up to 7 years; on the other hand, older children and men, that is, the youth and prime age, succumb for the most part to the spasm from dryness. But if in spasm caused by dryness those signs happen to supervene which are similar to such as occur in cases of phrenitis, namely the belief that one is picking and plucking nap from the clothes and gathering bits of wool, and the constant raising of the hands to the face, if these signs appear in men in a case of spasm, then you may conclude that they will succumb also to epilepsy and apoplexy and in this way die.

III 26 And the others, you must infer from all the signs as they have been described individually for each case

Ἰστέον ⟨ὅτι⟩ ἄλλο ἐστὶ τὸ ξυντεκμαίρεσθαι καὶ ἄλλο σημείωσις. τὸ γὰρ ξυντεκμαίρεσθαι τὸ μετὰ λόγου σημειοῦσθαι. ὁ δὲ λόγος αὐτὴν τὴν οὐσίαν ἀνιχνεύει τοῦ πράγματος. ἡ δὲ ἁπλῶς σημείωσις τῇ πείρᾳ ἕπεται,
229 μὴ | δυναμένης αἰτίαν ἀποδοῦναι τῆς σημειώσεως. θαυμάσαι δὲ ἔστι τὴν μεγαλόνοιαν τοῦ Ἱπποκράτους, ὅτι διὰ δύο λέξεων τά τε καθόλου συμπεριέλαβε καὶ τὰ κατὰ μέρος· εἰρηκὼς γὰρ τὰ ἐφ' ἑκάστοις τὰ καθόλου ἐσήμανεν· εἰρηκὼς δὲ τὰ ἕκαστα τὰ κατὰ μέρος ἐδήλωσε. διὰ δὲ τοῦ ἐφ' ἑκάστοις περὶ τῶν καθόλου διηλέχθη οὕτως· διηλέχθη γὰρ περὶ οὔρων, περὶ διαχωρημάτων καὶ ἱδρώτων καὶ ἐμέτων καὶ τῶν τοιούτων. διὰ δὲ τοῦ ἐπάγειν ἕκαστα ἰδίᾳ γέγραπται περὶ τῶν κατὰ μέρος διηλέχθη καὶ ὅτι αἱ διαφοραὶ τούτων ἤδη ἐγράφησαν· παραδέδωκε γὰρ ἡμῖν οὔρου διαφοράς, οἷόν ἐστι τὸ κριμνῶδες, τὸ πιτυρῶδες καὶ νεφελῶδες καὶ ἐναιώρημα καὶ τὰ τοιαῦτα. ἀλλὰ καὶ διαχωρημάτων διαφορὰς παραδέδωκεν· ἐμνημόνευσε γὰρ τρύζοντος διαχωρήματος καὶ ὑφαίμου καὶ μέλανος καὶ τῶν τοιούτων. ἀλλὰ καὶ ἱδρώτων διαφορὰς παραδέδωκεν· ἔφη γάρ, ποῖοι κατὰ φύσιν εἰσὶν ἱδρῶτες καὶ ποῖοι παρὰ φύσιν καὶ ὅτι οἱ μὲν θερμοί εἰσιν ἱδρῶτες, οἱ δὲ ψυχροί, καὶ ἢ δι' ὅλου τοῦ σώματος γίνονται ἢ ἐν μέρει τοῦ σώματος. ἀλλὰ καὶ περὶ πτυέλου διηλέχθη διαφορᾶς ἀφρώδους καὶ ὑποπύου καὶ τῶν τοιούτων. ἀλλὰ καὶ ἐμέτου ἔφη διαφορὰς χολώδους καὶ φλεγματώδους καὶ συναναμεμιγμένων τούτων καὶ τὰ τοιαῦτα. σκόπει οὖν μεγαλόνοιαν ἀνδρός, πόσα διὰ δύο λέξεων ἐσήμανεν. ἐκ τούτων οὖν ἁπάντων τῶν ἤδη εἰρημένων σημείων προγνώσῃ τοὺς τεθνηξομένους καὶ σωθησομένους ἐπὶ τῶν ὀξέων νοσημάτων.

III 27 [25: 230,5 A. = II 188,6 L.] Χρὴ δὲ τὸν μέλλοντα ὀρθῶς προγινώσκειν τούς τε περιεσομένους καὶ τὰ ἑξῆς.

Εἰπὼν ὀρθῶς προγινώσκειν ἐσήμανε τὸ ἀκριβῶς καὶ τὸ ἀεὶ καὶ ὡς ἐπίπαν προγινώσκειν· τὸν γὰρ τοιοῦτον οὐ λήσῃ ὅπῃ τρέψηται τὸ νόσημα, ἀλλὰ γινώσκει[ν] καὶ τοὺς ἀπολλυμένους καὶ τοὺς περισῳζομένους τῇ ἀκριβεῖ προγνώσει. |

230 III 28 [25: 230,7 A. = II 188,9 L.] Τὰ σημεῖα ἐκμανθάνοντα ταῦτα πάντα δύνασθαι κρίνειν

Ἀντὶ τοῦ ἐκμελετᾶν τὸ μανθάνειν εἶπεν, ὅτι 'δεῖ σε ἀεὶ ἐκμελετᾶν καὶ

27 sq. οὐ – νόσημα] Hipp. Progn. 20: pp. 221,14–222,1 A. = II p. 170,9 L. *item cit. supra*, p. 244,27 sq.

1 Ἰστέον *om.* L   ὅτι *add. Dietz*   2 οὐσίαν] φύσιν MP   6 συμπαρέλαβε MP   7 δὲ^{II}] γὰρ L   9 διαχώρησιν MP   10 ἐπαγαγεῖν MP*; sed cf. e.g. supra, pp. 284,29; 286,1*   ἰδίᾳ γέγραπται] *fort.* διαγέγραπται *restituendum est*   11 ἐγράφη P: ἐγεγράφησαν M   παραδέδωκα L: παρέδωκε MP: *corr. Dietz*   γὰρ] δὲ L   12 καὶ^{II} *om.* L   14 διαχωρήματα MP   μελάνων MP   15 παρέδωκεν MP   18 διαφορὰς M: *exspectaveris* διαφορῶν   19 ὑποπτύου MP   *ante* ἐμέτου *add.* περὶ MP   διαφορᾶς *codd.*: *corr. Dietz*   22 τῶν *om.* MP   23 σωθησομένους] ἐσομένους MP   24 τὸ μέλλον MP   25 *post* περιεσομένους *add.* καὶ τεθνηξομένους L (καὶ ἀποθανουμένους *aut* καὶ ἀπολ(λ)υμένους *praeb. codd. Hipp.*)   27 λήσει ... τρέψεται *Hipp.; sed cf. supra, p. 244,27sq.*   28 γινώσκειν *codd.*: *correxi*   31 δύνασαι MP

Note that inference (from symptoms) is one thing and interpretation of symptoms another. For to infer (from symptoms) is to interpret them logically. Logic tracks down the very essence of the matter. Simple interpretation of symptoms, on the other hand, relies on trial, not being able to give the reason for the interpretation. And one must admire the great mind of Hippocrates, because with two words he included both the general and the particular; for by saying for each case he denoted the general, and saying individually he indicated the particular. And by means of for each case he discussed the general in this way; for he has talked about urines, about feces and sweats and vomits and the like. And by going on to say as each has been described individually he discussed the particular and (means) that the varieties of these have already been described; for he has given us varieties of urine, such as the meal-like, the bran-like and cloudy and suspended and so on. He has also given varieties of feces; for he has mentioned the noisy feces and the blood-shot and the black and the like. He has given too varieties of sweats, saying which sweats are normal and which abnormal, and that some sweats are hot, others cold, and that they occur either throughout the body or in a part of the body. And he has discussed the varieties of spit, frothy and purulent and so on. And he has given varieties of vomit, bilious and phlegmatic and a blend of these and so on. Consider, then, the great mind of the man, how much he indicated by means of two words. From all these signs, then, which have been mentioned already, you will prognose who will die and who will be saved in cases of acute diseases.

III 27 For the one who is going to prognose correctly those who will survive it is necessary, etc.

By prognose correctly he means to prognose accurately and constantly and in general; for the direction that the disease takes will not escape such a one, but he will know by accurate prognosis both who will die and who will survive.

III 28 To understand fully all these signs and be able to judge them

He used understand in the sense "to work at studiously", (meaning) that 'You should always work studiously at these signs which I have

ἔχειν κατὰ νοῦν τὰ σημεῖα ταῦτα τὰ ὑπ' ἐμοῦ λεχθέντα· ἐὰν γὰρ ἀείσε ἐκμελετᾷς αὐτά, δύνασαι καὶ κρίνειν, ποίας εἰσὶ δυνάμεως, εἴτε ἀγαθὰ εἴτε κακά· τὰ ἀγαθὰ ἀγαθά ἐστι καὶ τὰ κακὰ κακά ἐστιν'.

III 29 [25: 230,8 A. = II 188,10 L.] Ἐκλογιζόμενον τὰς δυνάμεις αὐτῶν πρὸς ἀλλήλας

Τὸ λεγόμενον ἐνταῦθα τοιοῦτόν ἐστιν, ὅτι οὐ δεῖ προσέχειν τῷ ἀριθμῷ τὰ σημεῖα, ἀλλὰ τῷ ἀξιώματι καὶ τῇ δυνάμει τῶν σημείων· πολλάκις γὰρ ἓν σημεῖον ἀγαθόν ἐστι, πολλὰ δὲ κακά, καὶ περιγίνεται τὸ ἓν σημεῖον διὰ τὴν ἰσχύν. οὕτως γοῦν πολλάκις εἰσερχόμενος εἰς τὸν ἄρρωστον εὑρίσκω αὐτὸν εὔσφυκτον καὶ τῇ εὐσφυξίᾳ εὔπνουν, πολλὰ δὲ σημεῖα κακὰ ἐν τοῖς κενουμένοις, τυχὸν δι' οὔρων καὶ ὑποχωρημάτων καὶ ἱδρώτων· καὶ λέγω ὅτι διὰ τὴν ἰσχὺν τῆς εὐσφυξίας περιγίνεται ὁ ἄνθρωπος. καὶ ἰδοὺ ἓν σημεῖον τὸ κῦρος εἶχε παρὰ τὰ πολλά. ἔστι δ' ὅτε σημειούμεθα καὶ ἐκ τῶν κενουμένων καὶ ἐκ τῶν ἐνεργειῶν. καὶ ἀναγκαιότεραι αἱ ἐκ τῶν ἐνεργειῶν σημειώσεις ἤπερ τῶν κενουμένων, ἐπειδὴ αἱ ἐνέργειαι ὑπὸ δυνάμεων ἐπιτελοῦνται. καὶ αἱ δυνάμεις τριτταί εἰσιν, ἢ ψυχικαὶ ἢ ζωτικαὶ ἢ φυσικαί. καὶ αἱ μὲν ψυχικαὶ σημειώσεις τιμιώτεραί εἰσι καὶ τῷ ἀξιώματι καὶ τῇ δυνάμει τῶν ζωτικῶν. καὶ πάλιν αἱ ζωτικαὶ τιμιώτεραί εἰσι τῶν φυσικῶν. διὰ τοῦτο οὖν ὁ Ἱπποκράτης λέγει ὅτι δεῖ τὰς σημειώσεις οὐ τῷ ἀριθμῷ προσέχειν, ἀλλὰ τῷ ἀξιώματι.

III 30 [25: 230,11 A. = II 188,14 L.] Εὖ μέντοι χρὴ εἰδέναι περί τε τῶν τεκμηρίων καὶ τῶν ⟨ἄλλων⟩ σημείων

Παρακελεύεται ὁ Ἱπποκράτης τὸν ἰατρὸν καὶ τῷ λόγῳ κεχρῆσθαι καὶ τῇ πείρᾳ. ταῦτα δὲ ἔφη καὶ ὡς δογματικὸς καὶ ὡς ἐμπειρικός· διὰ γὰρ τοῦ εἰπεῖν αὐτὸν ὅτι χρὴ εἰδέναι καὶ περὶ τῶν τεκμηρίων τὸ ἐπιστημονικὸν ἐδήλωσε τοῦ λόγου· διὰ δὲ τοῦ εἰπεῖν καὶ τῶν ἄλλων |
231 σημείων τὸ στοχαστικὸν τῆς πείρας ἐδήλωσε. δεῖ οὖν τὸν ἰατρὸν καὶ δογματικὸν εἶναι καὶ ἐμπειρικόν.

III 31 [25: 231,2 A. = II 190,1 L.] Ἐπειδὴ καὶ ἐν Λιβύῃ καὶ ἐν Δήλῳ καὶ ἐν Σκύθῃσι φαίνεται τὰ προγεγραμμένα ἀληθεύοντα σημεῖα

Ἀποροῦσί τινες λέγοντες ὅτι «Πῶς ὁ Ἱπποκράτης, βραχυλόγος ὤν, ἐνταῦθα φαίνεται πολλῷ λόγῳ κεχρημένος; ἤδη γὰρ ἀνωτέρω εἰπὼν ὅτι

32–292,2 ἀρκεσθῆναι] *cf.* Gal. In Hipp. Progn. comm. III 45: CMG V 9,2 pp. 376,25–377,6   33 εἰπὼν] Hipp. Progn. 25: p. 231,1 A. = II p. 188,16 L.

1 κατὰ νοῦν] κατ' ἐμοῦ MP   ταῦτα *om.* MP   2 εἴτε[II]] ἢ L   4 Εἰσλογιζόμενον L: Ἐκλογιζόμενοι MP: *sec. plur. codd. Hipp. correxi*   7 τὰ σημεῖα] *cf. infra, lin. 19*   9 εἰς] πρὸς MP   τὸν *om.* MP   13 ἔσχε MP   καὶ *om.* L   16 ἢ[I et II] *om.* MP   ἢ[III]] καὶ M: *om.* P   22 ἄλλων *supplevi, cf. lin. 26*   25 καὶ *om.* MP   27 τῆς] καὶ L   29 ἐπεὶ *Hipp.*   30 σκύθοισι L: σκυθίησι MP: *corr. Dietz*   *post* φαίνεται *add.* καὶ MP   30 sq. ἀληθεύοντα σημεῖα *om.* MP   33 πολὺν λόγον MP   ὅτι *om.* MP

mentioned and keep them in mind; for if you always work studiously at them, you will be able to judge their power, whether they are good or bad; the good are good and the bad are bad'.

III 29 Calculating their powers by comparison with one another

What he is saying here is as follows, that one should not pay attention to the number of signs, but to their importance and power; for frequently, when there is one good sign and many bad, the one sign prevails on account of its strength. Thus, at any rate, I often come to the patient and find him with a good pulse and, thanks to this goodness of pulse, he is breathing easily, but there are many bad signs in the evacuations, namely in the urines and feces and sweats; and I say that the person will survive because of the strength of the good pulse. So you see that one sign has had more weight than many. Sometimes we take symptoms both from the evacuations and from the functions. And the interpretations of symptoms from the functions are more compelling than those from the evacuations, since the functions are brought to pass by faculties. And the faculties are three in number, psychic or vital or natural. And psychic symptoms are more valuable than the vital because of their importance and power. And again the vital are more valuable than the natural. For this reason, then, Hippocrates says that one should not pay attention to the number of symptoms, but to their importance.

III 30 However, one should be fully aware concerning sure signs and the other symptoms

Hippocrates is exhorting the doctor to use both reason and trial. And he said these things as both a Dogmatic and an Empiric; for by his saying one should be aware concerning sure signs he indicated knowledge from reasoning; and by saying and the other symptoms he indicated guesswork based on trial. It is necessary, then, for the doctor to be a Dogmatic and an Empiric.

III 31 Since the signs described before hold true in Libya and in Delos and in Scythia

Some raise a problem saying, "How is it that Hippocrates, a man of few words, seems to be using a lot of words here? For having

ἐν παντὶ ἔτει καὶ πάσῃ ὥρᾳ ἠδύνατο εἰπεῖν καὶ 'ἐν πάσῃ χώρᾳ τὰ αὐτά ἐστι σημεῖα' καὶ ἐν τούτῳ ἀρκεσθῆναι, ἀλλὰ πολυλογίᾳ ἐχρήσατο καὶ ἑκάστην χώραν ἐμνημόνευσε, Λιβύην καὶ Δῆλον καὶ Σκυθίαν.» καὶ λέγομεν ὅτι ἐπίτηδες τοῦτο πεποίηκεν ἀποκρουόμενος ἀπορίαν μεγίστην· ἵνα γὰρ μήτις ἀπορήσῃ αὐτῷ ὅτι «⟨Τί⟩ οὖν; καὶ ἐν τῇ θερμοτάτῃ χώρᾳ καὶ ἐν τῇ ψυχροτάτῃ τὰ αὐτὰ σημεῖά ἐστι, τὰ ἀγαθὰ ἀγαθὰ καὶ τὰ κακὰ κακά;», ταύτην οὖν τὴν ἀπορίαν προανακρουόμενος παραδειγματικῶς ἐμνημόνευσε καὶ τῆς θερμοτάτης χώρας καὶ τῆς ψυχροτάτης καὶ τῆς εὐκράτου, ὅτι ἐπὶ πάσης χώρας τὰ ἀγαθὰ σημεῖα ἀγαθά ἐστι καὶ τὰ κακὰ κακά ἐστι. καὶ διὰ τοῦ μνημονεῦσαι Λιβύης τὴν θερμοτάτην χώραν ἐδήλωσε, διὰ δὲ τῆς Σκυθίας τὴν ψυχροτάτην, διὰ δὲ τῆς Δήλου τὴν εὔκρατον.

III 32 [25: 231,6 A. = II 190,6 L.] Ποθεῖν δὲ χρὴ οὐδενὸς νοσήματος τοὔνομα καὶ τὰ ἑξῆς.

Ἴσως τις ἀπορεῖ ὅτι «Ὁ Ἱπποκράτης πάντα προθέμενος παραδοῦναι τὰ ὀξέα νοσήματα, οὔτε γὰρ τοῦ συνόχου ἐμνημόνευσεν οὔτε τοῦ καύσου, καίτοι καὶ αὐτῶν ὀξέων νοσημάτων ὄντων.» προσαπολογεῖται ὁ Ἱπποκράτης λέγων ὅτι 'Οὐ περὶ τὴν ὀνομασίαν τῶν νοσημάτων σπουδάζω ζητεῖν, ⟨...⟩ ὅτι τοῦ δεῖνος νοσήματος ὀνομαστὶ οὐκ ἐμνημόνευσα· ἀλλὰ δεῖ σκοπεῖν, ἐάν τι τῶν ἀναγκαίων παρέλειπα σημείων· περὶ γὰρ σημείων ὁ λόγος, οὐ περὶ ὀνομάτων.' ἔστι δὲ εἰπεῖν ὅτι καὶ τούτων τῶν νοσημάτων ἐμνημόνευσε δυνάμει, κἂν μὴ ὀνομαστί. καὶ σύνοχον μὲν ἐμνη-
282 μόνευσεν, ἡνίκα ἔλεγεν· Οἵ τε γὰρ | εὐηθέστατοι τῶν πυρετῶν τεταρταῖοι παύονται, ὁ δὲ σύνοχος ἐντὸς τῆς τετάρτης κρίνεται. ἀλλὰ καὶ τοῦ καύσου ἐμνημόνευσεν ἐν οἷς ἔλεγεν ὅτι 'τινὰ τῶν νοσημάτων τῇ ἑβδόμῃ κρίνεται', ὁ δὲ καῦσος τῇ ἑβδόμῃ κρίνεται πάντως. ἢ εἰπὲ ὅτι τοῦτο πεποίηκεν, ἐπειδὴ ἐγίνωσκεν ὅτι οὐ παντὶ ἔθνει ἡ αὐτὴ ὀνομασία ἐστίν, ἀλλ' ἑτέρως ὠνόμασται καὶ ἀλληνάλλως κέχρηνται τοῖς ὀνόμασι τῶν νοσημάτων· ἄλλως γὰρ παρὰ Σύροις καὶ ἄλλως παρ' Αἰγυπτίοις καὶ ἄλλως παρὰ Ῥωμαίοις. καὶ διὰ τοῦτο τῶν μὲν ὀνομάτων κατεφρόνησε, τῶν δὲ πραγμάτων καὶ αὐτῶν τῶν σημείων φροντίδα καὶ σπουδὴν ἐποιήσατο. ἐν οἷς σὺν θεῷ ἥ τε παροῦσα πραγματεία πληροῦται καὶ τὰ σχόλια τοῦ Προγνωστικοῦ. δόξα τῷ θεῷ. ἀμήν.

22 ἔλεγεν] Hipp. Progn. 20: p. 220,11–221,1 A. = II p. 168,8sq. L. 24 ἔλεγεν] Hipp. Progn. 20: p. 221,3 A. = II p. 168,11sq. L.

5 ὅτι – οὖν] ὁτιοῦν L: Τί *addidi* 6 εἰσὶ MP 7 προνοούμενος L 10 τοῦ] τὸ MP 11 δήλω MP 13 καὶ τὰ ἑξῆς *om.* MP 14 Ὁ Ἱπποκράτης *post* προθέμενος *trsp.* MP πάντα *om.* L 16 καίτοι – ὄντων *om.* MP αὐτῶν *coni. Dietz*: αὐτὰ τῶν *codd.*: *fort.* αὐτὰ τῶν ... ὄντα *scr. Steph.* προαπολογεῖται MP 18 *lacunam indicavi* 19 ἀνάγκων L παρέλειπε P: παρέλιπεν M 20 περὶ] τῶν MP 21 κἂν] καὶ MP 22 τε] δὲ MP γὰρ *om.* MP *post* πυρετῶν *add.* καὶ ἐπὶ σημείων ἀσφαλεστάτων βεβότες *ex Hipp.* MP 25 ἑβδόμῃ[I]] τετάρτῃ MP 26 *post* ὀνομασία *add.* τῶν ὀνομάτων L 27 ὀνομάζεται L 28 γὰρ *om.* MP

said earlier in every year and every season, he could have said also 'in every region the signs are the same' and have been satisfied with this, but he used many words and mentioned each region, Libya, Delos and Scythia." And we say that he does this for a purpose, to anticipate a serious objection; for in order that no one would raise the problem to him, "What then? (Do you mean) that the signs are the same both in the hottest and coldest region, the good being good and the bad being bad?"– in order, then, to forestall this problem, he mentioned for examples the hottest region and the coldest and the temperate, (to indicate) that in every region the good signs are good and the bad are bad. And by mentioning Libya he indicated the hottest region, by Scythia the coldest and by Delos the temperate.

III 32 One should not miss the name of any disease, etc.

Perhaps someone will raise the problem, "Hippocrates, in spite of his proposal to give us all the acute diseases, has not mentioned either unintermittent fever or causus, although these are acute diseases." Hippocrates replies to this, 'It is not my concern to investigate the names of the diseases, . . . that I have not mentioned such-and-such a disease by name; rather, you should examine whether I have left out any of the important signs; for the discussion is about signs, not names.' And one can say that he mentioned even these diseases in effect, though not by name. He mentioned unintermittent fever, when he said, The mildest fevers end on the fourth, for the unintermittent comes to crisis by the fourth. And he mentioned the causus as well where he said 'some diseases reach crisis on the seventh', for causus invariably comes to crisis on the seventh. Or you may say that he has done it (this way), since he knew that not all nations use the same names, but things are named differently and one uses one name for a disease and another a different name; for one is used by the Syrians, another by the Egyptians and another by the Romans. This is why he thought little of names and gave his concern and attention to the (underlying) realities and the signs themselves. Here, with God's help, is completed the present treatise, the commentary on the Prognosticon. Glory to God. Amen.

INDICES

I. Index grammaticus

* = exempla; → = vide

1. Articulus

a) *in periphrasi*

b) *cum adverbiis et pronominibus interrogativis*

2. Adiectiva

a) *declinatio*

b) *comparatio*

3. Pronomina

4. Praepositiones

5. Adverbia

6. Particulae

7. Verbi coniugatio

8. Verba auxiliaria

9. Verbi tempora

a) *perfectum pro praesenti*

b) *perfectum pro aoristo*

c) *imperfectum pro aoristo*

10. Verbi modi

a) *indicativus*

b) *coniunctivus*

c) *optativus*

11. Constructio

a) *casus*

ἐπιμιμνῄσκεσθαι c. dat. 262,13 πένεσθαι c. dat. 34,2 χρῆσθαι c. acc. 140,38

b) *congruentia*

neutr. pl. c. verbo pl.* 26,16 28,1.7 30,15 32,2 42,11 48,4 62,14.18 70,9 72,1.28 102,2 104,4

c) *verba c. praepos.*

ἰᾶσθαι ἐκ 60,28 μεταλαμβάνειν ἐκ 150,21 παρηγορεῖσθαι ἐκ 182,24 χαρακτηρίζεσθαι ἀπό 134,2

d) *participia*

nom. absol.*: αἱ σάρκες ... γυμναὶ οὖσαι, ἑτοίμως διαφαίνεται τὸ χρῶμα 102,11 στερισκόμενοι (sc. οἱ πόδες) ... καταβάλλονται αἱ ἐν αὐτοῖς φυσικαὶ δυνάμεις 148,29 ὠθούμενον τὸ διάφραγμα ... στενοχωρεῖται ὁ πνεύμων 156,25 sim. 164,27 178,2 190,10 208,17 212,37 224,39 – gen. absol. pro nom. subiecti*: εἰσελθόντος τοῦ Ἐρασιστράτου ... ἐπέβαλε τὴν χεῖρα 58,32 σημειουμένου αὐτοῦ ἔνευσε τῷ μετ' αὐτοῦ 60,5 εὖ ἐνεργουσῶν τῶν αἰσθήσεων δηλοῦσι τὸν ἐγκέφαλον κτλ. 68,1 sim. 70,6 78,9 98,20 106,1 110,21 182,30 – discrepantia casus: ἐπί τινων ἐξ ἀρχῆς τοῦτο πάσχοντας 96,25 διὰ πλημμελῆ βλάβην τῆς καθεκτικῆς δυνάμεως, πλέον κατέχουσα τοῦ δέοντος 170,27 sim. 172,1.9.19 ἐπὶ μεγίστῃ... θερμότητι, ἐξυπεροπτῶσαν καὶ οἷον ἀποτεφρουμένην 194,32 – discrepantia generis: τῶν ... σεμνὸν βίον διαγόντων γυναικῶν 68,26 τριττῶν γὰρ ὄντων ... δυνάμεων 284,10

II. Index nominum

sch. = in scholiis (pp. 36,32 – 52,39) quae ad Stephanum non pertinent; → = vide

III. Index verborum

exempla tantum exhibens

sch. = in scholiis (pp. 36,32–52,39) quae ad Stephanum non pertinent; → = vide

Bei Fragen zur Produktsicherheit wenden Sie sich bitte an:
If you have any questions regarding product safety,
please contact:

Walter de Gruyter GmbH
Genthiner Straße 13
10785 Berlin
productsafety@degruyterbrill.com